Understanding
Nursing Research

BUILDING AN EVIDENCE-BASED PRACTICE

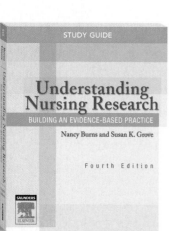

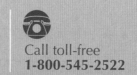

Understanding Nursing Research

BUILDING AN EVIDENCE-BASED PRACTICE

Fourth Edition

Nancy Burns, PhD, RN, FAAN
Jenkins Garrett Professor (retired)
School of Nursing
University of Texas at Arlington
Arlington, Texas

Susan K. Grove, PhD, APRN, BC, ANP, GNP
Associate Dean and Graduate Advisor
School of Nursing
University of Texas at Arlington
Arlington, Texas

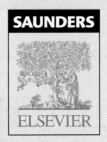

SAUNDERS

ELSEVIER

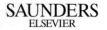

11830 Westline Industrial Drive
St. Louis, Missouri 63146

Understanding Nursing Research, 4th edition

ISBN-13: 978-1-4160-2640-2
ISBN-10: 1-4160-2640-1

Notice

Previous editions copyrighted 1995, 1999, 2003

ISBN-13: 978-1-4160-2640-2
ISBN-10: 1-4160-2640-1

Acquisitions Editor: Lee Henderson
Developmental Editor: Maureen Iannuzzi
Publishing Services Manager: Jeff Patterson
Design Direction: Bill Drone

Working together to grow
libraries in developing countries

www.elsevier.com | www.bookaid.org | www.sabre.org

ELSEVIER   BOOK AID International   Sabre Foundation

Printed in China
Last digit is the print number: 9   8   7   6   5   4   3   2   1

CONTRIBUTOR

Bonnie Raingruber, RN, PhD, CS
Professor of Nursing
Director of the Center
for Health and Human Services Research
California State University, Sacramento
Sacramento, California;

Nurse Researcher
University of California Davis Medical Center
Sacramento, California
Review and revision of portions of Chapter 13,
Critiquing Research Studies

CONSULTANT

Lioness Ayres, PhD, RN
Assistant Professor of Nursing
The University of Iowa
Iowa City, Iowa
Review of chapters for qualitative/quantitative
balance and accuracy

REVIEWERS

Judith W. Alexander, PhD, APRN, BC, CNAA
Associate Professor
College of Nursing
University of South Carolina
Columbia, South Carolina

Linda Amankwaa, PhD, RN
Albany State University
Albany, Georgia

Paula L. Antognoli, PhD, RN, CNAA
West Texas A&M University
Canyon, Texas

Angelina A. Arcamone, MSN, RN
Department of Nursing
Thomas Jefferson University
Philadelphia, Pennsylvania

Elizabeth Wenhold Black, RN, MSN, CSN, CS
Gwynedd-Mercy College
Gwynedd Valley, Pennsylvania

Penny S. Boyer, MS, RN
Associate Professor of Nursing
Hartwick College
Oneonta, New York

Kimberly Ferren Carter, PhD, RN
Radford University School of Nursing
Radford, Virginia

Dana Charles Clark, EdD, RN
Luzerne County Community College
Nanticoke, Pennsylvania

Ruth Davidhizar, DNS, RN, ARNP, BC, FAAN
Dean of Nursing
Bethel College
Mishawaka, Indiana

Joseph T. DeRanieri, PhD, RN, CPN, BCECR
Assistant Professor
Thomas Jefferson University
Philadelphia, Pennsylvania

Holli A. DeVon, PhD, RN
Assistant Professor
College of Nursing
Marquette University
Milwaukee, Wisconsin

Gloria Duke, PhD, RN
Associate Dean, Research & Outreach
The University of Texas at Tyler
College of Nursing & Health Sciences
Tyler, Texas

Jacqueline Fawcett, PhD, FAAN
College of Nursing and Health Sciences
University of Massachusetts Boston
Boston, Masachusetts

Carol Heinrich, PhD, RN
East Stroudsburg University
East Stroudsburg, Pennsylvania

Nikole Anderson Hicks, MSN, RNC
Kentucky Christian College
Grayson, Kentucky

Janet T. Ihlenfeld, PhD, RN
Professor
Department of Nursing
D'Youville College
Buffalo, New York

Kimberly A. Johnston, EdD, MSN, RNC, EdC
Chairperson and Associate Professor
Department of Nursing
Kutztown University
Kutztown, Pennsylvania

Linda W. Johnston, PhD, RN
University of South Carolina Aiken
Aiken, South Carolina

Rebecca Keele, PhD, APRN, BC
New Mexico State University
Las Cruces, New Mexico

Min-Shik Kim, DrPH, CS, APRN
Gannon University
Villa Maria School of Nursing
Erie, Pennsylvania

Patricia E. Kizilay, EdD, ARNP-BC, FAAP
Seton Hall University
South Orange, New Jersey

Mary L. Koehn, PhD, ARNP, FACCE
Assistant Professor
School of Nursing
Wichita State University
Wichita, Kansas

Barbara Ann Konopka, RN, MSN, CCRN, CEN
Instructor, Nursing
Pennsylvania State University
Dunmore, Pennsylvania

Suzanne Langer, PhD, CRNP, FAAN
Associate Professor
Department of Nursing
Thomas Jefferson University
Philadelphia, Pennsylvania

Sharon Martin, APRN, MSN
Saint Joseph's College
Standish, Maine

Margot L. Nelson, PhD, RN
Professor and Chair
Department of Nursing
Augustana College
Sioux Falls, South Dakota

Linda K. Niedringhaus, PhD, RN
Elmhurst College
Deicke Center for Nursing Education
Elmhurst, Illinois

Mary E. Norton, EdD, APN-C
Professor and Chair
Department of Graduate Nursing
Felician College
Lodi, New Jersey

Priscilla O'Connor, PhD, APRN, BC
Emerita
The College of New Jersey
Ewing, New Jersey

Kay L. Palmer, RN, MSN, CRRN
Old Dominion University
Norfolk, Virginia

Sheila P. Patros, PhD, RN
Eastern Kentucky University
Richmond, Kentucky

Barbara J. Patterson, PhD, MSN, RN
Widener University
Chester, Pennsylvania

Kelly Ruppel, PhD, RN
Associate Professor
MacMurray College
Jacksonville, Illinois

Sheryl J. Samuelson, PhD, RN
Millikin University
Decatur, Illinois

Ann Christy Seckman, MSN, RN
Clarkson College
Omaha, Nebraska

Sheila Donnaud Smith, PhD, RNC
Assistant Professor
Director, Edna Horn Gay Learning Center
Lamar University
Beaumont, Texas

Tish Smyer, DNSc, RN
Coordinator, RN Upward Mobility Option
College of Nursing
South Dakota State University
Brookings, South Dakota

Pam Springer, PhD, RN
Boise State University
Boise, Idaho

Susan K. Steele, DNS, APRN, AOCN®
Louisiana State University Health Sciences Center
New Orleans, Louisiana

Jill D. Steuer, PhD, RN, CNS
Associate Professor
Director, MSN Program
Capital University School of Nursing
Columbus, Ohio

Karen A. Stevens, PhD, MSN, FNP
Department of Nursing
Bowie State University
Bowie, Maryland

Diane M. Tomasic, EdD, RN
West Liberty State College
West Liberty, West Virginia

Patti Urso, PhD, RN, ANP, FNP, APRN, BC
University of Hawaii at Hilo
Hilo, Hawaii

Elizabeth A. Van Wynen, EdD, RN, CNA, BC
Joint Practice Clinician
Englewood Hospital and Medical Center
Clinical Associate Professor of Nursing
University of Medicine and Dentistry New Jersey,
Ramapo College of New Jersey,
Englewood Hospital and Medical Center
Englewood, New Jersey

Kathleen O. Vito, DNSc, RN
Director of Graduate Nursing Program
LaSalle University
Philadelphia, Pennsylvania

Evelyn Yeaw, PhD, RN
Professor
College of Nursing
University of Rhode Island
Kingston, Rhode Island

PREFACE

Research is a major force in nursing, and the evidence generated from research is changing practice, education, and health policy. Our aim in developing this essentials research text, *Understanding Nursing Research*, is to create an excitement about research in undergraduate students. The text emphasizes the importance of baccalaureate-educated nurses' being able to read, critique, and synthesize research so this evidence can be used to make changes in practice. A major goal of professional nursing and health care is the delivery of evidence-based care. By making nursing research an integral part of baccalaureate education, we hope to facilitate the movement of research into the mainstream of nursing. We also hope this text increases student awareness of the knowledge that has been generated through nursing research and that this knowledge is relevant to their practice. Only through research can nursing truly be recognized as a profession with documented effective outcomes for the patient, family, nurse provider, and health care system. Because of this expanded focus on evidence-based practice, we have subtitled this edition *Building an Evidence-Based Practice*.

Developing a fourth edition of *Understanding Nursing Research* has provided us with an opportunity to clarify and refine the essential content for an undergraduate text. The text is designed to assist undergraduate students in overcoming the barriers they frequently encounter in understanding the language used in nursing research. The revisions in this fourth edition are based on our own experiences with the text and input from dedicated reviewers, inquisitive students, and supportive faculty from across the country who provided us with many helpful suggestions.

Chapter 1, "Discovering Nursing Research," introduces the reader to nursing research, the history of research, and the significance of research evidence for nursing practice. The discussion of research methodologies and their importance in generating an evidence-based practice for nursing has been expanded. The historical information about nursing research has been updated to reflect current trends and events in the profession.

Chapter 2, "Introduction to the Quantitative Research Process," presents the steps of the quantitative research process in a concise manner and introduces students to the focus and findings of quantitative studies. Extensive, recent examples of descriptive, correlational, quasi-experimental, and experimental studies are provided, which reflect the quality of current nursing research.

Chapter 3, "Introduction to the Qualitative Research Process," provides detail on the common qualitative research methodologies, such as phenomenology, grounded theory, ethnography, and historical research. Suggestions are provided to assist students in experiencing collecting and analyzing qualitative data under the direction of their faculty.

Chapter 4, "Research Problems, Purposes, and Hypotheses," clarifies the difference between a problem and a purpose. Example problem and purpose statements are included from current qualitative, quantitative, and outcome studies.

Chapter 5, "Review of the Literature," provides a background for reading, critiquing, and summarizing research literature to determine the current knowledge in a selected area for use in nursing practice. This chapter details the process for accessing online sources and relevant practice information from the Internet.

Chapter 6, "Understanding Theory and Research Frameworks," has been revised to provide a clear and simplified explanation of the importance of frameworks in research and provides guidelines for critiquing frameworks in published studies.

Chapter 7, "Examining Ethics in Nursing Research," includes a detailed discussion of the use of ethics in research and the regulations that govern the research process. Detailed content and websites are provided to promote the students' understanding of the Health Insurance Portability and Accountability Act (HIPAA), the U.S. Department of Health and Human Services Protection of Human Subjects, and the Federal Drug Administration Regulations.

Chapter 8, "Clarifying Research Designs," addresses descriptive, correlational, quasi-experimental, and experimental designs and criteria for critiquing these designs in studies.

Chapter 9, "Outcomes Research," is included for the first time in this text. The inclusion of this chapter was stimulated by the increased numbers of outcome studies appearing in nursing and other health care journals.

Chapter 10, "Populations and Samples," includes detailed sections on sampling methods used in both quantitative and qualitative research.

Chapter 11, "Measurement and Data Collection in Research," has been updated to reflect current knowledge in the literature.

Chapter 12, "Understanding Statistics in Research," includes the following essential topics: processing data analysis; understanding the reasoning behind statistics; describing, predicting, and testing hypotheses using statistics; examining relationships using statistics; interpreting statistical outcomes; and judging statistical suitability.

Chapter 13, "Critiquing Research for Nursing Practice," summarizes and builds on the critique content provided in previous chapters and offers direction for conducting critiques of quantitative and qualitative studies. New to this chapter is the critique of a current qualitative study.

Chapter 14, "Building an Evidence-Based Practice," has been significantly updated to reflect the current trends in health care to provide evidence-based care. The levels of research evidence are discussed and demonstrated in a figure to assist nurses in determining when evidence is ready for use in practice. The chapter includes theories to assist nurses and agencies in moving toward evidence-based care.

A variety of changes have been made throughout the fourth edition of this text. Strategies designed to assist the reader in linking research findings to practice are increased; an example of such strategies is selecting study examples with which students as beginning clinicians can easily relate. Research examples have been updated throughout to include recently published quantitative, qualitative, and outcomes nursing studies.

This fourth edition of *Understanding Nursing Research* is appropriate for use in a variety of undergraduate research courses for both RN and general students because it provides an introduction to quantitative, qualitative, and outcomes research methodologies. This text not only will assist students in reading research literature, critiquing published studies, and summarizing research evidence to make changes in practice, but can also serve as a valuable resource for practicing nurses in critiquing studies and implementing research evidence in their clinical settings.

Learning Resources to Accompany Understanding Nursing Research, 4th edition

The ancillary package to accompany *Understanding Nursing Research* has been expanded for both the instructor and the student, to allow a maximum level of flexibility in course design and student review.

Instructor's Electronic Resource

The entire Instructor's Electronic Resource is available both online and on CD-ROM. The Instructor's Electronic Resource consists of an *Instructor's Resource Manual*, Test Bank, PowerPoint Lecture Slides, Electronic Image Collection, and Complimentary Research Article Library, and additional learning activities on the Evolve Resources website.

Instructor's Resource Manual

The *Instructor's Resource Manual* presents chapter focus, key terms, learning objectives, learning activities, and higher-level critique activities for each chapter in the main text. The chapter focus states the concepts to which the reader will be introduced when reading the chapter. Relevant outcomes are developed for undergraduate students. Instructors can select the outcomes that are most appropriate for their particular curricula and courses. The learning activities are a selection of individual and group assignments provided for use in or out of class to facilitate the learning of research content. Higher-level critique exercises are included for each chapter, based on the studies provided in the appendix of the *Manual*. Answer guidelines, with text page references, are provided for each exercise. The *Instructor's Resource Manual* can be saved, revised, and printed to custom-fit specific classes and individual teaching styles.

Test Bank

The Test Bank is made up of approximately 600 multiple-choice questions, including the topic, learning outcome, cognitive level, correct answer, rationale, and text reference. It is available in both ExamView and ParTest format and can be saved, revised, and printed to custom-fit the needs of the individual instructor.

PowerPoint Lecture Slides

The PowerPoint Lecture Slides contain approximately 800 slides, including important illustrations from the textbook. Slide presentations can be customized by revising or changing the order of existing slides. This teaching aid is provided to facilitate lecture preparation and presentation.

Electronic Image Collection

The electronic image collection consists of all images from the text. This collection can be used in classroom lectures to reinforce student learning.

Research Article Library

A collection of research articles, taken from leading nursing journals, can be found in the appendix of the *Instructor's Resource Manual* and in the *Evolve Learning Resources*.

Additional Learning Activities

Two additional learning activities are available on Evolve and may be activated by the instructor for the student's use:

- Critiquing Exercises are a selection of critical-thinking exercises based on supplied research articles and include answer guidelines for the instructor.
- Ideas for Research Projects

Companion Student CD

Four hundred interactive Review Questions are provided on the Companion CD-ROM that accompanies this text. The multiple-choice questions include rationales for both correct and incorrect answers, as well as a textbook page reference.

Evolve Resources for Students

This edition is web-enhanced, and students are prompted to the *Evolve* website for further practice. As students log onto the text's website, they will find open-book quizzes, crossword puzzles, bonus review questions, WebLinks, and, when activated by the instructor, critiquing exercises and ideas for research projects.

- The Open-Book Quizzes are composed of critical thinking questions in multiple-choice and fill-in-the-blank formats. Answers and text references are provided.
- Crossword Puzzles offer a fun review of the material in each chapter.
- Bonus Review Questions aid the student in reviewing and focusing the chapter material.
- Websites related to and organized by chapter are provided in the WebLinks component.

Study Guide

The *Study Guide*, available as a companion to the text, includes three recently published nursing studies that can be used in classroom discussions, as well as to address the study guide questions. The *Study Guide* provides exercises that target comprehension of the meaning of concepts used in each chapter. Exercises, including fill-in-the-blank, matching, and multiple-choice questions, encourage students to validate their understanding of the chapter content.

Critique activities provide students with opportunities to apply their new research knowledge to evaluate the quantitative and qualitative studies provided in the back of the *Study Guide*. For students who enjoy a little fun with their learning, crossword puzzles related to chapter content are provided.

Acknowledgments

Developing this essentials research text was a 2-year project, and there are many people we would like to thank. We express our appreciation to Dean Elizabeth Poster and Associate Deans Dr. Carolyn Cason, Dr. Jennifer Gray, and Dr. Beth Mancini of The University of Texas at Arlington School of Nursing. We extend our thanks to the faculty of the School of Nursing, for their endless support and encouragement. We also would like to thank other nursing faculty members across the world who are using our book to teach research and have spent valuable time to send us ideas and to identify errors in the text. Special thanks to the students who have read our book and provided honest feedback on its clarity and usefulness to them. We would also like to recognize the excellent reviews of the many colleagues, listed on the following pages, who helped us make important revisions in the text.

In conclusion, we would like to thank the people at Elsevier who helped produce this book. We thank the following individuals who have devoted extensive time to the development of this fourth edition, the instructor's ancillary materials, student study guide, and all of the web-based components. These individuals include Lee Henderson, Editor; Maureen Iannuzzi, Senior Developmental Editor; Jeanne Genz, Project Manager; and Amy Shehi, Multimedia Producer.

Nancy Burns,
PhD, RN, FAAN

Susan K. Grove,
PhD, APRN, BC, ANP, GNP

CONTENTS

Understanding Nursing Research

BUILDING AN EVIDENCE-BASED PRACTICE

Discovering Nursing Research

Chapter Overview

Learning Outcomes

After completing this chapter, you should be able to:

1. Define research and nursing research.
2. Describe the link between research and the development of an evidence-based practice for nursing.
3. Identify your role in research as a professional nurse.
4. Describe the development of nursing research from the time of Florence Nightingale into the twenty-first century.
5. Describe the ways of acquiring nursing knowledge (tradition, authority, borrowing, trial and error, personal experience, role modeling, intuition, reasoning, and research) that you use in practice.
6. Identify the type of research—quantitative, qualitative, or outcomes—conducted in published nursing studies.

Key Terms

STUDY TOOLS

Be sure to visit www.Evolve/Burns/Understanding for additional examples and self-tests. Also, a review of this chapter's concepts and practice exercises can be found in Chapter 1 of the Study Guide for *Understanding Nursing Research: Building an Evidence-Based Practice*, 4th edition.

Welcome to the world of nursing research. You may think it strange to consider research a "world," but it is a truly new way of experiencing reality. Entering a new world requires learning a unique language, incorporating new rules, and using new experiences to learn how to interact effectively within that world. As you become a part of this new world, your perceptions and methods of reasoning will be modified and expanded. For example, research involves questioning, and you will be encouraged to ask such questions as these: Why is this nursing intervention being used? Would another intervention be more effective? What research has been conducted in this area? What is the quality of the studies conducted to determine the effectiveness of this intervention? Do the findings from the studies conducted on this nursing intervention provide sound evidence for use in practice? How can you use the research evidence most effectively in your practice?

Because research is a new world to many of you, we have developed this textbook to facilitate your entry into and understanding of this world and its contribution to the delivery of quality nursing care. This first chapter provides a broad explanation of the world of nursing research. The importance of nursing research in developing an evidence-based practice and your role in research are addressed. The past, present, and future of nursing research are explored, including the scientific accomplishments in the profession over the last 150 years. The ways of acquiring knowledge in nursing are discussed, including the significance of research in developing nursing knowledge. The chapter concludes with a discussion of the common research methodologies used in generating nursing knowledge: quantitative, qualitative, and outcomes research.

What Is Nursing Research?

The word **research** means "to search again" or "to examine carefully." More specifically, research is a diligent, systematic inquiry or study that validates and refines existing knowledge and develops new knowledge. Diligent, systematic study indicates planning, organization, and persistence. The ultimate goal of research is the development of a research body of knowledge for a discipline or profession, such as nursing.

Defining nursing research requires determining the relevant knowledge needed by nurses. Because nursing is a practice profession, research is essential to develop and refine knowledge that can be used to improve clinical practice. Practicing nurses, such as yourself, need to be able to read research reports, identify effective interventions for practice, and implement these interventions to promote positive outcomes for patients and families. For example, extensive research has been done to determine the most effective technique for administering medications through an intramuscular (IM) injection. Two integrative reviews of the research have been conducted to develop guidelines for administering IM injections (Beyea & Nicoll, 1995; Rodger & King, 2004). **Integrative review of research** involves critiquing studies on a selected topic or practice problem, such as safe administration of IM injections; summarizing the study findings; and drawing conclusions about what is known and not known about the selected topic (Whittemore, 2005). This summary of current research knowledge is used to generate evidence-based guidelines for practice (Forrest & Miller, 2004). The guidelines for IM injections are based on the most current research evidence and identify the best needle size and length to use for administering different types of medications; the safest injection site (ventrogluteal site) for many medications; and the best injection technique to deliver a medication, minimize patient discomfort, and prevent physical damage (Beyea & Nicoll, 1995; Greenway, 2004; Rodger & King, 2000). These guidelines can direct you in giving IM injections with positive outcomes of accurate delivery of medication and absence of harm to the patient.

Extensive research is needed to develop sound empirical knowledge that can be synthesized into evidence for use in nursing practice. This research evidence might be synthesized to develop guidelines, standards, protocols, or policies to direct the implementation of a variety of nursing interventions. The ultimate goal of nursing is providing evidence-based practice that promotes high-quality outcomes for patients, families, health care providers, and the health care system. **Evidence-based practice** is the conscientious integration of best research evidence with clinical expertise and patient values and needs in the delivery of high-quality, cost-effective health care (Brown, 1999; Melnyk & Fineout-Overholt, 2005). Qualitative, quantitative, and outcomes research are essential to generate research evidence for specific nursing goals:

- Promoting an understanding of patients' and families' experiences with health and illness (a common focus of qualitative research)
- Implementing effective nursing interventions to promote patient health (a common focus of quantitative research)
- Providing high-quality, cost-effective care within the health care system (a common focus of outcomes research)

For example, research related to the administration of IM injections has been critiqued, summarized, and developed into evidence-based guidelines to direct the administration of medications by an IM route to infants, children, and adults in a variety of practice settings. The outcomes from using these evidence-based guidelines in practice include (1) adequate administration of medication to promote patient health, (2) minimal patient discomfort, and (3) no physical damage to the patient, all of which promote high-quality, cost-effective care.

Nursing research also is needed to generate knowledge about nursing education, nursing administration, health care services, characteristics of nurses, and nursing roles. The findings from these studies indirectly influence nursing practice and thus add to nursing's body of knowledge. Research is needed to provide high-quality learning experiences for nursing students. Through research, the best methods for delivering distance nursing education can be developed and refined. Nursing administration and health services studies are needed to improve the quality and cost-effectiveness of the health care delivery system. Studies of nurses and nursing roles can influence nurses' productivity, job satisfaction, and retention. In this era of nursing shortage, additional research is needed to determine effective ways to recruit individuals into and retain them in the profession of nursing. This type of research could have a major impact on the quality and number of nurses providing care to patients and families in the future.

In summary, nursing research is needed to generate knowledge that will directly and indirectly influence nursing practice. In this book, **nursing research** is defined as a scientific process that validates and refines existing knowledge and generates new knowledge that directly and indirectly influences nursing practice.

Why Is Research Important in Generating an Evidence-Based Practice for Nursing?

Nursing research is essential for the development of empirical knowledge that enables nurses to provide evidence-based nursing care (Brown, 1999; Melnyk & Fineout-Overholt, 2005). Broadly, the nursing profession is accountable to society for providing high-quality, cost-effective care for patients and families. Thus, the care provided by nurses must be constantly evaluated and improved on the basis of new and refined research knowledge. Through nursing research, empirical knowledge can be developed to improve nursing care, patient outcomes, and the health care delivery system. For example, nurses need research knowledge to improve their decision making in prioritizing and organizing their nursing care. A solid research base is needed to document the effectiveness of selected nursing interventions in treating particular patient problems and promoting positive patient and family outcomes. In addition, nurses need to use research findings to determine the best way to deliver health care services to ensure that the greatest number of people receive care. Accomplishing these goals will require you to critique, summarize, and use research evidence that provides description, explanation, prediction, and control of phenomena in your clinical practice.

Description

Description involves identifying and understanding the nature of nursing phenomena and sometimes the relationships among these phenomena (Chinn & Kramer, 1999). Through research, nurses are able to (1) describe what exists in nursing practice, (2) discover new information, (3) promote understanding of situations, and (4) classify information for use in the discipline. For example, Arslanian-Engoren and Scott (2003) conducted a qualitative study to describe the experience of surviving prolonged mechanical ventilation. The findings from this study provide nurses insight into the psychosocial needs of patients being weaned from ventilators. The implications for practice include expanding the involvement of the family in the weaning process and supporting patients in their expression of religious and spiritual beliefs. Research focused on description is essential groundwork for studies that will provide explanation, prediction, and control of nursing phenomena.

Explanation

Explanation clarifies the relationships among phenomena and identifies the reasons why certain events occur. For example, Pronk, Goodman, O'Connor, and Martinson (1999) studied the relationships between modifiable health risks (physical inactivity, obesity, and smoking) and health care charges and found that adverse health risks translate into significantly higher health care charges. Thus, managed health care systems, nurses, and consumers seeking to improve societal health and reduce health care costs need to promote modification of health risks (U.S. Department of Health and Human Services [USDHHS], 2000). Accordingly, more explanatory research is being conducted to link sedentary behaviors to obesity and diabetes in adults (Hu, Li, Colditz, Willett, & Manson, 2003) and quality of life to obesity in children and adolescents (Schwimmer, Burwinkle, & Varni, 2003). These studies illustrate how explanatory research is useful in identifying relationships among nursing phenomena, which is the basis for conducting research for prediction and control.

Prediction

Through **prediction**, the probability of a specific outcome can be estimated in a given situation (Chinn & Kramer, 1999). Predicting an outcome does not necessarily enable the nurse to modify or control the outcome. With predictive knowledge, however, nurses may be able to anticipate the effects that nursing interventions would have on patients and families. For example, Defloor (2000) conducted a study to determine the effects of position and type of mattress on skin pressure in persons lying in bed. The researcher found that use of the 30-degree semi-Fowler position and a polyethylene-urethane mattress produced a significant reduction in interface pressure between the mattress and skin. However, this type of study does not determine whether reducing interface pressure will decrease the incidence of pressure ulcers. Further research is needed to determine whether controlling the position and type of mattress will decrease the incidence of pressure ulcer development in patients on bed rest. Predictive studies isolate independent variables that require additional research to ensure their manipulation results in successful outcomes, as measured by designated dependent variables (Omery, Kasper, & Page, 1995).

Control

If the outcome of a situation can be predicted, the next step is to control or manipulate the situation to produce the desired outcome. **Control** can be described as the ability to write a prescription to produce the desired outcome. Currently, nurses prescribe specific interventions in their care plans to assist patients and families in achieving their health goals. These care plans need to reflect the most current evidence-based interventions to produce high-quality, cost-effective outcomes for patients and their families. For example, Chouinard and Robichaud-Ekstrand (2005) conducted a study that implemented a prescribed intervention to promote smoking cessation in patients with cardiovascular disease. The researchers found that an inpatient smoking cessation program with telephone follow-up in the home significantly increased the smoking abstinence rate in cardiovascular patients. Thus, implementing this intervention manipulated or controlled the situation to produce the positive outcome of smoking abstinence.

In summary, studies that document the effectiveness of specific nursing interventions make it possible to implement evidence-based care that will produce the best outcomes for patients and their families. The quality of research conducted in nursing affects not only the quality of care delivered but also the power of nurses in making decisions about the health care delivery system. A limited number of studies have developed knowledge that is useful for prediction and control in nursing practice. However, the extensive number of nursing studies conducted in the last two decades has greatly expanded the scientific knowledge available to you for describing, explaining, predicting, and controlling phenomena within your nursing practice.

What Is Your Role in Nursing Research?

Now that you have been introduced to the world of nursing research, what do you think will be your research role? You may believe that you have no role in research, that research is the responsibility of other nurses. However, generating a scientific knowledge base and using this research evidence in practice requires the participation of all nurses in a variety of research activities. Some nurses are producers of research and conduct studies to generate and refine the knowledge needed for nursing practice. Others are consumers of research and use research findings to improve their nursing practice.

Professional nursing organizations, such as American Nurses Association (ANA) (1989) and the American Association of Colleges of Nursing (AACN) (1999), have published position statements that identify the participation of nurses in research based on their educational preparation. Nurses with an associate degree in nursing (ADN), a bachelor of science degree in nursing (BSN), a master of science degree in nursing (MSN), a doctorate degree, and post-doctorate education each have a clearly designated role in research (ANA, 1989) (Figure 1-1). The researcher role a nurse assumes expands with his or her advanced education and expertise. Thus, nurses with a BSN degree have a significant role in critiquing and synthesizing research findings from the nursing profession and other disciplines for use in practice. These nurses also are important members of the health care teams that plan and implement research-based changes in nursing care and in the health care system (AACN, 1999). In addition, nurses with a BSN also provide valuable assistance in identifying research problems and collecting data for studies.

Nurses with an MSN are provided with the educational preparation to lead health care teams in making essential changes in nursing practice and in the health care system that are based on research. MSN-prepared nurses also conduct focused, initial studies in collaboration with other nurse scientists (ANA, 1989). Doctorally prepared nurses assume a major role in the conduct of research and in the generation of nursing knowledge in a selected area of interest. These nurse scientists often coordinate research teams that include MSN- and BSN-prepared nurses to facilitate the conduct of high-quality studies in a variety of health care agencies. The postdoctorally prepared nurse usually assumes a full researcher role and has a funded program of research. These scientists often are identified as experts in selected areas and provide mentoring of new nurse researchers. The maximum preparation of post-

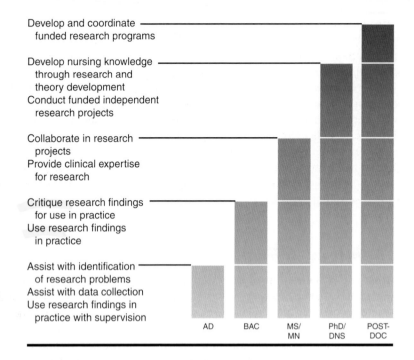

Figure 1-1. Research participation at various levels of education preparation. (American Nurses Association. [1989]. Education for participation in nursing research. Kansas City, MO: Author. Reprinted with permission.)

doctorate education provides a background for doing all the research activities identified for the other levels of educational preparation (see Figure 1-1).

This textbook was developed to encourage you to be a consumer of research. It provides content to assist you in reading research reports, critiquing these reports, and summarizing the findings for use in practice. Nursing's scientific knowledge base is rapidly expanding with the generation of new findings by nurses and other health care professionals using a variety of research methods. You can learn about these relevant research findings by reading research in clinical journals; attending professional conferences and meetings; and examining the findings of the extensive health care studies, evidence-based guidelines, and protocols that are provided on the Internet.

Reading research reports requires an understanding of the research process, which is detailed throughout this book. A **critique** of research involves careful examination of all aspects of a study to judge its strengths, limitations, meaning, and significance. Conducting critiques of studies is a major focus of this textbook, with critique activities highlighted in each chapter. The findings from multiple studies on a specific topic need to be summarized to determine their potential use in practice. This book provides direction for reading, critiquing, and summarizing the research literature as a basis for making changes in your practice. We hope that this book will increase your understanding of research and facilitate your implementation of an evidence-based practice.

Nursing's Participation in Research: Past to Present

Nursing's participation in research has changed drastically over the last 150 years and holds great promise for the twenty-first century. Initially, nursing research evolved slowly, from the investigations of Nightingale in the nineteenth century to the studies of nursing education in the 1930s and 1940s and the research of nurses and nursing roles in the 1950s and 1960s. In the 1970s through the 1990s, an increasing number of nursing studies focused on clinical problems and produced findings that had a direct impact on practice. Clinical research continues to be a major focus for the twenty-first century, with the goal of developing an evidence-based practice for nursing. Reviewing the history of nursing research enables you to identify the accomplishments and understand the need for further research. Table 1-1 outlines the key historical events that have influenced the development of research in nursing.

Florence Nightingale

Nightingale's (1859) initial research focused on the importance of a healthy environment in promoting patients' physical and mental well-being. She studied aspects of the environment such as ventilation, cleanliness, purity of water, and diet to determine the influence on patients' health (Herbert, 1981). However, Nightingale is most noted for her collection and analysis of soldier morbidity and mortality data during the Crimean War. This research enabled her to change the attitudes of the military and society toward the care of the sick. The military began to view the sick as having the right to adequate food, suitable quarters, and appropriate medical treatment. These interventions drastically reduced the mortality rate from 43% to 2% in the Crimean War (Cook, 1913). Nightingale also used research knowledge to make significant changes in society, such as testing public water, improving sanitation, preventing starvation, and decreasing morbidity and mortality (Palmer, 1977).

Nursing Research: 1900s through 1970s

The *American Journal of Nursing* was first published in 1900, and late in the 1920s and 1930s, case studies began appearing in this journal. A **case study** involves an in-depth analysis and a systematic description of one patient or a group of similar patients to promote understanding of health care interventions. Case studies are one example of the practice-related research that has been conducted in nursing over the last century.

Nursing educational opportunities expanded with Teachers College at Columbia University offering the first educational doctoral program for nurses in 1923 and Yale University offering the first master's degree in nursing in 1929. In 1950 the ANA initiated a 5-year study on nursing functions and activities. In 1959 the findings from this study were used to develop statements on functions, standards, and qualifications for professional nurses. During that time, clinical research began expanding as nursing specialty groups, such as community health, psychiatric–mental health, medical-surgical, pediatrics, and obstetrics, developed standards of care. The research conducted by the ANA and specialty groups provided the basis for the nursing practice standards that currently guide professional practice (Gortner & Nahm, 1977). The increase in research activity during the 1940s prompted the publication of the first research journal, *Nursing Research*, in 1952.

Table 1-1	Historical Events Influencing Research in Nursing
Year	Event
1850	Nightingale, first nurse researcher
1900	*American Journal of Nursing* first published
1923	Teachers College at Columbia University offers the first educational doctoral program for nurses
1929	First Master's in Nursing Degree is offered at Yale University
1932	The Association of Collegiate Schools of Nursing is organized
1950	American Nurses Association (ANA) study of nursing functions and activities
1952	*Nursing Research* first published
1953	Institute of Research and Service in Nursing Education established
1955	American Nurses Foundation established to fund nursing research
1963	*International Journal of Nursing Studies* first published
1965	ANA sponsored first nursing research conferences
1967	*Image* (Sigma Theta Tau Journal) first published, now entitled *Image—The Journal of Nursing Scholarship*
1970	ANA Commission on Nursing Research established
1972	ANA Council of Nurse Researchers established
1973	First Nursing Diagnosis Conference was held
1978	*Research in Nursing & Health* first published *Advances in Nursing Science* first published
1979	*Western Journal of Nursing Research* first published
1982-1983	Conduct and Utilization of Research in Nursing (CURN) Project (published)
1983	*Annual Review of Nursing Research* first published
1985	National Center for Nursing Research (NCNR) was established within the National Institutes of Health
1987	*Scholarly Inquiry for Nursing Practice* first published
1988	*Applied Nursing Research* first published *Nursing Science Quarterly* first published
1989	Agency for Health Care Policy and Research (AHCPR) was established Clinical practice guidelines were first published by the AHCPR
1992	*Healthy People 2000* was published by U.S. Department of Health and Human Services *Clinical Nursing Research* first published
1993	NCNR was renamed the National Institute of Nursing Research (NINR) *Journal of Nursing Measurement* first published
1994	*Qualitative Health Research* first published
1999	AHCPR renamed Agency for Healthcare Research and Quality (AHRQ)
1999	American Association of Colleges of Nursing position statement on nursing research
2000	*Healthy People 2010* was published by U.S. Department of Health and Human Services *Biological Research for Nursing* first published
2004	*Worldviews on Evidence-Based Nursing* first published
2005	NINR identified mission and funding priorities for 2000 to 2005
2005	AHRQ identified mission and funding priorities

In the 1950s and 1960s, nursing schools began introducing research and the steps of the research process at the baccalaureate level, and MSN-level nurses were provided a background for conducting research. In 1953 the Institute for Research and Service in Nursing Education was established at Teachers College of Columbia University, which provided learning experiences in research for doctoral students (Gortner & Nahm, 1977).

In the 1960s an increasing number of clinical studies focused on quality care and the development of criteria to measure patient outcomes. Intensive care units were developed, which promoted the investigation of nursing interventions, staffing patterns, and cost-effectiveness of care (Gortner & Nahm, 1977). An additional research journal, the *International Journal of Nursing Studies*, was published in 1963. In 1965 the ANA sponsored the first of a series of nursing research conferences to promote the communication of research findings and the use of these findings in clinical practice.

In the late 1960s and 1970s, nurses were involved in the development of models, conceptual frameworks, and theories to guide nursing practice. The nursing theorists' work provided direction for future nursing research. In 1978, Chinn began publishing the journal *Advances in Nursing Science*, which included nursing theorists' work and related research. Another event influencing research during the 1970s was the establishment of the ANA Commission on Nursing Research in 1970. In 1972 the commission established the Council of Nurse Researchers to advance research activities, provide an exchange of ideas, and recognize excellence in research. The commission also influenced the development of federal guidelines concerning research with human subjects and sponsored research programs nationally and internationally (See, 1977).

The communication of research findings was a major issue in the 1970s (Barnard, 1980). Sigma Theta Tau, the international honor society for nursing, sponsored national and international research conferences; the chapters of this organization sponsored many local conferences to communicate research findings. *Image*, now entitled *Image—The Journal of Nursing Scholarship*, was first published in 1967 by Sigma Theta Tau and includes research articles and summaries of research conducted on selected topics. Two additional research journals were first published in the 1970s: *Research in Nursing & Health* in 1978 and *Western Journal of Nursing Research* in 1979.

Nursing Research: 1980s and 1990s

The conduct of clinical research was the focus of the 1980s, and clinical journals began publishing more studies. One new research journal was published in 1987, *Scholarly Inquiry for Nursing Practice*, and two in 1988, *Applied Nursing Research* and *Nursing Science Quarterly*. Although the body of empirical knowledge generated through clinical research increased rapidly in the 1980s, little of this knowledge was used in practice. During 1982 and 1983 the materials from a federally funded project, Conduct and Utilization of Research in Nursing (CURN), were published to facilitate the use of research to improve nursing practice (Horsley, Crane, Crabtree, & Wood, 1983). In 1983 the first volume of the *Annual Review of Nursing Research* was published (Werley & Fitzpatrick, 1983). These volumes include experts' reviews of research organized into four areas: nursing practice, nursing care delivery, nursing education, and the nursing profession. These summaries of current research knowledge encourage the use of research findings in practice and provide direction for future research. Publication of the *Annual Review of Nursing Research* continues today, with leading expert nurse scientists providing summaries of research in their areas of expertise.

Qualitative research was introduced in the late 1970s, with the first studies appearing in nursing journals in the 1980s. The focus of qualitative research was holistic, with the intent to discover meaning and gain new insight and understanding of phenomena relevant to nursing. The number of qualitative researchers and studies expanded greatly in the 1990s, with qualitative studies appearing in most of the nursing research and clinical journals. In 1994 a journal focused on disseminating qualitative research, *Qualitative Health Research*, was first published. However, quantitative research has been and continues to be the most frequently used research methodology in conducing nursing research. In the 1990s, more new research journals were added, with *Clinical Nursing Research* first published in 1992 and the *Journal of Nursing Measurement* in 1993.

Another priority of the 1980s was to obtain increased funding for nursing research. Most of the federal funds in the 1980s were designated for medical studies involving the diagnosis and cure of diseases. However, the ANA achieved a major political victory for nursing research with the creation of the National Center for Nursing Research (NCNR) in 1985. The purpose of this center is to support the conduct and dissemination of knowledge developed through basic and clinical nursing research, training, and other programs in patient care research (Bauknecht, 1985). Under the direction of Dr. Ada Sue Hinshaw, the NCNR became the National Institute of Nursing Research (NINR) in 1993. During the 1990s the NINR (1993) focused its support on five research priorities: community-based nursing models, effectiveness of nursing interventions in human immunodeficiency virus and acquired immunodeficiency syndrome (HIV/AIDS), cognitive impairment, living with chronic illness, and biobehavioral factors related to immunocompetence. The NINR web site (http://ninr.nih.gov/ninr/about.html) provides the most current information on the institute's research priorities and activities.

Outcomes research emerged as an important methodology for documenting the effectiveness of health care services in the 1980s and 1990s. This effectiveness research evolved from the quality assessment and quality assurance functions that originated with the professional standards review organizations (the PSROs) in 1972. William Roper, director of the Health Care Finance Administration (HCFA), promoted outcomes research during the 1980s to determine quality and cost-effectiveness of patient care. In 1989 the Agency for Health Care Policy and Research (AHCPR) was established to facilitate the conduct of outcomes research (Rettig, 1991). AHCPR also had an active role in communicating research findings to health care practitioners and was responsible for publishing the first clinical practice guidelines in 1989. These guidelines included a synthesis of the latest research findings with directives for practice developed by health care experts in a variety of areas. Several of these evidence-based guidelines were published in the 1990s and provided standards for practice in nursing and medicine. The Healthcare Research and Quality Act of 1999 reauthorized the AHCPR, changing its name to the Agency for Healthcare Research and Quality (AHRQ). This significant change positioned the AHRQ as a scientific partner with the public and private sectors to improve the quality and safety of patient care. The AHRQ web site (http://www.ahrq.gov) provides the most current information on this agency and includes current guidelines for clinical practice.

Nursing Research: Twenty-First Century

The vision for nursing in the twenty-first century is the development of a scientific knowledge base that enables nurses to implement an evidence-based practice (Brown, 1999; Melnyk &

Fineout-Overholt, 2005). This vision is consistent with the mission of NINR, which is to "support clinical and basic research to establish a scientific basis for the care of individuals across the lifespan—from management of patients during illness and recovery to the reduction of risks for disease and disability, the promotion of healthy lifestyles, promoting quality of life in those with chronic illness, and care for the individuals at the end of life" (http://www.nih.gov/ninr). NINR is seeking expanded funding for nursing research and is encouraging a variety of methodologies (quantitative, qualitative, and outcomes research) to be used to generate essential knowledge for nursing practice. The expansion of biological research and the movement toward evidence-based practice in nursing has resulted in the publication of two new research journals, *Biological Research for Nursing* in 2000 and *Worldviews on Evidence-Based Nursing* in 2004.

The AHRQ has been designated as the lead agency supporting research designed to improve the quality of health care, reduce its cost, improve patient safety, decrease medical errors, and broaden access to essential services. AHRQ conducts and sponsors research that provides evidence-based information on health care outcomes, quality, cost, use, and access. This research information is needed to promote effective health care decision making by patients, clinicians, health system executives, and policy makers.

The focus of health care research and funding is expanding from the treatment of illness to include health promotion and illness prevention interventions. *Healthy People 2010*, published by the USDHHS (2000), increased the visibility of and identified priorities for health promotion research. In the twenty-first century, nurses could play a major role in the development of interventions to promote health and prevent illness in individuals, families, and communities (ANA, 2004). To ensure an effective research enterprise in nursing, the discipline must (1) create a research culture; (2) provide high-quality educational programs (baccalaureate, master's, doctorate, and postdoctorate) to prepare a workforce of nurse scientists; (3) develop a sound research infrastructure; and (4) obtain sufficient funding for essential research (AACN, 1999).

Acquiring Knowledge in Nursing

Some key questions that might be asked about knowledge include the following: What is knowledge? How is knowledge acquired in nursing? Is most of nursing's knowledge based on research? **Knowledge** is essential information acquired in a variety of ways, expected to be an accurate reflection of reality, and incorporated and used to direct a person's actions (Kaplan, 1964). During nursing education, an extensive amount of knowledge is acquired from classroom and clinical experiences. You had to learn, synthesize, incorporate, and apply this knowledge so that you could practice as a nurse.

The quality of your nursing practice depends on the quality of the knowledge that you acquired. Thus, you need to question the quality and credibility of new information that you hear or read. For example, what were the sources of the knowledge that you acquired during your nursing education? Were the nursing interventions taught based on research or tradition? Which interventions were based on research, and which need further study to determine their effectiveness? Nursing has historically acquired knowledge through traditions, authority, borrowing, trial and error, personal experience, role modeling, intuition, and reasoning. Only in the last decade have many of the research findings been included in nursing textbooks or instructors' lectures. This section introduces different ways of acquiring knowledge in nursing. Some nursing actions are based on sound scientific knowledge, but others need to be questioned, studied, and revised to reflect current research findings.

Traditions

Traditions include "truths" or beliefs that are based on customs and trends. Nursing traditions from the past have been transferred to the present by written and oral communication and role modeling, and they continue to influence the practice of nursing. For example, many of the policy and procedure manuals in hospitals contain traditional ideas. Traditions can positively influence nursing practice because they were developed from effective past experiences.

However, traditions also can narrow and limit the knowledge sought for nursing practice. For example, nursing units are frequently organized and run according to set rules or traditions that may not be efficient or effective. Often these traditions are neither questioned nor changed because they have existed for years and are frequently supported by people with power and authority. Many traditions have not been tested for accuracy or efficiency through research, and even those not supported through research tend to persist. For example, many patients with cardiac conditions are required to take basin baths throughout their hospitalization despite findings from nursing research that "the physiologic costs of the three types of baths (basin, tub, and shower) are similar; differences in responses to bathing seem more a function of subject variability than bath types; and many cardiac patients can take a tub bath or shower earlier in their hospitalization" (Winslow, Lane, & Gaffney, 1985, p. 164). Nursing's body of knowledge needs to have an empirical rather than a traditional base if nurses are to have a powerful impact on health care and patient outcomes.

Authority

An **authority** is a person with expertise and power who is able to influence opinion and behavior. A person is given authority because it is thought that she or he knows more in a given area than others do. Knowledge acquired from an authority is illustrated when one person credits another as the source of information. Nurses who publish articles and books or develop theories are frequently considered authorities. Students usually view their instructors as authorities, and clinical nursing experts are considered authorities within the clinical practice setting. Authorities maintain many customs or traditional ways of knowing; however, as with tradition, much of the knowledge acquired from authorities has not been validated by research. Although the knowledge may be useful, it needs to be questioned and verified through research.

Borrowing

Some nursing leaders have described part of nursing's knowledge as information borrowed from disciplines such as medicine, sociology, psychology, physiology, and education (McMurrey, 1982). **Borrowing** in nursing involves the appropriation and use of knowledge from other fields or disciplines to guide nursing practice. Nursing has borrowed in two ways. For years, some nurses have taken information from other disciplines and applied it directly to nursing practice. This information was not integrated within the unique focus of nursing. For example, some nurses have used the medical model to guide their nursing practice, thus focusing on the diagnosis and treatment of disease. This type of borrowing continues today as nurses use advances in technology to become highly specialized and focused on the detection and treatment of disease.

The second way of borrowing, which is more useful in nursing, involves integrating information from other disciplines within the focus of nursing. Because disciplines share knowledge, it is sometimes difficult to know where the boundaries exist between nursing's knowledge base and that of other disciplines. However, borrowed knowledge has been inadequate for answering many questions generated in nursing practice.

Trial and Error

Trial and error is an approach with unknown outcomes that is used in a situation of uncertainty in which other sources of knowledge are unavailable. Because each patient responds uniquely to a situation, there is uncertainty in nursing practice. Hence, nurses must use trial and error in providing nursing care. However, trial and error frequently involves no formal documentation of effective and ineffective nursing actions. With this strategy, knowledge is gained from experience, but often it is not shared with others. The trial-and-error approach to acquiring knowledge also can be time-consuming because multiple interventions may be implemented before one is found to be effective. There also is a risk of implementing nursing actions that are detrimental to patients' health. If studies are conducted on nursing interventions, selection and implementation of interventions can be based on scientific knowledge rather than chance.

Personal Experience

Personal experience involves gaining knowledge by being personally involved in an event, a situation, or a circumstance. Personal experience enables the nurse to gain skills and expertise by providing care to patients and families in clinical settings. Learning that occurs from personal experience enables the nurse to cluster ideas into a meaningful whole. For example, you may read about giving an injection or be told how to give an injection in a classroom setting, but you do not "know" how to give an injection until you observe other nurses giving injections to patients and actually give several injections yourself.

The amount of personal experience affects the complexity of a nurse's knowledge base. Benner (1984) described five levels of experience in the development of clinical knowledge and expertise: (1) novice, (2) advanced beginner, (3) competent, (4) proficient, and (5) expert. Novice nurses have no personal experience in the work they are to perform, but they have some preconceptions and expectations about clinical practice that they obtained during their education. These preconceptions and expectations are challenged, refined, confirmed, or refuted by personal experience in a clinical setting. The advanced beginner nurse has just enough experience to recognize and intervene in recurrent situations. For example, the advanced beginner is able to recognize and intervene in managing patients' pain. Competent nurses are able to generate and achieve long-range goals and plans because of years of personal experience. The competent nurse also is able to use personal knowledge to take conscious, deliberate actions that are efficient and organized. From a more complex knowledge base, the proficient nurse views the patient as a whole and as a member of a family and community. The proficient nurse recognizes that each patient and family responds differently to illness and health. The expert nurse has an extensive background of experience and is able to identify accurately and intervene skillfully in a situation. Personal experience increases the ability of the expert nurse to grasp a situation intuitively with accuracy and speed. Benner's (1984) qualitative research provides an increased understanding of how knowledge is acquired through personal experience. Additional research is needed to clarify the dynamics of expert nursing practice and to determine methods that will facilitate meaningful personal experiences for nursing students and new graduates.

Role Modeling

Role modeling is learning by imitating the behaviors of an expert. In nursing, role modeling enables the novice nurse to learn through interactions with or examples set by highly competent, expert nurses. Role models include admired teachers, expert clinicians, researchers, or persons who inspire others through their examples (Rempusheski, 1992). An intense form of role modeling is **mentorship,** in which the expert nurse serves as a teacher, sponsor, guide, and counselor for the novice nurse. The knowledge gained through personal experience is greatly enhanced by a high-quality relationship with a role model or mentor. Many new graduates enter internship programs provided by clinical agencies so that expert nurses can mentor them during the novices' first few months of employment.

Intuition

Intuition is an insight into or understanding of a situation or event as a whole that usually cannot be explained logically (Rew & Barrow, 1987). Because intuition is a type of knowing that seems to come unbidden, it may also be described as a "gut feeling" or a "hunch." Because intuition cannot be explained scientifically with ease, many people are uncomfortable with it. Some even believe that it does not exist. However, intuition is not the lack of knowing; rather, it is a result of "deep" knowledge (Benner, 1984). The knowledge is so deeply incorporated that it is difficult to bring it to the surface consciously and express it in a logical manner. Some nurses can intuitively recognize when a patient is experiencing a health crisis. Using this intuitive knowledge, they can assess the patient's condition and contact the physician for medical intervention.

Reasoning

Reasoning is the processing and organizing of ideas in order to reach conclusions. Through reasoning, people are able to make sense of both their thoughts and experiences. This type of logical thinking is often evident in the oral presentation of an argument in which each part is linked to reach a logical conclusion. The science of logic includes inductive and deductive reasoning. **Inductive reasoning** moves from the specific to the general; particular instances are observed and then combined into a larger whole or a general statement (Chinn & Kramer, 1999). An example of inductive reasoning follows:

PARTICULAR INSTANCES

A headache is an altered level of health that is stressful.

A terminal illness is an altered level of health that is stressful.

GENERAL STATEMENT

Therefore it can be induced that all altered levels of health are stressful.

Deductive reasoning moves from the general to the specific or from a general premise to a particular situation or conclusion (Chinn & Kramer, 1999). A **premise** or proposition is a statement of the proposed relationship between two or more concepts. An example of deductive reasoning follows:

PREMISES

All human beings experience loss.

All adolescents are human beings.

CONCLUSION

Therefore it can be deduced that all adolescents experience loss.

In this example, deductive reasoning is used to move from the two general premises about human beings and adolescents to the conclusion that "All adolescents experience loss." However, the conclusions generated from deductive reasoning are valid only if they are based on valid premises. Research is a means to test and confirm or refute a premise or proposition so that valid premises can be used as a basis for reasoning in nursing practice.

Acquiring Knowledge through Nursing Research

Acquiring knowledge through traditions, authority, borrowing, trial and error, personal experience, role modeling, intuition, and reasoning is important in nursing. However, these ways of acquiring knowledge are inadequate in providing a scientific knowledge base for nursing practice. The knowledge needed for practice is both specific and holistic, as well as process-oriented and outcomes-focused (ANA, 2003); thus, a variety of research methods are needed to generate this knowledge. This section introduces quantitative, qualitative, and outcomes research methods that have been used to generate knowledge for nursing practice.

Introduction to Quantitative and Qualitative Research

Quantitative and qualitative research complement each other because they generate different kinds of knowledge that are useful in nursing practice. Familiarity with these two types of research will help you identify, understand, and critique these studies in journals and books. Quantitative and qualitative research methodologies have some similarities; both require researcher expertise, involve rigor in implementation, and generate scientific knowledge for nursing practice. Some of the differences between the two methodologies are presented in Table 1-2.

A majority of the studies conducted in nursing have used quantitative research methods. **Quantitative research** is a formal, objective, systematic process in which numerical data are

Table 1-2	Quantitative and Qualitative Research Characteristics	
Characteristic	Quantitative Research	Qualitative Research
Philosophical origin	Logical positivism	Naturalistic, interpretive, humanistic
Focus	Concise, objective, reductionistic	Broad, subjective, holistic
Reasoning	Logistic, deductive	Dialectic, inductive
Basis of knowing	Cause-and-effect relationships	Meaning, discovery, understanding
Theoretical focus	Theory testing	Theory development

used to obtain information about the world. The quantitative approach toward scientific inquiry emerged from a branch of philosophy called *logical positivism*, which operates on strict rules of logic, truth, laws, and predictions. Quantitative researchers hold the position that "truth" is absolute and that a single reality can be defined by careful measurement. To find truth, the researcher must be objective, which means that values, feelings, and personal perceptions cannot enter into the measurement of reality. Quantitative research is conducted to test theory by describing variables, examining relationships among variables, and determining cause-and-effect interactions between variables (Burns & Grove, 2005).

Qualitative research is a systematic, subjective approach used to describe life experiences and situations and to give them meaning (Munhall, 2001). This research methodology evolved from the behavioral and social sciences as a method of understanding the unique, dynamic, holistic nature of human beings. The philosophical base of qualitative research is interpretive, humanistic, and naturalistic and is concerned with understanding the meaning of social interactions by those involved. Qualitative researchers believe that "truth" is both complex and dynamic and can be found only by studying people as they interact with and in their sociohistorical settings (Munhall, 1989; 2001). Nurses' interest in conducting qualitative research began in the late 1970s; currently, an extensive number of qualitative studies are conducted using a variety of qualitative research methods. Qualitative research is conducted to promote understanding of human experiences and situations and to develop theories that describe these experiences and situations. Because human emotions are difficult to quantify (i.e., assign a numerical value to), qualitative research seems to be a more effective method of investigating emotional responses than quantitative research (see Table 1-2).

Several types of quantitative and qualitative research have been conducted to generate nursing knowledge for practice. These types of research can be classified in a variety of ways. The classification system for this book (Table 1-3) includes the most common types of quantitative and qualitative research conducted in nursing. The quantitative research methods are classified into four categories: descriptive, correlational, quasi-experimental, and experimental. Descriptive research is conducted to explore new areas of research and to describe situations as they exist in the world. Correlational research is conducted to examine relationships and to develop and refine explanatory knowledge for nursing practice. Quasi-experimental and experimental studies are conducted to determine the effectiveness of nursing interventions in predicting and controlling the outcomes desired for patients and families. (These types of research are discussed in detail in Chapter 2.)

The qualitative research methods included in this text are phenomenological, grounded theory, ethnographical, and historical research (see Table 1-3). Phenomenological research is

Table 1-3	Classification System for Nursing Research Methods

I. Types of Quantitative Research
Descriptive research
Correlational research
Quasi-experimental research
Experimental research

OBJECTIVE

II. Types of Qualitative Research
Phenomenological research
Grounded theory research
Ethnographical research
Historical research

III. Outcomes Research

an inductive descriptive approach used to describe an experience as it is lived by an individual, such as the lived experience of chronic pain. Grounded theory research is an inductive research technique that is used to formulate, test, and refine a theory about a particular phenomenon. Grounded theory research initially was developed by Glaser and Strauss (1967) and was used to formulate a theory about the grieving process. Ethnographical research was developed by the discipline of anthropology for investigating cultures through an in-depth study of the members of the culture. Health practices vary among cultures, and these practices need to be recognized in delivering care to patients, families, and communities. Historical research is a narrative description or analysis of events that occurred in the remote or recent past. Through historical research, past mistakes are examined to facilitate an understanding of and an effective response to present situations (Munhall, 2001). (Qualitative research methods are the focus of Chapter 3.)

Introduction to Outcomes Research

The spiraling cost of health care has generated many questions about the quality and effectiveness of health care services and the patient's outcomes related to these services. Consumers want to know what services they are purchasing and if these services will improve their health. Health care policymakers want to know whether the care is cost effective and high in quality. These concerns have promoted the conduct of **outcomes research**, which focuses on examining the result of care or determining the changes in health status for the patient (Doran, 2003; Rettig, 1991). Four essential areas that require examination through outcomes research are the following: (1) patient responses to medical and nursing interventions; (2) functional maintenance or improvement of physical functioning for the patient; (3) financial outcomes achieved with the provision of health care services; and (4) patient satisfaction with the health outcomes, care received, and health care providers (Jones, 1993). Nurses are playing an active role in conducting outcomes research by participating in multidisciplinary research teams that examine the outcomes of health care services. This knowledge provides a basis for improving the quality of care nurses deliver in practice.

KEY CONCEPTS

- Research is defined as diligent, systematic inquiry to validate and refine existing knowledge and generate new knowledge.
- Nursing research is defined as a scientific process that validates and refines existing knowledge and generates new knowledge that directly and indirectly influences nursing practice.
- Evidence-based practice is the conscientious integration of best research evidence with clinical expertise and patient values and needs in the delivery of high-quality, cost-effective health care.
- Nightingale was the first nurse researcher who developed empirical knowledge to improve practice in the nineteenth century.
- The conduct of clinical research continues to be a major focus in the twenty-first century, with the goal of developing a research- or evidence-based practice for nursing.
- Quantitative research is a formal, objective, systematic process using numerical data to obtain information about the world. This research method is used to describe, examine relationships, and determine cause and effect.
- Qualitative research is a systematic, subjective approach used to describe life experiences and give them meaning. Knowledge generated from qualitative research will provide meaning and understanding of specific emotions, values, and life experiences.
- A third research method is outcomes research, which focuses on examining the result of care or in determining the changes in health status for the patient.

TIPS FOR FURTHER STUDY

- Review the sources on giving IM injections so you might use this evidence in your practice (Beyea & Nicoll, 1995; Greenway, 2004; Rodger & King, 2000).
- Visit the National Institute of Nursing Research (NINR) website http://ninr.nih.gov/ninr/about.html) and review the mission statement, strategic plan, and history for this agency.
- Search the Agency for Healthcare Research and Quality (AHRQ) website (http://www.ahrq.gov) and review the mission, strategic plan, and research findings provided by this agency.
- Read *Healthy People 2010: Understanding and Improving Health* to expand your understanding of the U.S. goals for health.
- For help in defining the Key Terms in this chapter, complete the "Relevant Terms" exercises in Chapter 1 of your *Study Guide* and the Crossword Puzzle for Chapter 1 at www.evolve/Burns/understanding.
- To practice identifying the research methods used by different types of research, complete the "Making Connections" exercises in Chapter 1 of your *Study Guide* and the "Matching" exercises in the Open-Book Quiz at www.evolve/Burns/understanding.

REFERENCES

American Association of Colleges of Nursing. (1999). Position statement: Nursing research. *Journal of Professional Nursing, 15*(4), 253–257.

American Nurses Association. (1989). *Education for participation in nursing research*. Kansas City, MO: Author.

American Nurses Association (2003). *Nursing's social policy statement* (2nd ed.). Washington, DC: Author.

American Nurses Association (2004). *Nursing: Scope and standards of practice*. Washington, DC: Author.

Arslanian-Engoren, C., & Scott, L. D. (2003). Issues in pulmonary nursing. The lived experience of survivors of prolonged mechanical ventilation: A phenomenological study. *Heart & Lung: The Journal of Acute and Critical Care, 32*(5), 328–334.

Barnard, K. E. (1980). Knowledge for practice: Directions for the future. *Nursing Research, 29*(4), 208–212.

Bauknecht, V. L. (1985). Capital commentary: NIH bill passes, includes nursing research center. *American Nurse, 17*(10), 2.

Benner, P. (1984). *From novice to expert: Excellence and power in clinical nursing practice.* Menlo Park, CA: Addison-Wesley.

Beyea, S. C., & Nicoll, L. H. (1995). Administration of medications via the intramuscular route: An integrative review of the literature and research-based protocol for the procedure. *Applied Nursing Research, 8*(1), 23–33.

Brown, S. J. (1999). *Knowledge for health care practice: A guide to using research evidence.* Philadelphia: Saunders.

Burns, N., & Grove, S. K. (2005). *The practice of nursing research: Conduct, critique, and utilization* (5th ed.). Philadelphia: Saunders.

Chinn, P. L., & Kramer, M. K. (1999). *Theory and nursing: A systematic approach* (5th ed.). St. Louis: Mosby.

Chouinard, M.C., & Robichaud-Ekstrand, S. (2005). The effectiveness of a nursing inpatient smoking cessation program in individuals with cardiovascular disease. *Nursing Research, 54*(4), 243–254.

Cook, E. (1913). *The life of Florence Nightingale* (Vol. 1). London: Macmillan.

Defloor, T. (2000). The effect of position and mattress on interface pressure. *Applied Nursing Research, 13*(1), 2–11.

Doran, D. M. (2003). *Nursing sensitive outcomes: The state of the science.* Sudbury, MA: Jones and Bartlett.

Forrest, J. L., & Miller, S. A. (2004). Part I: The anatomy of evidence-based publications: Article summaries and systematic reviews. *The Journal of Dental Hygiene, 78*(II), 343–348.

Glaser, B. G., & Strauss, A. L. (1967). *The discovery of grounded theory: Strategies for qualitative research.* Chicago: Aldine.

Gortner, S. R., & Nahm, H. (1977). An overview of nursing research in the United States. *Nursing Research, 26*(1), 10–33.

Greenway, K. (2004). Using the ventrologluteal site for intramuscular injection. *Nursing Standard, 18*(25), 39–42.

Herbert, R. G. (1981). *Florence Nightingale: Saint, reformer or rebel?* Malabar, FL: Robert E. Krieger.

Horsley, J. A., Crane, J., Crabtree, M. K., & Wood, D. J. (1983). *Using research to improve nursing practice: A guide, CURN Project.* New York: Grune & Stratton.

Hu, F. B., Li, T. Y., Colditz, G. A., Willett, W. C., & Manson, J. E. (2003). Television watching and other sedentary behaviors in relation to risk of obesity and type 2 diabetes mellitus in women. *Journal of the American Medical Association, 289*(14), 1785–1791.

Jones, K. R. (1993). Outcomes analysis: Methods and issues. *Nursing Economics, 11*(3), 145–152.

Kaplan, A. (1964). *The conduct of inquiry;* Methodology for behavioral science. San Francisco: Chandler.

McMurrey, P. H. (1982). Toward a unique knowledge base in nursing. *Image, 14*(1), 12–15.

Melnyk, B. M., & Fineout-Overholt, E. (2005). *Evidence-based practice in nursing & healthcare: A guide to best practice.* Philadelphia: Lippincott Williams & Wilkins.

Munhall, P. L. (1989). Philosophical ponderings on qualitative research methods in nursing. *Nursing Science Quarterly, 2*(1), 20–28.

Munhall, P. L. (2001). *Nursing Research: A qualitative perspective* (3rd ed.). Boston: Jones and Bartlett.

National Institute of Nursing Research (NINR) (September 23, 1993). *National nursing research agenda: Setting nursing research priorities.* Bethesda, MD: National Institutes of Health.

National Institute of Nursing Research (2006). *About the NINR.* Retrieved January 16, 2006, from http://ninr.nih.gov/ninr/about.html

Nightingale, F. (1859). *Notes on nursing: What it is, and what it is not.* Philadelphia: Lippincott.

Omery, A., Kasper, C. E., & Page, G. G. (1995). *In search of nursing science.* Thousand Oaks, CA: Sage Publications.

Palmer, I. S. (1977). Florence Nightingale: Reformer, reactionary, researcher. *Nursing Research, 26*(2), 84–89.

Pronk, N. P., Goodman, M. J., O'Connor, P. J., & Martinson, B. C. (1999). Relationship between modifiable health risks and short-term healthcare charges. *Journal of the American Medical Association, 282*(23), 2235–2239.

Rempusheski, V. F. (1992). A researcher as resource, mentor, and preceptor. *Applied Nursing Research, 5*(2), 105–107.

Rettig, R. (1991). History, development, and importance to nursing of outcomes research. *Journal of Nursing Quality Assurance, 5*(2), 13–17.

Rew, L., & Barrow, E. M. (1987). Intuition: A neglected hallmark of nursing knowledge. *Advances in Nursing Science, 10*(1), 49–62.

Rodger, M. A., & King, L. (2000). Drawing up and administering intramuscular injections: A review of the literature. *Journal of Advanced Nursing, 31*(3), 574–582.

See, E. M. (1977). The ANA and research in nursing. *Nursing Research, 26*(3), 165–171.

Schwimmer, J. B., Burwinkle, T. M., & Varni, J. W. (2003). Health-related quality of life of severely obese children and adolescents. *Journal of the American Medical Association, 289*(14), 1813–1819.

U. S. Department of Health and Human Services, (2000). *Healthy people 2010: Understanding and improving health.* Washington DC: U.S. Dept of Health and Human Services.

Werley, H. H., & Fitzpatrick, J. J. (1983). *Annual review of nursing research* (Vol. 1). New York: Springer.

Whittemore, R. (2005). Combining evidence in nursing research: Methods and implications. *Nursing Research, 54*(1), 56–62.

Winslow, E. H., Lane, L. D., & Gaffney, F. A. (1985). Oxygen uptake and cardiovascular responses in control adults and acute myocardial infarction patients during bathing. *Nursing Research, 34*(3), 164–169.

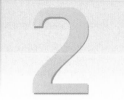

Introduction to the Quantitative Research Process

Chapter Overview

Learning Outcomes

After completing this chapter, you should be able to:

1. Define terms relevant to the quantitative research process: basic research, applied research, rigor, and control.

2. Compare and contrast the problem-solving process, nursing process, and research process.

3. Read research reports.

4. Identify the steps of the quantitative research process in descriptive, correlational, quasi-experimental, and experimental published studies.

5. Conduct an initial critique of a research report.

Key Terms

 STUDY TOOLS

Be sure to visit www.Evolve/Burns/Understanding for additional examples and self-tests. Also, a review of this chapter's concepts and practice exercises can be found in Chapter 2 of the Study Guide for *Understanding Nursing Research: Building an Evidence-Based Practice*, 4th edition.

What do you think of when you hear the word *research?* Frequently, the idea of experimentation comes to mind. Typical features of an **experiment** include randomizing subjects into groups, collecting data, and conducting statistical analyses. Frequently, an experiment is thought to be conducted to "prove" something, such as the effectiveness of a particular drug for treating an illness. These ideas are associated with quantitative research. Quantitative research includes specific steps that are detailed in research reports. Reading and critiquing quantitative studies require learning new terms, understanding the steps of the quantitative research process, and applying a variety of analytical skills.

This chapter provides an introduction to quantitative research and a background for reading a research report. Relevant terms are defined, and the problem-solving process and the nursing process are presented as a basis for understanding the quantitative research process. The steps of the quantitative research process are introduced, and a descriptive correlational study is presented as an example to promote understanding of the process. Also included are a discussion of the critical thinking skills needed for reading research reports and guidelines for conducting an initial critique of these reports. The chapter concludes with the identification of the steps of the research process from published quasi-experimental and experimental studies.

What Is Quantitative Research?

Quantitative research is a formal, objective, rigorous, systematic process for generating information about the world. Quantitative research is conducted to describe new situations, events, or concepts in the world. Some examples follow:

Describing the spread of bird flu and its potential influence on global health

Examining the relationship among the variables minutes of exercise per day, types of foods consumed, and children's weight

Determining the effectiveness of treatments such as herbal medicines on the health of patients and families

The classic experimental designs to test the effectiveness of treatments were originated by Sir Ronald Fisher (1935). He is noted for adding structure to the steps of the research process with such ideas as the hypothesis, research design, and statistical analysis. Fisher's studies provided the groundwork for what is now known as experimental research.

Throughout the years, a number of other quantitative approaches have been developed. Campbell and Stanley (1963) developed quasi-experimental approaches to study the effects of treatments under less controlled conditions. Karl Pearson developed statistical approaches for examining relationships between variables, which increased the conduct of correlational research. The fields of sociology, education, and psychology are noted for their development and expansion of strategies for conducting descriptive research. A broad range of quantitative research approaches is needed to develop knowledge for nursing practice. This section introduces the different types of quantitative research and provides definitions of terms relevant to the quantitative research process.

Types of Quantitative Research

Four types of quantitative research are included in this textbook:

- Descriptive
- Correlational
- Quasi-experimental
- Experimental

The type of research conducted is influenced by the current knowledge of a research problem. When little knowledge is available, descriptive studies often are conducted. As the knowledge level increases, correlational, quasi-experimental, and experimental studies are conducted.

Descriptive Research

Descriptive research is the exploration and description of phenomena in real-life situations; it provides an accurate account of characteristics of particular individuals, situations, or groups (Kerlinger & Lee, 2000). Through descriptive studies, researchers discover new meaning, describe what exists, determine the frequency with which something occurs, and categorize information. The outcomes of descriptive research include the description of concepts, identification of relationships, and development of hypotheses that provide a basis for future quantitative research.

Correlational Research

Correlational research involves the systematic investigation of relationships between or among variables. To do this, the researcher measures the selected variables in a sample and then uses correlational statistics to determine the relationships among the variables. Using correlational analysis, the researcher is able to determine the degree or strength and type (positive or negative) of a relationship between two variables. The strength of a relationship varies, ranging from −1 (perfect negative correlation) to +1 (perfect positive correlation), with 0 indicating no relationship. The positive relationship indicates that the variables vary together—that is, both variables either increase or decrease together. For example, research has shown that the more people smoke, the more lung damage they experience. The negative relationship indicates that the variables vary in opposite directions; thus, as one variable increases, the other will decrease. As an example, research has shown that an increase in the number of years of smoking is correlated with a decrease in life span. The primary intent of correlational studies is to explain the nature of relationships in the real world, not to determine cause and effect. However, correlational studies are the means for generating hypotheses to guide quasi-experimental and experimental studies that do focus on examining cause-and-effect relationships.

Quasi-Experimental Research

The purpose of quasi-experimental research is to examine causal relationships or to determine the effect of one variable on another. Quasi-experimental studies involve implementing a treatment and examining the effects of this treatment using selected methods of measurement (Cook & Campbell, 1979). Quasi-experimental studies differ from experimental studies by the level of control achieved by the researcher. Quasi-experimental studies usually lack a certain amount of control over the manipulation of the treatment, management of the setting, or selection of the subjects. When studying human behavior, especially in clinical settings, researchers frequently are unable to randomly select the subjects or to manipulate or control certain variables related to the subjects or the setting. Thus, nurse researchers conduct more quasi-experimental studies than experimental studies.

Experimental Research

Experimental research is an objective, systematic, highly controlled investigation for the purpose of predicting and controlling phenomena in nursing practice. In an experimental study, causality between the independent and the dependent variables is examined under highly controlled conditions (Kerlinger & Lee, 2000). Experimental research is considered the most powerful quantitative method because of the rigorous control of variables. The three main characteristics of experimental studies are (1) controlled manipulation of at least one treatment variable (independent variable); (2) exposure of some of the subjects to the treatment (experimental group), and no exposure of the remaining subjects (control group); and (3) random assignment of subjects to either the control or experimental group. Control in an experimental study is strengthened by random selection of subjects and the conduct of the study in a laboratory or research facility. The degree of control achieved in experimental studies varies according to the population studied, the variables examined, and the environment of the study.

Defining Terms Relevant to Quantitative Research

Understanding quantitative research requires comprehension of several important terms:

- Basic research
- Applied research
- Rigor
- Control

Basic Research

Basic research (or pure research) is scientific investigation that involves the pursuit of "knowledge for knowledge's sake" or for the pleasure of learning and finding truth (Miller, 1991). Basic scientific investigation seeks new knowledge about health phenomena with the hope of establishing general principles. The purpose of basic research is to generate and refine theory; thus, the findings frequently are not directly useful in practice (Wysocki, 1983). Basic nursing research on physiological variables might include laboratory investigations in animals or humans to develop principles regarding physiological functioning or pathologic processes or the effects of treatments on physiological and pathological functioning. These studies might focus on increasing understanding of oxygenation, perfusion, fluid and electrolyte balance, acid-base status, eating and sleeping patterns, and comfort status, as well as pathophysiology of the immune system (Bond & Heitkemper, 1987).

RESEARCH EXAMPLE Basic Research

Graves, Hitt, Pariza, Cook, and McCarthy (2005) conducted basic research to examine the effect of a diet supplemented with 0.5% conjugated linoleic acid (CLA) on muscle mass in mice with cancer. In this laboratory study, the tumor-bearing mice were experiencing cancer cachexia, or progressive weight loss, skeletal muscle wasting, fatigue, and anorexia. CLA supplementation was the independent variable or treatment implemented to determine its effect on the dependent or outcome variable of the gastrocnemius muscles mass in mice with and without cancer.

CRITIQUE

Basic research often is implemented in laboratories with animals to examine the effect of proposed interventions. Dietary CLA supplementation was identified as a potential treatment for cachexia and was implemented in tumor-bearing mice. Basic research usually precedes or is the basis for applied research. Thus, the basic research study by Graves et al. (2005) provides a basis for studying the effects of the CLA dietary supplement on weight loss and skeletal muscle wasting in cancer patients.

IMPLICATIONS FOR PRACTICE

Graves et al. (2005) found that CLA seems to preserve muscle mass in tumor-bearing mice by reducing the catabolic effects of tumor necrosis factor on skeletal muscle. This study increases current understanding of the biology of cancer cachexia and contributes to the development of dietary treatments to reduce the loss of skeletal muscle mass with cancer. Additional applied research is needed to determine if the CLA dietary supplement preserves muscle mass and maintains weight of cancer patients.

Applied Research

Applied research (or practical research) is scientific investigation conducted to generate knowledge that will directly influence or improve clinical practice. The purpose of applied research is to solve problems, make decisions, or predict or control outcomes in real-life practice situations. The findings from applied studies also can be invaluable to policymakers as a basis for making changes to address health and social problems (Miller, 1991). Many of the studies conducted in nursing are applied because researchers have chosen to focus on clinical problems and the testing of nursing interventions to improve patient outcomes. Applied research also is used to test theory and validate its usefulness in clinical practice. Often the new knowledge discovered through basic research is examined for usefulness in practice by applied research, making these approaches complementary (Wysocki, 1983).

RESEARCH EXAMPLE Applied Research

Olney (2005) conducted an applied study to determine the effects of massage on the blood pressure, heart rate, and anxiety level of patients with the diagnosis of hypertension. A pretest-posttest design was used to examine the effects of a 10-minute back massage (treatment or independent variable) given three times a week for 10 sessions on the systolic and diastolic blood pressures, heart rate, and anxiety level (outcomes or dependent variables) of the experimental group. The comparison group relaxed for 10 minutes in the same environment three times a week for 10 sessions.

CRITIQUE

Olney's (2005) quasi-experimental study addressed the effects of an intervention on the treatment of hypertension, which is one of the most common diseases in the United States. This is applied research, because the study focuses on a clinical practice problem of hypertension and the findings can be applied directly to practice. Nurses can use these study findings to develop a massage intervention for the treatment of patients with hypertension to significantly lower both systolic and diastolic blood pressures. Nurses are in a unique position to use back massage to improve patients' outcomes in the hospital. Home health nurses can teach family members to use back massage for patients in their homes to improve their blood pressure.

(continues)

IMPLICATIONS FOR PRACTICE

Olney (2005) found that the 10-minute back massage significantly lowered both the systolic and diastolic blood pressures of patients with hypertension. However, the experimental and comparison groups were not significantly different for heart rate or anxiety level. The researcher recommends that additional studies be conducted with a larger sample over a longer period of time to determine the long-term effects of massage on blood pressure, heart rate, and anxiety level.

Rigor in Quantitative Research

Rigor is the striving for excellence in research, and it requires discipline, adherence to detail, and strict accuracy. A rigorously conducted quantitative study has precise measuring tools, a representative sample, and a tightly controlled study design. To critique the rigor of a study, the reasoning and precision used in conducting the study must be examined. Logical reasoning, including deductive and inductive reasoning, is essential to the development of quantitative studies. The research process includes specific steps that are developed with meticulous detail and are logically linked. These steps, such as design, measurement, sample, data collection, and statistical analysis, need to be examined for weaknesses and errors.

Another aspect of rigor is precision, which encompasses accuracy, detail, and order. Precision is evident in the concise statement of the research purpose and detailed development of the study design. But the most explicit example of precision is the measurement or quantification of the study variables. For example, a researcher might use a cardiac monitor to measure and record the heart rate of subjects during an exercise program, rather than palpating a radial pulse for 30 seconds and recording it on a data collection sheet.

Control in Quantitative Research

Control involves the imposing of rules by the researcher to decrease the possibility of error, thereby increasing the probability that the study's findings are an accurate reflection of reality. The rules used to achieve control in research are referred to as design. Thus, quantitative research includes various degrees of control, ranging from uncontrolled to highly controlled, depending on the type of study (Table 2-1). Descriptive and correlational studies often are designed with little or no researcher control because subjects are examined as they

Table 2-1   Control in Quantitative Research

Type of Quantitative Research	Researcher Control	Research Setting
Descriptive	Uncontrolled	Natural or partially controlled
Correlational	Uncontrolled or partially controlled	Natural or partially controlled
Quasi-experimental	Partially controlled	Partially controlled
Experimental	Highly controlled	Laboratory or research unit

exist in their natural setting, such as home, work, or school. Quasi-experimental studies focus on determining the effectiveness of a treatment (independent variable) in producing a desired outcome (dependent variable) in a partially controlled setting. Thus, these studies are conducted with more control in the selection of subjects, implementation of the treatment, and measurement of the dependent variables. However, experimental studies are the most highly controlled type of quantitative research conducted to examine the effect of treatments on dependent variables. Experimental studies often are conducted on subjects in experimental units in health care agencies or on animals in laboratory settings (see Table 2-1).

Extraneous Variables

Through control, the researcher can reduce the influence of extraneous variables. Extraneous variables exist in all studies and can interfere with obtaining a clear understanding of the relationships among the study variables. For example, if a study focused on the effect of relaxation therapy on perception of incisional pain, the researchers would have to control the extraneous variables (such as type of surgical incision and time, amount, and type of pain medication administered following surgery) to prevent their influence on the patient's perception of pain. Selecting only patients with abdominal incisions who are hospitalized and intravenously receiving only one type of pain medication after surgery would control some of these extraneous variables. Thus, a study can be designed to decrease the influence of extraneous variables through the selection of subjects (sampling) and the research setting. Controlling extraneous variables enables the researcher to accurately determine the effect of an independent or treatment variable on a dependent or outcome variable.

Sampling

Sampling is a process of selecting subjects who are representative of the population being studied. Random sampling usually provides a sample that is representative of a population because each member of the population is selected independently and has an equal chance or probability of being included in the study. In quantitative research, both random and nonrandom samples are used. Descriptive studies often are conducted with nonrandom or nonprobability samples, in which the subjects are selected on the basis of convenience. Correlation and quasi-experimental studies include either nonrandom or random sampling methods, but having a randomly selected sample strengthens highly controlled experimental studies. A randomly selected sample is very difficult to obtain in nursing research, so quantitative studies often are conducted with convenience samples. To increase the control and rigor of a study and to decrease the potential for bias (slanting of findings away from what is true or accurate), the subjects who are part of a convenience sample often are randomly assigned to the treatment group or to the control (no treatment) group in quasi-experimental and experimental studies.

Research Settings

The setting is the location in which a study is conducted. There are three common settings for conducting research: natural, partially controlled, and highly controlled (see Table 2-1). A natural setting, or field setting, is an uncontrolled, real-life situation or environment

(Miller, 1991). Conducting a study in a natural setting means that the researcher does not manipulate or change the environment for the study. Descriptive and correlational studies often are conducted in natural settings. A **partially controlled setting** is an environment that is manipulated or modified in some way by the researcher. An increasing number of nursing studies are being conducted in partially controlled settings. Olney (2005) conducted her study in a partially controlled environment so that the effects of extraneous variables would have limited impact on the study outcomes. The experimental group received the back massage, and the comparison group was provided relaxation in the same controlled environment to decrease the effects of extraneous variables such as noise, temperature, and comfort of the bed. A **highly controlled setting** is an artificially constructed environment developed for the sole purpose of conducting research. Laboratories, research or experimental centers, and test units in hospitals or other health care agencies are highly controlled settings in which experimental studies often are conducted. This type of setting reduces the influence of extraneous variables, which enables the researcher to examine accurately the effect of one variable on another. Graves et al. (2005) conducted their study with mice in a laboratory setting, which is a highly controlled setting that is under the direction of the researcher.

Problem-Solving and Nursing Processes: Basis for Understanding the Quantitative Research Process

Research is a process, and it is similar in some ways to other processes. Therefore, the background acquired early in nursing education in problem solving and the nursing process also is useful in research. A **process** includes a purpose, a series of actions, and a goal. The purpose provides direction for the implementation of a series of actions to achieve an identified goal. The specific steps of the process can be revised and reimplemented in order to reach the end point or goal. The problem-solving process, nursing process, and research process are presented in Table 2-2. Relating the research process to problem solving and the nursing process may be helpful in understanding the steps of the quantitative research process.

Table 2-2   Comparison of the Problem-Solving Process, Nursing Process, and Research Process

Problem-Solving Process	Nursing Process	Research Process

Data collection	Assessment
	    Data collection
	    Data interpretation
		Knowledge of nursing world
		    Clinical experiences
		    Literature review

Problem definition	Nursing diagnosis	Problem and purpose identification

Plan
    Setting goals
    Identifying solutions
	Plan
	    Setting goals
	    Planned interventions
		Methodology
		    Design
		    Sample
		    Measurement methods
		    Data collection
		    Data analysis

Implementation	Implementation	Implementation
Evaluation and revision	Evaluation and modification	Outcomes, communication and synthesis of study findings to develop evidence-based practice

Comparing Problem Solving with the Nursing Process

The **problem-solving process** involves the systematic identification of a problem, determination of goals related to the problem, identification of possible approaches to achieve those goals (planning), implementation of selected approaches, and evaluation of goal achievement. Problem solving frequently is used in daily activities and in nursing practice. For example, you use problem solving when you select your clothing, decide where to live, and turn a patient with a fractured hip.

The **nursing process** is a subset of the problem-solving process. The steps of the nursing process are assessment, diagnosis, planning, implementation, evaluation, and modification (see Table 2-2). Assessment involves the collection and interpretation of data for the development of nursing diagnoses. These diagnoses guide the remaining steps of the nursing process, just as the step of identifying the problem directs the remaining steps of the problem-solving process. The planning step in the nursing process is the same as in the problem-solving process. Both processes involve implementation (putting the plan into action) and evaluation (determining the effectiveness of the process). If the process is ineffective, all steps are reviewed and revised (modified) as necessary. The process is implemented until the problems/diagnoses are resolved and the identified goals are achieved.

Comparing the Nursing Process with the Research Process

The nursing process and the research process have important similarities and differences. The two processes are similar because they both involve abstract, critical thinking and complex reasoning (Miller & Babcock, 1996). Using these processes, new information can be identified, relationships can be discovered, and predictions can be made about phenomena. In both processes, information is gathered, observations are made, problems are identified, plans are developed (methodology), and actions are taken (data collection and analysis) (Whitney, 1986). Both processes are reviewed for effectiveness and efficiency; the nursing process is evaluated, and outcomes are determined in the research process (see Table 2-2). Implementing the two processes expands and refines the user's knowledge. With this growth in knowledge and critical thinking, the user is able to implement increasingly complex nursing processes and studies.

The research and the nursing processes also have definite differences. Knowledge of the nursing process will assist you in understanding the research process. However, the **research process** is more complex than the nursing process. It requires an understanding of a unique language and involves the rigorous application of a variety of research methods (Burns, 1989; Burns & Grove, 2005). The research process also has a broader focus than that of the nursing process, in which the nurse focuses on a specific patient and family. During the research process, the researcher focuses on groups of patients and their families. In addition, researchers must be knowledgeable about the world of nursing to identify problems that require study. This knowledge is obtained from clinical and other personal experiences and by conducting a review of the literature.

The theoretical underpinnings of the research process are much stronger than those of the nursing process. All steps of the research process are logically linked to each other, as well as to the theoretical foundations of the study. The conduct of research requires greater precision, rigor, and control than are needed in implementation of the nursing process. The outcomes from research frequently are shared with a large number of nurses and other health care professionals through presentations and publications. In addition, the outcomes from several studies can be synthesized to provide sound evidence for nursing practice (Brown, 1999; Melnyk & Fineout-Overholt, 2005; Whittemore, 2005).

Identifying the Steps of the Quantitative Research Process

The **quantitative research process** involves conceptualizing a research project, planning and implementing that project, and communicating the findings. Figure 2-1 identifies the steps of the quantitative research process that usually are included in a research report. This figure indicates the logical flow of the process as one step builds progressively on another. The steps of the quantitative research process are briefly reviewed here; they are discussed in detail in Chapters 4 to 8 and 10 to 12. The descriptive correlational study conducted by Hulme and Grove (1994) on the symptoms of female survivors of child sexual abuse is used as an example to introduce the steps of the quantitative research process.

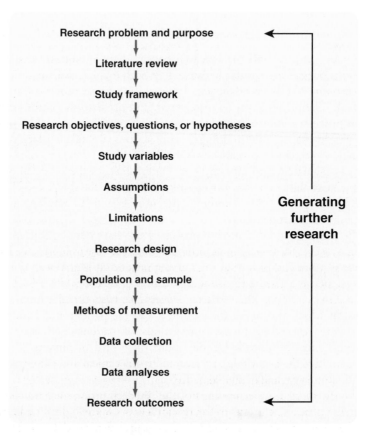

Figure 2-1. Steps of the quantitative research process.

Research Problem and Purpose

A research **problem** is an area of concern in which there is a gap in the knowledge base needed for nursing practice. The problem statement in a study usually identifies an area of concern for a particular population that requires investigation. Research is then conducted to generate essential knowledge that addresses the practice concern, with the ultimate goal of providing an evidence-based practice in nursing (Melnyk & Fineout-Overholt, 2005). The research **purpose** is generated from the problem and identifies the specific goal or aim of the study. The goal of a study might be to identify, describe, or explain a situation; predict a solution to a situation; or control a situation to produce positive outcomes in practice. The purpose includes the variables, population, and often the setting for the study. Chapter 4 presents a detailed discussion of the research problem and purpose.

RESEARCH EXAMPLE   Problem and Purpose

Hulme and Grove (1994) identified the following problem and purpose for their study of female survivors of child sexual abuse.

Research Problem

The actual prevalence of child sexual abuse is unknown but is thought to be high. Bagley and King (1990) were able to generalize from compiled research that at least 20% of all women in the samples surveyed had been victims of serious sexual abuse involving unwanted or coerced sexual contact up to the age of 17 years. Evidence indicates that the prevalence is greater for women born after 1960 than before (Bagley, 1990).

The impact of child sexual abuse on the lives of the girl victims and the women they become has only lately received the attention it deserves…the knowledge generated from research and theory has slowly forced the recognition of the long-term effects of child sexual abuse on both the survivors and society as a whole…. Recently, Brown and Garrison (1990) developed the Adult Survivors of Incest (ASI) Questionnaire to identify the patterns of symptoms and the factors contributing to the severity of these symptoms in survivors of childhood sexual abuse. This tool requires additional testing to determine its usefulness in identifying symptoms and contributing factors of adult survivors of incest and other types of child sexual abuse. (pp. 519–520)

Research Purpose

Thus, the purpose of this study was twofold: "(a) to describe the patterns of physical and psychosocial symptoms in female sexual abuse survivors using the ASI Questionnaire, and (b) to examine relationships among the symptoms and identified contributing factors." (Hulme & Grove, 1994, p. 520)

Literature Review

Researchers conduct a **literature review** to generate a picture of what is known and not known about a particular problem. Relevant literature includes only those sources that are pertinent to or highly important in providing the in-depth knowledge needed to study a selected problem. The literature review indicates whether adequate knowledge exists to make changes in practice or whether additional research is needed. Chapter 5 describes the process for reviewing the literature.

Hulme and Grove's (1994) review of the literature covered relevant theories and studies related to child sexual abuse and its contributing factors and long-term effects.

Theorists indicated that…the act of child sexual abuse can be explained as an abuse of power by a trusted parent figure, usually male, on a dependent child, violating the child's body, mind, and spirit. The family, which normally functions to nurture and protect the child from harm, is viewed as not fulfilling this function, leaving the child to feel further betrayed and powerless. Acceptance of the immediate psychological trauma of child sexual abuse has given impetus for acknowledging the long-term effects.

Studies of both nonclinical and clinical populations have lent support to these theoretical developments. When compared with control groups consisting of women who had not been sexually abused as children, survivors of child sexual abuse consistently have higher incidence of depression and lower self-esteem. Other psychosocial long-term effects encountered include suicidal plans, anxiety, distorted body image, decreased sexual satisfaction, poor general social adjustment, lower positive affect, negative personality characteristics, and feeling different from significant others…. The physical long-term effects suggested by research include gastrointestinal problems such as ulcers, spastic colitis, irritable bowel syndrome, and chronic abdominal pain; gynecological disorders; chronic headache; obesity; and increased lifetime surgeries.

Studies of contributing factors that may affect the traumatic impact of child sexual abuse are less in number and less conclusive than those that identify long-term effects. However, poor family functioning, increased age difference between the victim and perpetrator, threat or use of force or violence, multiple abusers, parent or primary caretaker as perpetrator, prolonged or intrusive abuse, and strong emotional bond to the perpetrator with betrayal of trust may all contribute to the increased severity of the long-term effects. (pp. 521–522)

Study Framework

A **framework** is the abstract, theoretical basis for a study that enables the researcher to link the findings to nursing's body of knowledge. In quantitative research, the framework is a testable theory that has been developed in nursing or in another discipline, such as psychology, physiology, or sociology. A **theory** consists of an integrated set of defined concepts and relational statements that present a view of a phenomenon and can be used to describe, explain, predict, or control the phenomenon. The relational statements of the theory, not the theory itself, are tested through research. A study framework can be expressed as a map or a diagram of the relationships that provide the basis for a study, or the framework can be presented in narrative format. Chapter 6 provides a background for understanding and critiquing study frameworks.

The framework for Hulme and Grove's (1994) study is Browne and Finkelhor's (1986) theory of Traumagenic Dynamics in the Impact of Child Sexual Abuse and is depicted in a map.

As shown in the illustration below child sexual abuse is at the center of the adult survivor's existence. Arising from the abuse are four trauma-causing dynamics: traumatic sexualization, betrayal, powerlessness, and stigmatization. These traumagenic dynamics lead to behavioral manifestations and collectively indicate a history of child sexual abuse. The behavioral manifestations were operationalized as physical and psychosocial symptoms for the purposes of this study. Penetrating the core of the adult survivors are the contributing factors, including the characteristics of the child sexual abuse and other factors occurring later in the survivor's life, that affect the severity of behavioral manifestations (Follette, Alexander, & Follette, 1991). The contributing factors examined in this study were age when the abuse began, duration of the abuse, and other victimizations. Other victimizations included past or present physical and emotional abuse, rape, control by others, and prostitution. (pp. 522–523)

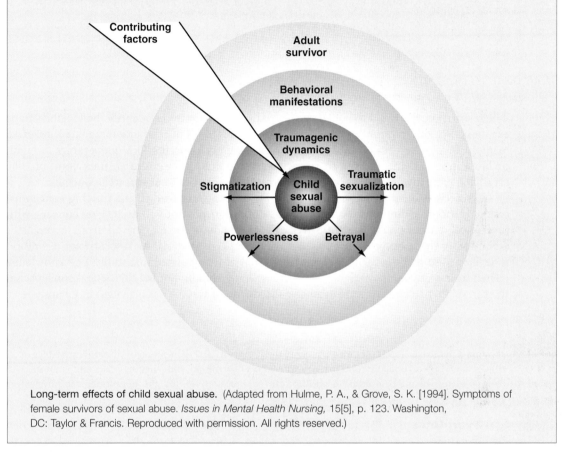

Long-term effects of child sexual abuse. (Adapted from Hulme, P. A., & Grove, S. K. [1994]. Symptoms of female survivors of sexual abuse. *Issues in Mental Health Nursing,* 15[5], p. 123. Washington, DC: Taylor & Francis. Reproduced with permission. All rights reserved.)

Research Objectives, Questions, and Hypotheses

Investigators formulate research objectives, questions, or hypotheses to bridge the gap between the more abstractly stated research problem and purpose and the study design and plan for data collection and analysis. Objectives, questions, and hypotheses are narrower in focus than the purpose and often specify only one or two research variables, identify the relationship between the variables, and indicate the population to be studied. Some descriptive studies include only a research purpose, whereas others include a purpose and either objectives or questions to direct the study. Some correlational studies include a purpose and specific questions or hypotheses. Quasi-experimental and experimental studies need to include hypotheses to direct the conduct of the studies and the interpretation of findings. Chapter 4 provides guidelines for critiquing objectives, questions, and hypotheses in research reports.

Hulme and Grove (1994) developed the following research questions to direct their study:

1. What patterns of physical and psychosocial symptoms are present in women 18 to 40 years of age who have experienced child sexual abuse?
2. Are there relationships among the number of physical and psychosocial symptoms, the age when the abuse began, the duration of abuse, and [the] number of other victimizations? (p. 523)

Study Variables

The research purpose and the objectives, questions, or hypotheses identify the variables to be examined in a study. **Variables** are concepts at various levels of abstraction that are measured, manipulated, or controlled in a study. More concrete concepts like temperature, weight, or blood pressure are referred to as variables in a study. The more abstract concepts like creativity, empathy, or social support sometimes are referred to as research concepts.

Researchers operationalize the variables or concepts in a study by identifying conceptual and operational definitions. A **conceptual definition** provides a variable or concept with theoretical meaning (Burns & Grove, 2005), and it is either derived from a theorist's definition of the concept or developed through concept analysis. An **operational definition** is developed so that the variable can be measured or manipulated in a study. The knowledge gained from studying the variable will increase understanding of the theoretical concept that the variable represents. A more extensive discussion of variables is provided in Chapter 4.

Hulme and Grove (1994) provided conceptual and operational definitions of the study variables—physical and psychosocial symptoms, age when the abuse began, duration of abuse, and victimizations—identified in their purpose and/or research questions. Only the definitions for physical symptoms and victimizations are presented as examples.

Physical Symptoms
Conceptual definition
Physical symptoms are "behavioral manifestations that result directly from the traumagenic dynamics of child sexual abuse" (Hulme & Grove, 1994, p. 522).

Operational definition
ASI Questionnaire was used to measure physical symptoms.

Victimizations
Conceptual definition
Experiences of any of multiple forms of abuse, including "past and present physical and emotional abuse, rape, control by others, and prostitution" (p. 523), in an adult survivor of child abuse.

Operational definition
ASI Questionnaire was used to measure victimizations.

Assumptions

Assumptions are statements that are taken for granted or are considered true, even though they have not been scientifically tested. Assumptions often are embedded (unrecognized) in thinking and behavior, and uncovering these assumptions requires introspection and a strong knowledge base in a research area. Sources of assumptions are universally accepted truths (e.g., "all humans are rational beings"), theories, previous research, and nursing practice (Myers, 1982).

In studies, assumptions are embedded in the philosophical base of the framework, study design, and interpretation of findings. Theories and research instruments are developed on the basis of assumptions that may or may not be recognized by the researcher. These assumptions influence the development and implementation of the research process. The recognition of assumptions by the researcher is a strength, not a weakness. Assumptions influence the logic of the study, and their recognition leads to more rigorous study development. Williams (1980) reviewed published nursing studies and other health care literature to identify 13 commonly embedded assumptions in health care research:

1. People want to assume control of their own health problems.
2. Stress should be avoided.
3. People are aware of the experiences that most affect their life choices.
4. Health is a priority for most people.
5. People in underserved areas feel underserved.
6. Most measurable attitudes are held strongly enough to direct behavior.
7. Health professionals view health care in a different manner than do lay persons.
8. Human biological and chemical factors show less variation than do cultural and social factors.
9. The nursing process is the best way of conceptualizing nursing practice.
10. Statistically significant differences relate to the variable or variables under consideration.
11. People operate on the basis of cognitive information.
12. Increased knowledge about an event lowers anxiety about the event.
13. Receipt of health care at home is preferable to receipt of care in an institution. (p. 48)

Hulme and Grove (1994) did not identify assumptions for their study, but the following assumptions seem to provide a basis for this study: (1) the child victim bears no responsibility for the sexual contact; (2) survivors can remember and are willing to report their past child sexual abuse; and (3) behavioral manifestations (physical and psychological symptoms) indicate altered health and functioning.

Limitations

Limitations are restrictions in a study that may decrease the credibility and generalizability of the findings. **Generalization** is the extension of the implications of the research findings from the sample to a larger population. For example, the findings from studying adult female survivors of child sexual abuse might be extended from this sample studied to all women who have survived child sexual abuse. The two types of limitations are theoretical and methodological. **Theoretical limitations** restrict the abstract generalization of the findings and are reflected in the study framework and the conceptual and operational definitions of the variables. Theoretical limitations might include (1) a concept that lacks clarity of definition in the theory used to develop the study framework; (2) the unclear relationships among some concepts in the theorist's work; (3) a study variable that lacks a clear link to a concept in the framework; and (4) an objective, question, or hypothesis that lacks a clear link to a relationship (or proposition) expressed in the study framework.

Methodological limitations can limit the credibility of the findings and restrict the population to which the findings can be generalized. Methodological limitations result from such factors as unrepresentative sample, weak design, single setting, limited control over treatment implementation, instruments with limited reliability and validity, limited control over data collection, and improper use of statistical analyses.

Hulme and Grove (1994) identified the following methodological limitation.

…[T]his study has limited generalizability due to the relatively small nonprobability sample… (p. 528). Additional replications drawing from various social classes and age groups are needed to improve the generalizability of Brown and Garrison's (1990) findings and establish reliability and validity of their tool. (p. 529)

Research Design

Research **design** is a blueprint for the conduct of a study that maximizes control over factors that could interfere with the study's desired outcome. The type of design directs the selection of a population, procedures for sampling, methods of measurement, and plans for data collection and analysis. The choice of research design depends on the researcher's expertise, the problem and purpose of the study, and the intent to generalize the findings. Sometimes the design of a study indicates that a pilot study was conducted. A **pilot study** frequently is defined as a smaller version of a proposed study, and it is conducted to refine the methodology. Researchers often develop the pilot study in a manner similar to that for the proposed study, using similar subjects, the same setting, the same treatment, and the same data collection and analysis techniques. Prescott and Soeken (1989), however, believe a pilot study can be conducted to develop and refine any of the steps in the research process. The reasons for conducting pilot studies are to:

1. Determine whether the proposed study is feasible. (For example: Are the subjects available? Does the researcher have the time and money to do the study?)
2. Develop or refine a research treatment.
3. Develop a protocol for the implementation of a treatment.
4. Identify problems with the design.
5. Determine whether the sample is representative of the population or whether the sampling technique is effective.
6. Examine the reliability and validity of the research instruments.
7. Develop or refine data collection instruments.
8. Refine the data collection and analysis plans.

9. Give the researcher experience with the subjects, setting, methodology, and methods of measurement.

10. Implement data analysis techniques (Prescott & Soeken, 1989; Van Ort, 1981).

Designs have been developed to meet unique research needs as they emerge; thus, a variety of descriptive, correlational, quasi-experimental, and experimental designs have been generated over time. In descriptive and correlational studies, no treatment is administered, so the purpose of the study design is to improve the precision of measurement. Quasi-experimental and experimental study designs usually involve treatment and control groups, and focus on achieving high levels of control as well as precision in measurement. A study's design usually is described in the methodology section of a research report.

Hulme and Grove (1994) used a descriptive correlational design to direct their study. The diagram of the design, presented in the illustration below, indicates the variables described and the relationships examined. The findings generated from correlational research provide a basis for generating hypotheses for testing in future research.

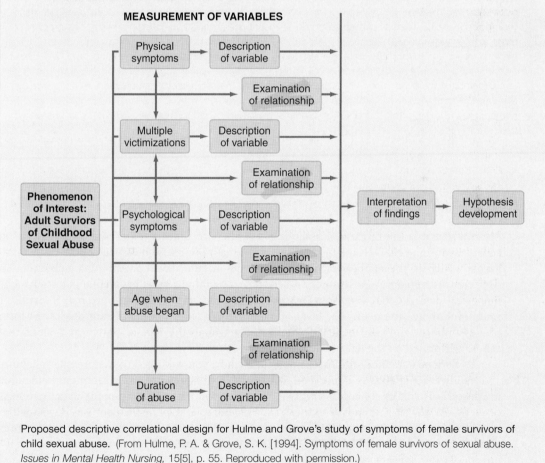

Proposed descriptive correlational design for Hulme and Grove's study of symptoms of female survivors of child sexual abuse. (From Hulme, P. A. & Grove, S. K. [1994]. Symptoms of female survivors of sexual abuse. *Issues in Mental Health Nursing,* 15[5], p. 55. Reproduced with permission.)

Population and Sample

The **population** is all elements (individuals, objects, or substances) that meet certain criteria for inclusion in a study (Kerlinger & Lee, 2000). A **sample** is a subset of the population that is selected for a particular study, and the members of a sample are the subjects. Sampling defines the process of selecting a group of people, events, behaviors, or other elements with which to conduct a study. Chapter 10 provides a background for critiquing populations and samples in research reports.

> In the following excerpt, the sampling method, setting, sample size, population, sample criteria, and sample characteristics are identified for the study conducted by Hulme and Grove (1994).
>
> The convenience sample [sampling method] was obtained by advertising for subjects at three state universities in the southwest [setting]. Despite the sensitive nature of the study, 22 [sample size] usable interviews were obtained. The sample included women between the ages of 18 and 39 years ($\overline{X}$ = 28 years, SD = 6.5 years) who were identified as survivors of child sexual abuse [population] [sample criteria]. The majority of these women were white (91%) and students (82%). A little more than half (54%) were single, seven (32%) were divorced, and three (14%) were married. Most (64%) had no children. A small percentage (14%) was on some form of public assistance and only 14% had been arrested. Although 27% of the subjects had step family members, the parents of 14 subjects (64%) were still married. Half the fathers were working class or self-employed; the rest were professionals. Mothers were either working class or self-employed (50%), homemakers (27%), or professionals (11%). Most subjects (95%) had siblings, and 36% knew or suspected their siblings also had been abused [sample characteristics]. (pp. 523–524)

Methods of Measurement

Measurement is the process of assigning "numbers to objects (or events or situations) in accord with some rule" (Kaplan, 1964, p. 177). A component of measurement is instrumentation, which is the application of specific rules to the development of a measurement device or instrument. An instrument is selected to examine a specific variable in a study. The numerical data generated with an instrument may be at the nominal, ordinal, interval, or ratio level of measurement. The level of measurement, with nominal being the lowest form of measurement and ratio being the highest, determines the type of statistical analysis that can be performed on the data.

To critique a method of measurement in a study, you will need to examine its reliability and validity. Reliability is concerned with how consistently the measurement technique measures a variable or concept. Validity is the extent to which the instrument actually reflects or measures what it is supposed to measure. For example, if an instrument was developed to measure chronic pain, the validity is the extent to which the instrument actually measures chronic pain and the reliability is how consistently it measures chronic pain. Chapter 11 introduces the concept of measurement and explains the different types of reliability and validity.

> Hulme and Grove (1994) used the ASI Questionnaire to measure the study variables.
>
> The ASI Questionnaire contains 10 sections: demographics; family origin; educational history, occupational history and public assistance; legal history; characteristics of the child sexual abuse (duration, perpetrator, pregnancy, type, and threats); past and present other victimizations; past and present physical symptoms; past and present psychosocial symptoms; and relationship with own children. Each section is followed by a response set that includes space for 'other'. Content validity was established by Brown and Garrison (1990) using an in-depth review of 132 clinical records.... For this descriptive correlational study...content validity of the tool was examined by asking an open-ended question: "Is there additional information you would like to share?" (p. 524)

Data Collection

Data collection is the precise, systematic gathering of information relevant to the research purpose or the specific objectives, questions, or hypotheses of a study. To collect data, the researcher must obtain permission from the setting or agency where the study is to be conducted. Consent also must be obtained from all research subjects to indicate their willingness to participate in the study. Frequently, the researcher asks the subject to sign a consent form, which describes the study, promises the subject confidentiality, and indicates that the subject can withdraw from the study at any time. The research report should document permission from an agency to conduct a study and consent from the subject to participate in the study (see Chapter 7).

During data collection, investigators will use a variety of techniques for measuring study variables, such as observation, interview, questionnaires, or scales. In an increasing number of studies, nurses measure physiological variables with high-technology equipment. Researchers collect and systematically record date on each subject, organizing the data in a way that facilitates computer entry. Data collection is usually described in the "Methodology" section of a research report under the subheading of "Procedures."

> Hulme and Grove (1994) identified the following procedure for data collection.
>
> Although the tool can be self-reporting, it was administered by personal interview to allow for elaboration of 'other' responses. The interviews lasted about one hour and were conducted in a private room provided by The University of Texas at Arlington. Each interview started with a discussion of the study benefits and risks and included signing a consent form. Risks included possible painful memories, anger, and sadness during the interview as well as emotional and physical discomfort after the interview. Sources of public and private counseling were provided to assist subjects with any difficulties experienced related to the study. (pp. 524–525)

Data Analysis

Data analysis is conducted to reduce, organize, and give meaning to the data. Analysis techniques conducted in quantitative research include descriptive and inferential analyses (see Chapter 12) and some sophisticated, advanced analyses (Burns & Grove, 2005). Investigators base their choice of analysis techniques primarily on the research objectives, questions, or hypotheses, and the level of measurement achieved by the research instruments. The data analysis process is described in the "Results" section of the research report; this section usually is organized by the research objectives, questions, or hypotheses.

Hulme and Grove (1994) used frequencies, percents, means, standard deviations, and Pearson correlations to answer their research questions.

Results

The first research question focused on patterns of physical and psychosocial symptoms. Six physical symptoms occurred in 50% or more of the subjects: insomnia, sexual dysfunction, overeating, drug abuse, severe headache, and two or more major surgeries.... Eleven psychosocial symptoms occurred in 75% or more of the subjects: depression, guilt, low self-esteem, inability to trust others, mood swings, suicidal thoughts, difficulty in relationships, confusion, flashbacks of the abuse, extreme anger, and memory lapse.... Self-injurious behavior was reported by eight subjects (33%). (pp. 527–528)

The second research question focused on the relationships among the number of physical and psychosocial symptoms and three contributing factors (age abuse began, duration of abuse, and other victimizations). There were five significant correlations among study variables: physical symptoms with other victimizations ($r = 0.59$, $p = 0.002$), physical symptoms with psychosocial symptoms ($r = 0.56$, $p = 0.003$), age abuse began with duration of abuse ($r = -0.50$, $p = 0.009$), psychosocial symptoms with other victimizations ($r = 0.40$, $p = 0.033$), and duration of abuse with psychosocial symptoms ($r = 0.40$, $p = 0.034$). (p. 528)

Research Outcomes

The results obtained from data analyses require interpretation to be meaningful. **Interpretation of research outcomes** involves examining the results from data analysis, forming conclusions, considering the implications for nursing, exploring the significance of the findings, generalizing the findings, and suggesting further studies. The research outcomes are presented in the "Discussion" section of a research report.

Hulme and Grove (1994) provided the following discussion of their findings, with implications for nursing and suggestions for further study.

Discussion

While this study may have limited generalizability due to the relatively small nonprobability sample, the findings do support previous research.... In addition, the findings support Browne and Finkelhor's (1986) framework that a wide range of behavioral manifestations (physical and psychosocial symptoms) comprise the long-term effects of child sexual abuse. (p. 528)

Brown and Garrison's (1990) ASI Questionnaire was effective in identifying patterns of physical and psychosocial symptoms in women with a history of child sexual abuse.... As data on the behavioral manifestations (physical and psychosocial symptoms) and the effect of each of the contributing factors accumulate, hypotheses need to be formulated to further test Browne and Finkelhor's (1986) framework explaining the long-term effects of child sexual abuse.... With additional research, the ASI Questionnaire might be adapted for use in clinical situations. This questionnaire might facilitate identification and delivery of appropriate treatment to female survivors of child sexual abuse in clinical settings. (pp. 529–530)

Reading Research Reports

Understanding the steps of the research process and learning new terms related to those steps will assist you in reading research reports. A **research report** summarizes the major elements of a study and identifies the contributions of that study to nursing knowledge. Research reports are presented at professional meetings and conferences and are published in journals and books. These reports often are overwhelming to nursing students and new graduates. Maybe you have had difficulty locating research articles or understanding the content of these articles. Research reports usually are written to communicate with other researchers, not with clinicians. Thus, the style of the report often is technical, and the report sometimes is filled with jargon, which is very confusing to students and practicing nurses. We would like to help you overcome some of these barriers and assist you in understanding the research literature by (1) identifying sources that publish research reports, (2) describing the content of a research report, and (3) providing tips for reading the research literature.

Sources of Research Reports

The most common sources for nursing research reports are professional journals. Research reports are the major focus of the following nursing research journals: *Advances in Nursing Science, Applied Nursing Research, Clinical Nursing Research: An International Journal, Journal of Nursing Scholarship, Nursing Research, Qualitative Nursing Research, Research in Nursing & Health, Scholarly Inquiry for Nursing Practice: An International Journal,* and *Western Journal of Nursing Research*. Two of these journals, *Applied Nursing Research* and *Clinical Nursing Research*, have focused on communicating research findings to practicing nurses. Thus the journals include less detail on the framework, methodology, and the statistical results of a study and more on discussion of the findings and the implications for practice. Many of the nursing clinical specialty journals also place a high priority on publishing research findings. Table 2-3 identifies the clinical journals in which research reports constitute 50% or more of the journal content. More than 95 nursing journals are published in the United States, and many of them include research articles (Swanson, McCloskey, & Bodensteiner, 1991).

Some research reports, such as those for complex qualitative studies, are lengthy and might be published as books or as chapters in books. Research reports of master's degree candidates are presented as theses. Doctoral candidates produce dissertations summarizing their research projects. Before publication, many research reports are presented at local, national, and international nursing and health care conferences. Often, brochures for conferences will indicate whether research reports are part of the program. The findings from many studies are now communicated through the Internet as journals are placed online, and selected Web sites include the most current health care research.

Content of Research Reports

At this point, you may be overwhelmed by the seeming complexity of a research report. You will find it easier to read and comprehend these reports if you understand each of the component parts. A research report often includes six parts: (1) "Abstract," (2) "Introduction," (3) "Methods," (4) "Results," (5) "Discussion," and (6) "References. These parts are described in this section, and the study by Olney (2005) that examined the effects of back massage on

Table 2-3	Journals That Focus on Research Articles
Journal	**Research Content (%)**
Research Journals	
Applied Nursing Research	100
Image—The Journal of Nursing Scholarship	70
Nursing Research	80
Research in Nursing & Health	100
Scholarly Inquiry for Nursing Practice	60
Western Journal of Nursing Research	90
Clinical Journals	
American Journal of Alzheimer's Care & Related Disorders and Research	60
Birth	70
Cardiovascular Nursing	60
Computers in Nursing	70
Heart & Lung: The Journal of Acute and Critical Care	50
Issues in Comprehensive Pediatric Nursing	100
Issues in Mental Health Nursing	67
Journal of Child and Adolescent Psychiatric and Mental Health Nursing	75
Journal of Continuing Education in Nursing	50
Journal of Holistic Nursing	50
Journal of National Black Nurses' Association	75
Journal of Nursing Education	80
Journal of Pediatric Nursing: Nursing Care of Children and Families	50
Journal of Transcultural Nursing	87
Maternal-Child Nursing Journal	75
Nursing Diagnosis	80
Public Health Nursing	75
Rehabilitation Nursing	50
The Diabetes Educator	75

Data from Swanson, E. A., McCloskey, J. C., & Bodensteiner, A. (1991). Publishing opportunities for nurses: A comparison of 92 U.S. journals. *Image—The Journal of Nursing Scholarship*, *23*(1), 33–38.

the blood pressure, heart rate, and anxiety level of persons with hypertension is presented as an example.

Abstract

The report usually begins with an **abstract**, which is a clear, concise summary of a study (Crosby, 1990). Abstracts range from 100 to 250 words and usually include the study purpose, design, setting, sample size, major results, and conclusions. Researchers hope their abstracts will concisely convey the findings from their study and capture your attention so that you will read the entire report.

Usually, four major content sections of a research report follow the abstract: "Introduction," "Methods," "Results," and "Discussion." The content covered in each of these sections is outlined in Table 2-4 and is briefly discussed in the following sections.

RESEARCH EXAMPLE Abstract

Olney (2005) developed the following clear, concise abstract, which conveys the critical information about her study.

Abstract

Hypertension, one of the most pervasive disease processes in the United States, can lead to target organ damage [research problem]. Although there is no one cause of primary hypertension, the theory of an unchecked long-term stress response continues to be a valid argument. Conversely, eliciting the relaxation response may alter the course of the unchecked stress response [framework]. Massage therapists have suggested that their therapy elicits the relaxation response and therefore can decrease blood pressure (BP) and hypertension. This preliminary study tested the effects of a regularly applied back massage on the BP [dependent or outcome variable] of patients with clinically diagnosed hypertension [research purpose]. In this experimental, pretest-posttest study [design], a 10-minute back massage was given to the experimental group ($n = 8$), three times a week for 10 sessions [treatment or independent variable]. The control group ($n = 6$) relaxed in the same environment for 10 minutes, three times a week for 10 sessions. Analysis of variance determined systolic BP changed significantly, $F_{(1,12)} = 17.90$, $p = .001$, between groups over time as did the diastolic BP, $F_{(1,12)} = 8.34$, $p = .014$. Effect size was 2.25 for systolic pressure and 1.56 for diastolic pressure (alpha of .05 and power of .80) [data analysis]. This preliminary study suggests that regular massage may lower BP in hypertensive persons [study findings]. (p. 98)

Table 2-4	Components of an Abstract

Introduction
Statement of the problem, with background and significance
Statement of the purpose
Brief literature review
Identification of the framework
Identification of the research objectives, questions, or hypotheses (if applicable)

Methods
Identification of the research design
Description of the treatment or intervention (if applicable)
Description of the sample and setting
Description of the methods of measurement (including reliability and validity)
Discussion of the data collection process

Results
Description of the data analysis procedures
Presentation of results in tables, figures, or narrative organized by the purpose(s) and/or objectives, questions, or hypotheses

Discussion
Discussion of major findings
Identification of the limitations
Presentation of conclusions
Implications of the findings for nursing practice
Recommendations for further research

Introduction

The "Introduction" section of a research report identifies the nature and scope of the problem being investigated and provides a case for the conduct of the study. You should be able to clearly identify the significance of conducting the study to generate knowledge for nursing practice. Olney's (2005) study was significant because it generated knowledge to assist persons with a chronic illness (hypertension) to promote their health and prevent additional problems, such as target organ damage. The purpose of this study was clearly stated in the abstract.

Depending on the type of research report, the literature review and the framework may be separate sections or part of the introduction. The literature review documents the current knowledge of the problem investigated and includes the sources that were used to develop the study and interpret the findings. For example, Olney (2005) summarized literature that focused on the concepts of stress, anxiety, hypertension, lifestyle modification, relaxation, and massage. A research report also needs to include a framework, but only about half of the published studies identify one (Moody et al., 1988). Olney (2005) identified her framework as the stress adaptation model and included the concepts of stress and anxiety contributing to the chronic condition of hypertension and the use of biofeedback methods to promote stress reduction and decrease BP. The framework concepts were briefly identified, defined, and interrelated to provide a basis for the study. However, the framework might have been more clearly expressed in this study and linked to the study purpose, hypotheses, and findings. A model or map sometimes is developed to clarify the logic within the framework, but one was not included in this study.

The literature review and framework are presented in a way that emphasizes the importance of and provides support for the study being reported. Investigators often end the introduction by identifying the objectives, questions, or hypotheses that they used to direct the study.

> Because this was a quasi-experimental study, Olney (2005) identified the following hypotheses:
>
> 1. Systolic and diastolic BP will change significantly over time in the experimental group when compared to the control group.
> 2. Heart rates will change significantly in the experimental group when compared to the control during the 10-min massage or relaxation period.
> 3. Anxiety scores in the experimental group will change significantly over time when compared to the control group (p. 100).

Methods

The "Methods" section of a research report describes how the study was conducted and usually includes the study design, treatment (if appropriate), sample, setting, methods of measurement, and data collection process. This section of the report needs to be presented in enough detail so that the reader can critique the adequacy of the study methods to produce reliable findings (Tornquist, Funk, Champagne, & Wiese, 1993).

Olney (2005) identified her design as an experimental pretest-posttest design. She also included the subsection "Sample," which described the population, sampling method, sample criteria, sample size, sample characteristics, and setting of the study.

"Measures" was another subsection of the study methodology that detailed the instruments used to measure the dependent variables of BP, heart rate, and anxiety. The OMRON BP monitor device was used to measure systolic and diastolic BP; heart rate was measured by a Finger Pulse Oximeter, and anxiety was measure with the State Trait Anxiety Inventory. The subsection "Procedure" detailed the treatment group procedure of back massage and the control group procedure of relaxation. The protection of subjects' rights and the informed consent process were also covered in the "Procedure" subsection.

Results

The "Results" section presents the outcomes of the statistical tests used to analyze the study data and the significance of these outcomes. The research purpose or objectives, questions, and hypotheses formulated for the study are used to organize this section. Researchers identify the statistical analyses conducted to address the purpose or each objective, question, or hypothesis, and present the specific results obtained from the analyses in tables, figures, or narrative of the report (Burns & Grove, 2005). Focusing more on the summary of the study results and their significance than on the statistical results can help to reduce the confusion that may be caused by the numbers.

Olney (2005) conducted statistical analyses to address her study hypotheses. The analyses were comprehensive and clearly presented using table, figures, and narrative. Analysis of variance (ANOVA) was used to test differences between the two groups for BP, heart rate, and anxiety level. Results indicated a significant difference in both systolic and diastolic BP from the treatment to the control group but no significant difference in heart rate or anxiety level. Thus, the first hypothesis was support but hypotheses 2 and 3 were not supported by the study results.

Discussion

The "Discussion" section ties together the other sections of the research report and gives them meaning. This section includes the major findings, limitations of the study, conclusions drawn from the findings, implications of the findings for nursing, and recommendations for further research.

Olney (2005) discussed her findings in detail, and compared and contrasted them with the findings of previous research. She also included a separate section on the implications for nursing practice and research. The implications for practice included the use of massage to decrease systolic and diastolic BP in patients with hypertension. Olney (2005) combined her discussion of study limitations with her recommendations for further research. She recommended additional research with the following features: (1) a larger more diverse sample, (2) a design that examines the impact of the relationship between nurse and participants, (3) hiring others to implement the treatment and collect data to prevent bias, and (4) extension of the study to examine the long-term effects of massage over weeks and months.

The conclusions drawn from a research project can be useful in at least three different ways. First, the intervention or treatment tested in a study can be used with patients to improve their care and promote a positive health outcome. Second, reading research reports might change your view of a patient's situation or give you greater insight into the situation. Last, studies heighten your awareness of the problems experienced by patients and assist you in assessing and working toward solutions for these problems.

References

A "References" section that includes all sources cited in the research report follows the "Discussion" section. The reference list includes the studies and theories that provide a basis for the conduct of the study. These sources provide an opportunity to read about the research problem in greater depth. We strongly encourage you to read the Olney (2005) article to identify the sections of a research report and to examine the content in each of these sections. This researcher detailed a rigorously conducted quasi-experimental study, provided findings that are supportive of previous research, and identified conclusions that provide sound evidence to direct the care of patients with hypertension.

Tips for Reading Research Reports

When you start reading research reports, you may be overwhelmed by the new terms and complex information presented. We hope that you will not be discouraged but will see the challenge of examining new knowledge generated through research. You probably will need to read the report slowly two or three times; you can use the glossary at the end of this book to review the definitions of unfamiliar terms. We recommend that you read the abstract first and then the "Discussion" section of the report. This approach will enable you to determine the relevance of the findings to you personally and to your practice. Initially, your focus should be on research reports you believe can provide relevant knowledge for your practice.

Reading a research report requires the use of a variety of critical thinking skills, such as skimming, comprehending, and analyzing, to facilitate an understanding of the study (Miller & Babcock, 1996). **Skimming a research report** involves quickly reviewing the source to gain a broad overview of the content. Try this approach: First, familiarize yourself with the title and check the author's name. Next, scan the "Abstract" or "Introduction" and the "Discussion" section. Knowing the findings of the study will provide you with a standard for evaluating the rest of the article (Tornquist et al., 1993). Then read the major headings and perhaps one or two sentences under each heading. Finally, reexamine the conclusions and implications for practice from the study. Skimming enables you to make a preliminary judgment about the value of a source and a determination about reading the report in depth.

Comprehending a research report requires that the entire study be read carefully. During this reading, focus on understanding major concepts and the logical flow of ideas within the study. You may wish to highlight information about the researchers, such as their education, their current positions, and any funding they received for the study. As you read the study, steps of the research process also might be highlighted. Record any notes in the margin so that you can easily identify the problem, purpose, framework, major variables, study design, treatment, sample, measurement methods, data collection process, analysis techniques, results, and study outcomes. Also record any creative ideas or questions you have in the margin of the report.

We encourage you to highlight the parts of the article that you do not understand and ask your instructor or other nurse researchers for clarification. Your greatest difficulty in reading the research report probably will be in understanding the statistical analyses. Information in Chapter 12 should help you comprehend the analyses. Basically, you must identify the particular statistics used, the results from each statistical analysis, and the meaning of the results. Statistical analyses are conducted to describe variables, examine relationships among variables, or determine differences among groups. The study purpose or specific objectives, questions, or hypotheses indicate whether the focus is on description, relationships, or differences. Therefore, you need to link each analysis technique to its results and then to the study purpose or objectives, questions, or hypotheses presented in the study.

The final reading skill, **analyzing a research report**, involves determining the value of the report's content. Break the content of the report into parts, and examine the parts in depth for accuracy, completeness, uniqueness of information, and organization. Note whether the steps of the research process build logically on each other or whether steps are missing or incomplete. Examine the discussion section of the report to determine whether the researchers have provided a critical argument for using the study findings in practice. Using the skills of skimming, comprehending, and analyzing while reading research reports will increase your comfort with studies, allow you to become an informed consumer of research, and expand your knowledge for making changes in practice. These skills for reading research reports are critical for conducting a comprehensive research critique. Chapter 13 focuses on the guidelines for critiquing quantitative and qualitative studies.

Practice Reading Quasi-Experimental and Experimental Studies

Knowing the parts of the research report—introduction, methods, results, and discussion—provides a basis for reading research reports of quantitative studies. The critical thinking skills of skimming, comprehending, and analyzing can be applied to your reading of the example quasi-experimental and experimental studies provided here.

Quasi-Experimental Study

Quasi-experimental studies are conducted to determine the effect of a treatment or independent variable on the dependent or outcome variables. Quasi-experimental studies lack the control of the design, sample, or setting that might be used in an experimental study.

RESEARCH EXAMPLE Quasi-Experimental Study

Hastings-Tolsma, Yucha, Tompkins, Robson, and Szeverenyi (1993) conducted a quasi-experimental study of the effects of warm and cold applications on the resolution of IV infiltrations. Read this article and identify the steps of the quantitative research process implemented in the conduct of this study. Then review the content outlined in this textbook with your ideas in mind.

(continues)

RESEARCH EXAMPLE *(continued)*

Steps of the Research Process

1. Research Problem

It has been estimated that as many as 80% of hospitalized patients receive intravenous (IV) therapy each day (Millam, 1988). IV infiltration, or extravasation, occurs in as many as 23% of all IV infusion failures (MacCara, 1983) and is second only to phlebitis as a cause of IV morbidity (Lewis & Hecker, 1991). The resulting tissue injury depends on the clinical condition of the patient, the nature of the infusate, and the volume infiltrated, and may range from little apparent injury to serious damage. In addition, considerable patient suffering, prolonged hospitalization, and significant costs may be incurred. Despite the frequency and potential severity of injury, little is known about how to treat IV infiltration effectively once it is identified. (Hastings-Tolsma et al., 1993, p. 171)

2. Research Purpose

The purpose of this research was "to determine the effect of warm versus cold applications on the pain intensity and the speed of resolution of the extravasation of a variety of commonly used intravenous solutions." (p. 172)

(Extravasation is the leaking of IV fluid from the vein into the surrounding tissues, resulting in swelling, pain, and tissue damage.)

3. Review of Literature

The literature review included relevant, current sources based on the year of publication of the study (1993), with the sources ranging from 1976 to 1991. The journal article was received by the journal editor in April 1992 and was accepted for publication in January 1993. The signs and symptoms of IV infiltration were identified, and the tissue damage that occurs with IV infiltration was described. The effects of the pH and osmolarity of different types of IV solutions on IV infiltration were also discussed. The literature review concluded with a description of the effects of a variety of treatments, including warm and cold applications, on the resolution of IV infiltrations. Hastings-Tolsma et al. (1993, p. 172) concluded that "examination of warm and cold application with less toxic infiltrates has not been studied carefully under controlled conditions."

4. Framework

Hastings-Tolsma and colleagues (1993) did not identify a framework for their study. They did identify relevant concepts (IV therapy, nature of infusate, vessel damage, extravasation, tissue damage, treatment, and resolution) and discuss the relationships among these concepts in their literature review. A possible map for their study framework is presented in Figure 2-2. The map indicates that the more IV therapy patients receive, the more likely they are to experience vessel damage that leads to extravasation or IV infiltration. The nature of the IV infusate (solution) also affects the severity of the vessel damage and extravasation. Extravasation leads to tissue damage, and the greater the extravasation, the greater the tissue damage. The treatment with warm and cold applications has an unknown effect on the extravasation and tissue damage. If the extravasation and tissue damage are decreased by either the cold or the warm treatment, then the patient experiences resolution of the extravasation.

5. Research Questions

(a) What are the differences in tissue response as measured by pain, erythema, induration, and interstitial fluid volume between warm versus cold applications to infiltrated IV sites? (b) What is the effect of warm

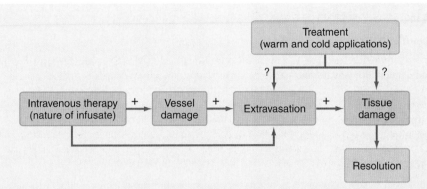

Figure 2-2. Proposed framework map for Hastings-Tolsma, Yucha, Tompkins, Robson, and Szeverenyi's (1993) study of the effect of warm and cold applications on the resolution of intravenous infiltrations.

versus cold applications in the resolution of infiltrated solutions of varying osmolarity when pH is held constant? (Hastings-Tolsma et al., 1993, pp. 172–173)

Hypotheses might have been more appropriate to direct this quasi-experimental study.

6. Variables

The independent variables were temperature applications (warm and cold) and osmolarity of the IV solution. The dependent variables were pain, erythema, induration, and interstitial fluid volume.

Independent Variable: Temperature Applications
Conceptual definition
Topical warm and cold applications to the sites of extravasation to promote reabsorption of infusate and resolution of the infiltration.

Operational definition
Warm (43° C) or cold (0° C) topical applications using a thermostatic pad to the sites of IV infiltration.

Independent Variable: Osmolarity of the IV Solution
Conceptual definition
Osmolar concentration, expressed in osmoles per liter of solution.

Operational definition
IV solutions of 50% saline (154 mOsm), normal saline (308 mOsm), or 3% saline (1027 mOsm) infiltrated at subject's IV site.

Dependent Variable: Pain
Conceptual definition
Sensation of discomfort caused by tissue damage and inflammatory response.

(continues)

RESEARCH EXAMPLE *(continued)*

Operational definition

Pain measured with the Analogue Chromatic Continuous Scale (ACCS), a self-report, one-dimensional visual analogue scale for quantifying pain intensity.

Dependent Variable: Erythema

Conceptual definition

Redness at the IV infiltration site as a result of inflammatory response.

Operational definition

Indelible ink used to mark the borders of erythema; then a centimeter ruler used to measure the widest perpendicular widths, and the two widths multiplied to estimate surface area of erythema.

Dependent Variable: Induration

Conceptual definition

Swelling at the IV infiltration site created by the IV solution, tissue damage, and inflammatory response.

Operational definition

Indelible ink used to mark the borders of induration; then a centimeter ruler used to measure the widest perpendicular widths, and the two widths multiplied to estimate the surface area of induration.

Dependent Variable: Interstitial Fluid Volume

Conceptual definition

Amount of fluid that leaks from the damaged blood vessel into the surrounding tissues.

Operational definition

Magnetic resonance imaging (MRI) was used to quantify the amount of infiltrate remaining at the IV site.

7. Design

The design most closely resembled an interrupted time series, with each subject receiving both warm and cold applications (treatment) to an IV site infiltrated by one of three types of solutions (50% saline, normal saline, or 3% saline) (treatment). The dependent variables were pain, erythema, induration, and interstitial fluid volume. They were measured at various times before and after the infiltration of the three IV solutions and the warm and cold applications.

8. Sample

The sample was composed of 18 healthy adult volunteers. All participants were nonpregnant and taking no medications.... Of the 18 participants studied, 78% were female ($n = 14$) and 22% were male ($n = 4$), and they ranged in age from 20 to 45 years with a mean age of 35 years ($SD = 7$). All subjects were Caucasian. The Health Science Center Institutional Review Board for the Protection of Human Subjects approved the research. After the study was explained to interested individuals, written informed consent was obtained from volunteers. All individuals were offered financial compensation for their participation. (Hastings-Tolsma et al., 1993, p. 173)

9. Procedures

All measurements were taken in the Health Science Center's Department of Radiology NMR Laboratory. After obtaining written informed consent, participants were taken to the MR imaging suite where infiltrations and subsequent measurements were made…. Total data collection time was approximately 32 hours. One of three solutions was infiltrated into the cephalic vein of the forearm: 50% saline (154 mOsm), normal saline (308 mOsm), or 3% saline (1027 mOsm). These solutions were selected because of the varying osmolarity range, as well as relatively common clinical use. Solutions were infiltrated sequentially so that each participant was given a different solution in the order of recruitment into the study. Randomization was used to determine right or left arm, as well as which application, warm or cold, would be used. (Hastings-Tolsma et al., 1993, p. 174)

10. Results

Warm and cold treatments to the infiltrated IV sites using three solutions revealed significant differences in tissue response as measured by the interstitial fluid volume…. For all three solutions, the volume remaining was always less with warm than with cold application, $F_{(1,15)} = 46.69$, $p = .001$. There was no difference in pain with warm or cold applications…. Surface area measurement failed to demonstrate the presence of erythema with any of the solutions…. Surface induration reflected a significant decrease over time, $F_{(2,16)} = 14.38$, $p = .001$, although accurate measurement of the infiltrate was nearly impossible after the first or second imaging period as the borders were so poorly defined…. There was no significant effect of warmth or cold on surface area. (Hastings-Tolsma et al., 1993, p. 175)

11. Discussion

This section includes the study conclusions, recommendations for further research, and implications of the findings for nursing practice.

These findings demonstrate that the application of warmth to sites of IV infiltration produces faster resolution of the extravasation than does cold, as monitored over 1 hour…. It is interesting to note that cold appeared to have a more immediate dramatic effect on the increase in interstitial edema than warmth when applied to the hyperosmolar infiltrate. Presumably this is due to osmosis of fluid from the plasma and surrounding tissues into the area of infiltration….

Other factors that might influence accurate assessment and treatment of infiltrations need to be examined. These should include the use of larger amounts of extravasate and other more varied and caustic solutions, as well as other treatments such as elevation, differing IV site placement, differing gauge needles, and the study of patients of varying ages and clinical conditions…. (p. 176)

The nurse generally has responsibility for IV therapy and criteria for accurate assessment and appropriate intervention clearly are needed. Findings from this research support the use of warm application to sites of infiltration of noncaustic solutions of varying osmolarity, but raise questions about the adequacy of currently used indicators of IV infiltrations. Continued scientific scrutiny should contribute to the development of standards useful in the assessment and treatment of IV extravasation. (Hastings-Tolsma et al., 1993, p. 177)

Experimental Study

The purpose of experimental research is to examine cause-and-effect relationships between independent and dependent variables under highly controlled conditions. The planning and implementation of experimental studies are highly controlled by the researcher, and often these studies are conducted in a laboratory setting on animals or objects. Few nursing studies are "purely" experimental.

RESEARCH EXAMPLE Experimental Study

McCarthy, Lo, Nguyen and Ney (1997) conducted an experimental study of the effects of protein density of food on food intake and nutritional status of tumor-bearing rats. Read this study, identify the steps of the quantitative research process, and then compare your findings with those presented in this section.

Steps of the Research Process

1. Research Problem

Anorexia and weight loss are significant concerns to cancer patients and their loved ones.... The progressive decline[s] in food intake and body weight are powerful negative prognostic indicators of survival in cancer patients.... The loss of lean body mass is a major aspect of the nutritional decline of cancer patients. The literature presents a uniform emphasis on increasing dietary protein intake with the expectation of preserving lean body mass of cancer patients.... However, it has been shown that healthy animals will reduce their food intake when protein density of their food is increased.... It is not known if this response to increased protein density of food will occur in hypophagic tumor-bearing rats.

It also should be noted that tumor growth is associated with depressed serum levels of insulin associated with depressed serum levels of insulin-like growth factor 1(IGF-1).... It is not known if serum levels of insulin or IGF-1 will improve in hypophagic tumor-bearing rats fed a diet of increased protein density. (McCarthy et al., 1997, pp. 130–132)

2. Research Purpose

The purpose of this laboratory study "was to determine (a) if increasing the protein density of food would affect food and total protein intake of tumor-bearing rats and (b) if increased protein intake would alter serum levels of insulin and IGF-1, two hormones requisite to protein synthesis and tissue anabolism" (McCarthy et al., 1997, p. 132).

3. Review of Literature

The literature review included current sources, based on the publication of the study in 1997, with publication dates that ranged from 1975 to 1995. A total of 31 (80%) of the 39 sources were published in the preceding 5 years (1991 to 1996). This article was submitted for publication in 1996, accepted for publication in October 1996, and published in April of 1997. The literature review included mainly studies focused on causes of tumor-induced anorexia and weight loss in cancer patients, impact of high-calorie and high-density protein diets on healthy animals, and the link between tumor growth and serum levels of insulin and IGF-1.

4. Framework

This study has an implied framework that is a combination of physiological and pathological theories about nutrient utilization, tumor development, body response to tumor development, anorexia, nutritional treatment of anorexia, and body response to nutritional supplementation.

5. Variables

The independent variable was a high-density protein diet. The dependent variables were serum insulin, serum IGF-1, food intake, protein intake, and body weight.

Independent Variable: High-Density Protein Diet

Conceptual definition

Nutritional supplement to promote increased intake, nutrient utilization, and weight stabilization with cancerous conditions.

Operational definition

Isocaloric diet containing 40% casein protein (TD#93331, Harlan Tecklad, Madison, WI). (The specific ingredients of this diet are provided in a table in the article.)

Dependent Variables: Serum Insulin and IGF-1

Conceptual definition

Sensitive markers indicating nutritional status and playing an important role in protein metabolism and tissue anabolism.

Operational definitions

Analysis of serum insulin was done using a radioimmunoassay (RIA).... Serum IGF-1 was determined by RIA after the IGF binding proteins were removed by high-performance chromatography under acid conditions. (McCarthy et al., 1997, p. 133)

Dependent Variables: Food Intake and Protein Intake

Conceptual definition

Nutrients consumed by healthy and tumor-bearing animals.

Operational definitions

Food intake was operationalized as the number of grams of food eaten by both the healthy and the tumor-bearing rats. Protein intake was operationalized as the number of milligrams of protein consumed by the healthy and the tumor-bearing rats.

Dependent Variable: Body Weight

Conceptual definition

Body mass of healthy and of tumor-bearing rats.

Operational definitions

Body weight in grams of healthy and of tumor-bearing rats at days 0, 15, 18, 24, and 27 of the experiment.

6. Design

This study has an experimental design that included four groups: (1) 15 healthy rats in the control group on a regular diet, (2) 15 healthy rats in a group on 40% protein diet, (3) 15 tumor-bearing rats on a regular diet, and (4) 15 tumor-bearing rats on 40% protein diet, with repeated measures of three of the five dependent variables.

The experimental period lasted for 27 days. For the first 15 days, all animals were maintained on a semi-purified rodent diet containing 20% casein protein.... After day 15 of tumor growth, one half of the tumor-bearing and one half of the healthy controls were switched to an isocaloric diet containing 40% casein protein. The dependent variables of serum insulin and serum IGF-1 were measured on day 27, and the other dependent variables of food intake, protein intake, and body weight were measured at day[s] 0, 15, 18, 24, and 27. (McCarthy et al., 1997, p. 133)

7. Sample and Setting

A total of 60 randomly selected male Buffalo rats, weighing between 100 and 120 grams were housed individually and maintained on a 12-hour light-dark cycle commencing at 6:00 am. Food and water were freely available. The animals were conditioned to the housing for 5 days before the start of the experiment and were

(continues)

RESEARCH EXAMPLE *(continued)*

treated at all times in a manner consistent with Department of Health, Education, and Welfare *Guidelines for the Care and Use of Laboratory Animals*.... The animals were matched according to weight and a total of 30 were randomly selected for tumor implant, leaving 30 healthy animals as controls. (McCarthy et al., 1997, pp. 132–133)

8. Data collection

The food was placed in conical dishes inside a metal cup to catch any spillage. The dishes were weighed each morning on a portable electric digital scale which was zeroed before each weighing.... The rats were weighed daily and at the end of the experiment the tumors were excised and weighed.... On day 27 of tumor growth, animals were lightly anesthetized with ether fumes and exsanguinated by cardiac puncture between 8 and 10 AM to control for any circadian variations in plasma hormone levels. The blood was allowed to coagulate and serum samples for 48 animals were frozen at ~20° C (12 specimens were inadvertently destroyed). (McCarthy et al., 1997, p. 133)

9. Results

The extensive study results were presented in five figures and narrative of the article.

There was a significant main effect of tumor growth, $F_{(1,56)} = 26.6$, $p < .001$, diet, $F_{(1, 56)} = 4.1$, $p = .05$, and days, $F_{(4,224)} = 29.6$, $p < .001$, on the grams of food eaten by the rats.... Due to the effect of tumor growth on food intake, the tumor-bearing animals were consuming less protein than healthy controls by day 15, $F_{(1,59)} = 16$, $p < .001$. On day 18, 3 days after the diet switch, protein intake was significantly different by tumor, $F_{(1,59)} = 377$ ($p < .001$) and by diet, $F_{(1,59)} = 176$, $p < .001$...body weight of tumor-bearing rats was significantly less than [that of] controls over the course of the experiment, $F_{(1,56)} = 20.5$, $p < .001$...there was a significant effect of tumor growth on mean serum insulin, $F_{(1,4)} = 4.7$, $p = .03$, but no effect of diet.... Similarly, serum IGF-1 was significantly lower in tumor-bearing rats than [in] healthy controls, $F_{(1,47)} = 25.7$, $p < .001$, and was not affected by diet. (McCarthy et al., 1997, pp. 133–136)

10. Discussion

This section presented the study findings and suggestions for further research.

Increasing the protein density of food from the standard 20% formulation to 40% resulted in a decline in total grams of food intake, and an increase in total grams protein intake of both control and tumor-bearing rats. The increased protein intake of tumor-bearing animals fed the 40% protein diet did not affect the nutrient status of these animals as indicated by body weight, or serum levels of total protein, insulin, or IGF-1, nor did it affect tumor size in the tumor-bearing animals.... These data suggest that the lower serum levels of IGF-1 and insulin in hypophagic tumor-bearing animals are not the direct results of their reduced food, or in this case, protein intake.... Increasing the protein density of food resulted in a decrease in food intake in both healthy control and tumor-bearing animals. (p. 136)

The regulation of food intake in humans is more complex than in animals which are maintained on standardized diets and feeding schedules. There is a need for studies to determine the effects of high calorie or high protein nutrition supplements on the total caloric and protein intake and, specifically, meal taking, of cancer patients. There is some evidence that use of nutritional supplements by patients with head and neck cancers results in a significant decline in food-derived calories and protein, though the caloric and protein density of the supplements produces a net increase in total calorie and protein intake.... However, there is little evidence that increased nutritional intake affects morbidity and mortality in weight-losing cancer patients.... Clearly, there is a need for further study of the metabolic impact of nutritional interventions, as well as the impact of calorie and/or protein dense nutritional supplements on meal taking and food appetite of cancer patients. (McCarthy et al., 1997, p. 137)

Conducting an Initial Critique of a Research Report

Being able to read research reports and identify the steps of the research process should enable you to conduct an initial critique of a report. Throughout this book you'll find boxes, entitled "Critique Guidelines," that furnish questions you will want to consider in your critique of various research elements.

CRITIQUE GUIDELINES   Quantitative Research

The following questions are important in conducting an initial critique of a quantitative research report.

1. Was a quantitative or a qualitative study conducted?
2. If the research was quantitative, was the study descriptive, correlational, quasi-experimental, or experimental?
3. Was the setting for the study natural, partially controlled, or highly controlled?
4. Were the steps of the study clearly identified?
5. Can you identify the following sections in the research report: problem, purpose, literature review, framework, variables, definitions of variables, design, treatment (if appropriate), sample, measurement methods, data collection, data analysis, and outcomes?
6. Were any of the steps of the research process missing?
7. Were the steps of the study logically linked? Use the following criteria to decide: The study problem and purpose provide a basis for the literature review and the framework presented. The purpose and framework provide a basis for the objectives, questions, or hypotheses identified. The objectives, questions, or hypotheses provide a basis for the study design, measurement, data collection, and data analysis. The findings from the study are linked to the framework and to previous studies cited in the literature review.

KEY CONCEPTS

- Quantitative research is the traditional research approach in nursing and includes descriptive, correlational, quasi-experimental, and experimental types of research.
- Basic, or pure, research is a scientific investigation that involves the pursuit of "knowledge for knowledge's sake," or for the pleasure of learning and finding truth.
- Applied, or practical, research is a scientific investigation conducted to generate knowledge that will directly influence or improve clinical practice.
- Conducting quantitative research requires rigor and control.
- A comparison of the problem-solving process, the nursing process, and the research process shows the similarities and differences in these processes and provides a basis for understanding the research process.
- The quantitative research process involves conceptualizing a research project, planning and implementing that project, and communicating the findings. The following steps of the quantitative research process are briefly introduced in this chapter.

- The research problem is an area of concern in which there is a gap in the knowledge needed for nursing practice. The research purpose is generated from the problem and identifies the specific goal or aim of the study.
- The review of relevant literature is conducted to generate a picture of what is known and unknown about a particular topic.
- The study framework is the theoretical basis for a study that guides the development of the study and enables the researcher to link the findings to nursing's body of knowledge.
- Research objectives, questions, or hypotheses are formulated to bridge the gap between the more abstractly stated research problem and purpose and the study design and plan for data collection and analysis.
- Study variables are concepts, at various levels of abstraction, that are measured, manipulated, or controlled in a study.
- Assumptions are statements that are taken for granted or are considered true even though they have not been scientifically tested.
- Limitations are theoretical or methodological restrictions in a study that may decrease the generalizability of the findings.
- Research design is a blueprint for conducting a study that maximizes control over factors that could interfere with the study's desired outcomes.
- The population is all of the elements that meet certain criteria for inclusion in a study. A sample is a subset of the population that is selected for a particular study; the members of a sample are the subjects.
- Measurement is the process of assigning numerical values to objects, events, or situations in accord with some rule. Methods of measurement are identified to measure each of the variables in a study.
- The data collection process involves the precise, systematic gathering of information relevant to the research purpose or the objectives, questions, or hypotheses of a study.
- Data analyses are conducted to reduce, organize, and give meaning to the data and to address the research purpose and/or objectives, questions, and hypotheses.
- Research outcomes include the conclusions or findings, generalization of findings, implications for nursing, and suggestions for further research.
- Reading research reports involves skimming, comprehending, and analyzing the report.
- The guidelines for conducting an initial critique of a quantitative study are provided.

TIPS FOR FURTHER STUDY

- Read the study by Olney (2005) and practice your skills in reading a research report (skimming, comprehending, and analyzing). To test your understanding of how to read a research report as well as other issues in this chapter, try the Bonus Review Questions at www.evolve/Burns/understanding.
- Ready the study by Graves et al. (2005) and identify the steps of the quantitative research process. For additional practice in identifying these steps, complete the "Key Ideas: Steps in the Research Process" section in Chapter 2 of your *Study Guide*.
- Conduct an initial critique on the Olney (2005) and Graves et al. (2005) studies using the guidelines in this chapter.

REFERENCES

Bagley, C. (1990). Development of a measure of unwanted sexual contact in childhood, for use in community mental health surveys. *Psychology Reports, 66*(2), 401–402.

Bagley, C. & King, K. K. (1990). *Child sexual abuse: The search for healing.* New York: Travistock/Routledge.

Bond, E. F., & Heitkemper, M. M. (1987). Importance of basic physiologic research in nursing science. *Heart & Lung: The Journal of Acute and Critical Care, 16*(4), 347–349.

Brown, B. E., & Garrison, C. J. (1990). Patterns of symptomatology of adult women incest survivors. *Western Journal of Nursing Research, 12*(5), 587–600.

Brown, S. J. (1999). *Knowledge for health care practice: A guide to using research evidence.* Philadelphia: Saunders.

Browne, A., & Finkelhor, D. (1986). Initial and long-term effects: A review of the research. In D. Finkelhor (Ed.), *A sourcebook on child sexual abuse* (pp. 143–179). Beverly Hills, CA: Sage.

Burns, N. (1989). The research process and the nursing process: Distinctly different. *Nursing Science Quarterly, 2*(4), 157–158.

Burns, N., & Grove, S. K. (2005). *The practice of nursing research: Conduct, critique, and utilization* (5th ed.). Philadelphia: Saunders.

Campbell, D. T., & Stanley, J. C. (1963). *Experimental and quasi-experimental designs for research.* Chicago: Rand McNally.

Cook, T. D., & Campbell, D. T. (1979). *Quasi-experimentation: Design and analysis issues for field settings.* Chicago: Rand McNally.

Crosby, L. J. (1990). The abstract: An important first impression. *Journal of Neuroscience Nursing, 22*(3), 192–194.

Fisher, Sir R. A. (1935). *The designs of experiments.* New York: Hafner.

Follette, N. M., Alexander, P. C., & Follette, W. C. (1991). Individual predictors of outcome in group treatment for incest survivors. *Journal of Consulting and Clinical Psychology, 59*(1), 150–155.

Graves, E., Hitt, A., Pariza, M. W., Cook, M. E., & McCarthy, D. O. (2005). Conjugated linoleic acid preserves gastrocnemius muscle mass in mice bearing the colon-26 adenocarcinoma. *Research in Nursing & Health, 28*(1), 48–55.

Hastings-Tolsma, M. T., Yucha, C. B., Tompkins, J., Robson, L., & Szeverenyi, N. (1993). Effect of warm and cold applications on the resolution of IV infiltrations. *Research in Nursing & Health, 16*(3), 171–178.

Hulme, P. A., & Grove, S. K. (1994). Symptoms of female survivors of child sexual abuse. *Issues in Mental Health Nursing, 15*(5), 519–532.

Kaplan, A. (1964). *The conduct of inquiry: Methodology for behavioral science.* San Francisco: Chandler.

Kerlinger, F. N., & Lee, H. B. (2000). *Foundations of behavioral research* (4th ed.). Fort Worth, TX: Harcourt.

Lewis, G. B., & Hecker, J. F. (1991). Radiological examination of failure of intravenous infusions. *British Journal of Surgery, 78*(4), 500–501.

MacCara, M. E. (1983). Extravasation: A hazard of intravenous therapy. *Drug Intelligence & Clinical Pharmacy, 17*(10), 713–717.

McCarthy, D. O., Lo, C., Nguyen, H., & Ney, D. M. (1997). The effect of protein density of food on food intake and nutritional status of tumor-bearing rats. *Research in Nursing & Health, 20*(2), 131–138.

Melnyk, B. M., & Fineout-Overholt, E. (2005). *Evidence-based practice in nursing & healthcare: A guide to best practice.* Philadelphia: Lippincott.

Millam, D. A. (1988). Managing complications of I.V. therapy. *Nursing, 18*(3), 34–43.

Miller, D. C. (1991). *Handbook of research design & social measurement* (5th ed.). Newbury Park, CA: Sage.

Miller, M. A., & Babcock, D. E. (1996). *Critical thinking applied to nursing.* St. Louis: Mosby.

Moody, L. E., Wilson, M. E., Smyth, K., Schwartz, R., Tittle, M., & Van Cott, M. L. (1988). Analysis of a decade of nursing practice research: 1977–1986. *Nursing Research, 37*(6), 374–379.

Myers, S. T. (1982). The search for assumptions. *Western Journal of Nursing Research, 4*(1), 91–98.

Olney, C. M. (2005). The effect of therapeutic back massage in hypertensive persons: A preliminary study. *Biological Research for Nursing, 7*(2), 98–105.

Prescott, P. A., & Soeken, K. L. (1989). The potential uses of pilot work. *Nursing Research, 38*(1), 60–62.

Swanson, E. A., McCloskey, J. C., & Bodensteiner, A. (1991). Publishing opportunities for nurses: A comparison of 92 U.S. journals. *Image—The Journal of Nursing Scholarship, 23*(1), 33–38.

Tornquist, E. M., Funk, S. G., Champagne, M. T., & Wiese, R. A. (1993). Advice on reading research: Overcoming the barriers. *Applied Nursing Research, 6*(4), 177–183.

Van Ort, S. (1981). Research design: Pilot study. In S. D. Krampitz & N. Pavlovich (Eds.), *Readings for nursing research* (pp. 49–53). St. Louis: Mosby.

Whitney, F. W., & Roncoli, M. (1986). Turning clinical problems into research. *Heart & Lung: The Journal of Acute and Critical Care, 15*(1), 57–59.

Whittemore, R. (2005). Combining evidence in nursing research: Methods and implications. *Nursing Research, 54*(1), 56–62.

Williams, M. A. (1980). Editorial: Assumptions in research. *Research in Nursing & Health, 3*(2), 47–48.

Wysocki, A. B. (1983). Basic versus applied research: Intrinsic and extrinsic considerations. *Western Journal of Nursing Research, 5*(3), 217–224.

Introduction to the Qualitative Research Process

CHAPTER 3

Chapter Overview

Learning Outcomes

After completing this chapter, you should be able to:

1. Describe the scientific rigor associated with qualitative research.
2. Differentiate the purposes of the four types of qualitative research.
3. Compare and contrast the research processes used in phenomenological, grounded theory, ethnographic, and historical research.
4. Examine the data collection issues for a qualitative study, including the relationships between the researcher and the participants and the reflections of the researcher on the meaning of the data.

Key Terms

Bracketing, p. 81
Coding, p. 82
Emic approach, p. 70
Ethnographic research, p. 69
Ethnonursing research, p. 70
Etic approach, p. 70
External criticism, p. 74

Grounded theory research, p. 66
Historical research, p. 71
Internal criticism, p. 75
Phenomenological research, p. 63
Primary source, p. 74
Qualitative research, p. 61

Reflexive thought, p. 80
Researcher-participant relationship, p. 76
Rigor, p. 91
Secondary source, p. 74
Storytakers, p. 88
Storytelling, p. 88

STUDY TOOLS

Be sure to visit http://evolve.elsevier.com/Burns/understanding/ for additional examples and self-tests. Also, a review of this chapter's concepts and practice exercises can be found in Chapter 3 of the Study Guide for *Understanding Nursing Research: Building an Evidence-Based Practice*, 4th edition.

Qualitative research is a systematic, subjective approach used to describe life experiences and give them meaning (Leininger, 1985; Munhall, 1989, 2001; Silva & Rothbart, 1984). Qualitative research is not a new idea in the social or behavioral sciences (Baumrind, 1980; Glaser & Strauss, 1967; Kaplan, 1964; Scheffler, 1967). The nursing community's interest in qualitative research began in the late 1970s.

The terminology and the methods of reasoning used in qualitative research differ from those used in more traditional, quantitative research methods and reflect alternative philosophical orientations. The specific philosophical orientation of each approach directs the research method. Although each qualitative approach is unique, there are many commonalities.

This chapter introduces some of the qualitative research approaches commonly used in nursing and reviews their contributions to nursing knowledge. To facilitate comprehension of these methods, the assumptions underlying the qualitative approaches are explored. Also presented is a general overview of the following qualitative approaches: phenomenological research, grounded theory research, ethnographic research, and historical research. The methods used to collect, analyze, and interpret qualitative data are described. The content provides a background for you to use in reading and comprehending published qualitative studies and in applying study findings to your clinical practice.

The Evidence Base: Do Qualitative Studies Contribute?

Qualitative studies currently are not included in the review of studies for evidence-based practice. Current reviews focus on evidence from randomized clinical trials (RCTs) and place lesser value on other quantitative studies. These reviews have carefully established criteria for use by review groups that evaluate the quality of studies for the development of the evidence base. The particular evidence of interest in a review for evidence-based practice is that the study clearly shows that the treatment (or intervention) causes the outcomes. Hawker, Payne, Kerr, Hardey, and Powell (2002) argue that "evidence-based practice cannot be restricted to randomized trials: Evidence originates from a variety of sources. Some areas of interest are not suited to an RCT or other forms of quantitative investigation" (p. 1285). Many writers are now arguing that qualitative research findings have much to offer evidence-based practice (Green & Britten, 1998; Popay, Rogers, & Williams, 1998; Whittemore, 2005).

The problem is the absence of criteria for judging the quality of qualitative studies. The Cochrane Collection has organized a Cochrane Qualitative Research Methods Group for the purpose of establishing criteria for evaluating qualitative studies. This work group continues to experience difficulty because of the lack of availability of optimal search strategies (OSSs) and the lack of acceptable criteria for judging qualitative studies (Grant, 2004). Current search strategies are not effective in identifying the available qualitative studies on a selected topic.

Cesario, Morin, and Santa-Donato (2002), who are members of the Evidence-Based Clinical Practice Guideline Development Team of Women's Health, Obstetric and Neonatal Nurses (AWHONN), have created a scoring system designed to place qualitative studies within specific levels of evidence. Two guideline development teams evaluated the validity of the tool and improved it as indicated by their experiences using it. The criteria have been used by the AWHONN's Nursing Management of the Second Stage of Labor Evidence-Based Clinical Practice Guideline Development Team. Further pilot testing is planned to evaluate the reliability and validity of the tool for general use.

Nurse researchers who develop evidenced-based guidelines recognize the importance of including evidence from qualitative studies. Work is under way to make this important evidence available and incorporate it within the guidelines for practice.

Philosophical View of Qualitative Research

The qualitative approaches are based on a worldview that is holistic, and many incorporate the following beliefs:

1. There are multiple, constructed realities.
2. The knower and the known are inseparable
3. Inquiry is value-bound
4. All generalizations are bounded by time and context (Lincoln and Guba, 1985)

The reasoning process used in qualitative research involves perceptually putting pieces together to make wholes. From this process, meaning is produced. Because perception varies with the individual, many different meanings are possible (Munhall, 2001). But, it is still possible for the identified meanings to be wrong. There are better and worse interpretations of data (Ayres & Poirier, 1996).

Frameworks are used in a different sense in qualitative research, because the goal is not hypothesis testing. In some qualitative studies, theory development is one of the results of the study. Each type of qualitative research is guided by a particular philosophical stance. The philosophy directs the questions that are asked, the observations that are made, and how the data are interpreted (Munhall, 2001). The researcher does not always clearly state the philosophical stance on which the study is based; however, this can be identified by a careful reading of the literature review, the presentation of the problem, and the methods used (Sandelowski, 1993). These philosophical bases and their associated research methods, developed outside of nursing, probably will undergo evolutionary changes within nursing.

The findings from a qualitative study lead to understanding of a phenomenon in a particular situation and are not generalized in the same way in which quantitative studies are. However, apprehension of the meanings of a phenomenon in a particular situation gives insights that can be applied more broadly. The insights from qualitative studies can guide nursing practice and aid in the important process of theory development for building nursing knowledge (Schwartz-Barcott & Kim, 1986).

Qualitative research provides a process through which nurses can examine a phenomenon outside of traditional views. The earliest and perhaps most dramatic demonstration of the influence qualitative research can have on nursing practice was the 4-year study conducted by Glaser and Strauss (1965, 1968, 1971), who initiated the use of grounded theory research methods for health-related studies. Their study, which described the social environment of dying patients in hospitals, was reported in three books: *Awareness of Dying* (Glaser & Strauss, 1965), *Time for Dying* (Glaser & Strauss, 1968), and *Status Passage* (Glaser & Strauss, 1971). At the time Glaser and Strauss were conducting their studies, the traditional view was that people could not cope with knowing that they were dying. The environment of care was designed to protect the patient from that knowledge. Glaser and Strauss (1965, 1968, 1971) examined what that protective social environment meant for the patient. This study changed the perception of nurses, who saw that the traditional care of the dying created loneliness and isolation, rather than protection. Nurses began to see the patient in a new light and changed their methods of patient care. Kübler-Ross (1969), perhaps influenced by the work of Glaser and Strauss, began her studies of the dying, using an approach similar to that of phenomenology. From this new orientation to care for the dying, hospice care developed. Now, almost 40 years later, the environment of care for the dying has changed.

Approaches to Qualitative Research

Four common approaches to qualitative research used in nursing are presented in this chapter: phenomenological, grounded theory, ethnographic, and historical. In some ways, these approaches differ greatly. Ethnographic and historical research are broad and are the accepted methodologies for a discipline. The worldview of phenomenology is more unique and is controversial. However, in each approach, the purpose is to examine meaning, and the unit of analysis is a word or phrase, rather than a numerical value.

Each of these four approaches is based on a philosophical orientation that influences the interpretation of the data. Thus, it is critical to understand the philosophy on which the method is based. Each approach is discussed in relation to its philosophical orientation and nursing knowledge, and a nursing study is provided to illustrate each methodology.

Phenomenological Research

Phenomenology is both a philosophy and a research method. The philosophical positions taken by phenomenological researchers are very different from the positions that are common in nursing culture and research traditions (Barkway, 2001; Boyd, 2001a; Caelli, 2000; Crotty, 1996; Darbyshire, Diekelmann, & Diekelmann, 1998; Giorgi, 2000; Munhall, 1989). However, discussions of this philosophical stance, appearing more frequently in the nursing literature, are introducing these ideas to a broader audience (Anderson, 1989; Beck, 1994; Boyd, 2001b; Geanellos, 2000; Kvigne, Gjengedal, & Kirkevold, 2002; Leonard, 1989; Munhall, 1989; Salsberry, Smith, & Boyd, 1989; Walters, 1995). Phenomenology as a philosophy has been the basis for a number of approaches to research. Phenomenologists view the person as integrated with the environment. The world shapes the self, and the self shapes the world. Phenomenologists differ in their philosophical beliefs. The two phenomenological philosophers whose work is most commonly adhered to in phenomenological nursing research are Heidegger and Husserl, whose views of the person and the world in which that person exists differ (Johnson, 2000). Phenomena are the world of experience. Phenomena occur only when a person experiences them. An experience is considered unique to the individual.

There are two approaches to phenomenological research, descriptive and interpretative. The purpose of descriptive **phenomenological research** is to describe experiences as they are lived—in phenomenological terms, to capture the "lived experience" of study participants. To describe it, the researcher must experience the phenomenon in a naive way (Kvigne et al., 2002; Sadala & Adorno, 2002). This is true even for the researcher's experiences in collecting data for a study and analyzing the data.

Nursing Knowledge and Phenomenological Research

Phenomenology is the philosophical base for three nursing theories: Parse's (1981) Theory of Man-Living-Health, Paterson and Zderad's (1976) Theory of Humanistic Nursing, and Watson's (1985) Theory of Caring. These three nursing theories use interpretive phenomenology. The broad research question that interpretive phenomenologists ask is "What is the meaning of one's lived experience?" Being a person is self-interpreting; therefore, the only reliable source of information to answer this question is the person. Understanding human behavior or experience, which is a central concern of nursing, requires that the person interpret the action or experience for the researcher; the researcher must then interpret the explanation provided by the person. Boyd (2001a) suggests that the long-range goal should be that of "making phenomenology work well for us in nursing research," that is, of extrapolating nursing research methodology from phenomenology. Phenomenology invites this kind of effort and insists on an openness that can protect such ideas about method from being reduced to dogma (p. 93).

Hermeneutics is a research method based on Heidegger's philosophical perspective that is being used by nurse researchers. Hermeneutics uses textual analysis as its primary research approach. Textual analysis "emphasizes the social and historic influences on qualitative interpretation" (Byrne, 2001, p. 968) and exposes hidden meanings. Hermeneutics originally was used to interpret biblical texts, seeking to ascertain the authentic meanings in order to determine how to live the Christian life. Hermeneutics is used in nursing research to increase the understanding of human nature (Byrne, 2001). The method also has been adopted by some feminist researchers (Ceci, 2003; Finch, 2004; Fleming, Gaidys, & Robb, 2003; Mitchell, 2004).

RESEARCH EXAMPLE   **Phenomenological Study**

One of the most significant nursing studies conducted using the phenomenological method is Benner's (1984) work, a critical description of nursing practice presented in the book *From Novice to Expert: Excellence and Power in Clinical Nursing Practice*. This study was funded by a grant from the U.S. Department of Health and Human Services, Division of Nursing, at a time when external funding for qualitative research was rare.

Benner (1984) explored the experience of clinical practice. The researcher develops a research question that involves the consideration of two factors (expressed as questions): "(1) What are the necessary and sufficient constituents of this feeling or experience? (2) What does the existence of this feeling or experience indicate concerning the nature of the human being?" (Omery, 1983, p. 55). Benner's research question was whether there were "distinguishable, characteristic differences in the novice and expert descriptions of the same clinical incident. If so, how could these differences, if identifiable from the nurses' descriptions of the incidents, be accounted for or understood?" (Benner, 1984, p. 14).

Benner (1984) conducted paired interviews with both beginning and expert nurses. Twenty-one pairs of nurses were selected from three hospitals in which preceptors were used to orient new graduates. Each member of the pair, one a preceptor and one a new graduate, was interviewed separately about patient care situations they had experienced together. Interviews and participant observation were conducted with additional nurses, including 51 experienced nurse clinicians, 11 new nursing graduates, and 5 senior nursing students. Individual interviews, small group interviews, and participant observation were conducted at six hospitals. Before the interviews, participants were given written explanations of the kinds of clinical descriptions of interest to the researchers. Interviews were recorded on tape and transcribed.

Benner's (1984) data analysis was an interpretive strategy based on Heideggerian phenomenology. She describes the procedure as follows:

> The interviews and participant-observer records were read independently by the research team members, and interpretations of the data were compared and consensually validated. Each interpretation was accepted only if there was agreement in labeling and interpreting the major competency demonstrated and only if it was effective in describing skilled practice. (p. 16)*

Benner's (1984) structural explanation of her findings was presented as five stages of gaining experience in clinical practice, which describe the nurse in a particular clinical situation as a novice, an advanced beginner, competent, proficient, or expert. The stages identified are based on the Dreyfus Model of Skill Acquisition (Dreyfus & Dreyfus, 1982).

Stage 1: Novice

Beginners have had no experience of the situations in which they are expected to perform. To give them entry to these situations and allow them to gain the experience so necessary for skill development, they are taught about the situations in terms of objective attributes such as weight, intake and output, temperature, blood pressure, pulse, and other such objectifiable, measurable parameters of a patient's conditions—features of the task that can be recognized without situational experiences. Novices are also taught context-free rules to guide action in respect to different attributes. (pp. 20–21)

Stage 2: Advanced Beginner

Advanced beginners are ones who can demonstrate marginally acceptable performance, ones who have coped with enough real situations to note (or to have pointed out to them by a mentor) the recurring meaningful situational components.... Aspects, in contrast to the measurable, context-free attributes or the procedural lists of things to do that are learned and used by the beginner, require prior experience in actual situations for recognitions. Aspects include overall, global characteristics that can be identified only through prior experience. (p. 22)

Stage 3: Competent

Competence, typified by the nurse who has been on the job in the same or similar situations two to three years, develops when the nurse begins to see his or her actions in terms of long-range goals or plans of which he or she is consciously aware. The plan dictates which attributes and aspects of the current and contemplated future situation are to be considered most important and those which can be ignored. Hence, for the competent nurse, a plan establishes a perspective, and the plan is based on considerable conscious, abstract, analytic contemplation of the problem. (p. 26)

*From Benner, P. (1984). *From novice to expert: Excellence and power in clinical nursing practice.* Menlo Park, CA: Addison-Wesley. Reprinted by permission.

(continues)

RESEARCH EXAMPLE *(continued)*

Stage 4: Proficient

Characteristically, the proficient performer perceives situations as wholes rather than in terms of aspects, and performance is guided by maxims. Maxims are cryptic instructions passed on by experts. Maxims make sense only if the person already has a deep understanding of the situation. (p. 10)

Perception is the key word here. The perspective is *not* thought out but "presents itself" based upon experience and recent events. Proficient nurses understand a situation as a whole because they perceive its meaning in terms of long-term goals. (p. 27)

Stage 5: Expert

The expert performer no longer relies on an analytic principle (rule, guideline, maxim) to connect her or his understanding of the situation to an appropriate action. The expert nurse, with an enormous background of experience, now has an intuitive grasp of each situation and zeros in on the accurate region of the problem without wasteful consideration of a large range of unfruitful, alternative diagnoses and solutions. (p. 32)

Benner (1984) also identified seven domains of practice: (1) the helping role, (2) the teaching-coaching function, (3) the diagnostic and patient-monitoring function, (4) effective management of rapidly changing situations, (5) administering and monitoring therapeutic interventions and regimens, (6) monitoring and ensuring the quality of health care practices, and (7) organizational and work role competencies. Nursing competencies representative of each domain were identified.

A bibliography of more recent phenomenological studies in nursing can be found on the Evolve website. If you are using CINAHL, type the search terms phenomenological and study to search for current phenomenological studies, many of which are available in full text.

Grounded Theory Research

Grounded theory research is an inductive technique that emerged from the discipline of sociology. The term *grounded* means that the theory that developed from the research has its roots in the data from which it was derived.

Philosophical Orientation

Grounded theory is based on symbolic interaction theory, which holds many views in common with phenomenology. George Herbert Mead (1934), a social psychologist, was a leader in the development of symbolic interaction theory. This theory explores how people define reality and how their beliefs are related to their actions. Reality is created by attaching meanings to situations. Meaning is expressed in such symbols as words, religious objects, and clothing. These symbolic meanings are the basis for actions and interactions. However, symbolic meanings are different for each individual, and we cannot completely know the symbolic meanings for another individual. In social life, meanings are shared by groups and are communicated to new members through socialization processes. Group life is based on consensus and shared meanings. Interaction may lead to redefinition and new meanings and can result in the redefinition of self. Because of its theoretical importance, the interaction is the focus of observation in grounded theory research (Chenitz & Swanson, 1986).

Grounded theory has been used most frequently to study areas in which little previous research has been conducted and to gain a new viewpoint in familiar areas of research. However, because of the high quality of theory generated through this method, further theory testing usually is not needed to enhance its usefulness.

Nursing Knowledge and Grounded Theory Research

Artinian (1988) has identified four qualitative modes of nursing inquiry within grounded theory: descriptive mode, discovery mode, emergent fit mode, and intervention mode. Each mode is used for different purposes: The descriptive mode provides rich detail and must precede all other modes. This mode, ideal for the beginning researcher, answers such questions as the following: "What is going on?" "How are activities organized?" "What roles are evident?" "What are the steps in a process?" "What does a patient do in a particular setting?" The discovery mode leads to the identification of patterns in a person's life experiences and relates the patterns to each other. Through this mode, a theory of social process referred to as substantive theory is developed; the theory explains a particular social world. The emergent fit mode is used when substantive theory has been developed to extend or refine this existing theory. This mode enables the researcher to focus on a selected portion of the theory, to build on previous work, or to establish a research program around a particular social process. The intervention mode is used to test the relationships in the substantive theory. The fundamental question for this mode is "How can I make something happen in a way that brings about a new and desired state of affairs?" This mode demands deep involvement on the part of the researcher and practitioner.

 RESEARCH EXAMPLE Grounded Theory Study

One significant study using a grounded theory approach that is relevant to clinical nursing practice is Fagerhaugh and Strauss's (1977) study of the politics of pain management. This study emerged from the previous work of Glaser and Strauss in the care of the dying (Glaser & Strauss, 1965, 1968; Strauss & Glaser, 1970) and chronically ill (Strauss, 1975; Strauss, Corbin, Fagerhaugh, Glaser, Maines, Suczek, et al., 1984). The study of pain involved 5 researchers and 2 years of systematic observations in 20 wards, 2 clinics, and 9 hospitals. The purposes of the study were to (1) develop an approach to pain management that was radically different from established approaches and (2) develop a substantive theory about what happens in hospitals when people are confronted with pain and attempt to deal with it (Fagerhaugh & Strauss, p. 13). The research questions were "Under what conditions is pain encountered by staff?" and "How will it be handled?" (Fagerhaugh & Strauss, p. 13).

In their study on pain, Fagerhaugh and Strauss (1977) observed a variety of situations in which pain was a common phenomenon. The clinical settings studied included an intensive care unit for severe burns, a cardiac care unit, an obstetrics ward, a physical rehabilitation unit, a neurology and neurosurgery unit, a routine surgery unit, a medical ward, an x-ray department, an emergency department, a kidney transplantation unit, and a cancer ward. The following excerpt is from the report of the grounded theory study on pain. It focuses on a description of the sampling process and demonstrates the care and detailed thought that must go into the development of sampling categories.

On all these wards we made "internal comparisons" along the theoretical dimensions. That is, we continued our theory-directed sampling: for instance, high-pain regimens versus low-pain regimens; experienced

(continues)

RESEARCH EXAMPLE *(continued)*

inflicters of regimen pain versus new inflicters; delivering mothers who had the fathers supporting their efforts to endure pain versus those who had no such supporting or controlling agents. Meanwhile, we were also looking at an activity that spanned separate wards and which would maximize variables as they related to pain infliction. We followed a number of personnel who drew blood from patients. We observed some who were very experienced, some who were not; some who were able to work in a leisurely fashion, some who were not; some who met "first-time" patients, others who met patients very experienced at this particular procedure; some who encountered patients with much ongoing pain and some who did not; some who had recently had experiences with accusations of incompetence and some who had not. (p. 308)

The core categories that evolved in the study were pain work, pain trajectories, legitimation, balancing, and accountability. Pain work was further classified as follows: nurses relieving pain, nurses handling pain expression, nurses diagnosing the meaning of pain, nurses inflicting pain, nurses minimizing or preventing pain, patients enduring pain, and the staff members controlling their own reactions to the patient's response to pain. The patient's cooperation in the pain work and negotiation between the staff and the patient were identified as important factors. An example of negotiation is described by Glasser (1973) as follows:

"This won't take long," I said to her…"it's not going to hurt…I think I can inject it right into the IV tubing and not have to stick you." She looked unconvinced. "Honestly I won't stick you unless I have to." (p. 130)

Pain trajectories were divided into expected and unexpected trajectories. For example, an expectant mother would have a very different pain trajectory from that experienced by a person with intractable back pain.

An unexpected trajectory—unexpected for a given ward, that is—carries a potential for staff and patient disturbance and ward upset. Both the sentimental order and the work order of the ward are threatened…. Patients with an unexpected or atypical trajectory tend to be labeled as "uncooperative" or "difficult," and relations between them and the staff are likely to grow progressively worse. (Fagerhaugh & Strauss, 1977, pp. 22–23)

The researchers also concluded that the pain trajectory was influenced by the patients' illnesses, their previous experience with pain, the medical care they were receiving, and their social history. The researchers observed that nursing and medical staff members seldom knew anything about the patient's pain trajectory other than their own observations.

Assessing and legitimizing pain also were important factors. Staff often suspected that patients claimed to have more pain than they really had or that patients claimed they had pain when they really had none. This left patients in the position of attempting to convince the staff that they were actually having the pain they claimed to have (legitimizing). Staff members and patients often were involved in the process of balancing priorities during pain work. Decisions were based on what the staff considered to be most important.

The staff members may not always agree among themselves, and the balancing done by the patient may not agree with the staff's. Patient and staff may even opt for opposite choices, disagreeing over the value of living a bit longer versus enduring terrible pain. They may be balancing quite different considerations. The staff may be balancing more work versus quicker pain relief, while the patient may be balancing pride in not complaining about pain versus difficulty of enduring it without more medication. (p. 25)

In terms of accountability, the researchers found that staff members did not consider pain work a major priority, and they tended to be more concerned with controlling patients' expression of pain than the experience of pain.

Fagerhaugh and Strauss (1977) showed in their study that grounded theory research examines a much broader scope of dimensions than can be examined with quantitative research. Such findings can be intuitively verified by your own experiences. The clear, cohesive description of the phenomenon can allow greater understanding of the phenomenon and thus lead to more control of nursing practice.

Fagerhaugh and Strauss (1977) concluded the following from their study:

> Genuine accountability concerning pain work could only be instituted if the major authorities on given wards or clinics understood the importance of that accountability and its implications for patient care. They would then need to convert that understanding into a commitment that would bring about necessary changes in written and verbal communication systems. This kind of understanding and commitment can probably come about only after considerable nationwide discussion, such as now is taking place about terminal care, but that kind of discussion seems to lie far in the future. (p. 27)

This ground-breaking study set in motion two decades of research, policy changes, and, ultimately, changes in clinical guidelines for practice related to the management of pain. Nurses are now held accountable not only for actions for relieving pain but for assessing the effectiveness of actions taken to relieve pain.

A bibliography of more recent grounded theory studies in nursing can be found on the Evolve website. If you are using CINAHL, type the search terms grounded theory and study to search for current grounded theory studies, many of which are available in full text.

Ethnographic Research

Ethnographic research was developed by anthropologists as a mechanism for studying cultures. The word *ethnography* means "portrait of a people." Many nurses involved in this type of research obtained their doctoral preparation in anthropology and have used anthropological techniques to examine cultural issues of interest in nursing. Although ethnography originated as the research methodology for the discipline of anthropology, it is now a part of the cultural research conducted by a number of other disciplines, including social psychology, sociology, political science, education, and nursing and also is used in feminist research. Ethnography has been associated with studies of primitive, foreign, or remote cultures. Such studies enabled the researcher to acquire new perspectives beyond his or her own ethnocentric perspective. Today, in nursing, the emphasis has shifted to obtaining cultural knowledge within the society to which a nurse researcher belongs (Germain & Munhall, 2001). Within nursing, one of the major contributions of ethnography may be to promote culturally specific care (Baillie, 1995).

Philosophical Orientation

The discipline of anthropology, which had its beginnings about the same time period as for nursing (in the mid-nineteenth century), provides a means to understand people, including their ways of living, believing, and adapting to changing environmental circumstances. Culture, the concept most central to anthropology, is "a way of life belonging to a designated group of people…a blueprint for living which guides a particular group's thoughts, actions, and sentiments…all the accumulated ways a group of people solve problems, which are reflected in the people's language, dress, food, and a number of accumulated traditions and customs" (Leininger, 1970, pp. 48–49). The purpose of anthropological research is to describe a culture by examining these various cultural characteristics.

Anthropologists study a people's origins, past ways of living, and ways of surviving through time. "The Australian aborigine, who lives in a non-technological society and a harsh natural environment, is as important an area of study in furthering a broad understanding of man as is contemporary Western man, who lives in a highly technological modern world" (Leininger, 1970, p. 7). Anthropologists may study cultures in remote parts of the world, in modern cities, and in modern rural areas. By comparing these cultures, they gain insights that increase our ability to predict the future directions of cultures and the forces that guide their destinies or that may provide opportunities to influence the direction of cultural development (Leininger, 1970).

Culture is both material and nonmaterial. Material culture consists of all created objects associated with a given group. Nonmaterial culture consists of other aspects of culture, such as symbolic referents, the network of social relations, and the beliefs reflected in social and political institutions. Symbolic meaning, social customs, and beliefs cannot be touched or stored in a museum; thus, they are not material, but they are essential elements of cultures. Cultures also have ideals that the people hold as desirable, even though they do not always live up to these standards. Anthropologists seek to discover the many parts of a whole culture and how these parts are interrelated so that a picture of the wholeness of the culture evolves (Leininger, 1970). Ethnographic research is used in nursing not only to increase ethnic cultural awareness but also to enhance the quality of health care for persons of all cultures. There are two basic research approaches in anthropology: emic and etic. The **emic approach** involves studying behaviors from within the culture; the **etic approach** involves studying behavior from outside the culture and examining similarities and differences across cultures.

Nursing Knowledge and Ethnographic Research

A group of nurse scientists influenced by Leininger's Theory of Transcultural Nursing, (Leininger, 1985) has developed an ethnographic research strategy for nursing. They refer to this strategy as **ethnonursing research**. Ethnonursing "focuses mainly on observing and documenting interactions with people of how these daily life conditions and patterns are influencing human care, health, and nursing care practices" (Leininger, 1985, p. 238). However, a number of nurse anthropologists not associated with the ethnonursing orientation also are providing important contributions to the nursing body of knowledge.

RESEARCH EXAMPLE   **Ethnographic Research**

A study of how nurses define medication error is titled "Rules outside the rules for administration of medication: A study in New South Wales, Australia is used to explain ethnographic research" (Baker, 1997). The purpose of this ethnomethodological study was to improve understanding of how nurses within the culture of hospital nursing practice define or redefine medication error.

In the brief literature review, Baker described Barker and McConnell's (1962) benchmark study reporting that the medication error rate for nurses was 1 in 10. The number of errors made was directly proportional to the number of medications administered by the nurse. These authors found that nurses were aware of only a few of the errors they made; of these recognized errors, they reported only a small number. Some studies found that as nurses became more experienced, they made fewer errors. Other studies indicated that experienced nurses made the same number of errors but reported fewer of them. A study by Frances (1980), which found that as nurses became more experienced, they seemed to redefine error, offered insight to Baker and raised a question that led her to conduct the present study: "If nurses do redefine error, what is the new definition?" (p. 155).

Baker (1997) spent 2 weeks in each of nine wards during morning, evening, and night shifts, and at times on weekends and public holidays. The total time spent in the wards was 18 weeks. She used participant observations, formal and informal interviews, written documents, and participation in shift reports. Some nurses did not wish to talk within the hospital, so arrangements were made to meet outside of the hospital. Shift reports proved to be a "rich source of data because nurses frequently account for their actions in asides during these formal reports" (p. 156). Baker discussed outcomes in three groups.

> The first group of findings are called situated and embodied logics. These are the practices adopted by nurses in order to accomplish certain goals in particular situations. Although they are situated, they and similar practices may be widespread. They include ways of managing the medication trolley, reading between lines of medication-order and administration sheets, and using the medication round for gathering information for other purposes. These situated and embodied logics help nurses to be orderly in the complex practice world.
>
> The second set of findings…[are] called the criteria for redefinition of error. This is a set of criteria nurses use to decide whether an incident is a "real" error. Of course every nurse is professionally obliged to report errors, but if an error can be redefined, a medication-related incident becomes a nonerror that does not need to be reported and no guilt is attached to it.
>
> The third set of findings [was] serendipitous and included the other uses to which nurses turn institutional rules with the purpose of making their own lives orderly. (p. 156)

The following criteria were used by nurses to decide whether incidents were errors.

1. If it's not my fault, it is not an error.
2. If everyone knows, it is not an error.
3. If you can put it right, it is not an error.
4. If a patient has needs that are more urgent than the accurate administration of medication, it is not an error.
5. A clerical error is not a medication error.
6. If an irregularity is carried out to prevent something worse, it is not an error.

To validate her conclusions, Baker shared the results of her analyses with the nurses who had participated in the study. They agreed with Baker's findings.

A bibliography of more recent ethnographic studies in nursing can be found on the Evolve website. If you are using CINAHL, type the search terms ethnographic and study to search for current ethnographic studies, many of which are available in full text.

Historical Research

Historical research examines events of the past. Many historians believe that the greatest value of historical knowledge is increased self-understanding; in addition, historical knowledge provides nurses with an increased understanding of their profession.

Philosophical Orientation

History is a science that dates back to the beginnings of humankind. The three primary questions of history are the following: "Where have we come from?" "Who are we?" "Where are we going?" Although the questions do not change, the answers do.

One of the assumptions of historical philosophy is that "there is nothing new under the sun." Because of this assumption, the historian can search throughout history for generalizations. For example, to answer the question "What causes wars?" a historian could search throughout history for commonalities in various wars and develop a theoretical explanation of the causes of wars. The questions a historian asks, the factors a historian looks for throughout history, and the nature of the explanation a historian gives in a study all are based on a specific worldview (Heller, 1982). Another assumption of historical philosophy is that it is possible to learn from the past. The philosophy of history is a search for wisdom in which the historian examines what has been, what is, and what ought to be. Historical philosophers have attempted to identify a developmental scheme for history to explain all events and structures as elements of the same social process.

Nursing Knowledge and Historical Research

Christy (1978) asks: "[H]ow can we in nursing today possibly plan where we are going when we don't know where we have been…[or] how we got here?" (p. 9). One criterion of a profession is that knowledge of the history of the profession is transmitted to those entering the profession. Until recently, historical nursing research has not been a valued activity, and few nurse researchers had the skills or desire to conduct it. Therefore, our knowledge of our past is sketchy. However, there is now a growing interest in the field of historical nursing research (Sarnecky, 1990).

Lusk (1997) suggests the following:

Topics should be significant, with the potential to illuminate or place a new perspective on current questions, thus contributing to scholarly understanding. Topics should also be feasible in terms of data and resource availability. Finally, topics should be intriguing and capable of sustaining a researcher's interest. (p. 355)

RESEARCH EXAMPLE   Historical Nursing Research

The researcher may spend much time reading related literature before making a final decision about the precise topic. In her doctoral dissertation, Waring (1978) used historical research to examine the idea of the nurse experiencing a "calling" to practice nursing. She described the extensive process of developing a precise topic as follows:

Originally my idea was to pursue concepts in the area of Puritan social thought and to relate concepts such as altruism and self-sacrifice to nursing. Two years after the formulation of this first idea, I finally realized that the topic was too broad. Reaching that point was slow and arduous but quite essential to the development of my thinking and the prospectus that developed as an outcome. When I first began the process, it seemed that I might have to abandon the topic "calling." Now, since the clarification and tightening up of my title and the clarification of my study thesis, I open volumes fearing that I will find yet another reference, once overlooked. It is only recently that I have become convinced that there was a needle in the haystack and that I had indeed found it. (pp. 18–19) [Waring's original title was "American Nursing and the Concept of the Calling."]

Developing Research Questions

After the topic has been clearly defined, the researcher will identify the questions to be examined during the research process. These questions tend to be more general and analytical than those found in quantitative studies.

Evans (1978), then a doctoral student, describes the research questions she developed for her historical study.

I propose to study the nursing student. Who was this living person inside the uniform? Where did she come from? What were her experiences as a nursing student? I use the word "experience" in terms of the dictionary definition of "living through." What did she live through? What happened to her and how did she respond, or react, as the case may be? What was her educational program like? We have a pretty good notion of what nurse educators and others thought about the educational program, but what about it from the students' point of view?

What were the functions of rituals and rites of passage such as bed check, morning inspection, and capping? What kind of person did the nursing student tend to become in order to successfully negotiate studenthood? What are the implications of this in terms of her own personal and professional development and the development of the profession at large? (p. 16)

Developing an Inventory of Sources

The next step is to determine whether sources of data for the study are available. Many of the materials for historical research are contained in private archives in libraries or are privately owned. Written permission must be obtained to gain access to library archives. Private materials often are difficult to ferret out, and when they are discovered, access may again be a problem.

Historical materials in nursing, such as letters, memos, handwritten materials, and mementos of significant leaders in nursing, are being discarded because no one recognizes their value. The same is true of materials related to the history of institutions and agencies with which nursing has been involved. Christy (1978) states, "It seems obvious that interest in the preservation of historical materials will only be stimulated if there is a concomitant interest in the value of historical research" (p. 9). Sometimes when such material is found, it is in such poor condition that much of the data are unclear or completely lost. Christy (1978) describes one of her experiences in searching for historical data as follows:

M. Adelaide Nutting and Isabel M. Stewart are two of the greatest leaders we have ever had, and their friends, acquaintances, and former students were persons of tremendous importance to developments in nursing and nursing education throughout the world. Since both of these women were historians, they saved letters, clippings, manuscripts—primary source materials of inestimable value. Their friends were from many walks of life: physicians, lawyers, social workers, philanthropists—supporters and nonsupporters of nursing and nursing interests. Miss Nutting and Miss Stewart crammed these documents into boxes, files, and whatever other receptacles were available and unfortunately some of these materials are this very day in those same old boxes.

When I began my research into the archives in 1966, the files were broken, rusty, and dilapidated. Many of the folders were so old and ill-tended that they fell apart in my hands, the ancient paper crumbled into dust before my eyes. My research was exhilaratingly stimulating, and appallingly depressing at the same time; stimulating due to the gold mine of data available, and depressing as I realized the lack of care provided for such priceless materials. In addition, there was little or no organization, and one had to go through each document, in each drawer, in each file, piece by piece. The boxes and cartons were worse, for materials bearing absolutely no relationship to each other were simply piled, willy-nilly, one atop the other. Is it any wonder that it took me eighteen months of solid work to get through them? (pp. 8–9)

Determining the Validity and Reliability of Data

The validity and reliability concerns in historical research are related to the sources from which data are collected. The most valued source of data is the primary source. A **primary source** is material most likely to shed true light on the information the researcher seeks. For example, material written by a person who experienced an event and letters and other mementos saved by the person being studied are primary source material. A **secondary source** is written by someone who previously read and summarized the primary source material. History books and textbooks are secondary source materials. Primary sources are considered more valid and reliable than secondary sources.

> The presumption is that an eyewitness can give a more accurate account of an occurrence than a person not present. If the author was an eyewitness, he is considered a primary source. If the author has been told about the occurrence by someone else, the author is a secondary source. The further the author moves from an eyewitness account, the less reliable are his statements. (Christy, 1975, p. 191)

Historical researchers use primary sources whenever possible. The historical researcher must consider the validity and reliability of primary sources used in the study. To determine this, the researcher uses principles of historical criticism.

> One does not merely pick up a copy of Grandmother's diary and gleefully assume that all the things Grandma wrote were the unvarnished facts. Grandmother's glasses may at times have been clouded, at other times rose-colored. The well-prepared researcher will scrutinize, criticize, and analyze before even accepting its having been written by Grandma! And even after the validity of the document is established, every attempt is made to uncover bias, prejudice, or just plain exaggeration on Grandmother's part. Healthy skepticism becomes a way of life for the serious historiographer. (Christy, 1978, p. 6)

Two strategies have been developed to determine the authenticity and accuracy of the source: external and internal criticism. **External criticism** is used to determine the validity of source material. The researcher needs to know where, when, why, and by whom a document was written. This may involve verifying the handwriting or determining the age of the paper on which it was written. Christy (1975) describes some difficulties she experienced in establishing the validity of documents:

> An interesting problem presented by early nursing leaders was their frugality. Nutting occasionally saved stationery from hotels, resorts, or steamship lines during vacation trips and used it at a later date. This required double checking as to her exact location at the time the letter was written. When she first went to Teachers College in 1907, she still wrote a few letters on Johns Hopkins stationery. I found this practice rather confusing in early stages of research. (p. 190)

Internal criticism is an examination of the reliability of the document. The researcher must determine possible biases of the author. To verify the accuracy of a statement, two independent sources that provide the same information are needed. In addition, the researcher must ensure that he or she understands the statements made by the writer, because words and their meanings change across time and across cultures. It also is possible to read into a document a meaning not originally intended by the author. This is most likely to happen when a researcher is seeking a particular meaning. Sometimes words can be taken out of context (Christy, 1975).

Collecting the Data

Data collection may require months or years of dedicated searching for pertinent material. Occasionally, one small source may open a door to an entire new field of facts. In addition, there is no clear, obvious end to data collection. The research guide developed in the planning stage of the study can be used by the researcher in making the decision to discontinue collection of data. These facets of data collection are described by Newton (1965) as follows:

> The search for data takes the researcher into most unexpected nooks and corners and adds facet after facet to the original problem. It may last for months or years or a decade. Days and weeks may be fruitless and endless references may be devoid of pertinent material. Again, one minor reference will open the door to the gold mine of facts. The search becomes more exciting when others know of it and bring possible clues to the investigator. The researcher cultivates persistence, optimism, and patience in his long and sometimes discouraging quest. But one real "find" spurs him on and he continues his search. Added to this skill is the training in the most meticulous recording of data with every detail complete, and the logical classification of the data. (p. 23)

Writing the Research Report

Historical research reports do not follow the traditional formalized style that is characteristic of much research. The studies are designed to attract the interest of the reader and may appear to be deceptively simple. The untrained eye may not recognize the extensive work that was required to write the paper. Christy (1975) explains as follows:

> The reader is never aware of the painstaking work, the careful attention to detail, ...[or] the arduous pursuit of clues endured by the writer of history. Perhaps that is why so many nurses have failed to recognize historiography as a legitimate research endeavor. It looks so easy. (p. 192)

A bibliography of more recent historical studies in nursing can be found on the Evolve website. If you are using CINAHL, type the search terms historical and study to search for current historical studies, many of which are available in full text.

Qualitative Research Methodology

This section presents a more detailed description of the methodologies commonly used in qualitative studies. In some ways the methods used are no different from those used in quantitative studies. The researcher must select a topic; state the problem or question; justify the significance of the study; design the study; identify sources of data, such as subjects; gain access to those sources of data; select subjects or other sources for study; gather data; describe, analyze, and interpret the data; and develop a written report of the results. There are, however, methods unique to qualitative studies and sometimes to specific types of qualitative research. An understanding of some of the unique methods used by qualitative researchers will help you appreciate the work involved in conducting such a study.

This section describes how participants (subjects) are selected, and how data are collected, managed, and analyzed. The achievement of rigor in qualitative research also is explored.

Selection of Participants

Subjects in qualitative studies are referred to as participants because the researcher and the participants cooperatively carry out the study. They provide assistance and guidance to the researcher, who could not be successful in carrying out the study without their help. Participants may volunteer to be involved in the study or be selected by the researcher because of their particular knowledge, experience, or views related to the study. Qualitative researchers use purposive sampling methods, rather than probability or convenience sampling methods. The researcher may select persons typical in relation to the phenomenon under study, or, to get diverse perspectives, the researcher may intentionally seek out people who are different in some way from other participants. The sampling technique of "snowballing," in which the researcher asks participants to suggest persons known to them who could provide information useful to the study, is commonly used.

Decisions regarding sample size are different from those in quantitative studies and are based on needs related to the purposes of the study. Usually the number of subjects is small relative to the number used in quantitative studies. In case studies, the researcher may use only one subject (Sandelowski, 1996). A study of 6 to 10 subjects is not unusual. However, studies seeking maximum variation to examine a complex phenomenon or to develop a theory may require larger samples.

The decision to stop seeking new subjects is made when the researcher ceases learning new information (informational redundancy) or when theoretical ideas seem complete (theoretical saturation) (Sandelowski, 1995).

The historical researcher seeks sources of information about the event being studied. These sources may include people who have experienced the event. But in most cases the sources are written documents or films. The researcher develops an inventory of sources and determines the validity and reliability of data from those sources.

Researcher-Participant Relationships

One of the important differences between quantitative and qualitative research lies in the relationship between the researcher and the participants of the study. The nature of this **researcher-participant relationship** has an impact on the collection and interpretation of data. Participants in qualitative research are not research subjects in the usual sense of the word; they are colleagues. The researcher must have the support and confidence of these persons to complete the research. Therefore, maintaining these relationships is very important. In ethnographic studies the researcher observes social behavior and may interact socially with the participants.

In various degrees the researcher influences the people being studied and, in turn, is influenced by them. The mere presence of the researcher may alter behavior in the setting. This involvement, considered a source of bias in quantitative research, is thought by qualitative researchers to be a natural element of the research process. The researcher's personality is a key factor in qualitative research. Skills in empathy and intuition are cultivated; the researcher must become closely involved in the subject's experience to interpret it. It is necessary for the researcher to be open to the perceptions of the participants, rather than to attach his or her own meaning to the experience. Participants may assist in determining research questions, guiding data collection, and interpreting results.

The ethnographic researcher must become very familiar with the culture being studied by active participation in it and by extensive questioning of participants. The process of becoming immersed in the culture involves gaining increasing familiarity with aspects of the culture, such as language, sociocultural norms, traditions, and other social dimensions, including family, communication patterns (verbal and nonverbal), religion, work patterns, and expression of emotion. Immersion also involves gradually increasing acceptance of the researcher into the culture. Although ethnographic researchers must be actively involved in the culture they are studying, they must avoid "going native," which will interfere with both data collection and analysis. In going native, the researcher becomes a part of the culture and loses the ability to observe clearly.

In addition to the role the qualitative researcher takes in the relationship, expectations of the study must be carefully considered. The researcher's aims and means need to be consistent with those of the participants. For example, if the researcher's desire is to change the behavior of the participants, this must also be their desire.

Data Collection Methods

The most common data collection methods used in qualitative studies are observing participants, interviewing participants, and examining written text. These three methods, as they are used in qualitative studies, are described in the following sections.

Observation

Observation is a fundamental method of gathering data for qualitative studies. The aim is to gather firsthand information in a naturally occurring situation. The researcher functions in the learning mode to answer the question "What is going on here?" It is important for the researcher to look carefully and to listen. In most cases the activities being observed are routine for the participants. The researcher focuses on the details of the routine. The process of activities may be as important to note as the discrete events. Unexpected events occurring during routine activities may be significant and are carefully noted. As in any observation process, the qualitative researcher will attend to some aspects of the situation while disregarding others. The researcher's focus on particular aspects of the situation may increase as insights about "what is going on" occur (Silverman, 1993).

Historians may observe film, videotapes, photographs, or artistic representations of historical events. The historical researcher must recognize that these sources are limited to information the photographer or artist selectively chooses to reveal. Important elements of the event may not have been photographed or may have been edited out. In some cases, film that has been edited out of finished products has been preserved and may be sought by historians. The breakdown of the Communist countries has provided a treasure trove of archived films that can be used to provide important historical insights into many aspects of people's lives, including health issues.

Various strategies may be used to record information about the observations. In some cases the researcher will take detailed handwritten notes while observing. In other cases the researcher may focus entirely on the observational experience to avoid missing something meaningful and may wait until after the observation period to make detailed notes. Another useful strategy is to videotape the events, so that careful observations and detailed notes can be taken at a later time.

Interviews

Differences exist between interviews conducted for a qualitative study and those conducted for a quantitative study. In qualitative studies, the interview format is more likely to be open-ended. Although the researcher defines the focus of the interview, there is no fixed sequence of questions. The questions addressed in interviews tend to change as the researcher gains insights from previous interviews and observations. Respondents are allowed, even encouraged, to raise important issues not addressed by the researcher. Interviews in qualitative studies range from semi-structured (fixed set of questions, no fixed responses) to unstructured (open-ended questions with probes).

During interviews for qualitative studies, the researcher and the participant are actively engaged in constructing a version of the world. The interviewer and interviewee have the common goal of making sense of the interviewee's experience (Ayres & Poirier, 1996). The researcher's goal is to obtain an authentic insight into the participant's experiences. Rather than occurring at a single point in time, dialogue between researcher and participant may continue at intervals across weeks or months. Use of recurring interviews can help to decrease the problems associated with fleeting relationships, in which respondents may have little commitment to the study or may provide only the information they believe the researcher wishes to hear (Silverman, 1993). Wimpenny and Gass (2000) compared the interviewing process in phenomenological and grounded theory research, to determine differences in interview technique. They examined interview methods used in both approaches to qualitative research in studies published between 1995 and 1998. They found that many qualitative researchers did not explicitly describe their data collection methods. Wimpenny and Gass (2000) concluded that in phenomenological and grounded theory research the interview method was not clearly linked to the qualitative approach being used.

Historical researchers may interview people who were participants in or observers of historical events. The focus of the interview may be to validate available information about the event, uncover heretofore unknown details about the event, or obtain the views about the event from persons who were not heard from previously. Historical events generally are considered to be constructed truths, rather than factual. Individual perspectives on an event may provide additional insight into the event, but they are not expected to provide the truth of an event, which will never be known (and perhaps does not exist). Another strategy for collecting historical data is to interview people and construct their biographies. In addition, the personal histories of a number of persons can be used to understand the evolving history of a region or institution.

Strategies used to record information from interviews include writing notes during the interview, writing detailed notes immediately after the interview, and recording the interview on tape.

Text as a Source of Qualitative Data

In qualitative studies, text is considered a rich source of data. The researcher may ask participants to write about a particular topic. In some cases these written narratives may be solicited by mail rather than in person. Text provided by participants may be a component of a larger study using a variety of sources of data. Text developed for other purposes, such as from patient records or procedure manuals, can be accessed for qualitative analysis. Published text from newspaper articles, magazine articles, books, or the Internet also can be used as qualitative data. Transcriptions of recorded interviews are commonly used in qualitative studies. In historical research, written descriptions of historical events, letters, and documents related to the event may be accessed for analysis. A historical study might examine the changing pattern of nursing practice in a selected area or of a nursing procedure by examining nursing textbooks and journal articles that describe a particular practice at different times. Notes taken during the reading of documents are important to the analysis process.

Data Management

Qualitative data analysis occurs concurrently with data collection, rather than sequentially as in quantitative research. Therefore, the researcher is attempting to simultaneously gather, manage, and interpret a growing bulk of data. Volumes of data are gathered during a qualitative study. The researcher must develop means of storing the data in an organized manner. Traditionally, qualitative data collection and analysis have been performed manually. The researcher records the data on small bits of paper or note cards that are then carefully coded, organized, and filed at the end of a day of gathering data. It is easy to lose data in the mass of paper. Keeping track of connections between various bits of data requires meticulous record keeping. Some qualitative researchers believe that a computer can be used to make management and analysis of qualitative data quicker and easier, without the risk of losing touch with the data. A computer assists such activities as processing, storing, retrieving, cataloging, and sorting, leaving the analysis up to the researcher.

Data Analysis

Qualitative data analysis occurs in three stages: description, analysis, and interpretation. The descriptive stage is more critical in qualitative studies than in quantitative ones. Researchers are encouraged to remain in the descriptive mode for as long as possible before moving on to analysis and interpretation. Because published qualitative studies tend not to describe the methodology in detail, many professionals believe that qualitative research is free-wheeling. According to Coffey and Atkinson (1996):

There still seem to be too many students and practitioners who believe implicitly that qualitative research can be done in a spirit of careless rapture, with no principled or disciplined thought whatsoever. They collect data with little thought for research problems and research design, and they think that they will know what to do with the data once those data are collected. [When they begin analysis] they find that things are not quite so simple. (p. 11)

Description

In the initial phases of a qualitative study, the researcher needs to become familiar with the data. This may involve reading and rereading notes and transcripts, recalling observations and experiences, listening to audiotapes, and viewing videotapes, until the researcher becomes immersed in the data. Audiotapes contain more than words; they contain feeling, emphasis, and nonverbal communication, which are as important to communication as words are. In phenomenological research, this immersion in the data is referred to as "dwelling with the data." The initial purpose of this immersion is to address the question "What is going on?" An important methodological technique in grounded theory research is the constant comparative process, in which every piece of data is compared with every other piece.

During data analysis, a dynamic interaction occurs between the researcher and his or her experience of the data, whether the data are communicated orally or in writing. During this process, referred to as **reflexive thought**, the researcher explores personal feelings and experiences that may influence the study and integrates this understanding into the study. The process requires a conscious self-awareness.

RESEARCH EXAMPLE   Qualitative Analysis

In a paper describing her experiences conducting a phenomenological study of caregiving behaviors, Drew (1989) reveals this interaction between herself as researcher and the data by describing the impact of participant relationships with her as she analyzes her data:

A session with a person who had been willing to talk about his or her experiences with caregivers, and who had invested energy into the interview session, often generated for me a sense of doing something worthwhile, as well as a feeling that I would be competent to analyze the transcribed material in a meaningful way. This sense of competency dispelled any doubts about being an intruder. I became relaxed, unself-conscious, and more self-assured. However, an encounter with a person with blunt affect, abrupt answers, and a paucity of responses left me feeling awkward and self-conscious. A sense of doubt about the validity of my project encroached as I attempted to elicit that person's thoughts. At the time, my immediate reaction was to think that I had obtained nothing from these individuals, when in fact, as I was to discover later, the "nothing" was something important that I was as yet unable to see.

It was at the point of discouragement about my interviewing skills that I became aware that I was mentally classifying interviews as either "good" or "bad," depending on my emotional response to the subjects. Good interviews were those in which I felt effective as an interviewer and was able to facilitate the person's recounting of experiences with caregivers. I enjoyed the interaction and felt that we connected on some level that produced meaningful discussion about the topic of relationships between patient and caregiver.

Bad interviews, on the other hand, were those in which I could not seem to get subjects to talk about how they had experienced their caregivers. There seemed to be no questions that I could devise with which to explore feelings, either positive or negative, with them. They gave no indications of awareness of their feelings, or of feelings in others. Whereas the subjects of the good interviews were people I experienced as open, curious, and thoughtful, those of the bad interviews were experienced as distrustful and elicited in me a sense of anxiety and frustration; it seemed I could not get through to them. I felt inadequate as an interviewer and was ready to discard these interviews. Frustration and anxiety arose because I felt that I was not getting the information that I needed for the study.

   Subsequently, I discovered that my feelings of frustration and inadequacy were causing me to overlook data and that when I could put them aside, new data that were rich in meaning became apparent.... This discovery was a powerful experience for me, affecting my approach to subsequent interviews and influencing analysis of data thereafter. (pp. 433–434)*

*From Drew, N. (1989). The interviewer's experience as data in phenomenological research. *Western Journal of Nursing Research, 11*(4), 431–439. Reprinted with permission of Sage Publications, Inc.

In some phenomenological research this critical thinking leads to **bracketing**, which is used to help the researcher avoid misinterpreting the phenomenon as it is being experienced by the participants. Bracketing is suspending or laying aside what the researcher knows about the experience being studied (Oiler, 1982). Other phenomenologists, especially those using Heideggerian phenomenology, do not bracket, but they do identify beliefs, assumptions, and preconceptions about the research topic. These are put in writing at the beginning of the study for self-reflection and external review. These procedures are intended to facilitate openness and new insights.

Transcribing Interviews

Tape-recorded interviews generally are transcribed word for word. Morse and Field (1995) provide the following instructions for transcribing a tape-recorded interview.

   Pauses should be indicated by using dashes, and ellipses should indicate gaps or prolonged pauses. All expressions, including exclamations, laughter, crying, and expletives, are included in the text and separated from the verbal text with square brackets. Type the interviews single-spaced with a blank line between each speaker. A generous margin on both sides of the page permits the left margin to be used for coding and the researcher's own critique of the interview style, and the right margin to be used for comments regarding the content.... Ensure that all pages are numbered sequentially and that each page is coded with the interview number and the participant number. (p. 131)

   Listening to recordings as soon as possible after an interview is recommended. Voice tone, inflection, and pauses of the researcher and the participant are important to note. While listening, the researcher is advised to read the written transcript of the tape and make notations of observations on the transcript (Morse & Field, 1995).

   Initial efforts at analysis focus on reducing the large volume of data acquired to facilitate examination. This may involve "selecting, focusing, simplifying, abstracting, and transforming the data" (Miles & Huberman, 1994, p. 10). During data reduction, the researcher begins to attach meaning to elements of the data; discovers classes of things, persons, events, and properties; and notes regularities in the setting or the people. The researcher then classifies the elements in the data, either by using an established classification system or by developing a new one.

Codes and Coding

Coding is a method of indexing or identifying categories in the data. A code is a symbol or abbreviation used to classify words or phrases in the data. Codes may be placed in the data when they are collected, entered into the computer, or examined at a later time. The purpose of coding is to facilitate the retrieval of data segments by coding category. Used in this manner, coding simplifies and reduces the data (Coffey & Atkinson, 1996; Miles & Huberman, 1994). Coffey and Atkinson (1996) point out that

> …[t]he nature of qualitative data means that data relating to one particular topic are not found neatly bundled together at exactly the same spot in each interview (and field-notes usually have even less predictable organization). The ability to locate stretches of data that, at least ostensibly, are "about" the same thing is a valuable aspect of data management. (p. 35)

Organizing data, selecting specific elements of the data for categories, and naming these categories will reflect the philosophical base of the study. Later in the study, coding may progress to the development of a taxonomy. For example, the researcher may develop a taxonomy of types of pain, types of patients, or types of patient education.

Morse and Field (1995) suggest that when selecting elements of the data to code, the researchers should note the following:

1. the kinds of things that are going on in the context being studied;
2. the forms a phenomenon takes; and
3. any variations within a phenomenon. (pp. 136–137)

Morse and Field suggest several innovative strategies for coding data. One approach is to use highlighter pens, with a different color for each major category. Another strategy, developed by Murdock (1971), is to assign each major category a number, which is inserted in the computerized text. With this approach, a word or phrase in the text could easily have several codes indicated by numbers. Knafl and Webster (1988) suggest using colored markers, paper clips, index cards, or self-adhesive stickers to identify categories of data. Codes often are written in the margins. Then data can be sorted by cutting the pages into sections according to codes. Each section can be taped or pasted onto an index card for filing. This procedure can be performed easily using computer programs for qualitative analysis, in which broad margins are available for coding. Computerized data can be sorted by code into separate files for each code, whereas identifiers such as data and source are retained.

Memoes—Reflective Remarks

While the researcher records notes, other thoughts or insights may emerge into his or her consciousness. These thoughts generally are included in the notes and are separated from the rest of the notes by ((double parentheses)). If needed, they may be extracted and used to construct memos later (Miles & Huberman, 1994).

Marginal Remarks

During review of the recorded notes, the researcher may recognize relationships or other relevant points. Such observations must be written down immediately. These remarks usually are placed in the right-hand margin of the notes. The remarks often connect the notes with other parts of the data or suggest new interpretations. Reviewing notes can become boring, which is a signal that thinking has ceased. Making marginal notes assists the researcher in "retaining a thoughtful stance" (Miles & Huberman, 1994).

Data Displays

One approach to describing qualitative data is use of data displays. Displays are highly condensed and are equivalent to the summary tables of statistical outcomes developed in quantitative research. These data displays allow the researcher to convey succinctly the main ideas of the research. Codes can be used to organize the display. The strategies for achieving displays are limited only by the imagination of the researcher. Displays can be developed relatively easily using computer spreadsheets, graphics programs, or desktop publishing programs. The sourcebook on qualitative analysis by Miles and Huberman (1994) contains additional information on data displays.

Marsh (1990) used a process-oriented matrix to test conclusions and an emergent theory from a qualitative study that examined healthy lifestyle changes. Seven people who had made or were making lifestyle changes were interviewed, with a focus on the process of lifestyle change. Marsh's emergent theory describing the process of lifestyle change is as follows.

An individual, aware of the need and desiring to alter his or her life-style, makes one or more attempts to change over time. The attempts result in relapse. A self-monitoring process mediates between awareness of the individual's need to change and his or her relapses in the process of change. At some point tension mounts over the need to change. This tension, labeled "readiness," is characterized by a combination of personal and environmental variables, such as low self-esteem or support from significant others. Following readiness, the individual experiences a profound self-revelation. The revelation is characterized by a dramatic self-insight, a coming to as if shaken by a new understanding of reality. The revelation is followed by a belief system change about personal power, following which the individual makes and sustains a health life-style change. An individual who experiences no revelation remains in the initial pattern of attempted change and relapse. Revelation appeared to be the emerging core variable of the life-style change process. (p. 45)

To evaluate the trustworthiness of the emergent theory, all of the data were examined for their fit in a matrix. Categories for the matrix were developed and decision rules established for inclusion of data within a category. Every subject was represented in the matrix. When a subject had made more than one lifestyle change, each change was represented separately in the matrix. The matrix is presented in Table 3-1 on pages 84–87.

Text continues on p. 88.

Table 3-1 Process-Oriented Matrix of Lifestyle Changes

Subject No.	Life-style Change	Problem Awareness	Relapse	Readiness	Revelation	Belief-system Change	Behavioral Outcome	Predicted Future Outcome
1	Overeating*	In 8th grade, I was conscious of being overweight. I need to do something for myself	I have no time to care for. I have character defects. I did not want to commit and fail	My husband was supportive. I got a friend to go to a meeting with me. People at group were honest. I want to live. Success of others in group was inspirational	I can use my power along with God's power to conquer the demon, overeating	I have strength in working with God; this gives me power, and I can use it	60-lb weight loss sustained for 4.5 months, confident of continued success	Will sustain
2	Overeating*	I feel uncomfortable and short of breath	I tried all new diets. My spouse supported my failure, both have poor will power	I got help from spouse. I got help from group	I realized, if that woman can do it, so can I	I no longer need to eat to be happy	75-lb weight loss sustained over 1 year	Will sustain
	Alcohol	None	None	I got support from spouse. I have low self-esteem. I got group support—I went willingly, with no expectations	It suddenly hit: "I didn't like me anymore"	I have personal power. I find support in group	Alcohol abstinence	Will sustain
	Smoking	I have a bad cough	I made two failed attempts	My father's health was bad. I had a bad cough. I really wanted to quit	None	I can do it by myself (strength from alcohol problem)	Sustained smoking cessation for several years	Will sustain

Table 3-1 Process-Oriented Matrix of Lifestyle Changes *(continued)*

Subject No.	Life-style Change	Problem Awareness	Relapse	Readiness	Revelation	Belief-system Change	Behavioral Outcome	Predicted Future Outcome
3	Overeating*	Eating is a sin I love it, I hate it At a group I was obsessive/compulsive over food	I had many, many failures Food controls me. I have little control I tried groups; I like the support but cannot keep with it	I have low self-esteem I am concerned for my child Group gives me hope and strength I have been depressed, I hate my life When I am depressed, I am okay; everything else is	None	None	Repeated relapses	Escalation of readiness
4	Overeating*	I was a fat slob and an introvert since I was a small child	I wanted a magic cure with no responsibility	I felt depressed and suicidal I have low life satisfaction I am a miserable, hurting person not in touch with self I have low self-esteem I joined group from fear of death I felt group inspiration, I am not alone	I realized I can control my life and it is okay to seek guidance from others "All of a sudden, everything was pulled together"	Asked my higher power for strength and help (higher power–God–inner self) Food controlled me; now I can control it; I am proud of me	Sustained 65-lb loss for 8 months Still needs group support, seeks reinforcement from others	Success if group support continued

(continues)

Table 3-1 Process-Oriented Matrix of Lifestyle Changes *(continued)*

Subject No.	Life-style Change	Problem Awareness	Relapse	Readiness	Revelation	Belief-system Change	Behavioral Outcome	Predicted Future Outcome
5	Smoking*	I was tired of it It was a hassle	I have no one to share the problem with, no pats on back, no group support I am a failure	I am joining groups to meet people in similar situation	None	None	Never received the group support I sought Another relapse	Success with right group
	Alcohol	I was sneaking I was hiding problem from family	None	I feel concern and love from little sister	I was shaken by my little sister's concern I suddenly knew I needed help	I want help at any cost Group support will help; joined group 3–4 years ago I am making written commitment	Reformed alcoholic, no backsliding, 3 years of sustained change	Will sustain
6	Smoking*	I was thinking about change I feel scared, angry I need a focus My body and health are changing It is filthy I am ambivalent	I made it convenient I quit in past, started again I want others to help	I am grasping a focus, letting others know; once you start, you need to keep going	None	None	Smoking cessation for 4 day Has not told family or friends, is afraid of failure	Relapse

Table 3-1 Process-Oriented Matrix of Lifestyle Changes *(continued)*

Subject No.	Life-style Change	Problem Awareness	Relapse	Readiness	Revelation	Belief-system Change	Behavioral Outcome	Predicted Future Outcome
7	Smoking*	It is expensive It is filthy I risk getting cancer of the mouth	I have made many attempts I am angry I do not want to give it up	I want group help Support of my son helps I am concerned for effect of my smoking on my grand-daughter and son	None	None	Relapse	Continued relapse
	Alcohol	I was hiding bottles I was a closet drinker	I tried quitting for 6 years I only have myself to blame	I have low self-esteem	I realized no one could do it for me; I could do it by myself	I am the only one who can do anything about it	Alcohol abstinence 6 years	Will sustain

*Change currently being made.

Reprinted from *Advances in Nursing Science, 12(3),* 51–52, with permission of Aspen Publishers, Inc. ©1990.

Counting

Qualitative researchers tend to avoid the use of numbers. However, when judgments of qualities are made, counting occurs. In describing a pattern, the researcher may observe that a particular pattern occurs frequently or more often. Something is considered important or significant. These judgments are made in part by counting. If counting will be part of the data analysis, the researcher needs to recognize and plan for this aspect of the process. Counting can help researchers to see what data they have, to verify a hypothesis, and to remain intellectually honest. Qualitative researchers work by insight and intuition; however, their conclusions can be wrong. It is easier to see confirming evidence than disconfirming evidence. Comparing insights by using numbers can be a good method of verification (Miles & Huberman, 1994).

Analysis

Analysis goes beyond description and uses specific methods to transform the data. Through this process, the researcher extends the data beyond the description. Using analysis, he or she identifies essential features and describes interrelationships among them (Wolcott, 1994). During analysis, the emphasis is on identifying themes and patterns in the data. Coding, used earlier for description, also can be used to expand, transform, and reconceptualize data, thus providing opportunities for more diverse analyses. Coffey and Atkinson (1996) suggest that by "reading through data extracts, one might discover particular events, key words, processes, or characters that capture the essence of a piece" (p. 31).

Memos

Memos are used to record insights or ideas related to notes, transcripts, or codes. Memos move the researcher toward theorizing and deal with conceptual rather than factual material. They may link pieces of data or use a specific piece of data as an example of a concept. The memo may be written to someone else involved in the study or to yourself. It is important to value these insights and write them down quickly. Whenever an idea emerges, even if it is vague and not well thought out, write it down immediately. Although you might think that the idea is so clear in your mind that it can be written later, such thoughts often are soon forgotten and cannot be retrieved. Memos need to be dated, titled according to their key concept, and connected by codes to the field notes or forms that generated the thoughts (Miles & Huberman, 1994).

Storytelling

During observation and interviewing the researcher may record stories shared by participants. Banks-Wallace (1998) describes a story as "an event or series of events, encompassed by temporal or spatial boundaries that are shared with others using an oral medium or sign language." **Storytelling** is the process or interaction used to share stories. People sharing a story (storytellers) and those listening to a story (**storytakers**) constitute the main elements of the storytelling process (Banks-Wallace, 1998, p. 17). Stories can promote understanding of a notable phenomenon. In some qualitative studies, the research may focus on gathering stories. Frank (2000) describes gathering narratives about illnesses. Gathering stories enables health care providers to develop storytelling as a powerful means to increase insight and to facilitate healthy behaviors of clients. For example, Nwoga (1997) studied how African American mothers use storytelling to educate their adolescent daughters about their sexuality. The stories used by these mothers, captured by Nwoga, could be useful in assisting other mothers struggling to help their daughters deal with sexuality issues.

Coffey and Atkinson (1996) discuss the importance of capturing stories in qualitative studies.

> The story is an obvious way for social actors, in talking to strangers (e.g., the researcher), to retell key experiences and events. Stories serve a variety of functions. Social actors often remember and order their careers or memories as a series of narrative chronicles, that is, as [a] series of stories marked by key happenings. Similarly, stories and legends are told and retold by members of particular social groups or organizations as a way of passing on a cultural heritage or an organizational culture. Tales of success or tales of key leaders/personalities are familiar genres with which to maintain a collective sense of the culture of an organization. The use of atrocity stories and morality fables is also well documented within organizational and occupational settings. Stories of medical settings are especially well documented (Atkinson, 1992; Dingwall, 1977). Here tales of professional incompetence are used to give warning of "what not to do" and what will happen if you commit mistakes.... Narratives are also a common genre from which to retell or come to terms with particularly sensitive or traumatic times and events. (p. 56). Sandelowski (1994) describes methods of analyzing stories in an article intriguingly titled "We are the stories we tell."

Narrative analysis is a qualitative means of formally analyzing stories. Using this method, the researcher "unpacks" the structure of the story. A story includes a sequence of events with a beginning, a middle, and an end. Stories have their own logic and are temporal in character (Coffey & Atkinson, 1996; Denzin, 1989). The structure also can be used to determine how people tell stories, how they shape the events they describe, how they make a point, how they "package" events and react to them, and how they communicate their stories to audiences. The structure used for narrative analysis as identified by Coffey and Atkinson (1996, p. 58) is as follows:

Structure	Question
Abstract	What is this about?
Orientation	Who? What? When? Where?
Complication	Then what happened?
Evaluation	So what?
Result	What finally happened?
Coda	Finish narrative

The abstract initiates the narrative by summarizing the point of the story or stating the proposition the narrative will illustrate. The orientation provides an introduction to the major events central to the story. The complication continues the narrative, describing complications in the event that makes it a story. Evaluation is the point of the narrative, followed by the result, which gives the outcome or resolution of events. The coda ends the story and provides a transition to other topics.

The narrative analysis can focus on social action embedded in the text or can examine the effect of the story. Stories serve a purpose. They may make a point or be moralistic.

They may be success stories, or may be a reminder of what not to do or how not to be, with guidance about how to avoid the fate described in the story. The purpose of the story can be the starting point for a more extensive narrative analysis. Narrative analysis may examine multiple accounts of key life events, leading to greater understanding of the impact of these events; it may assist in understanding the relationship between social processes and personal lives; or it may be used to elucidate cultural values, meanings, and personal experiences. Issues related to power, dominance, and opposition can be examined. Through stories, silenced groups can be given voice (Coffey & Atkinson, 1996). Poirier and Ayres (1997) use overreading as a method of analyzing narratives.

Coding is not used commonly in narrative analysis. Coding breaks data up into separate segments and is not useful in analyzing a story. The researcher can lose the sense that informants are providing an account or a narrative of events. However, Ayers, Kavanaugh and Knafl (2003) describe methods for using coding during narrative analysis.

Qualitative researchers may choose to communicate the findings of their study as a story. A story can be a powerful way to make a point. A story can be presented from a variety of perspectives: following chronological order, following the order in which the story was originally presented, focusing on progressive issues, focusing on only a critical or key event in the story, describing the plot and characters as one would stage a play, following an analytical framework, providing versions of an event from the stories of several viewers, or presenting the story as one would write a mystery story, thus appealing to problem solvers.

Interpretation

During interpretation, the researcher offers an interpretation of what is going on. The focus is on understanding and explaining findings beyond what can be stated with certainty (Coffey & Atkinson, 1996; Wolcott, 1994). Interpretation may focus on the usefulness of the findings for clinical practice or may move toward theorizing.

As the study progresses, relationships among categories, participants, actions, and events begin to emerge. The researcher will develop hunches about relationships that can be used to formulate tentative propositions. Statements or propositions can be written on index cards and sorted into categories or entered into the computer (Miles & Huberman, 1994).

Using information in the matrix in Table 3-1, Marsh (1990) made the following interpretations:

Subjects 1, 2, and 4 experienced revelation related to overeating, followed by a belief-system change. Each of these individuals had lost 60 to 75 pounds and had maintained the weight loss for 4.5 months to 1 year. Subject 3 experienced no revelation and had no success in weight loss. The matrix revealed patterns in the data that might have been overlooked. (p. 45)

For example, Marsh assumed that the "belief-system change" that occurred was a change in health beliefs. The matrix illustrated that the change was rather one of personal empowerment and involved beliefs about self, not about health.

As the data are collected and analyzed, the researcher gains increasing understanding of the dynamics in the process under study. This understanding might be considered a tentative theory. The first tentative theories often are vague and pieced together poorly; some are wrong. The best way to verify a tentative theory is to share it with others, particularly informants in the study situations. Informants have their own tentative theories that have never been clearly expressed. The tentative theory needs to be expressed as a map. Developing a good map of the tentative theory is difficult and requires some hard work.

The validity of predictions developed in a tentative theory must be tested; however, finding effective ways to test them is difficult. Predictions usually are developed near the end of the study. Because the findings often are context-specific, the predictions must be tested on the same or a similar sample. One strategy suggested is to predict outcomes expected at 6 months after the study. Six months later, these predictions can be sent to informants who participated in the study. The informants can be asked to respond to the accuracy of (1) the predictions and (2) the explanation of why the predicted events were expected to occur (Miles & Huberman, 1994).

People may easily identify patterns and themes from their observations. It often is difficult to find *real* additional evidence of a pattern while remaining open to disconfirming evidence. Any identified pattern should be subject to skepticism by the researcher and others (Miles & Huberman, 1994). Morse and Field (1995) state the following:

> The researcher must distinguish between representative cases and anecdotal cases. Representative cases appear with regularity and encompass the range of behaviors described within a category. The anecdotal case appears infrequently and depicts a small range of events that are atypical of the larger group.... Negative cases are those episodes that clearly refute an emergent theory or proposition. Negative cases are important because they help to clarify additional causal properties that influence the phenomena under study (Denzin, 1978). (p. 139)

Often during analysis, a conclusion seems plausible. It seems to fit; it makes good sense. When asked how he or she arrived at that point, the researcher may state that it "just feels right." These intuitive feelings are important in both qualitative and quantitative research. However, plausibility cannot stand alone. After plausibility must come systematic analysis. First, intuition yields insight; then careful examination of the data is done to verify the validity of that insight (Miles & Huberman, 1994).

Rigor in Qualitative Research

Scientific **rigor** is valued because it is associated with greater worth of research outcomes, and studies are critiqued as a means of judging rigor. Rigor is defined differently for qualitative research because the desired outcome is different from that in quantitative research (Burns, 1989; Dzurec, 1989; Morse, 1989; Sandelowski, 1986, 1993). In qualitative research, rigor is associated with openness, scrupulous adherence to a philosophical perspective, thoroughness in collecting data, and consideration of all of the data in the subjective theory development phase. Evaluation of the rigor of a qualitative study is based in part on the logic of the emerging theory and the clarity with which it sheds light on the studied phenomenon.

KEY CONCEPTS

- Qualitative research focuses on understanding the whole, which is consistent with the holistic philosophy of nursing. The qualitative approaches are based on a worldview that has the following beliefs: (1) there is not a single reality and (2) the meaning of what we know is defined by the situation or context.
- Each type of qualitative research is guided by a particular philosophy.
- Four common approaches to qualitative research used in nursing are presented in this chapter: phenomenological, grounded theory, ethnographic, and historical.
- Subjects in qualitative studies are referred to as participants.
- The relationship between the researcher and the individuals being studied is one of colleagues. The effectiveness of this relationship has an impact on the collection and interpretation of data.
- The most common data collection methods used in qualitative studies are observation, interviewing, and examination of textual data.
- Qualitative data analysis occurs concurrently with data collection, rather than sequentially as in quantitative research. Therefore, the researcher is attempting to simultaneously gather, manage, and interpret data.
- Qualitative data analysis occurs in three stages: description, analysis, and interpretation.
- In the initial phases of a qualitative study, the researcher needs to become familiar with the data. This may involve reading and rereading notes and transcripts, recalling observation and experiences, listening to audiotapes, and viewing videotapes, until the researcher becomes immersed in the data.
- During data analysis, a dynamic interaction occurs between the researcher's self and the data, whether the data are communicated orally or in writing. During this process, referred to as reflexive thought, the researcher explores personal feelings and experiences that may influence the study and integrates this understanding into the study. The process requires a conscious awareness of self.

TIPS FOR FURTHER STUDY

- If you have difficulty differentiating phenomenology from grounded theory, try the Review Questions on the CD-ROM included with this text and the Bonus Review Questions found at http://evolve.elsevier.com/Burns/understanding.
- For practice comparing and contrasting the research processes used in phenomenological, grounded theory, ethnographic, and historical research; see Chapter 3 of your *Study Guide*.
- For additional qualitative studies to examine, see your Evolve Learning Resources website.

REFERENCES

Anderson, J. M. (1989). The phenomenological perspective. In J. M. Morse (Ed.), *Qualitative nursing research: A contemporary dialogue* (pp. 15–26). Rockville, MD: Aspen.

Artinian, B. A. (1988). Qualitative modes of inquiry. *Western Journal of Nursing Research, 10*(2), 138–149.

Atkinson, P. (1992). The ethnography of a medical setting: Reading, writing and rhetoric. *Qualitative Health Research, 2*(4), 451–474.

Ayres, L., & Poirier, S. (1996). Focus on qualitative methods: Virtual text and the growth of meaning in qualitative research. *Research in Nursing & Health, 19*(2), 163–169.

Ayres, L., Kavanaugh, K., & Knafl, K. A. (2003). Within-case and across-case approaches to qualitative data analysis. *Qualitative Health Research 13*(6), 871.

Baillie, L. (1995). Ethnography and nursing research: A critical appraisal. *Nurse Researcher, 3*(2), 5–21.

Baker, H. M. (1997). Rules outside the rules for administration of medication: A study in New South Wales, Australia. *Image—The Journal of Nursing Scholarship, 29*(2), 155–158.

Banks-Wallace, J. (1998). Emancipatory potential of storytelling in a group. *Image—The Journal of Nursing Scholarship, 30*(1), 17–21.

Barker, K., & McConnell, W. (1962). The problems of detecting medication errors in hospitals. *American Journal of Hospital Pharmacy, 19*(8), 360–369.

Barkway, P. (2001). Michael Crotty and nursing phenomenology: Criticism or critique. *Nursing Inquiry, 8*(3), 191–195.

Baumrind, D. (1980). New directions in socialization research. *American Psychologist, 35*(7), 639–652.

Beck, C. T. (1994). Phenomenology: Its use in nursing research. *International Journal of Nursing Studies, 31*(6), 499–510.

Benner, P. (1984). *From novice to expert: Excellence and power in clinical nursing practice.* Menlo Park, CA: Addison-Wesley.

Boyd, C. O. (2001a). Philosophical foundation of qualitative research. In P.L. Munhall (Ed.), *Nursing research: A qualitative perspective* (pp. 65-98). Boston: Jones & Bartlett.

Boyd, C. O. (2001b). Phenomenology: The method. In P. L. Munhall (Ed.), *Nursing research: A qualitative perspective* (pp. 93–122). Boston: Jones & Bartlett.

Burns, N. (1989). Standards for qualitative research. *Nursing Science Quarterly, 2*(1), 44–52.

Byrne, M. (2001). Hermeneutics as a methodology for textual analysis, *AORN Journal, 73*(5), 968–970.

Caelli,K. (2003). The changing face of phenomenological research: Traditional and American phenology in nursing, *Qualitative Health Research, 10*(3), 366–377.

Ceci, C. (2003). Midnight reckonings: on a question of knowledge and nursing. *Nursing Philosophy, 4*(1), 61–76.

Cesario, S., Morin, K., & Santa-Donato, A. (2002). Evaluating the level of evidence of qualitative research.

Journal of Obstetrics and Gynecologic Neonatal Nursing, 31(6), 708–714.

Chenitz, W. C., & Swanson, J. M. (1986). Qualitative research using grounded theory. In W. C. Chenitz & J. M. Swanson (Eds.), *From practice to grounded theory: Qualitative research in nursing* (pp. 3–5). Menlo Park, CA: Addison-Wesley.

Christy, T. E. (1975). The methodology of historical research: A brief introduction. *Nursing Research, 24*(3), 189–192.

Christy, T. E. (1978). The hope of history. In M. L. Fitzpatrick (Ed.), *Historical studies in nursing* (pp. 3–11). New York: Teachers College Press.

Coffey, A., & Atkinson, P. (1996). *Making sense of qualitative data.* Thousand Oaks, CA: Sage.

Crotty, M. (1996). *Phenomenology and nursing research.* South Melbourne, Aus: Churchill Livingstone.

Darbyshire P., Diekelmann J., Diekelmann N. (1999). Reading Heidegger and interpretive phenomenology. A response to the work of Michael Crotty. *Nursing Inquiry, 6*(1), 17–25.

Denzin, N. K. (1978). *Sociological methods: A sourcebook* (2nd ed.). New York: McGraw-Hill.

Denzin, N. K. (1989). *Interpretive interactionism.* Newbury Park, CA: Sage.

Dingwall, R. (1977). Atrocity stories and professional relationships. *Sociology of Work and Occupations, 4*(4), 371–396.

Drew, N. (1989). The interviewer's experience as data in phenomenological research. *Western Journal of Nursing Research, 11*(4), 431–439.

Dreyfus, H., & Dreyfus, S. (1982). *Mind Over Machine. The power of human intuition and expertise in the era of the computer.* New York: Free Press.

Dzurec, L. C. (1989). The necessity for and evolution of multiple paradigms for nursing research: a poststructuralist perspective. *Advances in Nursing Science, 11*(4), 69–77.

Evans, J. C. (1978). Formulating an idea. In M. L. Fitzpatrick (Ed.), *Historical studies in nursing* (pp. 15–17). New York: Teachers College Press.

Fagerhaugh, S., & Strauss, A. (1977). *Politics of pain management: Staff-patient interaction.* Menlo Park, CA: Addison-Wesley.

Finch, L. P. (2004). Understanding patients' lived experiences: The interrelationship of rhetoric and hermeneutics. *Nursing Philosophy, 5*(3), 251–257.

Fleming, V., Gaidys, U., & Robb, Y. (2003). Hermeneutic research in nursing: developing a Gadamerian-based research method. *Nursing Inquiry, 10*(2), 113–120.

Frances, G. (1980). Nurses medication errors: A new perspective. *Supervisor Nurse, 11*(3), 11–13.

Frank, A. W. (2000). The standpoint of storyteller. *Qualitative Health Research, 10*(3), 354–365.

Geanellos, R. (2000). Exploring Ricoeur's hermeneutic theory of interpretation as a method of analyzing research texts. *Nursing Inquiry, 7*(2), 112.

Germain, C. P., & Munhall, P. L. (2001). Ethnography: the method, In P.L. Munhall (Ed.), *Nursing Research: A qualitative perspective* (pp. 277–306). Boston: Jones and Bartlett.

Giorgi, A (2000). The status of Husserlian phenomenology in caring research. *Scandinavian Journal of Caring Sciences. 14*(1), 3–10.

Glaser, B. G., & Strauss, A. (1971). *Status passage*. London: Routledge & Kegan Paul.

Glaser, B. G., & Strauss, A. (1965). *Awareness of dying*. Chicago: Aldine.

Glaser, B. G., & Strauss, A. (1967). *The discovery of grounded theory: Strategies for qualitative research*. Chicago: Aldine.

Glaser, B. G., & Strauss, A. (1968). *Time for dying*. Chicago: Aldine.

Glasser, B. G. (1973). *Ward 402*. New York: George Braziller.

Grant, M. J. (2004). How does your searching grow? A survey of search preferences and the use of optimal search strategies in the identification of qualitative research. *Health Information and Libraries Journal, 21*(1), 21–32.

Green, J., & Britten, N. (1998). Qualitative research and evidence based medicine. *British Medical Journal (International), 316*(7139), 1230–1232.

Hawker, S., Payne, S., Kerr, C., Hardey, M., & Powell, J. (2002). Appraising the evidence: Reviewing disparate data systematically. *Qualitative Health Research, 12*(9), 1284–1299.

Heller, A. (1982). *A theory of history*. London: Routledge & Kegan Paul.

Johnson, M. E. (2000). Heidegger and meaning: implications for phenomenological research, *Nursing Philosophy, 1*(2), 134–146.

Kaplan, A. (1964). *The conduct of inquiry: Methodology for behavioral science*. New York: Chandler.

Knafl, K. A., & Webster, D. C. (1988). Managing and analyzing qualitative data: A description of tasks, techniques, and materials. *Western Journal of Nursing Research, 10*(2), 195–218.

Kübler-Ross, E. (1969). *On death and dying*. New York: Macmillan.

Kvigne, K., Gjengedal, E., & Kirkevold, M. (2002). Gaining access to the life-world of women suffering from stroke: Methodological issues in empirical phenomenological studies. *Journal of Advanced Nursing, 40*(1), 61–68.

Leininger, M. M. (1970). *Nursing and anthropology: Two worlds to blend*. New York: Wiley.

Leininger, M. M. (1985). *Qualitative research methods in nursing*. Orlando, FL: Grune & Stratton.

Leonard, V. W. (1989). A Heideggerian phenomenologic perspective on the concept of the person. *Advances in Nursing Science, 11*(4), 40–55.

Lincoln, Y. S., & Guba, E. G. (1985). *Naturalistic Inquiry*. Beverly Hills, CA: Sage.

Lusk, B. (1997). Historical methodology for nursing research. *Image—The Journal of Nursing Scholarship, 29*(4), 355–359.

Marsh, G. W. (1990). Refining an emergent life-style-change theory through matrix analysis. *Advances in Nursing Science, 12*(3), 41–52.

Mead, G. H. (1934). *Mind, self and society*. Chicago: University of Chicago Press.

Miles, M. B., & Huberman, A. M. (1994). *Qualitative data analysis: An expanded sourcebook* (2nd ed.). Thousand Oaks, CA: Sage.

Mitchell, G. J. (2004). An emerging framework for human becoming criticism. *Nursing Science Quarterly, 17*(2), 103–109.

Morse, J. M. (1989). Qualitative nursing research: A free-for-all? In J. M. Morse (Ed.), *Qualitative nursing research: A contemporary dialogue* (pp. 14–22). Rockville, MD: Aspen.

Morse, J. M., & Field, P. A. (1995). *Qualitative research methods for health professionals* (2nd ed.). Thousand Oaks, CA: Sage.

Munhall, P. L. (1989). Philosophical ponderings on qualitative research methods in nursing. *Nursing Science Quarterly, 2*(1), 20–28.

Munhall, P. L. (Ed.). (2001). *Nursing research: A qualitative perspective*. Boston: Jones and Bartlett.

Murdock, G. (1971). *Outline of cultural materials*. New Haven, CT: Human Relations Area Files Press.

Newton, M. E. (1965). The case for historical research. *Nursing Research, 14*(1), 20–26.

Nwoga, I. (1997). *Mother-daughter conversations related to sex-role socialization and adolescent pregnancy*. Ph.D. dissertation, The University of Florida.

Oiler, C. (1982). The phenomenological approach in nursing research. *Nursing Research, 31*(3), 178–181.

Omery, A. (1983). Phenomenology: A method for nursing research. *Advances in Nursing Science, 5*(2), 49–63.

Parse, R. R. (1981). *Man-living-health: A theory of nursing*. New York: Wiley.

Patterson, J. G., & Zderad, L. T. (1976). *Humanistic nursing*. New York: Wiley.

Popay, J., Rogers, A., & Williams, G. (1998). Rationale and standards for the systematic review of qualitative literature in health services research. *Qualitative Health Research, 8*(3), 341–351.

Poirier, S., & Ayres, L. (1997). Endings, secrets, and silences: Overreading in narrative inquiry. *Research in Nursing & Health, 20*(6), 551–557.

Sadala, M. L., & Adorno, Role C. (2002). Phenomenology as a method to investigate the experience lived: A perspective from Husserl and Merleau Polty's thought. *Journal of Advanced Nursing, 37*(3), 282–293.

Salsberry, P. J., Smith, M. C., & Boyd, C. O. (1989). Dialogue on a research issue: Phenomenological research in nursing commentary and responses. *Nursing Science Quarterly, 2*(1), 9–19.

Sandelowski, M. (1986). The problem of rigor in qualitative research. *Advances in Nursing Science, 8*(3), 27–37.

Sandelowski, M. (1993). Rigor or rigor mortis: the problem of rigor in qualitative research revisited. *Advances in Nursing Science, 16*(2), 1–8.

Sandelowski, M. (1994). We are the stories we tell: narrative knowing in nursing practice. *Journal of Holistic Nursing, 12*(1), 23–33.

Sandelowski, M. (1995). Sample size in qualitative research. *Research in Nursing & Health, 18*(2), 179–183.

Sandelowski, M. (1996). One is the liveliest number: The case orientation of qualitative research. *Research in Nursing & Health, 19*(6), 525–529.

Sarnecky, M. T. (1990). Historiography: A legitimate research methodology for nursing. *Advances in Nursing Science, 12*(4), 1–10.

Scheffler, I. (1967). *Science & subjectivity.* Indianapolis: Bobbs-Merrill.

Schwartz-Barcott, D., & Kim, H. S. (1986). A hybrid model for concept development. In P. L. Chinn (Ed.), *Nursing research methodology: Issues and implementation* (pp. 91–101). Rockville, MD: Aspen.

Silva, M. C., & Rothbart, D. (1984). An analysis of changing trends in philosophies of science on nursing theory development and testing. *Advances in Nursing Science, 6*(2), 1–13.

Silverman, D. (1993). *Interpreting qualitative data: Methods for analyzing talk, text and interaction.* Thousand Oaks, CA: Sage.

Strauss, A. L. (1975). *Chronic illness and the quality of life.* St. Louis: Mosby.

Strauss, A. L., Corbin, J., Fagerhaugh, S., Glaser, B. G., Maines, D., Suczek, B., et al. (1984). *Chronic illness and the quality of life* (2nd ed.). St. Louis: Mosby.

Strauss, A.L., & Glaser, B. G. (1970). *Anguish.* Mill Valley, CA: Sociology Press.

Walters, A. J. (1995). The phenomenological movement: implications for nursing research, *Journal of Advanced Nursing, 22*(4), 791–799.

Waring, L. M. (1978). Developing the research prospectus. In M. L. Fitzpatrick (Ed.), *Historical studies in nursing* (pp. 18–20). New York: Teachers College Press.

Watson, J. (1985). *Nursing: Human science and human care: A theory of nursing.* Norwalk, CT: Appleton-Century-Crofts.

Whittemore, R. (2005). Combining evidence in nursing research: Methods and implications. *Nursing Research, 54*(1), 56–62.

Wimpenny, P., & Gass, J. (2000). Interviewing in phenomenology and grounded theory: Is there a difference? *Journal of Advanced Nursing, 31*(6), 1485–1492.

Wolcott, H. F. (1994). *Transforming qualitative data: Description, analysis, and interpretation.* Thousand Oaks, CA: Sage.

4

CHAPTER

Research Problems, Purposes, and Hypotheses

Chapter Overview

Learning Outcomes

After completing this chapter, you should be able to:

1. Identify research topics, problems, and purposes in published quantitative, qualitative, and outcomes studies.
2. Critique the significance of research problems and purposes in published studies.
3. Critique the feasibility of a study problem and purpose by examining the researcher's expertise; money commitment; availability of subjects, facilities, and equipment; and the study's ethical considerations.
4. Differentiate among the types of hypotheses (simple versus complex, nondirectional versus

directional, associative versus causal, and statistical versus research) in published studies.
5. Critique the quality of objectives, questions, and hypotheses presented in published studies.
6. Differentiate the types of variables in published studies.
7. Critique the conceptual and operational definitions of variables in published studies.

Key Terms

Conceptual definition, p. 128
Hypothesis, p. 118
  Associative hypothesis,
    p. 118
  Causal hypothesis, p. 120
  Complex hypothesis,
    p. 121
  Directional hypothesis,
    p. 123
  Nondirectional hypothesis,
    p. 122
  Null (statistical)
    hypothesis, p. 123
  Research hypothesis,
    p. 124

Simple hypothesis, p. 121
  Testable hypothesis,
    p. 124
Operational definition, p. 129
Problem statement, p. 99
Research objective, p. 112
Research problem, p. 98
Research purpose, p. 99
Research question, p. 115
Research topic, p. 97
Sample characteristics,
  p. 127
Variables, p. 125
  Confounding variables,
    p. 127

Demographic variables,
  p. 127
Dependent (response or
  outcome) variable,
  p. 126
Environmental variables,
  p. 127
Extraneous variables,
  p. 126
Independent (treatment or
  experimental) variable,
  p. 126
Research variables or
  concepts, p. 126

STUDY TOOLS

Be sure to visit http://evolve.elsevier.com/Burns/understanding/ for additional examples and self-tests. Also, a review of this chapter's concepts and practice exercises can be found in Chapter 4 of the Study Guide for *Understanding Nursing Research: Building an Evidence-Based Practice*, 4th edition.

We are constantly asking questions to gain a better understanding of ourselves and the world around us. This human ability to wonder and ask creative questions is the first step in the research process. By asking questions, clinical nurses and nurse researchers are able to identify significant research topics and problems that will generate research findings that can ultimately be used to make evidence-based changes in practice. A **research topic** is a concept or broad issue that is important to nursing, such as acute and chronic pain management, coping with illness, or health promotion. Each topic contains numerous potential research problems to guide quantitative, qualitative, and outcomes studies. For example, chronic pain management is a research topic that includes such potential problems as "What is chronic pain?" and "What is it like to live with chronic pain?" Qualitative research might be used to investigate these problems or areas of concern in nursing. Quantitative research might be used to study such problems as "How can chronic pain be accurately assessed?" and "What are effective interventions for managing chronic pain?" Outcomes research methodologies might be used to examine patient outcomes and the cost-effectiveness of care provided in a chronic pain management clinic.

The problem or area of concern provides the basis for developing the research purpose. The purpose or goal of a study guides the development of the objectives, questions, or hypotheses. The objectives, questions, or hypotheses bridge the gap between the more abstractly stated problem and purpose and the detailed design for conducting the study. Objectives, questions, and hypotheses include the variables, the relationships among the variables, and often the population to be studied.

This chapter includes content that will assist you in differentiating a problem from a purpose and critiquing the problems and purposes in published quantitative, qualitative, and outcomes studies. Objectives, questions, and hypotheses are discussed, and the different types of study variables are introduced. Also presented are guidelines that will assist you in critiquing the problems, purposes, objectives, questions, hypotheses, and variables in published quantitative, qualitative, and outcomes studies.

What Are Research Problems and Purposes?

A **research problem** is an area of concern where there is a gap in the knowledge base needed for nursing practice. Research is required to generate essential knowledge to address the practice concern, with the ultimate goal of providing evidence-based nursing care (Brown, 1999; Melnyk & Fineout-Overholt, 2005). In a published study, the research problem (1) identifies an area of concern for a particular population, (2) indicates the significance of the problem, (3) provides a background for the problem, and (4) outlines the need for additional study in a problem statement. Not all published studies include a clearly expressed problem, but the problem usually can be identified in the first or second paragraph of the article. The research problem from Wynd's (2005) study of the effect of guided health imagery on smoking cessation and long-term abstinence in adult smokers is presented as an example.

RESEARCH EXAMPLE   Problem and Purpose

Problem Significance

Despite a steady decline in cigarette smoking in the United States, 22% of the adults continue to smoke (Centers for Disease Control [and Prevention], 2005). A major priority for national health promotion activities is to reduce cigarette smoking prevalence to no more than 12% of all adults by the year 2010 (U.S. Department of Health and Human Services [USDHHS], 2000) (Wynd, 2005, p. 245).

Problem Background

Guided imagery has been clinically investigated with successful results for symptom management in patients undergoing surgery (Cupal & Brewer, 2001)...and experiencing chronic pain (Lewandowski, 2004).... Imagery was also used with women who experienced rape and other types of sexual assault to reevaluate and restructure traumatic situations into new and more positive images.... Short, Hall, Engel, and Nigg (2004) investigated the use of exercise imagery in 497 college students. Imagery was used to stimulate motivation to exercise, and the students imagined the actual exercise they wanted to accomplish (Wynd, 2005, p. 245).

Problem Statement

Although many people have suggested imagery as a clinical application for smoking cessation, little empirical research has been reported.... Additional studies are indicated to evaluate well-defined imagery interventions with longer follow-up periods (Wynd, 2005, p. 246).

Research Purpose

The study purpose was "to examine the effectiveness of guided health imagery for immediate smoking cessation and long-term abstinence in adult smokers" (Wynd, 2005, p. 245).

CRITIQUE

Research Problem

Wynd's (2005) study presents a clear, concise research problem that includes an area of concern and the following parts of a problem: (1) significance, (2) background, and (3) problem statement. In this example, the first paragraph clearly identifies the area of concern (prevalence of smoking) for a particular population (adult smokers). The prevalence of smoking in adults is a significant problem, because 22% are still smoking and smoking cessation is a federal priority identified in *Healthy People 2010* (USDHHS, 2000). The second paragraph provides a concise background regarding the effectiveness of guided imagery as a treatment for a variety of health care problems. The discussion of the problem concludes with a concise problem statement that indicates the gap in the knowledge needed for practice and provides a basis for the study conducted by Wynd.

This example research problem includes concepts such as cigarette smoking, imagery interventions, smoking cessation and abstinence, and health promotion. A variety of nursing interventions could be implemented to determine their effects on cigarette smoking. Thus, each problem provides the basis for generating a variety of research purposes. In this study, the knowledge gap regarding the effects of guided health imagery on smoking cessation and long-term abstinence provides clear direction for the formulation of the research purpose.

Research Purpose

The research purpose is a clear, concise statement of the specific aim or goal of a study. The goal of a study might be to identify, describe, or explain a situation or predict a solution to a problem. The purpose also includes the variables, the population, and often the setting for the study. A clearly stated research purpose can capture the essence of a study in a single sentence and is essential for directing the remaining steps of the research process (Creswell, 1994).

In a published study, the purpose often is presented after the problem or the literature review. In addition, the purpose frequently is reflected in the title of the study and is the first line of the study abstract. Wynd (2005) identified the purpose of her study in the article title and abstract and then after a discussion of the problem significance. The goal of this quasi-experimental study was to examine the effect of the nursing intervention guided health imagery (independent variable) on smoking cessation and long-term abstinence (dependent variables). The purpose was clearly stated and indicated the type of study conducted and included the study variables and population.

IMPLICATIONS FOR PRACTICE

The findings from Wynd's (2005) study indicated that at 24 months after the guided health imagery intervention, the smoking abstinence rates were significantly higher for the treatment group, at 26% abstinence, than for the placebo group, at 12% abstinence. Thus, Wynd concluded that guided health imagery is an effective intervention for the management of long-term smoking cessation and abstinence in adult smokers. Additional research is needed to determine if this intervention is effective with other adult smokers and can be used to manage cigarette smoking in practice.

Identifying the Problem and Purpose in Quantitative, Qualitative, and Outcomes Studies

Quantitative, qualitative, and outcomes research approaches enable nurses to investigate a variety of research problems and purposes. Examples of research topics, problems, and purposes for different types of quantitative, qualitative, and outcomes studies are presented in this section.

Problems and Purposes in Types of Quantitative Studies

Example research topics, problems, and purposes for the different types of quantitative research (descriptive, correlational, quasi-experimental, and experimental) are presented in Table 4-1. If little is known about a topic, the researcher usually starts with a descriptive study and progresses to quasi-experimental and experimental studies. An examination of the problems and purposes in Table 4-1 will reveal the differences and similarities among the types of quantitative research. The research purpose usually reflects the type of study that was conducted. The purpose of descriptive research is to identify and describe concepts or variables, identify possible relationships among variables, and delineate differences between or among groups.

Rambur, McIntosh, Val Palumbo, and Reinier (2005) conducted a descriptive study to compare job satisfaction and career retention for registered nurses (RNs) whose highest degree was Associate Degree in Nursing (ADN) or Bachelor of Science in Nursing (BSN). The RNs with a BSN had "significantly higher job satisfaction related to: (a) opportunity for autonomy and growth, (b) job stress and physical demands, and (c) job and organizational security" (Rambur et al., p. 185). Thus, these findings support the preparation of RNs with a BSN versus an ADN for greater individual and social return on the educational investment.

The purpose of correlational research is to examine the type (positive or negative) and strength of relationships among variables. In her correlational study, Reishtein (2005) found that of the three symptoms—dyspnea, fatigue, and sleep difficulty—studied, only dyspnea was significantly related to the other symptoms and to functional performance. Accordingly, management of chronic obstructive pulmonary disease (COPD) probably is best focused on relieving dyspnea to control the patients' symptom experience and improve their functional performance. Additional research is needed to identify the variables that will predict functional performance in patients with COPD.

Quasi-experimental studies are conducted to determine the effect of a treatment or independent variable on designated dependent or outcome variables. Artinian, Washington, and Templin (2001) examined the effects of two independent variables (home telemonitoring [HT] and community-based monitoring [CBM]) on the dependent variable blood pressure control in a population of African American women (see Table 4-1). Both the HT and the CBM groups had significantly lower systolic and diastolic blood pressure (BP) than the comparison group at a 3-month follow-up evaluation. With additional study, these two interventions— HT and CBM—might provide an effective way for nurses to monitor patients' BP, promote compliance in BP treatments, and improve hypertension control in minority patients.

Experimental studies are conducted in highly controlled settings, using a highly structured design to determine the effect of one or more independent variables on one or more dependent variables. Rasmussen and Farr (2003) conducted an experimental study of the effects of morphine and time of day on pain and beta-endorphin (BE) in groups of mice in a laboratory setting (see Table 4-1). In this basic research, the investigators found that morphine abolishes the BE response to pain but does not inhibit pain equally at all times of the day. Thus, morphine doses should be titrated to maximize pain control, with less medication. Additional research in humans is needed, however, before the findings will have implications for nursing practice.

Table 4-1	Quantitative Research: Topics, Problems, and Purposes	
Type of Research	Research Topic	Research Problem and Purpose
Descriptive research	Educational preparation, registered nurses, individual (job satisfaction) and social return on investment (career retention)	*Title of study:* "Education as a determinant of career retention and job satisfaction among registered nurses" (Rambur, McIntosh, Val Palumbo, & Reinier, 2005, p. 185) *Problem:* "As the current nursing shortage increases concerns about staff of health care facilities' ability to provide high quality care (Aiken, Clarke, Sloan, Sochalski, & Silber, 2002), many initiatives are being aimed at the recruitment and retention of the nursing workforce. The pressing need to educate more nurses should stimulate reconsideration of how limited resources for nursing education are spent as educational capacity is increased.... Although many studies have been aimed toward understanding the outcomes of baccalaureate and associate degree education for nurses, few studies have been focused on education as an individual or social return on investment or in years contributed to the profession" (Rambur et al., 2005, pp. 185–186). *Purpose:* The purpose of this study was "to compare job satisfaction and career retention in two cohorts of RNs, those whose highest degrees were the associate degree (AD) or the bachelor's degree (BS) in nursing" (Rambur et al., 2005, p. 185).
Correlational research	Symptoms (dyspnea, fatigue, and sleep difficulty) of chronic obstructive pulmonary disease (COPD) patients, functional performance, chronic illness	*Title of study:* "Relationship between symptoms and functional performance in COPD" (Reishtein, 2005, p. 39) *Problem:* "COPD has been estimated to affect 14 million people in the United States, limiting activity in 1,310,000 individuals. As the population ages, the prevalence of COPD is predicted to increase....Researchers have examined the link between symptoms and function....Two components of affected performance, physical performance and role performance, together can be considered aspects of functional performance....No researchers have explored the collective impact of the symptoms dyspnea, fatigue, and sleep difficulty on functional performance in patients with COPD" (Reishtein, 2005, pp. 39–40). *Purpose:* "Thus, the purpose in this study was to use the Theory of Unpleasant Symptoms to determine the interrelationships and relative contributions of three symptoms [dyspnea, fatigue, and sleep difficulty] to functional performance in people with COPD" (Reishtein, 2005, p. 40).

(continues)

Table 4–1	Purposes of the Literature Review in Qualitative Research *(continued)*	
Type of Research	Research Topic	Research Problem and Purpose
Quasi-experimental research	Blood pressure monitoring, hypertension management, home and community-based monitoring, blood pressure control, minority patients	*Title of study:* "Effects of home telemonitoring and community-based monitoring on blood pressure (BP) control in urban African Americans: A pilot study" (Artinian, Washington, & Templin, 2001, p. 191) *Problem:* "One in four adults has hypertension (HTN), which highlights the prevalence of HTN as a cardiovascular risk factor (American Heart Association, 1999)....According to the World Health Organization (WHO) (WHO Expert Committee, 1996), HTN is the second most common reason for physician office visits world-wide. African Americans have a higher prevalence and greater severity of HTN than do other minorities and whites....Although scientific evidence has established that there is an array of both nonpharmacologic and pharmacologic strategies that reduce BP, the rate of awareness, treatment, and control of HTN in the U.S. population is declining, increasing danger for African Americans in particular (JNC-VI-Joint National Committee on Detection, Evaluation, and Treatment of High Blood Pressure, 1997). Inadequate BP monitoring is an important factor that affects BP control....One way to improve HTN awareness and control is to facilitate access to care by realizing that the point of access need not be limited to a clinic, emergency department, or physician office. The need for tertiary alternative strategies to promote BP control is high" (Artinian et al., 2001, pp. 191–192). *Purpose:* Therefore, the purpose of this study was to determine the "effects of home telemonitoring and community-based monitoring on blood pressure control in urban African Americans" (Artinian et al., 2001, p. 191).
Experimental research	Pain management, analgesics, morphine, beta-endorphin (BE), circadian rhythm, animals	*Title of study:* "Effects of morphine and time of day on pain and beta-endorphin" (Rasmussen & Farr, 2003, p. 105) *Problem:* "Although narcotics have been used as analgesics for many years, clients still are experiencing pain.... Morphine is an important pharmacological modulator of pain and initiator of analgesia....Circadian (approximately 24 hours) rhythms influence the expression of pain and the body's responsiveness to analgesic mediations.... Endogenous opioids, such as morphine, activate the descending pain control system....Currently, the timing of the administration of morphine is not based on its circadian effects. Both PLRL [paw-licking response latency in mice] and BE are known to exhibit a circadian rhythm, or a rhythm that repeats once in a 24-hour period. Yet no well-controlled, time-based studies have been conducted to test the effects of morphine on pain response (PLRL) and plasma BE when administered at different times of day" (Rasmussen & Farr, 2003, pp. 105–107). *Purpose:* "The purpose of the study...was to investigate whether there were time-of-day differences in the effects of morphine on the pain tolerance threshold and the circadian plasma BE response to pain" (Rasmussen & Farr, 2003, p. 107).

Problems and Purposes in Types of Qualitative Studies

The problems formulated for qualitative research identify areas of concern that require investigation to gain new insights, expand understanding, or improve comprehension of the whole (Munhall, 2001). The purpose of a qualitative study indicates the focus of the study, which may be a concept such as pain, an event such as loss of a child, or a facet of a culture such as the healing practices of a specific Native American Indian tribe. In addition, the purpose often identifies the qualitative approach used and the basic assumptions for this approach (Creswell, 1994). Examples of research topics, problems, and purposes for the types of qualitative research—phenomenological, grounded theory, ethnographic, and historical—commonly conducted in nursing are presented in Table 4-2.

Phenomenological research is conducted to promote an understanding of human experiences from an individual researcher's perspective, such as older widows' lived experience of home care (Porter, 2005). Porter found that "home care must be understood as more than what providers do in the homes of service recipients. The older woman who lives alone should be viewed as one who experiences home care and intends to negotiate reliance upon her standby helpers" (p. 302). Porter's study provides insight into and promotes understanding of the growing problem of elderly needing care to promote their independence in their homes.

In grounded theory research, the problem identifies the area of concern and the purpose indicates the focus of the theory to be developed from the research (Munhall, 2001). For example, Draucker (2005, p. 155) conducted a grounded theory study "to begin development of a substantive theory of the processes of mental health services used by adolescents who are depressed and by their families." Draucker found that as mental health services were used by depressed adolescents and their families, they implemented the following actions when venturing through the system: (1) steering clear to avoid the treatment pitfalls; (2) holding back to manage the treatment pitfalls; and (3) letting it, the therapy, take hold to promote success with the treatment. Using mental health services is a complex interactive process that requires strategies to avoid pitfalls for depressed adolescents and their parents.

In ethnographic research, the problem and purpose identify the culture and the specific attributes of the culture that are to be examined, described, analyzed, and interpreted (Germain, 2001). Kauffman (1995) described the haven provided by a senior center for elderly African Americans in an inner city ghetto known for drug-related violence and crime. The study findings indicated that the elders' social interactions and mental health were improved by active participation in the center. The researcher encouraged policy makers and health care professionals to recognize the needs of inner city residents and to provide culturally competent health care to these individuals.

The problem and purpose in historical research focus on a specific individual, a characteristic of society, an event, or a situation in the past, as well as identifying the time period in the past that was examined by the study (Fitzpatrick, 2001). For example, Krisman-Scott (2000) conducted a historical study of disclosure of terminal prognosis from 1930 to 1990 (see Table 4-2). The study conclusions were that disclosure of terminal prognosis has slowly changed over time, from concealment in the 1930s to more general acceptance of disclosure today. The groundwork for the change took place in the 1950s and 1960s and culminated in the 1970s. This change is based on the expanding view of individual rights, perceptions of death, and health care providers' responsibilities.

Table 4-2	Qualitative Research: Topics, Problems, and Purposes	
Type of Research	**Research Topic**	**Research Problem and Purpose**
Phenomenological research	Elderly, widows, experience of home care, practice model, independent living, nursing care	*Title of study:* "Older widows' experience of home care" (Porter, 2005, p. 296) *Problem:* "Home care has undergone sweeping changes in reimbursement policies, access, and utilization, leading to uncertainty about its focus and goals.... Although there is little consensus about the goals of home care (Weissert et al., 2003), there is considerable consensus that home care refers to services provided to people at home and that most home-care clients are women....Unfortunately, few qualitative studies about home care have reinforced the pervasive dichotomies of formal-informal care and caregiver-care receiver that are embedded in standard definitions of home care" (Porter, 2005, p. 296). *Purpose:* The purpose of this phenomenological study was to "describe the experience of home care for older widows living alone in their own homes" (Porter, 2005, p. 296).
Grounded theory research	Depression, adolescents, families, processes of mental health service use, mental health treatment, theory development	*Title of study:* "Processes of mental health service use by adolescents with depression" (Draucker, 2005, p. 155) *Problem:* "Although depression is a serious mental health problem that affects the health and well being of many adolescents, few receive mental health treatment. Between 10% and 15% of children and adolescents in the United States show some symptoms of depression. The 1-year prevalence of major depression disorder (MDD) in adolescents is thought to be as high as 8.3%; the prevalence of dysthymic disorder is estimated to be 3% (U.S. Department of Health and Human Services [USDHHS], 1999). From 20% to 40% of depressed children have another depressive episode within 2 years, 70% will relapse in adulthood, and 20% to 40% of adolescents with depression will develop bipolar disorder (USDHHS, 1999)....Despite 2 decades of significant advancements in the development of psychotherapeutic and pharmacological approaches for children and adolescents with depression (Kazdin, 2004; March et al., 2004), only 20% of children with a serious emotional disturbance receive mental health specialty services; 40% receive some form of mental health intervention; and 40% to 60% of children and adolescents who receive treatment terminate it prematurely" (Draucker, 2005, p. 155). *Purpose:* "The purpose of this research is to begin development of a substantive theory to explain the processes by which adolescents with depression and their families use mental health services" (Draucker, 2005, p. 155).

Table 4–2	Qualitative Research: Topics, Problems, and Purposes *(continued)*	
Type of Research	Research Topic	Research Problem and Purpose
Ethnographic research	Inner-city ghettos, survival, elders, drug activity	*Title of study:* "Center as haven: Findings of an urban ethnography" (Kauffman, 1995, p. 231) *Problem:* "In underserved, inner-city ghettos known for drug-related violence and crime, active participation in community life is dangerous and even life-threatening. This is especially true for elders burdened with the infirmities of aging and lacking the means to provide for alternatives to social isolation. Few researchers have ventured into inner-city communities known for troublesome and dangerous public spaces…. Therefore, little is known about the social lives of people in these communities, in particular, vulnerable older people who are frequently victims of illegal drug activity" (Kauffman, 1995, p. 231). *Purpose:* "This urban ethnography was conducted over a period of three years in a predominantly African American inner-city ghetto. The main question to be answered was: How do elders survive in the midst of 'drug warfare' in an inner-city community known for its dangerous streets and public spaces?" (Kauffman, 1995, p. 231).
Historical research	Disclosure, terminal prognosis, dying, historical analysis	*Title of study:* "An historical analysis of disclosure of terminal status" (Krisman-Scott, 2000, p. 47) *Problem:* "In the last century the manner and place in which Americans experience death has changed. Sudden death has decreased and slow dying has increased….Often, in response to both avoidance and denial, the dying pretend to be unaware. This cycle of pretense, instead of being helpful, robs a person of the opportunity to make appropriate end-of-life decisions and maintain power and control over what remains of life….Nurses, for a variety of reasons, have for the most part avoided telling people they are close to death, even though secrecy creates serious problems in caring for the dying….The amount of information given to patients about illness, treatment, and prognosis has changed over time. Movement toward greater disclosure of health information to patients has occurred in the past 60 years" (Krisman-Scott, 2000, p. 47). *Purpose:* "The purpose of this study was to examine the concept of disclosure as it relates to terminal prognosis and trace its historical development and practice in the United States over the last 60 years" (Krisman-Scott, 2000, p. 47).

Problems and Purposes in Outcomes Research

Outcomes research is conducted to examine the end results of care. Table 4-3 includes the topics, problem, and purpose from an outcomes study by Rudy, Daly, Douglas, Montenegro, Song, and Dyer (1995). This study was conducted to determine the outcomes for patients who are chronically critically ill in the special care unit (SCU) compared with the intensive

Table 4-3	Outcomes Research: Topics, Problem, and Purpose	
Type of Research	Research Topic	Research Problem and Purpose
Outcomes research	Patient outcomes, special care unit, intensive care unit, chronically critically ill	*Title of study:* "Patient outcomes for the chronically critically ill: Special care unit versus intensive care unit" (Rudy, Daly, Douglas, Montenegro, Song, & Dyer, 1995) *Problem:* "The original purpose of intensive care units (ICUs) was to locate groups of patients together who had similar needs for specialized monitoring and care so that highly trained health care personnel would be available to meet these specialized needs. As the success of ICUs has grown and expanded, the assumption that a typical ICU patient will require only a short length of stay in the unit during the most acute phase of an illness has given way to the recognition that stays of more than one month are not uncommon.... These long-stay ICU patients represent a challenge to the current system, not only because of costs, but also because of concern for patient outcomes.... While ample evidence confirms that this subpopulation of ICU patients represents a drain on hospital resources, few studies have attempted to evaluate the effects of a care delivery system outside the ICU setting on patient outcomes, costs, and nurse outcomes" (Rudy et al., 1995, p. 324). *Purpose:* "The purpose of this study was to compare the effects of a low–technology environment of care and a nurse case management care delivery system (specific care unit, SCU) with the traditional high–technology environment (ICU) and primary nursing care delivery system on the patient outcomes of length of stay, mortality, readmission, complications, satisfaction, and cost" (Rudy et al., 1995, p. 324)

care unit (ICU). Common outcomes of cost, patient satisfaction, length of stay, complications, and readmissions were examined to determine the impact of care in these two units on the patients and the health care system. The findings from this 4-year study demonstrated that nurse case-managers in an SCU setting can produce patient outcomes as good as or better than those obtained in the traditional ICU environment, for long-term critically ill patients. In addition, caring for patients in the SCU was more cost-effective than caring for those in the ICU.

Determining the Significance of a Study Problem and Purpose

A research problem is significant in nursing when it has the potential to generate or refine relevant knowledge for practice. While critiquing the significance of the problem and purpose in a published study, you need to determine whether the knowledge generated in the study (1) influences nursing practice, (2) builds on previous research, (3) promotes theory testing or development, or (4) addresses current concerns or priorities in nursing (Burns & Grove, 2005; Moody, Vera, Blanks, & Visscher, 1989).

Influences Nursing Practice

The practice of nursing needs to be based on empirical knowledge or knowledge that is generated through research. Thus, studies that address clinical concerns and generate findings to improve nursing practice are considered significant. Several research problems and purposes have focused on the effects of nursing interventions or on ways to improve these interventions. For example, researchers have examined the effects of (1) pelvic muscle exercises on stress urinary incontinence (Johnson, 2001); (2) relaxation and music on pain after intestinal surgery (Good, Anderson, Ahn, Cong, & Stanton-Hicks, 2005); and (3) guided health imagery to promote smoking cessation (Wynd, 2005). These intervention-focused studies generated knowledge that can be used to improve the care provided to patients and their families.

Builds on Previous Research

A significant study problem and purpose are based on previous research. In a research article, the "Introduction" and "Literature Review" sections include relevant studies that provide a basis for the current study. Often, a summary of the current literature indicates what is known and not known in the area being studied. The gaps in the current knowledge base provide support for and document the significance of the study's purpose. The study by Wynd (2005), introduced earlier in this chapter, indicated what was known and not known about the effectiveness of treatments for smoking cessation. Guided imagery has been used as an effective treatment for other health problems, but what was not known was the effectiveness of this treatment in smoking cessation programs and long-term abstinence. The intent of Wynd's study was to generate additional knowledge about an effective treatment for cigarette smoking in adults.

Promotes Theory Testing or Development

Significant problems and purposes are supported by theory, and the study may focus on either testing or developing theory (Chinn & Kramer, 1998). For example, Steele and Porche (2005) conducted a study to test the theory of planned behavior by Ajzen (2002). A model of Ajzen's theory is presented in Figure 4-1. This theory was used to predict the intentions of rural southeastern Louisiana women to obtain a mammogram. The model indicates that behavioral belief strength influences attitude, normative belief strength influences subjective norm, and control belief strength influences perceived behavior control. Attitude, subjective norm, and perceived behavioral control are predictive of a person's intention, and intention is predictive of behavior. The researchers found that perceived behavior control was the most predictive of a woman's intention to get a mammogram, and attitude was the second greatest predictor. The woman's intention to get a mammogram was predictive of her behavior of obtaining the mammogram. Thus, Ajzen's theory was supported by the conduct of this study, and it can be used to explain the mammography intentions of rural women (Steele & Porche, 2005).

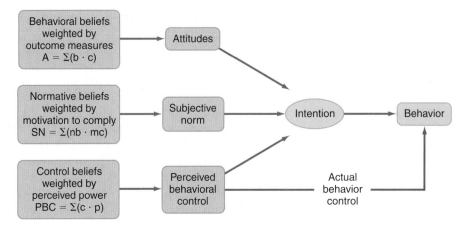

Figure 4-1. The theory of planned behavior (Ajzen, 2002).

Addresses Nursing Research Priorities

Since 1975, expert researchers, specialty groups, and funding agencies have identified a variety of nursing research priorities. Lindeman (1975) developed an initial list of research priorities for clinical practice that included nursing interventions focused on care of the elderly, pain management, and patient education. Nurses continue research in these areas today, with the goal of developing evidence-based nursing practice.

Many professional organizations have identified research priorities that are communicated through their websites. For example, the American Association of Critical-Care Nurses (AACN) published its most current research priorities on its website (http://www.aacn.org). The AACN identified five broad research areas: effective and appropriate use of technology to achieve optimal patient assessment, management, and/or outcomes; creating a healing, humane environment; processes and systems that foster the optimal contribution of critical care nurses; effective approaches to symptom management; and prevention and management of complications.

The American Organization of Nurse Executives (AONE) established the following research priorities for the year 2000: (1) workforce, (2) patient care advocacy, and (3) technology. The workforce topic includes research focused on diversity, composition, professional growth, accountability, and recruitment and retention. Patient care advocacy includes research to address such areas as relationships in the community, among health professionals, and in health care settings; efficient use of resources, new management methods, and techniques; and improvement in health care processes and outcomes across the continuum. In the area of technology, investigations need to examine the outcomes of technology adaptations, systems improvement and infrastructure changes to accommodate new technology, and leadership in managing technological change. AONE provides a discussion of its research priorities on its website (http://www.aone.org).

A major nursing research funding agency is the National Institute for Nursing Research (NINR). The NINR develops the National Nursing Research Agenda, which includes the following: identifying nursing research priorities, outlining a plan for implementing priority studies, and obtaining resources to support these priority projects. NINR has developed four goals to direct the institute's activities over 5 years (2000 to 2004). Goal 1 is to identify and support research opportunities that will achieve scientific distinction and produce significant contributions to health. The priority areas selected include the following: end-of-life and palliative care research, chronic illness experiences, quality of life and quality of care, health promotion and disease prevention, symptom management of illness and treatment, telehealth interventions and monitoring, and cultural and ethnic considerations in health and illness. Goal 2 is to identify and support future areas of opportunity to advance research on high-quality, cost-effective care and to contribute to the scientific base for nursing practice. The priorities related to this goal include research on the following: chronic illness and long-term care, health promotion and risk behaviors, cardiopulmonary health and critical care, neuro-function and sensory conditions, immune responses and oncology, and reproductive and infant health. Goal 3 is to communicate and disseminate research findings resulting from NINR-funded research, and Goal 4 is to enhance the development of nurse researchers through training and career development opportunities. Details about NINR mission, goals, and areas of funding are available on the Institute website (http://ninr.nih.gov/ninr/).

Another federal agency that is funding health care research is the Agency for Healthcare Research and Quality (AHRQ), formerly the Agency for Health Care Policy and Research (AHCPR). The purpose of the AHRQ is to enhance the quality, appropriateness, and effectiveness of health care services, as well as the access to such services, through the establishment of a broad base of scientific research and through the promotion of improvements in clinical practice and in the organization, financing, and delivery of health care services. A list of some of the current research-focused missions follows:

- Care Management Mission: To promote the receipt of effective, evidence-based, and patient-centered care for acute and chronic conditions through research, information dissemination, tool development, and promotion of policies
- Cost, Organization, and Socio-Economics Mission: To improve quality, efficiency, and effectiveness of health care by providing public and private decision makers with the information, tools, and assistance they need to improve the way they organize, finance, pay for, and regulate health care
- Data Development Mission: To develop and maintain data and tools to measure health care quality, efficiency, and effectiveness and to facilitate data use and translation into usable information by external and internal stakeholders to inform decision-making and quality improvement processes
- Health Information Technology (IT) Mission: To increase the development, diffusion, and adoption of health IT to improve the quality, safety, efficiency, and effectiveness of health care for all Americans
- Long-Term Care (LTC) Mission: To improve outcomes, quality, and evidence-based focused care provided in all LTC settings, transitions across settings, special service accommodation for the LTC population

- Patient Safety Mission: To decrease errors, risks, and/or hazards in health care and their harmful impact on patients
- Pharmaceutical Outcomes Mission: To improve health outcomes through the safe and effective use of pharmaceuticals
- Prevention Mission: To increase the adoption and the delivery (and use) of evidence-based clinical preventive services in the United States
- System Capacity and Emergency Preparedness Mission: To empower communities and health care systems to support all people by enhancing system capacity and preparing for urgent and emergent demands and needs
- Training Mission: To continue to foster the growth, dissemination, and translation of the field and science of health services research to achieve AHRQ's mission and address Department priorities in the transfer of health care research (see the AHRQ website [http://www.ahrq.gov]).

Expert researchers, professional organizations, and federal agencies have identified research priorities to direct the future conduct of health care research. In critiquing a study, you need to determine whether the problem and purpose are based on previous research, theory, and current research priorities. Whether the findings will have an impact on nursing practice also needs to be determined. These four elements, discussed in this section, document the significance of the study in developing and refining nursing knowledge.

Examining the Feasibility of a Problem and Purpose

In critiquing a study, begin by determining the feasibility of the problem and the purpose of the study. The feasibility of a study is determined by examining the researchers' expertise; money commitment; availability of subjects, facilities, and equipment; and the study's ethical considerations (Kahn, 1994; Rogers, 1987). The feasibility of Wynd's (2005) study of the effects of guided health imagery on smoking cessation and long-term abstinence is critiqued and presented as an example.

Researcher Expertise

The research problem and purpose studied need to be within the area of expertise of the researcher(s). Research reports usually identify the education of the researchers and their current positions, which indicate their expertise to conduct a study. Also examine the reference list to determine if the researchers have conducted additional studies in this area. Wynd (2005), for example, has a doctoral degree and is a professor and director of the PhD in Nursing Program at the University of Akron College of Nursing. The reference list includes three additional studies conducted by Wynd that focus on the treatment of cigarette smoking with guided imagery. Thus, this investigator has a strong background for conducting research in the area of guided imagery as a treatment for smoking in adults.

Money Commitment

The problem and purpose studied are influenced by the amount of money available to the researcher. The cost of a research project can range from a few dollars for a student's small study to hundreds of thousands of dollars for complex projects. In critiquing a study, one of the points that are analyzed is whether the researchers' financial resources were adequate to complete a quality study. Sources of funding for a study usually are identified in the article. For example, a study may have been funded by a federal research grant from the NINR or by a professional organization such as Sigma Theta Tau or the AACN. The researchers may have received financial assistance from companies that provided necessary equipment or support from the agency where they work. Receiving funding for a study indicates that it was reviewed by peers who chose to support the research financially. Wynd (2005) indicated that her study was funded by the University of Akron Faculty Research Grants Program.

Availability of Subjects, Facilities, and Equipment

Researchers need to have adequate sample size, facilities, and equipment to implement their study. Most published studies indicate the sample size and setting(s) in the "Methods" section of the research report. Often nursing studies are conducted in natural or partially controlled settings, such as a home, hospital unit, or clinic. Many of these facilities are easy to access, and the hospitals and clinics provide access to large numbers of patients. Wynd's (2005) study included 72 subjects who were recruited from a hospital outpatient clinic where adult smokers received routine health care. Thus, the potential subjects were easy to contact and obtain for participation in the study.

A review of the "Methods" section of the research article will determine if adequate, accurate equipment was available. Nursing studies frequently require a limited amount of equipment, such as a tape or video recorder for interviews, or physiological instruments, such as an electrocardiogram (ECG) or thermometer. Wynd (2005) conducted a quasi-experimental study that examined the effects of guided imagery on smoking cessation in adults. The study interventions or treatments included imagery exercises directed by a 20-minute audiotape cassette and counseling and education sessions. These interventions were implemented by the researcher and her trained assistants. The dependent or outcome variables were measured with self-report forms and scales that were completed by the subjects in their homes or at the clinic. Thus, with funding, the researcher had adequate resources to obtain the materials she needed for implementing the treatments and measuring the outcome variables.

Ethical Considerations

The purpose selected for investigation must be ethical, which means that the subjects' rights and the rights of others in the setting are protected (Burns & Grove, 2005). An ethical study confers more benefits than risks in its conduct and will generate useful knowledge for practice. Wynd's (2005) study carried very limited risks of time and fatigue and great potential for benefits if the subjects stopped smoking. The potential subjects were informed about the study, were asked to participate, and signed a consent form if they agreed to be in the study. Thus, this is an ethical study that protected the rights of the subjects and has a potential to improve patient outcomes.

CRITIQUE GUIDELINES Problems and Purposes in Published Studies

The problem and purpose must be clearly and concisely expressed in a published study. In addition, the significance and feasibility of the problem and purpose need to be examined. Ask yourself the following questions when critiquing the problem and purpose in a study.

1. Is the problem clearly and concisely expressed early in the study?
2. Is the problem sufficiently delimited in scope without being trivial?
3. Is the purpose clearly expressed?
4. Does the purpose narrow and clarify the focus or aim of the study?
5. Does the purpose identify the variables, population, and setting for the study?
6. Are the problem and purpose significant in generating nursing knowledge? Is the study based on previous research, theory, and current research priorities? Will the findings have an impact on nursing practice?
7. Was it feasible for the researchers to study the problem and purpose identified? Did the researchers have the expertise to conduct the study? Did they have adequate money, subjects, setting, and equipment to conduct the study? Was the purpose of the study ethical?

Examining Research Objectives, Questions, and Hypotheses in Research Reports

Research objectives, questions, and hypotheses evolve from the problem, purpose, and study framework, and direct the remaining steps of the research process. In a published study the objectives, questions, or hypotheses usually are presented after the "Literature Review" section and right before the "Methods" section. The content in this section is provided to assist you in identifying and critiquing objectives, questions, and hypotheses in published studies.

Research Objectives Implemented in Quantitative and Qualitative Studies

A **research objective** is a clear, concise, declarative statement that is expressed in the present tense. For clarity, an objective usually focuses on one or two variables and indicates whether they are to be identified or described. Sometimes the purpose of objectives is to identify relationships among variables or to determine differences between two or more groups regarding selected variables. The research objectives formulated for quantitative and qualitative studies have many similarities. However, the objectives directing qualitative studies commonly are broader in focus and include variables or concepts that are more complex and abstract than those of quantitative studies (Munhall, 2001).

RESEARCH EXAMPLE   Problem, Purpose, and Objectives from a Quantitative Study

A descriptive study by Steinkrauss, Lipman, Hendell, Gerdes, Thornton, & Stanley (2005) demonstrates the logical flow from research problem and purpose to research objectives in a quantitative study.

Research Problem

Hypoglycemia is a serious disorder in childhood and may cause a number of sequelae. One cause of hypoglycemia is congenital hyperinsulinism (HI). Children with HI are exposed to various degrees of hypoglycemia. Because of the risk of seizures and brain damage associated with hypoglycemia, infants and children with HI are at an increased risk of developmental delay.... Hypoglycemia in infants and children has been investigated for more than 50 years. **A universally accepted definition of hypoglycemia, however, does not exist.... Debate about the developmental consequences of hypoglycemia plagues researchers. One aspect of this debate relates to the issues of severity and duration of hypoglycemia and the effect of these two factors on development.** (Steinkrauss et al., 2005, pp. 109 & 112)

Research Purpose

The purpose of this study was to describe the effects of hypoglycemia on development in a group of children with HI (Steinkrauss et al., 2005, p. 109).

Research Objectives

The objectives of this study were expressed as specific aims, which are the same as research objectives.

The specific aims of this study were threefold: (a) to describe the frequency and extent of developmental delay in a cohort of children with HI, (b) to identify differences in developmental outcome among types of hyperinsulinism, and (c) to identify associations between hypoglycemia history and developmental outcome. (Steinkrauss et al., 2005, p. 113)

CRITIQUE

Steinkrauss et al. (2005) identified a significant problem of HI in children that can result in episodes of hypoglycemia that can be linked to developmental outcomes. The problem statement (**boldface** in the example) clearly indicates what is not known and provides a basis for the purpose and objectives of this study. The purpose clearly indicates this is a descriptive study that is focused on the effects of hypoglycemia on development (research variables) in children with HI (population). The study objectives build on the problem and purpose and provide more clarity regarding the focus of the study. The first objective focuses on description of the development delays in children with HI. The second objective focuses on determining the differences in developmental outcomes among the types of HI experienced by the children. The third objective focuses on the examination of a relationship between the two variables hypoglycemia history and development outcome. Thus, this study identified a significant problem and a feasible purpose for research. In addition, the study objective provided clear direction for the conduct of the study and the interpretation of the study results.

(continues)

IMPLICATIONS FOR PRACTICE

Steinkrauss et al. (2005) found that those infants presenting with HI in the first week of life and who were medically unresponsive to HI treatment were more likely to have developmental delays. Thus, these findings supported the link between HI, hypoglycemia, and developmental delays. The importance for clinical practice is the early recognition and control of hypoglycemia to decrease and/or prevent developmental delays in infants and children with HI.

RESEARCH EXAMPLE   Problem, Purpose, and Objectives in a Qualitative Study

A phenomenological study by Rehm and Rohr (2002) included objectives to direct their investigation of parents', nurses', and educators' perceptions of risks and benefits of school attendance by children who are medically fragile and technology-dependent. The problem, purpose, and objectives from this qualitative study are presented and critiqued.

Research Problem

Participation in school is an important activity for most children, providing opportunities for critical cognitive, social, and emotional growth. Advances in medical treatments and home-care regimens for serious childhood health conditions have resulted in a growing population of children who, though impaired in some activities of daily life, are capable of participating in a wide range of academic and social endeavors.... **The integration of medically fragile children, some of who are dependent on technology and specialized care, into the daily routines of school life pose many challenges for the children and their classmates, educators, families, and health-care providers. Few evaluations of the implications of school attendance by children who are medically fragile/technology-dependent (MFTD) have been published.** (Rehm & Rohr, 2002, p. 345)

Research Purpose

The purpose of this study was to explore family, child, and organizational consequences resulting from school attendance of children who are MFTD (Rehm & Rohr, 2002, p. 345).

Research Objectives

Specifics aims of this study included: (a) to learn how families, educators, and health-care providers ensure the safety and health of children who are MFTD in the school setting and (b) to describe their perceptions about the social and emotional consequences for the children, their peers, and their families resulting from school participation (Rehm & Rohr, 2002, p. 345).

CRITIQUE

In this phenomenological study, the problem statement (**boldface** in the example) indicated that little research has been conducted to determine the implications of school attendance by MFTD children, which provided a basis for the study purpose. The stated aims or objectives further clarify the focus of this qualitative study. The first objective focused on identification and description of how families, educators, and health care providers (populations) ensured the safety and health (study concepts) of MFTD children in the school setting. The second objective focused on description of the social and emotional consequences (study concepts) for the MFTD children, their peers, and their families. This study is concerned with concepts, rather than variables. The study concepts of safety, health, and social and emotional consequences are complex and abstract for the purpose of understanding everyday life experiences from the viewpoint of the affected children, families, and educators. Thus, Rehm and Rohr (2002) identified a significant research problem that included a clear problem statement indicating what was not known in this area of concern. The problem provided a basis for identifying a feasible, focused qualitative study purpose, and the objectives provided additional clarification of the study goals.

IMPLICATIONS FOR PRACTICE

Rehm and Rohr (2002) found that it was beneficial for children who are medically fragile and dependent on technology to attend school, both to increase their socialization and acquisition of skills and for a "break" for families providing their care. However, these investigators also identified associated risks, including difficulty in obtaining appropriate care, exposure to infection, and social isolation or teasing. The knowledge gained from this study can be used to influence policies and to plan nursing care and services to improve the quality of life for the MFTD children attending school and their families.

Research Questions Implemented in Quantitative and Qualitative Studies

A **research question** is a clear, concise interrogative statement that is worded in the present tense, includes one or more variables (or concepts), and is expressed to guide the implementation of quantitative and qualitative studies. The foci of research questions are description of variable(s) or concept(s), examination of relationships among variables, and determination of differences between two or more groups regarding selected variable(s). The research questions for quantitative studies are usually concisely and narrowly focused and inclusive of the study variables and population. The research questions directing qualitative studies often are limited in number, broadly focused, and inclusive of the variables or concepts to be studied. It is really a matter of choice whether researchers identify objectives or questions for their study.

RESEARCH EXAMPLE   Problem, Purpose, and Questions from a Quantitative Study

Webb and Beckstead (2002) conducted a quantitative study of stress-related influences on blood pressure in African American women. Research questions were developed to direct this comparative descriptive study. The flow from research problem and purpose to research questions is demonstrated in the following excerpts from this study.

(continues)

RESEARCH EXAMPLE *(continued)*

Research Problem

African American women residing in the United States have one of the highest rates of cardiovascular mortality and morbidity in the developed world (Gillum, 1996). A major cause of cardiovascular disease in this population is the high prevalence of essential hypertension. Hypertension develops earlier in life and average blood pressure is much higher in African American women than in Caucasian women.... **Despite the high prevalence of hypertension in African American women, they have been greatly under-represented in studies that have evaluated the influence of stress-related variables (anger, coping resources, and strain) on the development of hypertension. The few epidemiological studies that have included African American populations have evaluated traditional risk factors (physical activity and obesity) and often have focused on unemployed women from lower socioeconomic levels or older, less active women.** (Webb & Beckstead, 2002, pp. 383–385)

Research Purpose

The purpose of this study was to compare three groups of employed African American women who had varied blood pressure status on stress-related factors [anger, coping resources, and strain] (Webb & Beckstead, 2002, p. 385).

Research Questions

What percentage of a sample of working African American women has hypertension?

What is the relationship of blood pressure status to three stress-related variables, anger, coping resources, and strain?

Is there a significant difference in demographic and health-related variables among women with different blood pressure status (normotensive, diagnosed hypertension, elevated blood pressure)?

Is there a significant difference in anger, coping resources, and strain among women with different blood pressure status (normotensive, diagnosed hypertension, elevated blood pressure)? (Webb & Beckstead, 2002, pp. 385–386).

CRITIQUE

Webb and Beckstead (2002) conducted a study focused on a common health problem of hypertension in an understudied population of African American women. The problem statement (**boldface** in the example) indicated the knowledge deficit and provided a basis for the research purpose. The purpose clearly indicated the population but would have been clearer if it had included the specific variables studied (note that the variables are provided in brackets after the purpose). The problem and purpose did provide a basis for the research questions that clarified the specific areas of focus for the study. Question 1 focused on identification of the African American women with hypertension. Question 2 focused on the relationship of blood pressure status to the research variables anger, coping resources, and strain. Questions 3 and 4 focused on examining differences among three groups of women—normotensive, diagnosed with hypertension, or with elevated blood pressure—in demographic and health-related variables and in the research variables anger, coping resources, and strain. These questions were presented immediately before the "Methods" section of the research report and were used to direct the implementation of the study procedures, organize data analysis, and facilitate the interpretation of the findings.

IMPLICATIONS FOR PRACTICE

Webb and Beckstead (2002) found that the group with elevated blood pressure had significantly greater rational-cognitive coping resources than those observed for the normotensive or the hypertension-diagnosed groups. However, no significant differences were found between the groups for anger or personal strain. This study used a relatively small sample of employed African American women, and a majority of the women were normotensive (57%); these study characteristics limit the generalizability of the findings. In addition, the role of anger in the development and progression of hypertension remains uncertain. Further research is needed to determine if stress-related factors contribute to the development and influence the management of hypertension.

RESEARCH EXAMPLE   Questions from a Qualitative Study

The questions in qualitative studies identify the variables or concepts that will be examined and often clarify the focus of the study, which might be a lived experience, a health practice in a specific culture, or the history of a nursing intervention. Draucker (2005) conducted a grounded theory study of the use of mental health services by adolescents with depression and their families. The problem and purpose of this study are presented in Table 4-2. The researcher also stated questions to direct her study.

Research Questions

Thus, the following research questions were addressed in this study: (a) How do depressed adolescents and their families decide whether to use mental health services? (b) What are common processes of mental health service use by adolescents with depression and their families? and (c) Do service use processes differ for African American and Caucasian adolescents who are depressed and their families? (Draucker, 2005, p. 156).

CRITIQUE

Draucker (2005) clearly identified a significant problem, and the purpose was to develop a substantive theory of the processes of mental health service use by adolescents and their families (see Table 4-2). Thus, a grounded theory study was conducted to describe the processes of mental health services use by depressed adolescents and their families. The broadly but concisely stated questions provide direction for implementation of the study. The first two questions focus on description of whether to use and the process for using mental health services. The third question focuses on differences between two ethnic groups (African Americans and Caucasians) and their use of mental health services.

IMPLICATIONS FOR PRACTICE

Draucker (2005) found that the depressed adolescents and their families identified several treatment pitfalls associated with mental health services: (1) mental health clinicians would think them "crazy"; (2) the clinician would tell others their "business"; and (3) the clinician would "not have a clue" about what

(continues)

> **IMPLICATIONS FOR PRACTICE** *(continued)*
>
> they needed. To avoid these pitfalls, Draucker suggested, mental health care providers can implement the following strategies:
>
> - Convey to adolescents and their families that the clinician does not think the affected youth is "crazy" and that treatment will not be arbitrarily limited to drug therapies.
> - Give adolescents and their families full authority regarding the sharing of their information.
> - Design the treatment plan to consider the adolescent's age, ethnic background, and specific life circumstances.
>
> These findings provide the basis for initial theory development regarding the use of mental health services by depressed adolescents and their families.

Hypotheses

A **hypothesis** is a formal statement of the expected relationship(s) between two or more variables in a specified population. The hypothesis translates the research problem and purpose into a clear explanation or prediction of the expected results or outcomes of the study. A clearly stated hypothesis includes the variables to be manipulated or measured, identifies the population to be examined, and indicates the proposed outcomes for the study. Hypotheses also influence the study design, sampling method, data collection and analysis process, and interpretation of findings. In this section, types of hypotheses are described and a testable hypothesis is discussed.

Types of Hypotheses

Different types of relationships and numbers of variables are identified in hypotheses. A study might have one, four, or more hypotheses, depending on its complexity. The type of hypothesis developed is based on the purpose of the study. Hypotheses can be described using four categories: (1) associative versus causal, (2) simple versus complex, (3) nondirectional versus directional and (4) null versus research.

Associative versus Causal Hypotheses

The relationships identified in hypotheses are associative or causal. An **associative hypothesis** proposes relationships among variables that occur or exist together in the real world, so that when one variable changes, the other changes (Reynolds, 1971). Associative hypotheses usually are expressed using one of the following formats:

- Variable X is related to variables Y and Z in a specified population (predicts relationships among variables but does not indicate the types of relationships).
- An increase in variable X is associated with an increase in variable Y in a specified population (predicts a positive relationship).
- A decrease in variable X is associated with a decrease in variable Y in a specified population (predicts a positive relationship).

- An increase in variable X is associated with a decrease in variable Y in a specified population (predicts a negative relationship).
- Variables X and Y can be used to predict variable Z in a study (independent variables used to predict a dependent variable in a predictive correlational study).

Associative hypotheses identify relationships among variables in a study but do not indicate that one variable causes an effect on another variable.

RESEARCH EXAMPLE   Associative Hypotheses

Reishtein (2005) conducted a study of the relationship between symptoms and functional performance in COPD. The problem and purpose for this study are presented in Table 4-1. The following associative hypotheses were presented:

(1) Positive relationships exist among dyspnea, fatigue, and sleep difficulty in people with COPD;

(2) Dyspnea, fatigue, and sleep difficulty are related to functional performance; and

(3) Dyspnea, fatigue, and sleep difficulty, taken together, will explain more of the variance in functional performance in people with COPD than any of these symptoms alone (Reishtein, 2005, p. 40).

CRITIQUE

Hypothesis 1 predicts positive relationships or associations among the variables dyspnea, fatigue, and sleep difficulty for patients with COPD. A positive relationship means that the variables change together; thus, they will all increase together in value or all decrease together. These relationships are depicted in the following diagram.

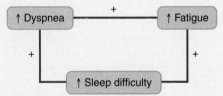

Hypothesis 2 predicts relationships between three variables—dyspnea, fatigue, and sleep difficulty—and the variable functional performance but does not identify the type of relationship. These relationships are shown in the following diagram.

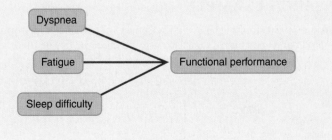

(continues)

CRITIQUE *(continued)*

Hypothesis 3 uses the independent variables dyspnea, fatigue, and sleep difficulty to predict the functional performance in COPD patients. This relationship can be diagrammed as follows.

Dyspnea + Fatigue + Sleep difficulty	⟶	Functional performance

These hypotheses clearly identify the study independent variables (dyspnea, fatigue, and sleep difficulty), dependent or outcome variable (functional performance), and population (COPD patients).

IMPLICATIONS FOR PRACTICE

The results from the study only partially support the hypotheses. Only dyspnea was related to the other symptoms of fatigue and sleep difficulty and to functional performance. Thus, managing dyspnea may be the best way to improve symptoms and functional performance in patients with COPD. Additional research is needed to recognize other symptoms that might be predictive of performance function in COPD patients and direct future management of this disease.

A **causal hypothesis** proposes a cause-and-effect interaction between two or more variables, which are referred to as independent and dependent variables. The independent variable (treatment or experimental variable) is manipulated by the researcher to cause an effect on the dependent variable. The researcher then measures the dependent variable (outcome or criterion variable) to examine the effect created by the independent variable. A format for stating a causal hypothesis is the following: The subjects in the experimental group, who are exposed to the independent variable, demonstrate greater change, as measured by the dependent variable, than do the subjects in the comparison or control group, who are not exposed to the independent variable.

RESEARCH EXAMPLE   Causal Hypothesis

Artinian et al. (2001, p. 191) studied the "effects of home telemonitoring and community-based monitoring on blood pressure control in urban African Americans." The following causal hypothesis was used to direct their study. The problem and purpose for this study are presented in Table 4-1.

Persons who participate in nurse-managed home telemonitoring (HT) plus usual care or who participate in nurse-managed community-based monitoring (CBM) plus usual care will have greater improvement in blood pressure (BP) from baseline to 3 months' follow-up than will persons who receive usual care only (Artinian et al., 2001, p. 191).

CRITIQUE

This hypothesis is clearly expressed according to the format for a causal hypothesis. The independent variables are the two types of nurse-managed BP monitoring, HT and CBM, and the dependent variable is BP control. The independent variables of HT and CBM were manipulated to determine their effect on the dependent variable of BP. The population is clearly identified as African Americans with hypertension, who were recruited from a family community center in Detroit (setting). The three study groups were the comparison group that received usual care and the two experimental group that received either HT or CBM and usual care. This hypothesis is diagrammed in the following figure, in which a causal arrow (➔) is used to show the causal relationships among the independent and dependent variables.

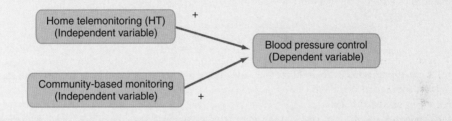

IMPLICATIONS FOR PRACTICE

The findings from this study supported the hypothesis, indicating that the two monitoring interventions (HT and CBM) were effective in improving BP control in hypertensive African Americans. With additional research, these interventions might be used to improve the management of hypertension in African Americans.

Simple versus Complex Hypotheses

A **simple hypothesis** states the relationship (associative or causal) between two variables. A **complex hypothesis** states the relationships (associative or causal) among three or more variables.

RESEARCH EXAMPLE Simple Hypothesis

Moser and Dracup (2000) studied the impact of cardiopulmonary resuscitation (CPR) training on the perception of control felt by the spouses of patients recovering from cardiac disease. These researchers stated two simple hypotheses to direct their study:

Hypothesis 1: "Higher levels of perceived control would be associated with less emotional distress in spouses" of patients recovering from cardiac disease.
Hypothesis 2: "Perceived control could be enhanced in spouses of cardiac patients by cardiopulmonary resuscitation (CPR) training" (Moser & Dracup, 2000, p. 271)

(continues)

CRITIQUE

Hypothesis 1 is a clearly stated associative, simple hypothesis. This hypothesis states a negative or inverse relationship between two variables, as shown in the following diagram.

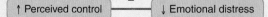

Hypothesis 2 is a causal, simple hypothesis predicting that the independent variable (CPR) causes an increase in the dependent variable (perceived control). The causal relationship in this hypothesis is depicted in the following diagram.

Cardiopulmonary resuscitation (CPR) training —+→ Perceived control

These hypotheses clearly indicate the expected outcomes of the study and identify the study variables and population.

IMPLICATIONS FOR PRACTICE

The study findings did support the hypotheses: CPR training significantly increased the perceived control in spouses of recovering cardiac patients. This perceived control is important for the spouses' psychological recovery when their partners have had a major cardiac event. These study findings support CPR training for spouses of cardiac patients to decrease their emotional distress, and future studies are needed to determine if the CPR training affects the outcomes for the cardiac patient.

A complex hypothesis predicts the relationship (associative or causal) among three or more variables. Artinian et al. (2001) stated a complex, causal hypothesis that includes two independent variables and one dependent variable. The hypothesis and the variables are identified in Table 4-4. Moore and Dolansky (2001, p. 93) conducted a quasi-experimental study "to test the effects of an early home recovery information intervention on physical functioning, psychological distress, and symptom frequency 1 month following coronary artery bypass graft surgery (CABG)." This complex, causal hypothesis is presented in Table 4-4 also, which includes the number and types of variables studied.

Nondirectional versus Directional Hypotheses

A nondirectional hypothesis states that a relationship exists but does not predict the nature of the relationship. If the direction of the relationship being studied is not clear in clinical practice or in the theoretical or empirical literature, the researcher has no clear indication of the nature of the relationship. Under these circumstances, nondirectional hypotheses are developed, such as the one by Reishtein (2005, p. 40) identified earlier in this section: "(2) Dyspnea, fatigue, and sleep difficulty are related to functional performance." This is an

Table 4-4	Complex, Causal Hypotheses and Their Variables		
Hypotheses		Independent Variables	Dependent Variables
"Persons who participate in nurse-managed home telemonitoring (HT) plus usual care or who participate in nurse-managed community-based monitoring (CBM) plus usual care will have greater improvement in blood pressure from baseline to 3 months' follow-up than will persons who receive usual care only" (Artinian, Washington, & Templin, 2001, p. 191).		Home telemonitoring Community-based monitoring	Blood pressure
"Both men and women who participated in the CHIP (Cardiac Home Information Program) intervention would have lower levels of psychological distress, higher levels of physical functioning, and fewer adverse symptoms than would women and men who did not participate in such a program" (Moore & Dolansky, 2001, p. 94).		Cardiac Home Information Program (CHIP)	Psychological distress Physical functioning Adverse symptoms

associative, complex, nondirectional hypothesis. It is associative because it predicts a relationship; complex because there are four variables (dyspnea, fatigue, sleep difficulty, and functional performance); and nondirectional because the nature of the relationships (positive or negative) among the variables is not indicated.

A **directional hypothesis** states the nature (positive or negative) of the interaction between two or more variables. The use of terms such as *positive, negative, less, more, increase, decrease, greater, higher,* or *lower* in a hypothesis indicates the direction of the relationship. Directional hypotheses are developed from theoretical statements (propositions), findings of previous studies, and clinical experience. As the knowledge on which a study is based increases, the researcher is able to make a prediction about the direction of a relationship between the variables being studied. For example, Reishtein stated a directional hypothesis: "...Positive relationships exist among dyspnea, fatigue, and sleep difficulty in people with COPD" (2005, p. 40). This is an associative, complex, directional hypothesis. It is associative because it predicts a relationship; complex because there are three variables (dyspnea, fatigue, and sleep difficulty); and directional because a positive relationship is predicted. A positive relationship indicates that the variables change together and can either increase or decrease together.

A causal hypothesis predicts the effect of an independent variable on a dependent variable, specifying the direction of the relationship. The independent variable either increases or decreases each dependent variable. Thus, all causal hypotheses are directional. Examine the causal hypotheses in Table 4-4, and note the effect of the independent variables on the dependent variables in these two studies.

Null versus Research Hypotheses

The **null hypothesis** (H_0), also referred to as a **statistical hypothesis**, is used for statistical testing and for interpreting statistical outcomes. Even if the null hypothesis is not stated, it is implied, because it is the converse of the research hypothesis (Kerlinger & Lee, 1999).

Some researchers state the null hypothesis because it is more easily interpreted on the basis of the results of statistical analyses. The null hypothesis also is used when the researcher believes there is no relationship between two variables and when theoretical or empirical information is inadequate to state a research hypothesis.

A null hypothesis can be simple or complex and associative or causal. An example of a simple, associative, null hypothesis is the following: "There is no relationship between the number of experiences performing a developmental assessment skill and learning of the skill" (Koniak, 1985, p. 85). Fahs and Kinney (1991) developed the following causal, null hypothesis to direct their study: "There is no difference in the occurrence of bruise at injection site with low-dose heparin therapy when administered in three different subcutaneous sites [abdomen, thigh, and arm]" (p. 204). No statistically significant difference in bruising was found at 60 and 72 hours after injection for the three sites. Thus, this null hypothesis was supported and provides direction for giving heparin in clinical practice.

A **research hypothesis** is the alternative hypothesis (H_1 or H_A) to the null hypothesis and states that a relationship exists between two or more variables. All of the hypotheses stated in previous sections of this chapter have been research hypotheses, except for the two null hypotheses given in the previous paragraph. Research hypotheses can be simple or complex, nondirectional or directional, and associative or causal (see the research hypotheses in Table 4-4 for examples).

Testable Hypothesis

A testable hypothesis is clearly stated and predicts a relationship between two or more variables. Hypotheses are clearer without specifying the presence or absence of a "significant difference," because determination of the level of significance is only a statistical technique applied to sample data. In addition, hypotheses should not identify methodological points, such as techniques of sampling, measurement, and data analysis (Kerlinger & Lee, 1999). Therefore, such phrases as "measured by," "in a random sample of," and "using ANOVA" (analysis of variance) are inappropriate because they limit the hypothesis to the measurement methods, sample, or analysis techniques identified for one study. In addition, hypotheses need to reflect the variables and population outlined in the research purpose and are expressed in the present tense, not the future tense. Expressing hypotheses in the present tense does not limit them to the study being conducted and enables them to be used in additional research.

The value of a hypothesis ultimately is derived from whether it is testable in the real world. A **testable hypothesis** is one that contains variables that are measurable or able to be manipulated. Thus, the independent variable must be clearly defined, often by a protocol, so that it can be implemented precisely and consistently as a treatment in the study. The dependent variable must be precisely defined to indicate how it will be accurately measured.

A testable hypothesis also needs to predict a relationship that can be "supported" or "not supported" as indicated by the data collected and analyzed. If the hypothesis states an associative relationship, correlational analyses are conducted on the data to determine the existence, type, and strength of the relationship between the variables studied. The hypothesis that states a causal link between the independent and dependent variables is evaluated using statistics that examine differences between the experimental and comparison or control groups, such as the *t*-test or ANOVA. It is the null hypothesis (stated or implied) that is tested to determine whether the independent variable produced a significant effect on the dependent variable.

The research objectives, questions, and hypotheses need to be clearly focused and concisely expressed in studies. Both objectives and questions are used in qualitative studies and descriptive and correlational quantitative studies, but questions are more common. Some correlational studies focus on predicting relationships and may include hypotheses. Quasi-experimental and experimental studies need to be directed by hypotheses.

CRITIQUE GUIDELINES   Research Objectives, Questions, and Hypotheses in Published Studies

You may find the following questions to be helpful during a critique of the objectives, questions, and hypotheses in a study.

1. Are the objectives, questions, or hypotheses formally stated in the study? If they were not stated, were they needed to direct the conduct of the study? If the study is quasi-experimental or experimental, hypotheses are needed to direct the study.
2. Are the objectives, questions, or hypotheses clearly focused and concisely expressed in the study? Do they clearly identify the variables and population to be studied?
3. Are the study objectives, questions, or hypotheses based on the purpose?
4. Are the variables and relationships among the variables identified in the objectives, questions, or hypotheses linked to the concepts and propositions in the study framework?
5. Are the hypotheses associative or causal, simple or complex, directional or nondirectional, and research or null?
6. Are the hypotheses testable in this study? Thus are they clearly stated in the present tense, with measurable dependent variables, and appropriate independent variables that can be consistently implemented during a study?

Understanding Study Variables

The research purpose and objectives, questions, and hypotheses include the variables or concepts to be examined in a study. **Variables** are qualities, properties, or characteristics of persons, things, or situations that change or vary. Variables also are concepts at different levels of abstraction that are concisely defined to promote their measurement or manipulation within a study (Chinn & Kramer, 1998). In this section, different types of variables are described, and conceptual and operational definitions of variables are discussed.

Types of Variables

Variables are classified into a variety of types to explain their use in research. Some variables are manipulated; others are controlled. Some variables are identified but not measured; others are measured with refined measurement devices. The types of variables presented in this section include independent, dependent, research, extraneous, and demographic.

Independent and Dependent Variables

The relationship between independent and dependent variables is the basis for formulating hypotheses for correlational, quasi-experimental, and experimental studies. An independent variable is a stimulus or activity that is manipulated or varied by the researcher to create an effect on the dependent variable. The independent variable is also called a treatment or experimental variable. A dependent variable is the outcome or response that the researcher wants to predict or explain. Changes in the dependent variable are presumed to be caused by the independent variable. The independent and dependent variables for the Artinian et al. (2001) and Moore and Dolansky (2001) studies are presented in Table 4-4 as an example.

Research Variables or Concepts

Qualitative studies and some quantitative (descriptive and correlational) studies involve the investigation of research variables or concepts. Research variables or concepts are the qualities, properties, or characteristics identified in the research purpose and objectives or questions that are observed or measured in a study. Research variables or concepts are used when the intent of the study is to observe or measure variables as they exist in a natural setting without the implementation of a treatment. Thus no independent variables are manipulated, and no cause-and-effect relationships are examined. Draucker (2005) conducted a qualitative study to describe the use of mental health services by depressed adolescents and their families. The problem and purpose of this study are presented in Table 4-4 and the research questions that guide this study were presented earlier in this chapter. Draucker used grounded theory methodology to investigate a single concept, processes of mental health services use (research concept), in an ethnically diverse (African American and Caucasian) population of depressed adolescents and their families.

Extraneous Variables

Extraneous variables exist in all studies and can affect the measurement of study variables and the relationships among these variables. Extraneous variables are of primary concern in quantitative studies because they can interfere with obtaining a clear understanding of the relational or causal dynamics within these studies. These variables are classified as recognized or unrecognized and controlled or uncontrolled. Some extraneous variables are not recognized until the study is in progress or is completed, but their presence influences the study outcome.

Researchers attempt to recognize and control as many extraneous variables as possible in quasi-experimental and experimental studies, and specific designs and sample criteria have been developed to control the influence of extraneous variables. Wynd (2005, p. 247) in her quasi-experiment study of the use of guided imagery for smoking cessation and long-term abstinence set the following sample criteria for inclusion in the study: "age 18 or older, smoking history of at least five cigarettes per day for a minimum of 1 year", and "considered 'healthy' in that they had no known type of smoking-related illness." These sample criteria ensure that the subjects were adults, had a smoking history, and were healthy. These sample criteria remove the impact of extraneous variables such as adolescent smokers less than 18 years of age, smoking less than one year, and illness on the outcomes of the study.

The extraneous variables that are not recognized until the study is in process, or are recognized before the study is initiated but cannot be controlled, are referred to as **confounding variables**. Sometimes extraneous variables can be measured during the study and controlled statistically during analysis. Analysis of covariance (ANCOVA) was used by Moore and Dolansky (2001) to control the effects of the extraneous variables of age, comorbidity, and presurgical cardiac functional status that might have influenced the outcomes from a Cardiac Home Information Program (CHIP), which was provided to patients who had coronary artery bypass graft (CABG) surgery. However, extraneous variables that cannot be controlled or measured are a design weakness and can hinder the interpretation of findings. As control in quasi-experimental and experimental studies decreases, the potential influence of confounding variables increases.

Environmental variables are a type of extraneous variable composing the setting in which the study is conducted. Examples of these variables include climate, family, health care system, and governmental organizations. If a researcher is studying humans in an uncontrolled or natural setting, it is impossible and undesirable to control all the extraneous variables. In qualitative and some quantitative (descriptive and correlational) studies, little or no attempt is made to control extraneous variables. The intent is to study subjects in their natural environment without controlling or altering that setting or situation. The environmental variables in quasi-experimental and experimental research can be controlled by using a laboratory setting or a specially constructed research unit in a hospital. Environmental control is an extremely important part of conducting an experimental study. For example, Rasmussen and Farr (2003) conducted an experimental study using rats in a laboratory setting (see Table 4-1 for the problem and purpose of this study). The laboratory controlled for many of the environmental variables, so they did not have an impact on the study outcome.

Demographic Variables

Demographic variables are characteristics or attributes of subjects that are collected to describe the sample. Some common demographic variables are age, education, gender, ethnic origin (race), marital status, income, job classification, and medical diagnosis. When a study is completed, the demographic data are analyzed to provide a picture of the sample and are called **sample characteristics**. A study's sample characteristics can be presented in table format or narrative. As discussed earlier in this chapter, Reishtein (2005) conducted a correlational study to examine the relationship between symptoms (dyspnea, fatigue, and sleep difficulty) and functional performance in COPD patients. The demographic variables examined in this study included: gender, race, age, oxygen usage, medications, and FEV_1 (forced expiratory volume) % predicted. Table 4-5 presents the demographic profile of the subjects in this study; this profile is also referred to as the sample characteristics for the study. The demographic variables are identified by the researcher when a proposal is developed for conducting the study. Once data are collected from the study subjects on these demographic variables and analyzed, the results are called sample characteristics that describe the sample.

Sample characteristics can also be presented in narrative format in the research report. For example, in a grounded theory study of use of mental health services by depressed adolescents and their families, Draucker (2005) described her sample using a narrative

Table 4-5	Demographic and Clinical Characteristics of Study Sample (*N* = 100)			
		Clinic *(n)*	Home *(n)*	Total (%)
Sex	Male	47	30	77
	Female	4	19	23
Race	White	31	49	80
	African-American	20	0	20
Age *M* (SD)		68.15 (9.23)	69.35 (11.47)	68.73 (10.34)
Oxygen usage	Never	24	31	55
	Some of the time	12	10	22
	All of the time	15	8	23
Medications	Prednisone	5	4	9
	Theophylline	13	7	20
	Both medications	3	2	5
	Neither medication	30	36	66
FEV_1% predicted *M* (SD)		40.45 (13.18)	42.19 (13.56)	41.17 (11.79)

From Reishtein, J. L. (2005). Relationships between symptoms and functional performance in COPD. *Research in Nursing & Health, 28*(1), 39–47.

format. The demographic variables for the study were gender, ethnicity or race, employment status, income, marital status, and parental status, as can be determined by reading through the following example. Draucker described her sample characteristics as follows:

> Data were collected from 63 participants, including 52 young adults, 4 parents, and 7 professionals. Of the young adults, 17 were male (9 African American and 8 Caucasian) and 35 were female (15 African American and 20 Caucasian). Almost half of the young adults (*n* = 23, 44%) were students, 13% (*n* = 7) were unemployed, and the rest reported a variety of occupations including retail sales, health care worker, food service worker, and entertainer. The majority (*n* = 47, 90%) reported incomes under $15,000 a year. Most (*n* = 47, 94%) were single. Five of the young adult participants had one child and three were pregnant. Of the parent participants, three were mothers (two Caucasian and one African American) and one was a father (Caucasian). Of the professional participants, three were men (one African American, one Caucasian, and one "other") and four were women (two African American and two Caucasian). Their professions were teacher and coach, case manager, youth mentor, choir director, youth minister and coach, social service program coordinator, and nurse. (Draucker, 2005, p. 157)

Conceptual and Operational Definitions of Variables

A variable is operationalized in a study by the development of conceptual and operational definitions. A **conceptual definition** provides the theoretical meaning of a variable (Chinn & Kramer, 1998) and often is derived from a theorist's definition of a related concept. In a published study, the framework includes concepts and their definitions, and the variables are selected to represent the concepts. Thus, the variables are conceptually defined, indicating the link with the concepts in the framework. An **operational definition** is derived from a set of procedures or progressive acts that a researcher performs to receive sensory impressions (such as sound, visual, or tactile impressions) that indicate the existence or degree of existence of a variable (Reynolds, 1971). Operational definitions need to be independent of time and setting so that variables can be investigated at different times and in different settings using the same operational definitions. An operational definition is developed so that a variable can be measured or manipulated in a concrete situation, and the knowledge gained from studying the variable will increase the understanding of the theoretical concept that this variable represents.

Two of the variables from the Wynd (2005) study, which was presented earlier in this chapter, are operationalized as an example. This quasi-experimental study had an independent variable of guided health imagery and a dependent variable of smoking cessation. The conceptual and operational definitions for these two variables are presented as follows.

RESEARCH EXAMPLE   Conceptual and Operational Definitions of Variables

Independent Variable: Guided Health Imagery

Conceptual definition.

A highly focused form of concentration that creates an alteration of sensations, awareness, and perceptions with the same biopsychosocial, integrative properties that allow people to process sensory information....The guided imagery intervention designed for use in this current study incorporated a higher-order, molar image of health for self-evaluation and restructuring of lifestyles (Wynd, 2005, p. 246).

Operational definition.

The guided health imagery intervention protocol consisted of: (a) raising awareness about imagery abilities by envisioning childhood bedrooms for memory; (b) deep diaphragmatic breathing practice with 5-second inhalations, and exhalations using the abdomen and diaphragm; (c) progressive muscle relaxation exercises involving tension followed by full relaxation of each muscle group from head to toe to achieve a relaxed, accepting frame of mind. Once relaxed and open to the guided health imagery visualization, the interventionist used a 20-minute audiotape that provided a guided health imagery exercise (Wynd, 2005, pp. 247–248).

Dependent Variable: Smoking Cessation

Conceptual definition.

A future-oriented, health-promoting behavior that results in a smoke free lifestyle and improved health.

Operational definition.

Smoking rates that were "monitored through use of self-report data and were validated by corroborating reports from friends and family members… Participants who varied in their answers from their significant contacts or could not be reached by telephone were considered ongoing smokers and were included in the resulting relapse rates" (Wynd, 2005, p. 247).

(continues)

CRITIQUE

The variables in the Wynd (2005) study were clearly identified and defined. The conceptual definitions for guided health imagery and smoking cessation were found in the framework section of the article so there was a clear link between the concepts in the framework and the study variables. The operational definitions were found in the methods section of the research report and the measurement of smoking cessation was in a section labeled measurement and the guided health imagery was in the intervention section. The conceptual definitions based on the framework provided direction for the development of the guided health imagery intervention and the measurement of the dependent variable smoking cessation. Findings from this study are presented earlier in this chapter.

The variables in quasi-experimental and experimental research are narrow and specific in focus and can be quantified (converted to numbers) or manipulated using specified steps that are often developed into a protocol. In addition, the variables are objectively defined to decrease researcher bias, as indicated in the previous example. The research variables or concepts in descriptive and correlational quantitative studies and qualitative studies usually are more abstract and broadly defined.

RESEARCH EXAMPLE   Conceptual and Operational Definitions of Research Concepts

In many qualitative studies, the focus of the study is to define the concept(s) being studied. For example, Draucker (2005) conducted her study to describe the process of mental health service use by adolescents with depression and their families.

Research Concept: Processes of Mental Health Service Use

Conceptual definition

The process of using mental health services was found to have two major themes of pitfalls of the treatment process and venturing through the system. The pitfalls of treatment identified by the adolescents were that the health professionals would think they were crazy, share their private information, and not have a clue about their illness. The venturing through the system involved steering clear of the treatment pitfalls, holding back to manage the treatment pitfalls, and letting therapy take hold to promote success of the treatment.

Operational definition

Data were collected by "open-ended interviews. The participants were asked to describe their perceptions of their experiences with depression as adolescents, with a special focus on any mental health treatment they might have received or considered. If the participant agreed to have an adult family member or caregiver participate, that person was contacted and interviewed about his or her experiences related to the child's depression" (Draucker, 2005, p. 157).

CRITIQUE

The research concept of processes of mental health service use was conceptually and operationally defined in the research report. The conceptual definition was in the "Discussion" section of the study because the focus was to develop a theory describing the concept processes of mental health service use. The operational definition of the research concept was found in the "Methods" section under "Data Collection," which described the face-to-face interviews with adolescents and their family members. The conceptual definition is consistent with the operational definition because open-ended interviews were used to generate the data that were synthesized to describe the processes of mental health service use.

CRITIQUE GUIDELINES Variables in Published Studies

Variables must be identified clearly and defined conceptually and operationally in a published study. Ask the following questions when critiquing the variables in a study.

1. Are the independent or dependent variables or research variables or concepts identified?
2. Are the variables that are manipulated or measured in the study consistent with the variables identified in the purpose or the objectives, questions, or hypotheses?
3. Are the variables reflective of the concepts identified in the study framework?
4. Are the variables clearly defined conceptually and operationally based on theory and previous research?
5. Is the conceptual definition of the variable consistent with the operational definition?
6. Were the essential demographic variables examined and summarized?
7. Were the extraneous variables identified and controlled as necessary in the study?
8. Are there uncontrolled extraneous variables that may have influenced the findings? Is the potential impact of these variables on the findings discussed?

KEY CONCEPTS

- The research problem is an area of concern where there is a gap in the knowledge base needed for nursing practice. The problem includes significance, background, and problem statement.
- The research purpose is a concise, clear statement of the specific goal or aim of the study.
- A significant problem and purpose influence nursing practice, build on previous research, promote theory development, and/or address current concerns or priorities in nursing.
- Study feasibility is evaluated by examining the researchers' expertise; money commitments; availability of subjects, facilities, and equipment; and the study's ethical considerations.
- Research objectives, questions, or hypotheses are formulated to bridge the gap between the more abstractly stated research problem and purpose and the detailed design and data analysis.
- A hypothesis is the formal statement of the expected relationship(s) between two or more variables in a specified population.
- Hypotheses can be described using four categories: (1) associative versus causal, (2) simple versus complex, (3) nondirectional versus directional, and (4) null versus research.

- Variables are qualities, properties, or characteristics of persons, things, or situations that change or vary.
- An independent variable is a stimulus or activity that is manipulated or varied by the researcher to create an effect on the dependent variable.
- A dependent variable is the response, behavior, or outcome that the researcher wants to predict or explain.
- Research variables or concepts are the qualities, properties, or characteristics that are observed or measured in a study.
- Demographic variables are characteristics or attributes of the subjects that are collected and analyzed to describe the study sample.
- A variable is operationalized in a study by developing conceptual and operational definitions.
- A conceptual definition provides the theoretical meaning of a variable and is derived from a theorist's definition of a related concept.
- Operational definitions indicate how a treatment or independent variable will be implemented and how the dependent variable will be measured.

TIPS FOR FURTHER STUDY

- Review problems, purpose, and variables by answering the Bonus Review Questions at http://evolve.elsevier.com/Burns/understanding. Then read the Good et al. (2005) study and identify the problem, purpose, and variables in the study.
- Access the website for the American Association of Critical Care Nurses and identify the research agenda for this organization.
- Evidence-based guidelines exist for the treatment of hypertension. Find the most current guidelines for hypertension diagnosis and treatment online.
- To strengthen your understanding of hypotheses, complete the "Making Connections: Objectives; Questions; and Hypotheses" section in Chapter 4 of your *Study Guide*. Then develop a null hypothesis for each of the research hypotheses presented in Table 4-4.

REFERENCES

Aiken, L. H., Clarke, S. P., Sloan, D. M., Sochalski, J., & Silber, J. H. (2002). Hospital nurse staffing and patient mortality, nurse burnout, and job dissatisfaction. *Journal of the American Medical Association, 288*(16), 1987–1993.

Ajzen, I., (2002). The theory of planned behavior: Home page. Retrieved October 21, 2005, from http://www-unix.oit.umass.edu/~aizen/index.html

American Heart Association. (1999). *1999 heart and stroke statistical update*. Dallas: Author, 1999.

Artinian, N. T., Washington, O. G., & Templin, T. N. (2001). Effects of home telemonitoring and community-based monitoring on blood pressure control in urban African Americans: A pilot study. *Heart & Lung: The Journal of Acute and Critical Care, 30*(3), 191–199.

Brown, S. J. (1999). *Knowledge for health care practice: A guide to using research evidence*. Philadelphia: Saunders.

Burns, N., & Grove, S. K. (2005). *The practice of nursing research: Conduct, critique, and utilization* (5th ed.). Philadelphia: Saunders.

Centers for Disease Control and Prevention. (2005). Cigarette smoking among adults—United States, 2003. *MMWR: Morbidity and Mortality Weekly Report, 54*(20), 509–513.

Chinn, P. L., & Kramer, M. K. (1999). *Theory and nursing: Integrated knowledge development* (5th ed.). St. Louis: Mosby.

Creswell, J. W. (1994). *Research design: Qualitative and quantitative approaches*. Thousand Oaks, CA: Sage.

Cupal, D. D., & Brewer, B. W. (2001). Effects of relaxation and guided imagery on knee strength, reinjury anxiety, and pain following anterior cruciate ligament reconstruction. *Rehabilitation Psychology, 46*(1), 28–43.

Draucker, C. B. (2005). Processes of mental health service use by adolescents with depression. *Image—The Journal of Nursing Scholarship, 37*(2), 155–162.

Fahs, P. S. S., & Kinney, M. R. (1991). The abdomen, thigh, and arm as sites for subcutaneous sodium heparin injections. *Nursing Research, 40*(4), 204–207.

Fitzpatrick, M. L. (2001). Historical research: The method. In P. L. Munhall (Ed.), *Nursing research: A qualitative perspective* (3rd ed.). (pp. 403–415). Boston: Jones and Bartlett.

Germain, C. P. (2001). Ethnography: The method. In P. L. Munhall (Ed.), *Nursing research: A qualitative perspective* (3rd ed.). (pp. 277–306). Boston: Jones and Bartlett.

Gillum, R. F. (1996). Epidemiology of hypertension in African American women. *American Heart Journal, 131*(2), 385–395.

Good, M., Anderson, G. C., Ahn, S., Cong, X., & Stanton-Hicks, M. (2005). Relaxation and music reduce pain following intestinal surgery. *Research in Nursing & Health, 28*(3), 240–251.

Johnson, V. Y. (2001). Effects of a submaximal exercise protocol to recondition the pelvic floor musculature. *Nursing Research, 50*(1), 33–41.

JNC-VI-National Committee on Detection, Evaluation, and Treatment of High Blood Pressure. (1997). *The sixth report of the Joint National Committee on prevention, detection, evaluation, and treatment of high blood pressure.* NIH Publication No. 98-4080. Bethesda, MD: National Institutes of Health.

Kahn, C. R. (1994). Picking a research problem: The critical decision. *The New England Journal of Medicine, 330*(21), 1530–1533.

Kauffman, K. S. (1995). Center as haven: Findings of an urban ethnography. *Nursing Research, 44*(4), 231–236.

Kazdin, A. E. (2004). Psychotherapy for children and adolescents. In M. J. Lambert (Ed.), *Handbook of psychotherapy and behavior change* (pp. 543–587). New York: Wiley.

Kerlinger, F. N., & Lee, H. B. (2000). *Foundations of behavioral research* (4th ed.). Atworth TX: Harcourt College.

Krisman-Scott, M. A. (2000). An historical analysis of disclosure of terminal status. *Journal of Nursing Scholarship, 32*(1), 47–52.

Koniak, D. (1985). Autotutorial and lecture-demonstration instruction: A comparative analysis of the effects upon students' learning of a developmental assessment skill. *Western Journal of Nursing Research, 7*(1), 80–100.

Lewandowski, W.A. (2004). Patterning of pain and power with guided imagery. *Nursing Science Quarterly, 17*(3), 233–241.

Lindeman, C. A. (1975). Delphi survey of priorities in clinical nursing research. *Nursing Research, 24*(6), 434–441.

March, J., Silva, S., Petrycki, S., Curry, J., Wells, K., Fairbank, J., Burns, B., et al. (2004). Fluoxetine, cognitive-behavioral therapy, and their combination for adolescents with depression: Treatment for adolescents with depression study (TADS) randomized control trial. *Journal of the American Medical Association, 292*(7), 807–820.

Melnyk, B. M., & Fineout-Overholt, E. (2005). *Evidence-based practice in nursing & healthcare: A guide to best practice.* Philadelphia: Lippincott Williams & Wilkins.

Moody, L., Vera, H., Blanks, C., & Visscher, M. (1989). Developing questions of substance for nursing science. *Western Journal of Nursing Research, 11*(4), 393–404.

Moore, S. M., & Dolansky, M. A. (2001). Randomized trial of a home recovery intervention following coronary artery bypass surgery. *Research in Nursing & Health, 24*(2), 93–104.

Moser, D. K., & Dracup, K. (2000). Impact of cardiopulmonary resuscitation training on perceived control in spouses of recovering cardiac patients. *Research in Nursing & Health, 23*(4), 270–278.

Munhall, P. L. (2001). *Nursing research: A qualitative perspective* (3rd ed.). Boston: Jones and Bartlett.

Porter, E. J. (2005). Older widows' experience of home care. *Nursing Research, 54*(5), 296–303.

Rambur, B., McIntosh, B., Palumbo, M.V., & Reinier, K. (2005). Education as a determinant of career retention and job satisfaction among registered nurses. *Journal of Nursing Scholarship, 37*(2), 185–192.

Rasmussen, N. A., & Farr, L. A. (2003). Effects of morphine and time of day on pain and beta-endorphin. *Biological Research for Nursing, 5*(2), 105–116.

Rehm, R. S., & Rohr, J. A. (2002). Parents', nurses', and educators' perceptions of risks and benefits of school attendance by children who are medically fragile/technology-dependent. *Journal of Pediatric Nursing, 17*(5), 345–353.

Reishtein, J. L. (2005). Relationship between symptoms and functional performance in COPD. *Research in Nursing & Health, 28*(1), 39–47.

Reynolds, P. D. (1971). *A primer in theory construction.* Indianapolis: Bobbs-Merrill.

Rogers, B. (1987). Research corner: Is the research project feasible? *American Association of Occupational Health Nurses Journal, 35*(7), 327–328.

Rudy, E. B., Daly, B. J., Douglas, S., Montenegro, H. D., Song, R., & Dyer, M. A. (1995). Patient outcomes for the chronically critically ill: Special care unit versus intensive care unit. *Nursing Research, 44*(6), 324–331.

Short, S. E., Hall, C. R., Engel, S. R., & Nigg, C. R. (2004). Exercise imagery and the stages of change. *Journal of Mental Imagery, 28*(1–2), 61–78.

Steele, S. K., & Porche, D. J. (2005). Testing the theory of planned behavior to predict mammography intention. *Nursing Research, 54*(5), 332–338.

Steinkrauss, L., Lipman, T. H., Hendell, C. D., Gerdes, M., Thornton, P. S., & Stanley, C. A. (2005). Effects of hypoglycemia on developmental outcome in children with congenital hyperinsulinism. *Journal of Pediatric Nursing, 20*(2), 109–118.

U.S. Department of Health and Human Services. (2000). *Healthy people 2010.* Washington, DC: U.S. Government Printing Office.

U.S. Department of Health and Human Services, Substance Abuse and Mental Health Services Administration, Center for Mental Health Services, National Institutes of Health, National Institute of Mental Health. (1999). *Mental health: A report of the Surgeon General.* Rockville, MD: Author.

Webb, M. S., & Beckstead, J. W. (2002). Stress-related influences on blood pressure in African American women. *Research in Nursing & Health, 25*(5), 383–393.

Weissert, W., Chernew, M., & Hirth, R. (2003). Titrating versus targeting home care services to frail elderly clients: An application of agency theory and cost-benefit analysis to home care policy. *Journal of Aging and Health, 15*(1), 99–123.

WHO Expert Committee. (1996). *Hypertension control.* Geneva: World Health Organization.

Wynd, C. A. (2005). Guided health imagery for smoking cessation and long-term abstinence. *Journal of Nursing Scholarship, 37*(3), 245–250.

Review of the Literature

Learning Outcomes

After completing this chapter, you should be able to:

1. Critique the literature review section of a
   published study.
2. Conduct a computerized search of the
   literature.

3. Write a literature review to promote the use
   of evidence-based knowledge in nursing
   practice.

134

Key Terms

STUDY TOOLS

Be sure to visit http://evolve.elsevier.com/Burns/understanding/ for additional examples and self-tests. Also, a review of this chapter's concepts and practice exercises can be found in Chapter 5 of the Study Guide for *Understanding Nursing Research: Building an Evidence-Based Practice*, 4th edition.

A wealth of information from nursing studies is available in the literature for clinicians and researchers. More research information appears every day, averaging 6000 new scientific articles daily. The number of nursing journals also is increasing dramatically, and a multitude of nursing research reports is available in full text electronically, as well as in print form. Thus, conducting a literature review is much more enlightening now than in the past.

A **review of literature** provides you with the current theoretical and scientific knowledge about a particular problem, and resulting in a synthesis of what is known and not known. You may keep current in your practice by regularly searching the literature for information on topics of particular interest. Increasingly, nurses in clinical practice are conducting small studies on their own units. If you plan to conduct such a study, however, be sure to first examine the literature for information about previous studies relevant to the clinical problem.

Computerized databases make literature searches easier than ever. When you conduct a literature review for information about clinical problems, synthesize the knowledge you have gathered in a written summary and share it with your colleagues.

This chapter provides essential information to assist you in searching the literature, critiquing the literature review sections of quantitative and qualitative studies, and synthesizing research evidence to guide practice. A literature review on the prediction and prevention of pressure ulcers is presented as an example of research knowledge that is ready for use in practice.

Understanding the Literature Review in Published Studies

Literature reviews in published studies provide a background for the problem studied. Such reviews include (1) a description of the current knowledge of a practice problem, (2) identification of the gaps in this knowledge base, and (3) the contribution of the present study to the building of knowledge in this area. The scope of a literature review must be both broad enough to allow the reader to become familiar with the research problem and narrow enough to include only the most relevant sources. Sources used need to be relevant and current. **Relevant studies** are those with a direct bearing on the problem of concern. **Current sources** are those published within five years prior to acceptance of the manuscript for publication.

To increase your understanding of the literature reviews presented in published studies, the following areas are addressed in this section:

- Sources included in a literature review
- Purpose of the literature review in quantitative studies
- Purpose of the literature review in qualitative studies

Sources Included in a Literature Review

Two main types of sources are cited in the review of literature for research: (1) theoretical and (2) empirical. The word *empirical* in this context refers to knowledge derived from research. In other words, the knowledge is based on data from research (data-based). Other types of published information, such as descriptions of clinical situations, educational literature, and position papers, are examined by the researcher in the process of reviewing the literature but are rarely cited in a research publication because of their subjectivity (Pinch, 1995). Sources in literature reviews may be either primary or secondary; as discussed later on, this is an important distinction.

Citation is the act of quoting a source, using it as an example, or presenting it as support for a position taken. A **periodical**, such as a journal, is published over time and is numbered sequentially for the years published. This sequential numbering is seen in the year, volume, issue, and page numbering of a journal. A **monograph**, such as a book on a specific subject, a record of conference proceedings, or a pamphlet, usually is a one-time publication and may be updated with a new edition. Periodicals and monographs are available in a variety of media, such as print, on-line, or CD-ROM.

Theoretical and Data-based Literature

Theoretical literature includes concept analyses, models, theories, and conceptual frameworks that support a selected research problem and purpose. Theoretical sources can be found in periodicals and monographs. In a published study, theoretical and conceptual sources are described and summarized to reflect the current understanding of the research problem and to provide a basis for the study framework. **Data-based literature** consists of reports of research and includes published studies, usually in journals or books, and unpublished studies, such as master theses and doctoral dissertations. Data-based publications are peer reviewed before being published. **Peer reviewed** means that scholars familiar with the topic of the research read the report and validate its accuracy and the appropriateness of the methodology used in the study. Thus, the paper is considered trustworthy. A **thesis** is a report of a research project completed by a postgraduate student as part of the requirements for a master's degree. A **dissertation** is a report of an extensive, usually original research project that is completed as the final requirement for a doctoral degree.

The data-based literature reviewed depends on the study problem and the type of research conducted. Research problems that have been studied frequently or are currently being investigated have a more extensive data-based literature than that available for new or unique problems. Descriptive studies usually are conducted in new areas of research, and fewer studies of this type are available for review than quasi-experimental or experimental studies.

Primary and Secondary Sources

The published literature includes primary and secondary sources. A **primary source** is written by the person who originated or is responsible for generating the ideas published. In data-based publications, a primary data-based source is written by the person(s) who conducted the research. A primary theoretical source is written by the theorist who developed the theory or conceptual content. A **secondary source** summarizes or quotes content from primary sources. Thus, authors of secondary sources paraphrase the works of researchers and theorists. The problem with secondary sources is that the author has interpreted the works of someone else, and this interpretation is influenced by that author's perception and bias. Sometimes errors and misinterpretations have been spread by authors using secondary sources rather than primary sources. Predominantly primary sources are cited in research reports. Secondary sources are used only if primary sources cannot be located or if the secondary source provides creative ideas or a unique organization of information not found in a primary source.

Purpose of the Literature Review in Quantitative Research

The review of literature in quantitative research is conducted to direct the planning and execution of a study. The major literature review is performed at the beginning of the research process (before the study is conducted). A limited review is conducted after the study is completed to identify studies published since the original literature review. The results of both reviews are included in writing the research report. The purpose of the literature review is similar for the different types of quantitative studies—descriptive, correlational, quasi-experimental, and experimental.

A quantitative research report cites relevant sources in its "Introduction," "Methods," "Results," and "Discussion" sections. The "Introduction" section uses relevant sources to summarize the background and significance of the research problem. The "Review of Literature" section includes both theoretical and data-based sources that document the current knowledge of the problem studied.

A quantitative study develops its "Framework" section (not always so labeled) from the theoretical literature and sometimes from data-based literature, depending on the focus of the study. The "Methods" section of the research report describes the design, sample, measurement methods, treatment, and data collection process. Information from the literature review may be cited in various parts of the "Methods" section to validate the methods used in the study. The "Results" section compares the analysis of the data in the present study with the results of previous studies. The "Discussion" section of the research report provides conclusions that are a synthesis of the findings from previous research and those from the present study.

Purpose of the Literature Review in Qualitative Research

In qualitative research the purpose and timing of the literature review vary according to the type of study to be conducted (Table 5-1). Phenomenologists believe that the literature should be reviewed *after* data collection and analysis, so that the information in the literature will not influence the researcher's openness (Munhall, 2001). For example, if a researcher decides to describe the phenomenon of dying, the review of literature will include Kübler-Ross' (1969) five stages of grieving. Knowing the details of these stages can influence the way the researcher views the phenomenon during data collection and analysis. If the literature review is delayed until after the data have been collected and analyzed, however, the information from the literature can be compared with findings from the present study to determine similarities and differences, without any bias from preknowledge.

Grounded theory researchers include a minimal review of relevant studies at the beginning of the research process. This review is merely a means of making the researcher aware of what studies have been conducted, but the information from these studies is not used to direct data collection or theory development for the current study. The researcher uses the literature primarily to explain, support, and extend the theory generated in the study (Munhall, 2001).

The review of literature in ethnographic research is similar to that in quantitative research. The literature is reviewed early in the research process to provide a general understanding of the variables to be examined in a selected culture. The literature usually is theoretical, because few studies typically have been conducted in the area of interest. From these sources a framework is developed for examining complex human situations in the selected culture (Munhall, 2001). The literature review also provides a background for conducting the study and interpreting the findings.

Historical researchers conduct an initial literature review to select a research topic and to develop research questions. Then the investigator develops an inventory of sources, locates these sources, and examines them; thus, the literature constitutes a major source of data in historical research. Because historical research requires an extensive review of literature that is sometimes difficult to locate, the researcher can spend months and even years locating and examining sources. The information gained from the literature is analyzed and organized into a report to explain how an identified phenomenon has evolved over a particular time period (Munhall, 2001).

Table 5-1	Purposes of the Literature Review in Qualitative Research
Type of Research	**Specific Purpose**
Phenomenological research	Compare and combine findings from the study with the literature to determine current knowledge of a phenomenon
Grounded theory research	Explain, support, and extend the theory generated in the study
Ethnographic research	Provide a background for conducting the study, as in quantitative research
Historical research	Develop research questions and provide a source of data in the study

Critiquing the Literature Review in a Published Study

The "Review of Literature" section of a research report must be identified and critiqued for quality. The literature review might be a clearly identified section in the report or part of the introduction. A good-quality literature review logically builds a case for the study being reported. Thus, reading the literature review provides a basic understanding of the study problem and evidence that the study conducted was appropriate as indicated by the current knowledge of this problem. This section provides guidelines for critiquing the literature review in a published study and an example literature review critique.

Guidelines for Conducting the Critique

Critiquing the literature review of a published study involves examining the quality of the content and sources presented. A correctly prepared literature review includes what is known and not known about the study problem and identifies the focus of the present study. Thus, the review provides a basis for the study purpose and often is organized according to the variables in the purpose statement. The sources cited must be relevant and current for the problem and purpose of the study. The reviewer must locate and review the sources or respective abstracts to determine whether these sources are relevant. To judge whether all of the relevant sources are cited, the reviewer must search the literature to determine the relevant sources. This is very time-consuming and usually is not done for critique of an article. However, you can review the reference list and determine the focus of the sources, the number of data-based and theoretical sources cited, and where and when the sources were published. Sources should be current up to the date the paper was accepted for publication. (Recall that a current source is one published within five years of the date accepted for publication.)

Sources cited should be comprehensive as well as current. How comprehensive the list of sources is depends on whether the problem studied has existed for years or is relatively new. Some problems have been studied for decades, and the literature review often includes landmark studies that were conducted years ago. **Landmark studies** are significant research projects that generate knowledge that influences a discipline and sometimes society as a whole. Such studies frequently are replicated or serve as the basis for the generation of additional studies. For example, Williams (1972) studied factors that contribute to skin breakdown, and the findings from this landmark study provided the basis for numerous studies on the prevention, care, and treatment of pressure ulcers. As of August 13, 2005, a CINAHL search using the keywords pressure ulcer and study yielded 912 studies. Many of these studies have been synthesized to provide guidelines for the prediction, care, and prevention of pressure ulcers in clinical practice (Barczak, Barnett, Childs, & Bosley, 1997; Bergstrom et al., 1994; Cullum, Deeks, Sheldon, Song, & Fletcher, 2001; Harrison, Wells, Fisher, & Prince, 1996; Lewis, Pearson, & Ward 2003; National Pressure Ulcer Advisory Panel, 1989; Panel for the Prediction and Prevention of Pressure Ulcers in Adults, 1992; Pressure Ulcer Consensus Group 2000; Rutledge, Donaldson, & Pravikoff, 2000; Whittemore, 1998). These syntheses are the basis for evidence-based practice. As a nurse, you are now held accountable for keeping up with current research-based knowledge in your area of practice.

The usefulness of a study for research-based knowledge depends on the quality of the study. This quality begins with the literature review. Critiquing the literature review section of a published study often is difficult for students because they are less familiar with the topic than are the authors of the article. In addition, the literature review sections frequently are too concise to present the current knowledge on selected topics because the review often is reduced to comply with space limitations for publication (Downs, 1999a, 1999b).

CRITIQUE GUIDELINES   The Literature Review

Ask the following questions to assess the quality of a literature review in a study. Your instructor may provide additional questions to guide you in assignments requiring critiquing a review of literature.

1. Identify the primary data-based sources cited in the review. How did you determine that they are primary data-based sources? What references cited are primary sources but are not data-based? How did you determine that they are not data-based? Are secondary sources cited?
2. Are the references current? What years would be current for the study being critiqued?
3. Are relevant studies identified and described? What criteria did you use to determine whether the studies are relevant?
4. Are relevant theories identified and described? What criteria did you use to determine whether the theories are relevant?
5. Are relevant landmark studies described? How did you determine that the studies you identified are landmark studies?
6. Are relevant studies critiqued? Identify the critique statements made.
7. Are the sources paraphrased to promote the flow of the content presented or are there too many direct quotes? Quote three paraphrased statements from the article.
8. Is the current knowledge about the research problem described? How did you determine that the knowledge is current?
9. Does the literature review identify the gap(s) in the knowledge base that provides a basis for the study conducted? Provide the statements made by the author that identify the gap in knowledge.
10. Is the literature review clearly organized, logically developed, and concisely written? Justify your conclusion.
11. Does the literature review logically build a case for the study being reported? Why or why not?

A Sample Critique

The review of literature from Oh, Suh, Hwang, and Seo's (2005) study of the effects of nasogastric tube feeding on serum sodium, potassium, and glucose levels is presented as an example for use in performing a critique.

RESEARCH EXAMPLE A Literature Review

The purpose of Oh and colleagues' (2005) study was to "examine whether significant alterations in serum sodium, potassium, and glucose levels occurred after tube feeding with iso-osmolar formula in acute brain infarction patients" (p. 141). The literature review is presented on page 142 of the research article, and the references are on page 146.

BACKGROUND OR LITERATURE REVIEW

The beneficial effects of enteral feeding for stimulating the growth and motility of the gastrointestinal tract and reducing infections and metabolic complications have been reported (Kirby et al., 1995; Minard & Kudsk, 1998; Rhoney, Parker, Formea, Yap, & Coplin, 2002). However, many studies have shown that nasogastric tube feeding often produces feeding intolerance and other complications, such as nausea, vomiting, diarrhea, constipation, regurgitation, aspiration, nasal mucosa ulcerations, tube obstruction or displacement, and water and electrolyte imbalance (Cataldi-Betcher et al., 1983; Pancorbo-Hidalgo et al., 2001). As proposed by many researchers, however, the incidence of such gastrointestinal, respiratory, and mechanical complications can be reduced by improving nasogastric feeding methods, i.e., by giving a bolus injection with a syringe, gravity infusion, or pump-controlled infusion, or by administering gastrostomy feedings (Norton et al., 1996; Rhoney et al., 2002).

With respect to the electrolyte imbalances induced by tube feeding, two early case studies showed that serum electrolyte imbalances occurred by tube feeding (Kubo et al., 1976; Walike, 1969). Since then, various studies have indicated that electrolyte imbalance was serious enough to produce problems with consciousness, heart failure, neuromuscular over-stimulation, hyperreflexia, vascular collapse, and sometimes death in patients with stroke or other health problems.

The prevalent electrolyte imbalances reported after nasogastric tube feeding are hypernatremia, hyponatremia, hyperkalemia, and hyperglycemia (Cataldi-Betcher et al., 1983; Gormican et al., 1973; Pancorbo-Hidalgo et al., 2001; Vanlandingham et al., 1981; Walike, 1969). However Woolfson and colleagues (1976) showed that nasogastric tube feeding produced metabolic complications only rarely. Such inconsistency in results might be related to uncontrolled disease-related variables and relatively small sample sizes. Therefore, a more systematic analysis excluding the influences of other extrinsic variables was necessary. As a way to exclude disease-related variables, we limited the sample to ischemic stroke (brain infarction) patients so that the metabolic effects of disease or medications could be consistent among participants. (p. 142).

References (p. 146)

Bowman, M., Eisenberg, P., Katz, B., & Metheny, N. (1989). Effect of tube-feeding osmolality on serum sodium levels. *Critical Care Nurse, 9*(1), 22–28.

Cataldi-Betcher, E., Seltzer, M., Slocum, B., & Jones, K. (1983). Complication occurring during enteral nutrition support: A prospective study. *Journal of Parenteral and Enteral Nutrition, 7*(6), 546–552.

Davalos, A., Ricart, W., Gonzales-Huix, F., Soler, S., Marrugat, J., Molins, A., et al. (1996). Effect of malnutrition after acute stroke on clinical outcome. *Stroke, 27*(6), 1028–1032.

Gormican, A., Liddy, E., & Thrush, L. (1973). Nutritional status of patients after extended tube feeding. *Journal of the American Dietetic Association*, 63(3), 247–253.

Kirby, D. F., Delegge, M.H., & Richard, F. C. (1995). American Gastroenterological Association technical review on tube feeding. *Gastroenterology, 108*(4), 1282–1303.

Kubo, W., Grant, M., Walike, B., Bergstrom, N., Wong, H., Hanson, R., et al., (1976). Fluid and electrolyte problems of tube-fed patients. *American Journal of Nursing, 76*(6), 912–916.

Mazighi, M., & Amarenco, R. (2001). Hyperglycemia: A predictor of poor prognosis in acute stroke. *Diabetes & Metabolism, 27*(6), 718–720.

(continues)

RESEARCH EXAMPLE *(continued)*

Minard, G., & Kudsk, K. A. (1998). Nutritional support and infection: Does the route matter? *World Journal of Surgery, 22*(2), 213–219.

Norton, B., Homer-Ward, M., Donnelly, M. T., Long, R. G., & Holmes, G. K. (1996). A randomized prospective comparison of percutaneous endoscopic gastrostomy and nasogastric tube feeding after acute dysphagic stroke. *British Medical Journal, 312*(7022), 16–21.

Pancorbo-Hidalgo, P. L., Garcia-Fernandez, F. P., & Ramirez-Perez, C. (2001). Complications associated with enteral nutrition by nasogastric tube in an internal medicine unit. *Journal of Clinical Nursing, 10*(4), 482–490.

Rhoney, D. H., Parker, Jr., D., Formea, C. M., Yap, C., & Coplin, W. M. (2002). Tolerability of bolus versus continuous gastric feeding in brain-injured patients. *Neurological Research, 24*(6), 613–620.

Sheldon, G. F., & Baker, C. (1980). Complication of nutritional support. *Critical Care Medicine, 8*(1), 35–37.

Suchner, U., Senftleben, U., Eckart, T., Scholz, M. R., Beck, K., Murr, R., et al. (1996). Enteral versus parenteral nutrition: Effects on gastrointestinal function and metabolism. *Nutrition, 12*(1), 13–22.

Vanlandingham, S., Simpson, S., & Daniel, P. (1981). Metabolic abnormalities in patients supported with enteral feeding. *Journal of Enteral Nutrition, 5*(4), 322–324.

Walike, J. W. (1969). Tube-feeding syndrome in head and neck surgery. *Archives of Otolaryngology, 89*(3), 533–536.

Woolfson, A., Saour, J., Ricketts, C., Pollard, B., Hardy, S., & Allison, S. (1976). Prolonged nasogastric tube feeding in critically ill and surgical patients. *Postgraduate Medical Journal, 52*(613), 678–682.

CRITIQUE

Primary data-based sources include the following:

> Bowman, M., Eisenberg, P., Katz, B., & Metheny, N. (1989). Effect of tube-feeding osmolality on serum sodium levels. *Critical Care Nurse, 9*(1), 22–28.

A search of CINAHL for the article determines that it is an data-based because it is categorized by CINAHL as "clinical research." An abstract, which would provide even better information, is not provided for this reference.

> Cataldi-Betcher, E., Seltzer, M., Slocum, B., & Jones, K. (1983). Complication occurring during enteral nutrition support: A prospective study. *Journal of Parenteral and Enteral Nutrition, 7*(6), 546–552.

The title indicates that it is a study and thus a data-based source.

> Gormican, A., Liddy, E., & Thrush, L. (1973). Nutritional status of patients after extended tube feeding. *Journal of the American Dietetic Association*, 63(3), 247–253.

> Kubo, W., Grant, M., Walike, B., Bergstrom, N., Wong, H., Hanson, R., et al. (1976). Fluid and electrolyte problems of tube-fed patients. *American Journal of Nursing*, 76(6), 912–916.

This source is classified as a case study by Oh and colleagues.

> Minard, G., & Kudsk, K. A. (1998). Nutritional support and infection: Does the route matter? *World Journal of Surgery*, 22(2), 213–219.

This reference is not available in CINAHL. However, a search of MedLine located the reference. An abstract did not clearly indicate whether or not this was a study; however, MedLine classified it as a "comparative study." Thus, this reference is a data-based source.

Norton, B., Homer-Ward, M., Donnelly, M. T., Long, R. G., & Holmes, G. K. (1996). A randomized prospective comparison of percutaneous endoscopic gastrostomy and nasogastric tube feeding after acute dysphagic stroke. *British Medical Journal, 312*(7022), 16–21.

The title reveals the reference as a study and thus a data-based source.

Pancorbo-Hidalgo, P. L., Garcia-Fernandez, F. P., & Ramirez-Perez, C. (2001). Complications associated with enteral nutrition by nasogastric tube in an internal medicine unit. *Journal of Clinical Nursing, 10*(4), 482–490.

Whether or not it is a data-based source is not clear from the title or the name of the journal. A search of CINAHL identifies the reference with an abstract in which the author indicates that it is a report of a clinical study.

Rhoney, D. H., Parker, D., Jr., Formca, C. M., Yap, C., & Coplin, W. M. (2002). Tolerability of bolus versus continuous gastric feeding in brain-injured patients. *Neurological Research, 24*(6), 613–620.

The journal title indicates that only studies are published in this journal. Thus, it can be classified as a primary data-based source.

Vanlandingham, S., Simpson, S., & Daniel, P. (1981). Metabolic abnormalities in patients supported with enteral feeding. *Journal of Enteral Nutrition, 5*(4), 322–324.

MedLine search reveals this is a descriptive study.

Walike, J. W. (1969). Tube-feeding syndrome in head and neck surgery. *Archives of Otolaryngology, 89*(3), 533–536.

This study was classified by Oh and colleagues as a case study and thus is a data-based source.
All primary sources were data-based studies.
Secondary sources included the following:

Kirby, D. F., Delegge, M. H., & Richard, F. C. (1995). American Gastroenterological Association technical review on tube feeding. *Gastroenterology, 108*(4), 1282–1303.

The Oh et al. (2005) study was accepted for publication in 2004. Studies cited from 1999 to 2004 would be considered current. The following references are current by these standards: Pancorbo-Hidalgo, Garcia-Fernandez, and Ramirez-Perez (2001) and Rhoney, Parker, Formca, Yap, and Coplin (2002). This does not mean that studies published earlier are not important; rather, it indicates that the authors searched the literature early in their project to guide the planning of the study and added more recent relevant studies before completing and submitting their paper for review.

Relevant studies have a direct bearing on the current research project. Criteria used to judge relevance in this case include whether the studies addressed enteral tube feedings, and whether complications that occur as a result of the tube feedings, including metabolic imbalances, were examined. All of the studies included in the literature review met these criteria.

Theories were not addressed in the literature review.

Landmark studies have influenced a discipline and sometimes society. This influence may be that the study triggers the initiation of additional research and the building of knowledge that changes practice. Landmark studies are often the first study conducted to address a clinical concern. In this light, two studies cited in the literature review could be considered landmark studies: Walike (1969) and Kubo, Grant, Walike, Bergstrom, Wong, Hanson, et al. (1976).

The studies are critiqued; however, the critique statements do not address a specific study and are subtle. The critique included the following phrases: "uncontrolled disease-related variables," "relatively

(continues)

CRITIQUE *(continued)*

small sample sizes," and "failure to exclude the influences of extrinsic variables." These phrases indicate weaknesses in the studies that would limit the validity of their findings.

There were no direct quotes from previous studies; neither were there paraphrased statements from studies. Rather, the study findings from all of the cited studies were synthesized. Thus, the authors did not discuss individual studies but instead merged the findings from all of the studies to identify what is currently known in this field of research.

Current knowledge about the research problem was described. This was determined by conducting a search for studies on the topic published in the five years prior to acceptance of the article that were not cited by the authors. None were found. The authors cite Kirby, Delegge, and Richard (1995), who synthesized the studies conducted in this field of research. A search for a more recent review of research in this field was conducted, and none was found.

The gap in the knowledge base identified by the authors was the inconsistency in identification and severity of metabolic abnormalities occurring as a result of long-term tube feeding. The authors stated:

> ...[V]arious studies have indicated that electrolyte imbalance was serious enough to produce problems with consciousness, heart failure, neuromuscular over-stimulation, hyperreflexia, vascular collapse, and sometimes death in patients with stroke or other health problems.
>
> The prevalent electrolyte imbalances reported after nasogastric tube feeding are hypernatremia, hyponatremia, hyperkalemia, and hyperglycemia (Cataldi-Betcher et al., 1983; Gormican et al., 1973; Pancorbo-Hidalgo et al., 2001; Vanlandingham et al, 1981; Walike, 1969). However Woolfson and colleagues (1976) reported that nasogastric tube feeding produced metabolic complications only rarely in their study.

The literature is organized, logical, and concise. Oh and colleagues begin by discussing literature validating the advantages of enteral feedings, studies showing better methods of providing tube feedings, and documentation of complications of tube feedings. Next, they discuss the inconsistency in research findings related to complications. Then they indicate how their study will contribute to the body of knowledge.

IMPLICATIONS FOR PRACTICE

The following study findings merit consideration regarding clinical practice (Oh, Suh, Hwang, & Seo, 2005):

> The mean levels of serum sodium before and after tube feedings were within normal ranges in this study. (p. 145)
>
> After tube feedings the incidence of hyponatremia decreased, and normal serum sodium level and hypernatremia increased. (p. 145)
>
> Changes in the incidence rate of hypernatremia, hyponatremia, and normal sodium levels after tube feedings were not statistically significant. (p. 145)
>
> The high incidence of hypokalemia in our study could have been related to the hyperglycemia of participants; 93% of our sample were hyperglycemic before tube feeding began. (p. 146)
>
> Our results indicated that nasogastric feeding with iso-osmolar formulas did not significantly affect levels of serum sodium and potassium. However, most patients were hyperglycemic before

starting tube feedings, and the percentage of hyperglycemic patients remained high after tube feedings, indicating that hyperglycemia could be induced during the acute stages of brain infarction regardless of tube feeding. Although the mechanism of hyperglycemia has not been clarified, the need for controlling blood glucose level in patients receiving enteral nutrition is evident. (p. 147)

Performing a Literature Review

A background in reading research reports and critiquing the literature review sections of published studies should provide assistance during a review of the literature in an area of interest. This section focuses on reviewing relevant literature to generate a picture of what is known and not known about a problem and to determine whether the knowledge is ready for use in practice. For example, maybe you have noted that many hospitalized patients are elderly, and far too many of them develop pressure ulcers during their hospital stay. Reviewing the research literature might provide possible solutions for this practice problem. Reviewing the literature requires that you be able to (1) use the library, (2) identify relevant research sources, and (3) locate these sources.

Using the Library

This section provides you with information about libraries and some tips on using them. There are three major categories of libraries: public, academic, and special (Strauch, Linton, & Cohen, 1989). The **public library** serves the needs of the community in which it is located and usually contains few research reports. The **academic library** is located within an institution of higher learning. It contains numerous research reports in journals and books and provides access to many other sources on-line. Most academic libraries have an **interlibrary loan department**, which can be useful when you cannot find a particular research report. This department frequently can locate and obtain books, booklets, conference proceedings, and articles from other libraries within 1 or 2 weeks.

The **special library** contains a collection of materials on a specific topic or specialty area, such as nursing or medicine. Large hospitals, health care centers, and health research centers have special libraries that contain sources relevant to health care providers and researchers. The most comprehensive collection of national and international nursing literature is available at the Center for Nursing Scholarship in Indianapolis. Specialty libraries, such as those in hospitals, often have a librarian who will assist nurses in conducting a literature search.

The process of using a library and searching the literature has changed dramatically as the use of computers has increased. Today, good libraries provide access to large numbers of electronic databases that supply a broad scope of the available literature nationally and internationally. Thus, library users are able to identify relevant sources quickly and also to print full-text versions of many of these sources immediately. Photocopies can be made from journals held by the library, and photocopies of articles not otherwise available often can be obtained through Interlibrary loan arrangements between your library and other libraries across the country.

It may not even be necessary to go to a library to use the services you need. Authorized users can access many library services at any time and location by using the Internet. Library consultations, database searching, Interlibrary loan services, full-text article downloads, and more often are available to faculty and student researchers, even those who live far from the university. The Internet can provide a link to the university library, through direct modem connections and through e-mail.

Computers also are available for users within the library. However, each library's computerized resources differ. Written documentation usually will provide step-by-step explanations of how to use electronic resources. When you use library services for the first time, ask the library personnel for an orientation to services offered, or search for orientation material available electronically. Library personnel in the reference department are familiar with the library's collections and operations and can provide assistance in using the computers to access electronic resources, as well as indexes, abstracts, and reference materials in the library. Common **library sources** for research reports include journals, books, conference proceedings, master theses, and doctoral dissertations (Strauch et al., 1989).

Identifying Relevant Research Sources

Once a problem in clinical practice is identified, the literature can be searched for studies related to this problem. Before you begin searching the literature, you should consider exactly what information you are seeking. A written plan of the search strategy can save considerable time. The plan should include selecting databases to search, selecting keywords, locating relevant literature, and storing the references using reference management software. Several electronic searches, not just one, may be required to obtain the studies needed.

Selecting Databases to Search

A **bibliographical database** is a compilation of citations. A citation provides the information necessary to locate a reference. For example, the author's name, year of publication, title, journal name, volume number, issue number, and page numbers all are needed to find a journal article. A database may consist of citations relevant to a specific discipline or may be a broad collection of citations from a variety of disciplines. The most relevant nursing database is CINAHL, accessible at http://www.cinahl.com, which contains citations of nursing literature published after 1955. Another database commonly used by nurse researchers is MEDLINE. The National Library of Medicine provides free access to MEDLINE through PubMed, available at http://www.ncbi.nih.gov/entrez/query.fcgi. For a variety of reasons, including the cost of receipt and storage and convenience to library users, many libraries are discontinuing subscriptions to paper versions of journals and, instead, subscribing to services that provide access to electronic versions. Libraries subscribe to vendors that, for a fee, provide software, such as Silver Platter, OVID, EBSCOhost, and PaperChase, which can be used to access multiple bibliographical databases. **Full-text databases** of journal articles are now available for some journals. This means that you can conduct a computer search on a topic, get a list of citations, identify the citations that seem useful, and select the full-text option to read the text online, print it, or save it as a computer file. What a time saver! CINAHL now provides access to the full text of some articles.

Selecting Keywords

Keywords are the major concepts or variables of a research problem or topic. These terms will be what you key in to begin a search. In most databases, phrases can be used, as well as single terms. As relevant studies are identified, they can be reviewed for other terms to be used as keywords. Alternative terms (synonyms) for concepts or variables also can be used as keywords. Most databases have a thesaurus that can be used to identify keyword search terms. The thesaurus can be accessed by logging on to the database. Truncating words may allow you to locate more citations related to that term. For example, various authors may have used intervene, intervenes, intervened, intervening, intervention, or intervenor. To capture all of these terms, a truncated term, such as interven, interven*, or interven$ (the form depends on the rule of the search engine you are using), can be used in a search. Also consider irregular plurals, such as woman becoming the plural women, as search terms. If an author is cited frequently, a search using the author's name can be performed. If the author's name is used, the term needs to be identified as an author term, not a keyword term.

List each search term that is used in a documented search plan. As new terms are discovered, add them to the list. For each search, record (1) the name of the database that is used, (2) the date the search is performed, (3) the exact search strategy that is used, (4) the number of articles that are found, and (5) the percentage of relevant articles that are found. You can even develop a table to record this information from multiple search strategies (Table 5-2). Save the results of each search on your computer's hard drive, a floppy disk, "flash (memory) stick," or a "zip disk" for later reference. Be sure to write the file name of the saved search results in the search record.

Using Reference Management Software

Reference management software can make it considerably easier to track the references that have been obtained through searches. This type of software can be used to conduct searches and to store the information on all search fields for each reference obtained in a search,

Table 5-2	Written Search Record			
Database Searched	Date of Search	Search Strategy	Number of Articles Found	Percentage of Articles Relevant
CINAHL				
MEDLINE				
Academic Search Premier				
Cochrane Library				

including the abstract. Once this is done, all of the needed citation information and the abstract are readily available electronically when the literature review is written. As you read each article, you can insert any comments into the reference file.

Reference management software has been developed to interface directly with the most commonly used word processing software. With such tools, the reference information can be organized using whatever citation style you stipulate. Citations can be inserted directly into a paper with just a keystroke or two. The two most commonly used software packages, along with the websites with information about them, are as follows:

- ProCite: http://www.isiresearchsoft.com/pc/PChome.asp
- EndNote: http://www.endnote.com

A trial version of either software package can be downloaded from the website and used to write one or two papers. In this way, you can judge each program's effectiveness in helping track and cite references and decide whether to purchase it.

In addition, a relatively new product, RefWorks, is available on the Internet. It can be accessed at www.refworks.com. RefWorks does not require that you purchase software to install on your computer. Rather, it operates directly from the Internet. References can be imported directly from a bibliographical database by selecting desired items from the search, saving them in a file, and uploading them to RefWorks.

Locating Relevant Literature

Within each bibliographic database, a search is initiated by performing a separate search of each keyword that has been identified. Search engines are unforgiving of misspellings, so key in terms carefully, and double-check for spelling errors when results are unexpectedly sparse. Most databases allow you to indicate quickly where in the database records you wish to search for the term: in the article titles, journal names, keywords, formal subject headings, or full text of the articles. Citations usually are listed with the most recent ones first.

Most databases provide abstracts of the articles in which the term is cited, allowing you to get some sense of their content, so that you may judge whether the term is useful in relation to your selected topic. If an important reference is found, it should be saved to a file. If full text of the reference is provided, you can save a PDF or HTML version of the file.

At this point, do not attempt to examine all of the listed citations. Instead, merely note the number of citations, or "hits," that were found in the search. In some cases, the number of hits may be far too large for you to examine all of them. For example, in August 2005, a search of an on-line database using the keyword coping yielded 12,528 hits. The keyword phrase social support yielded 4520 hits.

After a search has been completed, save the results as a file, and record the number of citations; then perform another search using the next keyword, and so on. When you have completed this activity, you should have some sense of the extent of available literature in your area of interest. At this point, you also should have enough information to plan more complex searches.

Performing Complex Searches

A **complex search** combines two or more concepts or synonyms in one search. Selection of the concepts or synonyms to combine may be based on the results of previous searches. The method of performing more complex searches varies with the bibliographical database, so when a particular database is used for the first time, it is best to look for instructions and consider consulting a librarian.

In some bibliographical databases, the word and is used to combine terms. In some databases, AND must be in uppercase. Sometimes quotation marks must be placed around the concepts—for example, "coping and social support". In others, just typing coping and social support will find the references needed. While using CINAHL and OVID software, you can perform searches for individual terms and then initiate a complex search by selecting the "combine" option at the top of the screen. A new screen appears, listing the previous searches you have performed. You may select two or more of the previous searches to combine. For example, you might wish to combine the concepts of coping and social support. In August 2005, selecting the "combine AND" option in CINAHL for the coping search and the social support search yielded 963 hits.

Searches for some topics may reveal that many hits are not useful because the selected search term includes another subject that is of no interest. For example, you may want to examine studies of coping but not those discussing coping in relation to support. To eliminate references with the term *support*, use as your search phrase coping NOT support.

A number of other complex operations can be used to search databases, but the search methods described here will get you started. Instructions about how to use search options should be available in the database you are using. Some databases provide an advanced search option in which separate boxes are available for inclusion of multiple terms. For example, you might wish to include an author's last name, one or more key terms, and a journal title in a single search.

Limiting the Search

Several strategies may be used to limit a search if, after performing complex searches, you still have too many hits. The limits that can be imposed vary with the database. In CINAHL, for example, a search may be limited to English language articles. You can limit the years of a search. For example, a search might be limited to articles published in the last 10 years. Searches can be limited to find only papers that are research, are reviews, are published in consumer health journals, include abstracts, or are available in full text.

When the combined search for coping and social support, described in the last section, was limited to research papers in English, there were 828 hits. In CINAHL, a search can be limited by clicking on the icon above the search history labeled "limit." The icon figure is a bull's-eye with a red arrow. Limiting the search to research papers in English published between 2000 and 2005 yielded 382 hits. A search limited to research papers in English with full text available yielded 159 hits.

Based on the titles, the hits that seem most relevant to a topic can be selected by clicking the box to the left of the reference in the list of citations (OVID software). Then the citations that have been selected can be either printed or saved to a file. Saving the citation to a file and then printing it with a word processing program takes considerably less paper than trying to print directly from the database. The full-text option can be selected for hits with full text available. These papers can be either printed or saved to files for printing later or reading later on the computer screen.

Selecting Search Fields

A **search field** is one of the various categories of information provided about an article by the bibliographical database. The fields vary with the bibliographical database. In CINAHL, selecting the "Search Fields" option at the top of the search page allows you to choose the search fields that you would like to be listed for the references you select. The following list explains the search fields available in CINAHL:

> **Accession number.** The number that is assigned to the citation when it was entered into the CINAHL database.
>
> **Special fields contained.** List of the special fields available for a particular citation. Special fields include abstracts and cited references.
>
> **Authors.** Names of the authors, last name first, then initials of first names. Author names are in blue and underlined. The underlining indicates that clicking on the name will result in a search listing all of the citations in the database in which that individual is an author. This option allows you to identify other publications by authors who are central to building the body of knowledge of the topic you have selected to study.
>
> **Institution.** The institution(s) at which the author(s) was affiliated at the time the article was published. This information might be useful if you wished to contact the author.
>
> **Title.** Title of the article.
>
> **Source.** Journal title, volume number, issue number, page numbers, year, month, and number of references.
>
> **Abbreviated source.** Abbreviated version of the journal title, volume number, issue number, page numbers, year, month, and number of references.
>
> **Document delivery.** The National Library of Medicine (NLM) serial identifier number. This number is useful if you plan to request delivery of the document by fax, e-mail, or postal delivery. In many cases, there is a rather large fee for this service.
>
> **Journal subset.** The categories to which the journal has been assigned. For example, the journal may be classified as a core nursing journal, a nursing journal, a peer-reviewed journal, or a U.S. journal.
>
> **Special interest category.** The categories of specialization to which the journal has been assigned. For example, the journal may be classified in the category of Oncologic Care.
>
> **CINAHL subject headings.** The key words from the CINAHL thesaurus, which have been assigned to the article. Examination of these subject headings across the references obtained in a search can suggest additional keywords to be added to the keyword list.
>
> **Instrumentation.** A list of measurement instruments used in the study.
>
> **Abstract.** An abstract of the study.
>
> **ISSN.** The International Standard Serial Number, an identifier number for the journal.
>
> **Publication type.** The type of article. For example, journal article, research journal article, dissertation. Also indicates the presence of tables, graphs, and charts.
>
> **Language.** The language in which the article is written. In many cases, articles that are not in English have English abstracts.
>
> **Entry month.** The month in which the citation was included in CINAHL.

> **Cited references.** List of full references for all citations included in the paper. These references can be valuable because they allow you to cross-check the completeness of your computer searches.

Cross-check by comparing the database-cited references list from articles you have obtained with the list of citations obtained from your searches. This is very easy to do if you are using reference-managing software. In many cases you will find treasures that would have been missed if you had relied only on the computer search. Some of the references, which may not be journals or books listed in the databases that have been searched, may provide clues to other databases that might offer additional useful sources. These references suggest new keywords for another computer search in the databases you have been using.

Linking

Linking moves you from one website to another. In citation databases such as CINAHL, linking allows you to choose the underlined phrase full text and go directly to a full-text electronic version of an article. This is possible because a link has been established between the database and an archive of full-text journal articles. In the coming years, nursing databases will provide links from one electronic article to another and eventually to electronic books. This type of linking will allow the user to click on a citation in the text or the reference list of an electronic article and be connected directly with the full text of the referenced article. The time required to locate and obtain a majority of articles on a selected topic will be greatly reduced. Currently, multiple archives of full-text nursing journal articles are available, but the various archives are not interconnected. Efforts are under way to develop linking capabilities across databases (Barber, 2001).

Searching Electronic Journals

A number of new nursing journals have been developed that are published only in electronic form; such a publication is referred to as an electronic journal. Because of the high costs of publishing and distributing a printed journal, a publishing company risks losing money unless there is a very large market for the journal. Most of the electronic journals are targeted to relatively small specialty audiences. These journals may have more current information on a topic than can be found in traditional journals, because articles submitted by authors are reviewed and published in electronic journals within 3 to 4 months. For articles submitted to printed journals, the time from submission to publication typically is 1 to 2 years (Fitzpatrick, 2001).

Many electronic journals have been established at universities by faculty members interested in a particular specialty area. In some cases, subscribing to the online journal may be the only way to gain access to the articles. Some electronic journals are listed in available bibliographic databases, and full-text articles from the electronic journal can be accessed through the database. However, many electronic journals are not yet in the bibliographic databases or may not be in the database you are using. Ingenta (http://www.ingenta.com) is a commercial website that allows the search of thousands of on-line journals from many disciplines.

Relevant articles from an electronic journal can be obtained by first locating the journal on the Internet and then scanning the titles of the published articles. Many libraries have contracts with the vendors that enable their affiliated users to have off-campus access to some of these journals and databases. Some contracts require that nonaffiliated users use the resources only within the library. Still other contracts require that all use of the resources occur in the library or other specified buildings or terminals. A list of the current electronic nursing journals is available at the following Web addresses:

- http://www.nursefriendly.com/nursing/linksections/nursingjournals.html
- http://www.healthweb.org (select "nursing" from list)
- http://www.healthweb.org/browse.cfm?categoryid=1727
- http://www.medbioworld.com

Many libraries provide lists of the electronic journals available to their affiliated users. If you are affiliated with the library, you may be able to obtain articles quite easily.

Searching the World Wide Web

It is unlikely that studies relevant to a topic can be found by searching the Web using general search engines; however, you may find other relevant information. One advantage of information obtained from the Web is that it is likely to be more current than material found in books. One disadvantage is that the information is uneven in terms of accuracy. There is no screening process for information placed on the Web. Thus, a considerable amount of misinformation can be found, as well as some gems that might not be found elsewhere. It is important to check the source of any information obtained on the Web so that its validity can be judged.

A wide range of search engines are available for conducting Web searches. Search engines vary in the following ways: (1) the approach used to search the Web, (2) the extent of the Web that is covered (most do not cover the entire Web, so you may need to use more than one engine), (3) the frequency with which the search engine updates the websites that are indexed, and (4) the ease with which they are used. New search engines appear on the scene almost daily, so identifying the best search engine in this book would not be particularly useful. Many university libraries provide a list of good search engines.

When a promising site is found, its location can be stored in the Web browser (using features called "favorites" in Internet Explorer, Google, or Mozilla Foxfire). Remember, however, that if a website will be used as a reference in a bibliography, the date it was visited and the address (URL [Uniform Research Locator]) it had at that time are required for proper citation.

Storing a website address on a browser simplifies return visits to check information. Additionally, many websites frequently are updated and can be regularly checked for new information. Sometimes clicking on a link (underlined or highlighted name) on one website will reveal other websites with helpful information. Following these links—**surfing the Web**—is an important part of a Web search. Information overload is one problem that may be encountered during such a search; you may find too much information and need to be selective about what you retrieve.

Although Web browsers store a history of the websites you have visited as you move from one to another, it is wise to store their locations in the browser to avoid having to retrace the steps back through the links. Also, websites often are changed or deleted, so it is a good idea to save a particularly useful Web page as a file. Text, graphics, or both may be saved from the

Web. If space on your hard drive is a problem, a "zip" (file compression) program can be used to store the file in a smaller form.

Metasearchers offer relatively new approaches to searching the Web. These programs perform a search by using multiple search engines, enabling a single search to cover more of the Web. Currently, our favorite metasearcher is Dogpile, which can be found at http://www.dogpile.com. Dogpile uses an innovative strategy for searching that increases the number of hits on a topic.

Systematically Recording References

The bibliographical information on a source should be recorded in a systematic manner, according to the format that will be used in the reference list. Many journals and academic institutions use the format developed by the American Psychological Association (APA) (2001). The reference lists in this book are presented using an APA format. Computerized lists of sources usually contain complete citations for references and should be filed for future use. You also can easily search a computerized database with a computer and obtain complete reference citations.

Sources that will be cited in a paper or recorded in a reference list should be cross-checked two or three times to prevent errors. Damrosch and Damrosch (1996) have identified some of the common errors that authors make when applying the APA format, and these authors provide guidelines for how to avoid such lapses in style. The sources cited in the reference list should follow the correct format for print and on-line full-text versions, as follows:

PRINT VERSION
> Plawecki, H. M. (1996). Improving a manuscript's chances for acceptance. *Journal of Holistic Nursing, 14*, 3.

ON-LINE FULL-TEXT VERSION
> Plawecki, H. M. (1996). Improving a manuscript's chances for acceptance. *Journal of Holistic Nursing, 14*, 3. Available: OVID File: Periodical Abstracts Research II Item: 02993150.

Clarifying Evidence for Best Practices through Literature Reviews

The process of reviewing the literature in preparation for conducting a study involves careful critique of the methodology and an examination of the existing literature. Findings from each research report are clarified by the reviewer and then paraphrased. **Paraphrasing** involves expressing an author's findings clearly and concisely in the reviewer's own words. A new study is then designed to improve the methodology and to strengthen the **evidence for best practices**. In recent years, it has become increasingly urgent that the literature also be reviewed to define the state of the science in a given area of practice through integrated literature reviews and meta-analyses.

Integrated Literature Reviews: State of the Science

An **integrative review of research** is conducted to identify, analyze, and synthesize the results from independent studies to determine the current knowledge (what is known and not known) in a particular area (Ganong, 1987; Hearn, Feuer, Higginson, & Sheldon, 1999; Jadad, Moher, & Klassen, 1998; Smith & Stullenbarger, 1991). For example, a group of nurses on a nursing unit may find a need for an integrated review regarding a particular patient care problem. If a review cannot be found in the literature, it may be necessary to perform one specific to the needs of the unit. The results may be used to guide the development of a protocol for the procedure or to create a critical pathway tool.

The studies are selected for inclusion in the review on the basis of their quality and their relationship to a selected practice problem. Initially, therefore, the studies are read and critiqued. Then the studies that are of the highest quality are selected, and their purposes, methods, results, and findings are compared. It may help to develop a table that includes essential information from each study so that comparisons can be made (Table 5-3) (Martin, 1997). It also may help to identify the findings that are common among the different studies and to compare and contrast the outcomes of these studies. Table 5-4 was developed as an

Table 5-3	Synthesizing Studies to Generate a Review of Literature					
Author(s) and Year	Purpose	Sample	Measurement	Treatment	Results	Findings
Allman, 1991						
Bergstrom, Braden, Laguzza, & Holman, 1987						
Berlowitz & Wilking, 1989						
Braden & Bergstrom, 1987						
Harrison, Wells, Fisher, & Prince, 1996						
Norton, 1989						
Norton, McLaren, & Exton-Smith, 1975						
Okamoto, Lamers, & Shurtleff, 1983						

Table 5-4	Comparison and Contrast Study Findings on the Prediction and Prevention of Pressure Ulcers		
Author(s) and Year	Finding 1	Finding 2	Finding 3
Allman, 1991			
Bergstrom, Braden, Laguzza, & Holman, 1987			
Berlowitz & Wilking, 1989			
Braden & Bergstrom, 1987			
Harrison, Wells, Fisher, & Prince, 1996			
Norton, 1989			
Norton, McLaren, & Exton-Smith, 1975			
Okamoto, Lamers, & Shurtleff, 1983			

example, using the studies conducted on the prediction and prevention of pressure ulcers in adults. The next step is integrating the findings from all of the studies. The type of reasoning used during the integration of findings is synthesis. **Synthesis of sources** involves compiling the findings from all of the selected studies and analyzing and interpreting those findings. Finally, the meanings obtained from all sources are combined, or **clustered**, to specify the current state of research-based knowledge for a particular area of clinical practice. A number of integrated reviews of research have been written on pressure ulcer prevention.[*]

Expert researchers and clinicians have developed publications that summarize nursing knowledge on a variety of topics. In 1983 the first volume of the *Annual Review of Nursing Research* was published. The integrative reviews of research included in these annual publications cover relevant topics about nursing practice, nursing care delivery, nursing education, and the nursing profession. Integrative reviews also have been published in a variety of clinical and research journals. The international Cochrane Collaboration (http://www.cochrane.org) and the Agency for Health Care Research and Quality (http://www.ahrq.gov) commission

---

[*]Anthony, 1996; Armstrong & Bortz, 2001; Carlson & King, 1990; Cooper, 1987; Draper & Denis, 1996; Hedrick-Thompson, 1992; Land, 1995; Panel for the Prediction and Prevention of Pressure Ulcers in Adults, 1992; Rutledge, Donaldson, & Pravikoff, 2000; Witko, 1998; & Whittemore, 1998.

systematic reviews on critical areas of health care. The journal *Evidence-Based Nursing* also participates in identifying clinical research for practice (Sermeus & Vanhaecht, 2000).

Meta-analyses

Meta-analyses go beyond the integrated review by performing statistical analyses using summative findings from multiple published studies. Using these strategies, it is possible to provide a global estimate of such measures as the mean number of days of hospitalization after a particular procedure or the reduction in the number of hours a patient spends in a coronary care unit resulting from a particular nursing intervention. The results from meta-analyses sometimes are referred to as **benchmarking** (Rudy, Lucke, Whitman, & Davidson, 2001). Meta-analyses are discussed in greater detail in Chapter 13.

Writing a Review of Literature

A well-prepared literature review documents the current knowledge on a selected topic and indicates the findings that are ready for use in practice. Often a detailed outline is developed to guide the writing of a literature review. The review of literature begins with an introduction, includes a presentation of relevant studies, and concludes with a summary of current knowledge (Burns & Grove, 2005). The headings and essential content of a literature review are briefly described as follows:

1. **Introduction.** The introduction indicates the focus or purpose of the review; describes the organization of sources; and indicates the basis for ordering the sources—for example, from least to most important or from least to most current. This section should be brief and interesting enough to capture the attention of the reader. The introduction may need to be rewritten several times in the course of developing other sections of the literature review.
2. **Data-based literature.** Data-based literature includes quality studies that are relevant for a selected evidence-based project. For each study, the purpose, sample size, design, and specific findings should be presented, with a scholarly but brief critique of the study's strengths and weaknesses. This critique should be clear and concise and include only the most relevant studies. The content from these sources is best paraphrased or summarized in your own words. If a direct quotation is used, it should be kept short to promote the flow of ideas. Long quotations often are unnecessary and interfere with the reader's train of thought.

    Ethical issues must be considered in presenting research sources (Gunter, 1981). The content from studies must be presented honestly and not distorted to support a selected utilization project. The weaknesses of a study need to be addressed, but it is not necessary to be highly critical of a researcher's work. The criticism should be focused on the content, be related in some way to the proposed project, and be stated as possible or plausible explanations, so that it is neutral and scholarly rather than negative and blaming. Additionally, the researcher's works that are cited in the literature review should be accurately documented.
3. **Summary.** The summary includes a concise presentation of the research knowledge about a selected topic, including what is known and not known.

RESEARCH EXAMPLE   Quantitative Summary

The Panel for the Prediction and Prevention of Pressure Ulcers in Adults (1992) has summarized the research literature related to the prevention of pressure ulcers in adults. The following excerpt presents key information from the panel's summary of risk assessment tools and risk factors.

Risk Assessment Tools and Risk Factors

Goal

Identify at risk individuals needing prevention and the specific factors placing them at risk.

Bed- and chair-bound individuals or those with impaired ability to reposition should be assessed for additional factors that increase risk for developing pressure ulcers. These factors include immobility, incontinence, nutritional factors such as inadequate dietary intake and impaired nutritional status, and altered level of consciousness. Individuals should be assessed on admission to acute care and rehabilitation hospitals, nursing homes, home care programs, and other health care facilities. A systematic risk assessment can be accomplished by using a validated risk assessment tool such as the Braden Scale or Norton Scale. Pressure ulcer risk should be reassessed at periodic intervals. All assessments of risk should be documented.

Rationale

To prevent pressure ulcers, individuals at risk must be identified so that risk factors can be reduced through intervention. The primary risk factors for pressure ulcers are immobility and limited activity levels (Allman, compiled, 1991; Berlowitz & Wilking, 1989; Norton, McLaren, & Exton-Smith, 1975; Okamoto, Lamers, & Shurtleff, 1983). Therefore, persons with impaired ability to reposition themselves or those whose activity is limited to bed or any chair should be assessed for their risk of developing a pressure ulcer. To determine the magnitude of risk, the degree to which mobility and activity levels are limited can be quantified. Both the Norton Scale (Norton et al., 1975) and the Braden Scale (Bergstrom, Braden, Laguzza, & Holman, 1987; Braden & Bergstrom, 1987) assess these factors.

Other risk factors for pressure ulcer development include incontinence, impaired nutritional status, and altered level of consciousness. Incontinence is assessed by the Moisture subscale of the Braden Scale (Braden & Bergstrom, 1987) and the Incontinence component of the Norton Scale. Nutritional factors are considered indirectly in the General Condition component of the Norton Scale (Norton, 1989) and the Nutritional Status subscale of the Braden Scale. Altered level of consciousness is assessed by the Norton Scale Mental Condition subscale, and the Braden Scale Sensory Perception subscale.

Numerous risk assessment tools exist; however, only the Braden Scale and the Norton Scale (original and modified) have been tested extensively. The Braden Scale has been evaluated in diverse sites that include medical-surgical units, intensive care units, and nursing homes. The Norton Scale has been tested with elderly subjects in hospital settings.

The reported sensitivity and specificity of these risk assessment tools have varied greatly. This variability probably reflects differences in study settings, populations, and outcome measures. The degree to which preventative interventions have been implemented in response to the findings of the risk assessments in these studies may have also contributed to the variability in their reported performance.

Despite the limitations of the Norton and Braden scales, their use ensures systematic evaluation of individual risk factors. No information is currently available to suggest that adaptations of these risk assessment tools or the assessment of any single risk factor or a combination of risk factors predict risk as well as the overall scores obtained by the tools.

The condition of an individual admitted to a health care facility is not static; consequently, pressure ulcer risk requires routine reexamination. The frequency with which such reevaluations need to be done is unknown. However, if an individual becomes bed- or chair-bound or develops difficulty with repositioning,

(continues)

RESEARCH EXAMPLE *(continued)*

pressure ulcer risk needs to be assessed. Accurate and complete documentation of all risk assessments ensures continuity of care and may be used as a foundation for the skin care plan. (Panel for the Prediction and Prevention of Pressure Ulcers in Adults, 1992, pp. 13–15)

IMPLICATIONS FOR PRACTICE

Once you have read and summarized the research literature, you will need to make a decision about whether the available knowledge is adequate to make a change in clinical practice. For example, what changes would you make in your practice after reading the summary of research literature on risk assessment tools and risk factors for prevention of pressure ulcers? Research has shown that the Braden (Braden & Bergstrom, 1987) and Norton scales (Norton, 1989) are effective in assessing patients at risk for developing pressure ulcers. In addition, both scales have been effective in assessing pressure ulcer risk in the elderly. Both scales might be submitted to your agency so that the administration and staff can select one for use in practice. The next step involves developing a plan to change practice based on research. The process for using research findings in practice is the focus of Chapter 13.

RESEARCH EXAMPLE   Qualitative

Lutz (2005) provides a literature review in the published report of a grounded theory study entitled "Abuse experiences, perceptions, and associated decisions during the childbearing cycle." The study was funded by grants from the National Institute for Nursing Research (9F31-NR07336, T32-NR07061) and a Woodrow Wilson-Johnson & Johnson Dissertation Grant in Women's Health from the Woodrow Wilson National Fellowship Foundation. "An earlier version of this article was awarded the Carol A. Lindeman Award for a New Researcher from the Western Institute of Nursing, presented at the 37th Annual Communicating Nursing Research Conference on April 23, 2004, in Portland, OR, and published in the conference proceedings: Communicating Nursing Research, 37, 101, 103–109." (p. 802) A brief literature is provided at the beginning of the study.

The prevalence of IPA [intimate partner abuse] during pregnancy among clinic-based samples ranges from 0.9% to 20.1%, with the majority of studies reporting a prevalence range of 3.9% to 8.3% (Gazmararian et al., 1996). IPA in pregnancy is associated with IPA in the postpartum (Gielen, O'Campo, Faden, Kass, & Zue, 1994; Harrykissoon, Rickert, & Wiemann, 2002; Hedin, 2000; Martin, Mackie, Kupper, Buesher, & Moracco, 2001; Stewart, 1994). IPA may be initiated or escalate in pregnancy and can negatively affect maternal and infant outcomes, women's general health, and health services utilization (Campbell, Pugh, Campbell, & Visscher, 1995; Curry, Perrin, & Wall, 1998; Dye, Tolliver, Lee, & Kenney, 1995; McFarlane, Parker, & Soeken, 1995). IPA may also be a significant risk factor for maternal mortality (Krulewitch, Pierre-Louis, de Leon-Gomez, Guy, & Green, 2001). The risk of being a victim of an attempted or completed homicide was at least 3 times higher for women abused in pregnancy in a multicenter study (McFarlane, Campbell, Sharps, & Watson, 2002).

Extant knowledge regarding IPA during pregnancy has been gained primarily through quantitative investigations focused on the incidence and prevalence of, correlates of, and maternal and infant health outcomes. Qualitative studies have revealed the complexities, contradictions, and meanings associated with

IPA (e.g., Brown, 1997; Campbell, Rose, Kub, & Nedd, 1998; Davis, 2002; Draucker & Madsen, 1999; Kearney, 2001; Landenburger, 1989; Merritt-Gray & Wuest, 1995; Moss, Pitula, Campell, & Halstead, 1997; Smith et al., 1995; Ulrich, 1991). Women's response to IPA has been depicted as a complex process with incremental alterations in perception. Reasons women gave for their partners' violence during pregnancy have also been explored (Campbell, Oliver, & Bullock, 1998). Four themes were identified: jealousy of the unborn child, pregnancy-specific violence not directed toward the unborn child, anger toward the unborn child, and anger against the woman or "business as usual." Campbell, Oliver, et al., (1998) suggested that women's attributions for IPA provide important information about women's risk, the risk for child abuse, and the presence of self-blame. Researchers have also studied women's understanding of IPA during the childbearing period, experiencing the phenomenon as loss of self, being controlled, and destruction (McCosker, Barnard, & Gerber, 2003) (Lutz, 2005, pp. 803–804).

Following a presentation of the study methods and findings, the discussion section relates the study findings to those of previous studies.

This investigation revealed the unique interrelationship between IPA and the childbearing cycle, supporting the findings of McCosker et al. (2003) that pregnancy cannot be considered solely as a time frame for studying IPA but must be viewed as a continuum in which abuse and childbearing coexist. Participants' focus on constructing a family influenced their perceptions of IPA and decision making regarding the abusive relationship and disclosing abuse. Despite IPA, the childbearing cycle strengthened bonds to the intimate male partner and commitment to family and imbued women with new hopes and dreams for the idealized family—normal components of maternal-role acquisition (Mercer, 1995; Rubin, 1984). Pregnancy was also seen as something to be endured and left many feeling trapped in the abusive relationship.

As found in other studies (Landenburger, 1989, 1993; Merritt-Gray & Wuest, 1995; Moss et al., 1997; Smith et al., 1995), IPA negatively affected women's self-image. The process of becoming a mother and forming a maternal identity was also negatively affected. Because of IPA, women perceived their experiences during the childbearing cycle as differing from accepting sociocultural mores. The discrepancy between personal experience and sociocultural myths and expectations left women feeling isolated, disappointed, saddened, embarrassed, ashamed, and stigmatized. Interventions such as encouraging a pregnant woman to leave or take steps toward leaving an abusive relationship contradict the process of becoming a mother and may ultimately intensify feelings of stigma and shame for women who are abused.

Studies have described the complex process that women go through to make sense of IPA and leave or change an abusive relationship (Brown, 1997; Campbell, Rose, et al., 1998; Fishwick, 1993; Landenburger, 1989, 1993; Merritt-Gray & Wuest, 1995; Ulrich, 1991). The current study revealed that the childbearing cycle adds more complexity to this process because of divergent expectations concerning pregnancy and IPA. The childbearing cycle compounded the stigma associated with IPA, intensified embarrassment, and compelled participants to guard their status as a woman who was abused. Pregnancy imbued women with hope that IPA would cease and resolve to stay in the relationship for their family. As found in other studies (Hassouneh-Phillips, 2001; Kearney, 2001; Moss et al., 1997), cultural, social, and religious values and expectations strongly influenced women's perceptions of the risks and costs of IPA. The sociocultural or religious group often conveyed sanctions against leaving a relationship, which underscores the importance of understanding a woman's sociocultural background.

According to participants in this investigation, certain events significantly altered the way in which the abusive relationship was perceived. Although severity of partner's abuse and property damage, serious injury, or a more serious type of physical abuse were described by Campbell, Rose, et al. (1998) as distinct pivotal event, in the current study, those events were subsumed under the label *perceived increased dangerousness*. Data also indicate that the period after birth up to 2 years later significantly altered women's

(continues)

RESEARCH EXAMPLE *(continued)*

perception of an abusive relationship. As suggested by Martin and colleagues (2001), these data support the idea that IPA assessment and intervention could be conducted with mothers in pediatric settings as part of routine pediatric care in the first 2 years of a child's life." (Lutz, 2005, pp. 820-821)

References

Brown, J. (1997). Working toward freedom from violence: The process of change in battered women. *Violence Against Women, 3*(1), 5-26.

Campbell, J. C., Oliver, C. E., & Bullock, L. C. F. (1998). The dynamics of battering during pregnancy: Women's explanations of why. In J. C. Campbell (Ed.), *Empowering survivors of abuse: Health care for battered women and their children* (Vol. 10, pp. 81-89). Thousand Oaks, CA: Sage.

Campbell, J. C., Pugh, I. C., Campbell, D., & Visscher, M. (1995). The influence of abuse on pregnancy intention. *Women's Health Issues, 5*(4), 214-223.

Campbell, J., Rose, L., Kub, J., & Nedd, D. (1998). Voices of strength and resistance: A contextual and longitudinal analysis of women's responses to battering. *Journal of Interpersonal Violence, 13*(6), 734-762.

Curry, M. A., Perrin, N., & Wall, E. (1998). Effects of abuse on maternal complications and birth weight in adult and adolescent women. *Obstetrics & Gynecology, 92*(4), 530-534.

Davis, R. E. (2002). Leave-taking experiences in the lives of abused women. *Clinical Nursing Research, 11*(3), 285-305.

Draucker, C. B., & Madsen, C. (1999). Women dwelling with violence. *Image: Journal of Nursing Scholarship, 31*(4), 327-332.

Dye, T. D., Tolliver, N. J., Lee, R. V., & Kenney, C. J. (1995). Violence, pregnancy and birth outcome in Appalachia. *Paediatric and Perinatal Epidemiology, 9*(1), 35-47.

Fishwick, N. J. (1993). Health care encounters of women in abusive relationships: A process of protecting personal integrity. Unpublished doctoral dissertation, Case Western Reserve University, St. Louis, MO.

Gazmararian, J. A., Lazorick, S., Spitz, A. M., Ballard, T. J., Saltzman, L. E., & Marks, J. S. (1996). Prevalence of violence against pregnant women. *JAMA: Journal of the American Medical Association, 275*(24), 1915-1920.

Gielen, A. C., O'Campo, P. J., Faden, R. R., Kass, N. E., & Zue, Z. (1994). Interpersonal conflict and physical violence during the childbearing year. *Social Science & Medicine, 39*(6), 781-787.

Harrykissoon, S. D., Rickert, V. I., & Wiemann, C. M. (2002). Prevalence and patterns of initimate partner violence among adolescent mothers during the postpartum period. *Archives of Pediatrics & Adolescent Medicine, 156*(4), 325-330.

Hassouneh-Phillips, D. (2001). American Muslim women's experiences of leaving abusive relationships. *Health Care for Women International, 22*(4), 415-432.

Hedin, L. W. (2000). Postpartum, also a risk period for domestic violence. *European Journal of Obstetrics & Gynecology & Reproductive Biology, 89*(1), 41-45.

Kearney, M. H. (2001). Enduring love: A grounded formal theory of women's experience of domestic violence. *Research in Nursing & Health, 24*(4), 270-282.

Krulewitch, C. J., Pierre-Louis, M. L., de Leon-Gomez, R., Guy, R., & Green, R. (2001). Hidden from view: Violent deaths among pregnant women in the District of Columbia, 1988-1996. *Journal of Midwifery and Women's Health, 46*(1), 4-10.

Landenburger, K. M. (1989). A process of entrapment in and recovery from an abusive relationship. *Issues in Mental Health Nursing, 10*(3/4), 209-227.

Landenburger, K. M. (1993). Exploration of women's identity: Clinical approaches with abused women. *AWHONN's Clinical Issues in Perinatal and Women's Health Nursing, 4*(3), 378-384.

Martin, S. L., Mackie, L., Kupper, L. L., Buesher, P. A., & Moracco, K. E. (2001). Physical abuse of women before, during, and after pregnancy. *Journal of the American Medical Association, 285*(12), 1581-1584.

McCosker, H., Barnard, A., & Gerber, R. (2003). A phenomenographic study of women's experiences of domestic violence during the childbearing years. *Online Journal of Issues in Nursing.* Retrieved September 21, 2004, from www.ana.org/OJIN/topic17/tpc17_6.htm

McFarlane, J., Campbell, J. C., Sharps, P., & Watson, K. (2002). Abuse during pregnancy and femicide: Urgent implications for women's health. *Obstetrics & Gynecology, 100*(1), 27-36.

McFarlane, Parker, B., & Soeken, K. (1995). Abuse during pregnancy: Frequence, severity, perpetrator, and risk factors of homicide. *Public Health Nursing, 12*(5), 284-289.

Mercer, R. T. (1995). *Becoming a mother.* New York: Springer.

Merritt-Gray, M., & Wuest, J. (1995). Counteracting abuse and breaking free: The process of leaving through women's voices. *Health Care for Women International, 16*(5), 399-412.

Moss, V. A., Pitula, C. R., Campbell, J. C., & Halstead, L. (1997). The experience of terminating an abusive relationship from an Anglo and African American perspective: A qualitative descriptive study. *Issues in Mental Health Nursing, 18*(5), 433-454.

Rubin, R. (1984). *Maternal identity and the maternal experience.* New York: Springer.

Smith, P. H., Tessaro, I., & Earp, J. A. L. (1995). Women's experiences with battering: A conceptualization from qualitative research. *Women's Health Issues, 5*(4), 173-182.

Stewart, D. E. (1994). Incidence of postpartum abuse in women with a history of abuse during pregnancy. *Canadian Medical Association Journal, 151*(1), 1601-1604.

Ulrich, Y. C. (1991). Women's reasons for leaving abusive spouses. *Health Care for Women International, 12*(4), 465-473.

Are there ways in which this study might influence your practice in situations involving abused pregnant women? Is it important information to share with colleagues who might be caring for abused pregnant women?

KEY CONCEPTS

- The review of literature in a research report is a summary of current knowledge about a particular practice problem and includes what is known and not known about this problem.
- The literature is reviewed to summarize knowledge for use in practice or to provide a basis for conducting a study.
- Through the use of electronic databases, a large volume of references can be located quickly.
- Keywords are the major concepts or variables that must be included in a search.
- A search should be initiated by performing a separate search of each keyword that has been identified.
- Reference management software should be used to track the references obtained through the searches.
- The literature review usually begins with an introduction, includes data-based sources, and concludes with a summary of current knowledge.

TIPS FOR FURTHER STUDY

- If you have difficulty differentiating between a primary and secondary source, practice by completing the "Making Connections" Primary and Secondary Sources page of your *Study Guide*, Chapter 5.
- Do you need practice selecting databases to search? Consult the Resources Appendix on http://www.evolve/Burns/understanding.

REFERENCES

Allman, R. M. (1991). Pressure ulcers among bedridden hospitalized elderly. Division of Gerontology/Geriatrics, University of Alabama at Birmingham. Unpublished data compiled.

American Psychological Association. (2001). *Publication manual of the American Psychological Association* (5th ed.). Washington, DC: Author.

Anthony, D. (1996). The treatment of decubitus ulcers: A century of misinformation in the textbooks. *Journal of Advanced Nursing, 24*(2), 309–316.

Armstrong, D., & Bortz, P. (2001). An integrative review of pressure relief in surgical patients. *AORN Journal, 73*(3), 645, 647–648.

Barber, D. (April, 2001). A guide to electronic journal archives. *Online Journal of Issues in Nursing, 5*(11), Manuscript 7. Retrieved February 19, 2002, from http://www. nursingworld.org/ojin/topic11_7.htm

Barczak, C. A., Barnett, R. I., Childs, E. J., & Bosley, L. M. (1997). Fourth national pressure ulcer prevalence survey. *Advances in Wound Care, 10*(4), 18–26.

Bergstrom, N., et al. (1994). *Treatment of pressure ulcers.* Clinical Practice Guideline No. 15. AHCPR Publication No. 95-0652. Rockville, MD: Agency for Health Care Policy and Research, Public Health Service, U.S. Department of Health and Human Services.

Bergstrom, N., Braden, B. J., Laguzza, A., & Holman, V. (1987). The Braden Scale for predicting pressure sore risk. *Nursing Research, 36*(4), 205–210.

Berlowitz, D. R., & Wilking, S. V. (1989). Risk factors for pressure sores. A comparison of cross-sectional and cohort-derived data. *Journal of the American Geriatrics Society, 37*(11), 1043–1050.

Braden, B., & Bergstrom, N. (1987). A conceptual schema for the study of the etiology of pressure sores. *Rehabilitation Nursing, 12*(1), 8–12.

Burns, N., & Grove, S. K. (2005). *The practice of nursing research: Conduct, critique, and utilization* (5th ed.). Philadelphia: Saunders.

Carlson, C. E., & King, R. B. (1990). Prevention of pressure sores. In J. J. Fitzpatrick, R. L. Taunton, & J. O. Benoliel (Eds.), *Annual review of nursing research* (Vol. 8, pp. 35–36). New York: Springer.

Cooper, D. M. (1987). Pressure ulcers: Unpublished research 1976-1986: Process to outcome. *Nursing Clinics of North America, 22*(2), 475–492.

Cullum, N., Deeks, J., Sheldon, T. A., Song, F., & Fletcher, A. W. (2001). Beds, mattresses and cushions for pressure sore prevention and treatment. *The Cochrane Library (Oxford), 2*(20), 1–10.

Damrosch, S., & Damrosch, G. D. (1996). Methodology corner. Avoiding common mistakes in APA style: The briefest of guidelines. *Nursing Research, 45*(6), 331–333.

Downs, F. S. (1999a). How much is enough? *Applied Nursing Research, 12*(3), 164–165.

Downs, F. S. (1999b). How to cozy up to a research report. *Applied Nursing Research, 12*(4), 215–216.

Draper, S., & Denis, N. (1996). Preventing heel pressure ulcers: A review of studies evaluating body support surfaces and heel devices. *Orthoscope, 2*(3), 5–6.

Fitzpatrick, J. J. (2001). Scholarly publishing: Current issues of cost and quality, fueled by the rapid expansion of electronic publishing. *Applied Nursing Research, 14*(1), 1–2.

Ganong, L. H. (1987). Integrative reviews of nursing research. *Research in Nursing & Health, 10*(1), 1–11.

Gunter, L. (1981). Literature review. In S. D. Krampitz & N. Pavlovich (Eds.), *Readings for nursing research* (pp. 11–16). St. Louis: Mosby.

Harrison, M. B., Wells, G., Fisher, A., & Prince, M. (1996). Practice guidelines for the prediction and prevention of pressure ulcers: Evaluating the evidence. *Applied Nursing Research, 9*(1), 9–17.

Hearn, J., Feuer, D., Higginson, I. J., & Sheldon, T. (1999). Issues in research: Systematic reviews. *Palliative Medicine, 13*(1), 75–80.

Hedrick-Thompson, J. K. (1992). A review of pressure reduction device studies. *Journal of Vascular Nursing, 10*(4), 3–5.

Jadad, A. R., Moher, D., & Klassen, T. P. (1998). Guides for reading and interpreting systematic reviews. *Archives of Pediatrics and Adolescent Medicine, 152*(8), 812–817.

Kübler-Ross, E. (1969). *On death and dying.* New York: Macmillan.

Land, L. (1995). A review of pressure damage prevention strategies. *Journal of Advanced Nursing, 22*(2), 329–337.

Landis, E. (1930). Micro-injection studies of capillary blood pressure in human skin. *Heart, 15,* 209–278.

Lewis, M., Pearson, A., & Ward, C. (2003). Pressure ulcer prevention and treatment: Transforming research findings into consensus based clinical guidelines. *International Journal of Nursing Practice, 9*(2), 92–102.

Lutz, (2005).

Martin, P. A. (1997). Ask an expert: Writing a useful literature review for a quantitative research project. *Applied Nursing Research, 10*(3), 159–162.

Munhall, P. L. (2001). *Nursing research: A qualitative perspective* (3rd ed.). Boston: Jones and Bartlett.

National Pressure Ulcer Advisory Panel (1989). *Pressure ulcers: Incidence, economics, risk assessment. Consensus development conference statement.* West Dundee, IL: S-N Publications.

Norton, D. (1989). Calculating the risk: Reflections on the Norton Scale. *Decubitus, 2*(3), 24–31.

Norton, D., McLaren, R., & Exton-Smith, A. N. (1975). *An investigation of geriatric nursing problems in hospital.* Edinburgh: Churchill Livingstone.

Oh, H., Suh, Y., Hwang, S., & Seo, W. (2005). Effects of nasogastric tube feeding on serum sodium, potassium, and glucose levels. *The Journal of Nursing Scholarship, 37*(2), 141–147.

Okamoto, G. A., Lamers, J. V., & Shurtleff, D. B. (1983). Skin breakdown in patients with myelomeningocele. *Archives of Physical Medicine Rehabilitation, 64*(1), 20–23.

Panel for the Prediction and Prevention of Pressure Ulcers in Adults. (1992). *Pressure ulcers in adults: Prediction and prevention.* Clinical practice guidelines. AHCPR Publication No. 92 047. Rockville, MD: Agency for Health Care Policy and Research, Public Health Service, U.S. Department of Health and Human Services.

Pinch, W. J. (1995). Synthesis: Implementing a complex process. *Nurse Educator, 20*(1), 34–40.

Pressure Ulcer Consensus Group (2000). *Pressure ulcer prevention guidelines.* Glasgow: Author.

Rudy, E. B., Lucke, J. F., Whitman, G. R., & Davidson, L. J. (2001). Benchmarking patient outcomes. *The Journal of Nursing Scholarship, 33*(2), 185–189.

Rutledge, D. N., Donaldson, N. E., & Pravikoff, D. S. (2000). Protection of skin integrity: Progress in pressure ulcer prevention since the AHCPR 1992 guideline. *Online Journal of Clinical Innovations, 3*(5), 1–67.

Sermeus, W., & Vanhaecht, K. (2000). WISECARE to support evidence in practice. *Applied Nursing Research, 13*(3), 159–161.

Smith, M. C., & Stullenbarger, E. (1991). A prototype for integrative review and meta-analysis of nursing research. *Journal of Advanced Nursing, 16*(11), 1272–1283.

Stoneberg, C., Pitcock, N., & Myton, C. (1986). Pressure sores in the homebound: One solution. *American Journal of Nursing, 86*(4), 426–428.

Strauch, K., Linton, R., & Cohen, C. (1989). *Library research guide to nursing: Illustrated search strategy and sources.* Ann Arbor, MI: Pierian Press.

Whittemore, R. (1998). Pressure-reduction support surfaces: A review of the literature. *Journal of Wound, Ostomy, and Continence Nursing, 25*(1), 6–25.

Williams, A. (1972). A study of factors contributing to skin breakdown. *Nursing Research, 21*(3), 238–243.

Witko, A. (1998). A review of the literature on pressure-reduction support surfaces: Something is missing. *Journal of Wound, Ostomy, and Continence Nursing, 25*(4), 177.

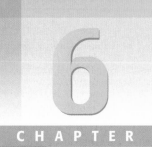

Understanding Theory and Research Frameworks

Chapter Overview

Learning Outcomes

After completing this chapter, you should be able to:

1. Describe the purpose of study frameworks.
2. Identify the elements of a study framework: concept, relational statement, conceptual model, theory, and conceptual map.
3. Develop a conceptual map of a framework presented in a published study.
4. Critique the framework in a study.

Key Terms

STUDY TOOLS

Be sure to visit http://evolve.elsevier.com/Burns/understanding for additional examples and self-tests. Also, a review of this chapter's concepts and practice exercises can be found in Chapter 6 of the Study Guide for *Understanding Nursing Research: Building an Evidence-Based Practice*, 4th edition.

Theory is essential to research as the initial inspiration that impels the researcher to embark on a research venture. When an idea for a study emerges, the researcher has a theory about what the study outcomes will be and why. That theory may not be formally stated or even written, but it is nonetheless a rudimentary theory. If a researcher tells you about the ideas of a study, you may question the use of a particular variable, or ask why particular study outcomes are expected. The explanation you receive is an expression of the researcher's theory about the study.

Sometimes the researcher has read a relevant theory and may have used these theoretical ideas in clinical practice. The researcher may have read studies that tested that theory. In this case, the theory may have inspired the researcher to put the theoretical claims to the test.

As a researcher develops a plan for conducting a quantitative study, the theory on which the study is based is expressed as the study framework. The framework spells out the logic that the researcher is using in planning the study. When the study is carried out, the researcher can then answer the question "Was my theory correct?" Thus, a study tests the accuracy of theoretical ideas. In explaining the study findings, the researcher will interpret those findings in relation to the theory. A researcher conducting a qualitative study would conduct their study, and in examining the study results would ask questions such as "How consistent were my findings with my expectations" or "How consistent were my findings with the literature?" An outcome of a qualitative study is sometimes a theory that emerges from the study findings.

An important part of critiquing the quality of a study is to identify and evaluate the framework. Understanding the theory on which a study is based also will help you determine whether it is appropriate to apply the study findings to your practice.

To assist you in learning about theories and how they are used in research, this chapter discusses what theories are and how they are tested, how a framework is developed, which strategies can be used to identify the framework in a published study, and how frameworks should be critiqued.

What Is a Theory?

Disciplines (such as Nursing) use theories to organize their body of knowledge and to establish what is known about a phenomenon. Formally, a **theory** is defined as an integrated set of defined concepts and statements that present a view of a phenomenon and can be used to describe, explain, predict, and control that phenomenon.

Theories Are Abstract

Theories are **abstract**, rather than concrete. *Abstract* means that the theory is the expression of an idea, apart from any specific instance. An abstract idea focuses on more general things.

Concrete refers to realities or actual instances—it focuses on the particular, rather than the general. For example, the word *anxiety* represents an abstract idea; a family member's pacing in an intensive care waiting room is a particular instance and thus is concrete.

The abstract ideas in theories can be tested through research to verify that they hold true in a concrete reality. As you will see shortly, Walker (1992) demonstrated that the abstract idea of the mother bonding with her newborn infant within a few hours or days did not hold true in actual instances observed in studies.

In some cases, theories are generated as a result of research. The specific instances discovered during the study are used by the researcher to develop more abstract (or general) ideas about the phenomenon of interest. Selye developed his theory of stress (1976) through specific instances demonstrated in multiple studies. Because Selye was a physician, he used case studies as specific instances of the phenomenon he was describing. The specific instances discovered during a qualitative study often are used to generate theory. Critical thinking is required to generate theory, to test theory, or to relate concrete realities to abstract ideas.

Theories Guide Nursing Practice

Theories have been developed in nursing to explain phenomena important to clinical practice. For example, nursing has a theory of uncertainty in illness (Mishel, 1988), a theory of health promotion behavior (Pender, Murdaugh & Parsons, 2001), and a theory of mother-infant attachment (Walker, 1992). Sometimes nurses use theories developed in other disciplines, such as psychology or biology, and apply them to nursing situations. Although nurses use these theories to guide their practice, in many cases the theories have not been tested to determine whether the nursing actions proposed by the theory actually have the effects claimed.

In their theory of mother-infant bonding, Klaus and Kennell (1976) suggested that bonding between a mother and her newborn child occurred within hours or days of birth. They proposed that if skin-to-skin physical contact between mother and child did not occur during this short time frame, bonding would not occur, and the relationship between mother and child would be permanently impaired. Nurses leaped on this idea and focused intensely on ensuring that early physical contact occurred between mother and newborn. However, research testing this theoretical notion demonstrated that it was not true (Walker, 1992). Mother and newborn, although kept apart because of illness or other circumstances, were able to bond.

This example supports the contention that theories should not be applied to clinical practice without first testing the ideas through research. In this case a theory of attachment, based on long-term studies of mothers and infants, emerged. These studies found that development of an attachment between mother and child was indeed critical but that the process occurred over a period of months rather than days. These findings, expressed as the Theory of Attachment (Walker, 1992), guide nurses in their care of mothers and their children.

Conceptual Models

Conceptual models are similar to theories and sometimes are referred to as theories. However, conceptual models are even more abstract than theories. A **conceptual model** broadly explains phenomena of interest, expresses assumptions, and reflects a philosophical stance. A **phenomenon** (the plural form is **phenomena**) is an occurrence or a circumstance that is observed, something that impresses the observer as extraordinary, or a thing that appears to and is constructed by the mind. Caring is a phenomenon. You provide caring as part of your nursing practice. How do you explain caring in your nursing practice? You can give a specific example of your caring for a patient, but can you make clear what caring is? Watson (1985) has developed a conceptual model of caring that expresses her philosophy of caring in nursing. Swanson (1991) developed a middle range theory of caring that is based on research. You might be interested in determining whether your ideas of caring are more consistent with Watson's model or Swanson's theory.

Assumptions are statements that are taken for granted or considered true, even though they have not been scientifically tested. For example, a fairly common assumption is that people who *are* poor *feel* poor. Do you think this assumption is true? **Philosophies** are rational intellectual explorations of truths or principles of being, knowledge, or conduct. A **philosophical stance** is a specific philosophical view held by a person or group of people. For example, a philosophical stance might hold that there is no single reality—that reality is different for each person. What do you think?

Although conceptual models vary in their level of abstraction and in the breadth of phenomena they explain, they all provide an overall picture of the phenomena they address. Conceptual models generally are not considered testable through research. However, theories derived from a conceptual model can be tested.

Most disciplines have several conceptual models, each with a distinctive vocabulary. A number of conceptual models have been developed in nursing. For example, Roy's model (Roy and Andrews, 1999) describes adaptation as the primary phenomenon of interest to nursing. Their model identifies the elements they consider essential to adaptation and describes how the elements interact to produce adaptation. Orem (2001) considers self-care to be the phenomenon that is central to nursing. Her model explains how nurses facilitate the self-care of clients. Rogers (Rogers, Malinski, & Barrett, 1994) sees human beings as the central phenomenon of interest to nursing, and Rogers' model is designed to explain the nature of human beings. A conceptual model may use the same or similar terms as those of other models but define them in different ways. For example, Roy, Orem, and Rogers all may use the term *health* but define it in different ways. How would you define health?

Middle Range Theories

Middle range theories are less abstract and more narrow in scope than conceptual models (or grand theories). They tend to be more closely linked to clinical practice and research than conceptual models and thus have a greater appeal to clinicians and clinical researchers. Middle range theories may emerge from the review of studies for the purpose of building evidence-based practice related to a particular clinical problem. Middle range theories also can be used as the framework of a study, thus contributing to the validation of the middle range theory (Liehr & Smith, 1999; Peterson & Bredow, 2004; Smith & Liehr, 2003).

Table 6-1 lists some of the middle range theories currently being used as frameworks in nursing studies.

Table 6-1	Middle Range Theories
Theory	**Author(s) of Relevant Study**
Acute pain	Good, 1998
Acute pain management	Huth & Moore, 1998
Adaptation to chronic pain	Dunn, 2001, 2004, 2005
Adapting to diabetes mellitus	Whittemore & Roy, 2002
Affiliated individuation as a mediator of stress	Acton, 1997
Balance between analgesia and side effects	Good & Moore, 1996; Good, 1998
Bureaucratic caring	Ray, 1989
Caregiver stress	Tsai, 2003; Dethloff, 2004
Caring	Swanson, 1991
Caring through relation and dialogue	Sanford, 2000
Chronic pain	Tsai, Tak, Moore, & Palencia, 2003
Chronic sorrow	Eakes, Burke, & Hainsworth, 1998
Coercion in the development of behavior	Patterson, 1982
Community empowerment	Hildebrandt, 1994
Connecting in cyberspace	Hrabe, 2001
Critical analysis of disparity	Crist, 2002
Culturing brokering	Jezewski, 1995
Cultural competence	Purnell, 2005
Cultural negotiation	Engebretson & Littleton, 2001
Dyspnea	Gift, 1992
Empathy	Olson & Hanchett, 1997
Entry into nursing home as a status passage	Chenitz, 1983
Experiencing transitions	Meleis, Sawyer, Im, Messias, & Schumacher, 2000
Facilitating growth and development	Kinney, 1990
Fulfillment	Kylma & Vehvilainen-Julkunen, 1995
Grief	Chapman & Pepler, 1998
Hazardous secrets and reluctantly taking charge	Burke, Kauffmann, Costello, & Dillon, 1991
Health belief	Champion, 1985
Health promotion	Pender, 1987
Health promotion for preterm infants	Mefford, 2004
Health-related quality of life	Wilson & Cleary, 1995
Home care	Smith, Pace, Kochinda, Kleinbeck, Koehler, & Popkess-Vawter, 2002
Homelessness-hopelessness	Tollett & Thomas, 1995

Table 6–1	Middle Range Theories—cont'd

Theory	Author(s) of Relevant Study
Hope	Morse & Doberneck, 1995
Illness constellation	Morse & Johnson, 1991
Informed caring	Swanson, 1993
Inner strength in women	Marsh, Beard, & Bailey, 2002; Roux, Dingley, & Bush, 2002
Interaction model of client behavior	Cox, 1982
Interpersonal perceptual awareness	Brooks & Thomas, 1997
Language, conflict, and ethnolinguistic theory	Cargile, Giles, & Clement, 1995
Maternal role attainment	Mercer, 1986
Meaning in suffering	Starck & McGovern, 1992
Mother-infant attachment theory	Bowlby, 1969, 1973
Multidimensional load and tolerance model	Rumpt, 2002 (Dutch)
Needs-driven dementia-compromised behavior model	Algase et al., 1996; Collins & Buettner, 2002
Negotiating partnerships	Powell-Cope, 1994
Negotiating uncertainty	Duff, 2002
Nurse expressed empathy and patient distress	Olson & Hanchett, 1997
Nurse midwifery care	Thompson et al., 1989
Nursing intervention outcomes model	Kreulen, 1994
Parental problem solving	Myers, 2002
Peaceful end of life	Ruland & Moore, 1998
Perimenopausal process	Quinn, 1991
Personal risking	Hitchcock & Wilson, 1992
Planned behavior	Ajzen, 1991
Postpartum depression	Beck, 1993
Precarious ordering	Wuest, 2001
Prevention as intervention	August-Brady, 2000
Psychological adaptation	Levesque et al., 1998
Quality of family caregiving	Phillips & Rempusheski, 1986
Quality of life of stroke survivors	Fairfax, 2002
Resilience	Polk, 1997
Self-care of elderly	Backman, 2003
Self-care management for vulnerable populations	Dorsey & Murdaugh, 2003; Jenerette, 2004
Self-efficacy	Bandura, 1982, 1989, 1997
Self-regulatory model	Leventhal et al., 1997
Self-transcendence	Reed, 1991
Sense of coherence	Antonovsky, 1987
Social learning theory	Bandura, 1986
Spiritual care in nursing	Mahlungulu & Uys, 2004

(continues)

Table 6-1	Middle Range Theories—cont'd
Theory	**Author(s) of Relevant Study**
Stress, appraisal, and coping	Lazarus & Folkman, 1984
Symptom management	University of California, San Francisco School of Nursing Symptom Management Group, 1994
Testicular self-examination (TSE) adoption	Fessenden, 2002
The Double ABC-X Model of family adaptation	McCubbin & Patterson, 1983
The urine control theory	Jirovec, Jenkins, Isenberg, & Baiardi, 1999
Transtheoretical model	Prochaska & Velicer, 1997
Uncertainty	Mischel, 1991
Uncertainty of illness	Deane & Degner, 1998
Unpleasant symptoms	Lenz, Pugh, Milligan, Gift, & Suppe, 1997
Well-being in adults with diabetes mellitus	Casalenuovo, 2002
Women's anger	Thomas, 1991

Practice Theories—Intervention Theories

Practice theories are even more specific than middle range theories. They are designed to theoretically propose specific approaches to particular nursing practice situations. Comfort Theory (Kolcaba, 1994) is an example of a practice theory. Practice theory sometimes is referred to as prescriptive theory. One form of this level of theory is intervention theory. Such theories direct the implementation of a specific nursing intervention and provide theoretical explanations of how and why the intervention is effective in addressing a particular patient care problem. These theories are tested through programs of research to validate the effectiveness of the intervention in addressing the problem. In some cases, practice theory emerges from the guidelines that direct evidence-based practice. Now, researchers are conducting studies to examine the feasibility of implementing the guidelines that have emerged from synthesis of findings in the research literature.

An example of an intervention theory is Simple Pleasures, in which a nursing intervention is designed for provision to persons with dementia (Colling & Buettner, 2002). The ideas for the intervention emerged from a middle range theory, the Need-Driven Dementia-Compromised Behavior Model. This theory challenged the view that behaviors such as vocalizing, aggression, wandering, and passivity in persons with dementia were "disruptive" and reinterpreted them as being the result of an interaction of environmental triggers and relatively stable individual characteristics. The theory proposes that the environmental triggers can be changed, resulting in changes in the behaviors of the person with dementia.

People with dementia in nursing homes often spend 60% to 80% of their time with nothing to do. Family visits decrease as the dementia increases. Boredom and inactivity are environmental triggers that lead to "disruptive behaviors." Rather than intentionally being disruptive, the person with dementia attempts to create his or her own activity. This occurs because nursing homes and other dementia care facilities do not have the funds to provide social recreational items. The unmet needs prompt the behavior. Simple Pleasures prescribes an intervention that causes changes in the environmental triggers, thus altering the behavior of the person with dementia. Volunteers visit, bringing items that can be used to increase activities, and provide socialization. Volunteers create suggested items including purses with small items inside that stimulate the person with dementia to investigate the contents of the purse, play a tetherball game, use sewing cards, arrange flowers that have been provided, or push a cart designed for wandering. Studies using these prescribed activities have demonstrated a significant decrease in "disruptive behaviors."

Framework

A **framework** is a brief explanation of a theory or those portions of a theory to be tested in a quantitative study. Every quantitative study has a framework. This is true whether the study is physiological or psychosocial. A clearly expressed framework is one indication of a well-developed quantitative study. Perhaps the researcher expects one variable to cause the other. In a well-thought-out quantitative study, the researcher explains abstractly in the framework why one variable is expected to cause the other. The idea is expressed concretely as a hypothesis to be tested through the study methodology.

Unfortunately, in some quantitative studies, the ideas that compose the framework remain nebulous and vaguely expressed. Although the researcher believes that the variables being studied are related in some fashion, this notion is expressed only in concrete terms. The researcher may make little attempt to explain why the variables are thought to be related. However, the rudiment of a framework is the expectation (perhaps not directly expressed) that there may be one or more important links among the study variables. Sometimes, rudimentary ideas for the framework are expressed in the introduction or literature review, in which linkages among variables found in previous studies are discussed, but then the researcher stops without fully developing the ideas as a framework. These are referred to as **implicit frameworks**. In most cases, a careful reader can extract an implicit framework from the text. Unfortunately, many nursing studies have implicit frameworks.

In qualitative studies, the approach to theorizing proceeds somewhat differently. In grounded theory research, for example, the first step in the research process is to identify (through the development of substantive codes) the critical concepts and processes that characterize the phenomenon. Subsequent analysis identifies the critical links among those concepts and processes, leading to the development of a grounded theory. In descriptive phenomenology, a similar process is undertaken except that no theory is developed—rather the "essential structure" (a conceptual framework) is developed from the data.

As the body of knowledge related to a phenomenon increases, the development of a framework to express the knowledge becomes easier. Accordingly, frameworks for quasi-experimental and experimental studies, which usually have a background of descriptive and correlational studies, generally are more easily and fully developed than frameworks for descriptive studies. Descriptive studies often examine multiple factors to understand a phenomenon not previously well studied. Theoretical work related to the phenomenon may be tentative or nonexistent. Therefore, the framework may not be as well developed.

In some studies the framework is derived from a well-tested theory that has been used as the framework for many quantitative studies. Most theories used as nursing research frameworks are from other fields and are based on theoretical works from psychology (e.g., the theory of stress and coping [Lazarus & Folkman, 1984]), physiology (e.g., The Theory of Biological Rhythms [Luce, 1970]), and sociology (e.g., The Health Belief Model [Becker, 1976]). In other quantitative studies, the framework is developed from newly proposed theory. In nursing, new theories often emerge from questions related to identified nursing problems. Additionally, new theories may arise from clinical insight suggesting that a relationship exists between or among elements important to desired nursing outcomes. These situations tend to be concrete, and they require that the researcher, using critical reasoning, express the concrete ideas in abstract language. New theories also may be developed from conceptual models or from elements of existing theories not previously related.

Elements of Theory

The first step in understanding theories is to become familiar with the elements related to theoretical ideas and their application. These elements include the concept, relational statement, and conceptual map.

Concept

A **concept** is a term that abstractly describes and names an object or phenomenon, thus providing it with a separate identity or meaning. For example, the term *anxiety* is a concept. The concept is the basic element of a theory. A published study should include identification and definition of all of the concepts important to the framework. Two terms closely related to concept are *construct* and *variable*. In conceptual models, concepts have very general meanings and sometimes are referred to as **constructs**. A construct associated with the concept of anxiety might be emotional responses. At a more concrete level, terms are referred to as variables and are narrow in their definition. A **variable** is more specific than a concept. The word *variable* implies that the term is defined so that it is measurable and suggests that numerical values of the term are able to vary ("vari-able") from one instance to another. A variable related to anxiety might be palmar sweating, because a specific method exists for assigning numerical values to varying amounts of palmar sweat. The linkages among constructs, concepts, and variables are illustrated in the following diagram.

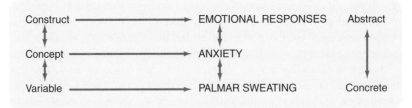

Defining Concepts

Defining concepts allows consistency in the way the term is used. A **conceptual definition** differs from the dictionary definition of a word. A conceptual definition is more comprehensive than a denotative (or dictionary) definition and includes associated meanings the word may have. A conceptual definition is referred to as connotative. Connotations of a term bring memories, moods, or images subtly or indirectly to mind. For example, a conceptual definition of *fireplace* might include the senses of hospitality and warm comfort that often are associated with fireplaces, whereas the dictionary definition is narrower and more specific: an open recess for holding a fire at the base of a chimney. Many terms commonly used in clinical nursing language have not been clearly defined. The use of these terms in theory or research requires thoughtful exploration of the connotative meanings that the terms have within nursing and a clear statement of their meaning within the particular theory or study.

The importance of going beyond the denotative, dictionary definition of a concept is illustrated in a study designed to explore the meaning of *caring* that was funded by the National Center for Nursing Research and conducted by Morse, Solberg, Neander, Bottorff, and Johnson (1990). The questions posed by these researchers illustrate the critical thought that must precede the development of a conceptual definition. Although the concept of caring is central to nursing, efforts to define it have been difficult. For example, the terms *caring*, *care*, and *nursing care* have different meanings. Caring may be an action such as "taking care of" or a concern such as "caring about." Caring may be viewed from the perspective of the nurse or that of the patient. The authors identified five categories of caring: (1) caring as a human trait, (2) caring as a moral imperative (ethically, one is obligated to provide it), (3) caring as an affect (feeling), (4) caring as an interpersonal relationship, and (5) caring as a therapeutic intervention. Caring has an effect on the subjective experience of the patient and on the physical response of the patient.

A number of questions about caring must be answered:

(1) "Is caring a constant and uniform characteristic, or may caring be present in various degrees within individuals?" (2) "Is caring an emotional state that can be depleted?" (3) "Can caring be nontherapeutic? Can a nurse care too much?" (4) "Can cure occur without caring? Can a nurse provide safe practice without caring?" (5) "What difference does caring make to the patient?" (Morse et al., 1990, pp. 9–11) Swanson and colleague's work (1991, 1993; Swanson, Jensen, Specht, Johnson, & Maas, 1997) has addressed some of these queries to clarify the conceptual meaning of care.

The authors' conclusion was that a clear conceptual definition of caring did not exist. The work of these authors generated considerable effort by others to develop further the conceptual definition of caring.

A related concept, *direct caregiving*, has been carefully examined by Swanson, Jensen, Specht, Johnson, and Maas (1997), who defined it to be " provision by a family care provider of appropriate personal and health care for a family member or significant other" (pp. 68-69). Caregiving addresses the care recipient's emotional, social, and physical needs. For direct caregiving to occur, the caregiver must have a sense of responsibility, filial obligation (in certain cases), adequate financial resources, good health, and family and relational/marital support. Social skills, spiritual support, the history of the relationship between caregiver and care recipient, and role acceptance also have been identified as important antecedents to direct caregiving (Swanson et al., 1977, p. 69).

Because of the significance of conceptual definitions, it is important that you identify the researcher's conceptual definitions of terms when you critique a study. In a quantitative study, each variable in the study must be associated with a concept, a conceptual definition, and a method of measurement. The links among the conceptual definitions, the variables in the study, and the related measurement methods are then determined. (These linkages are discussed in Chapter 4.)

CRITIQUE GUIDELINES Framework of the Study

The framework of a quantitative study must be critiqued within the context of the overall study. Therefore, use critical reasoning to critique the logical structure of the framework itself, and to address the following questions:

1. What are the concepts in the framework?
2. How are the concepts defined?
3. Are the conceptual definitions clear and adequate?
4. What are the variables in the study?
5. Is each study variable associated with a concept and its definition?
6. What measurement methods are used in the study?
7. Is each measurement method consistent with its associated concept and conceptual definition?

Critiquing a framework of a quantitative study requires that you go beyond the framework itself to examine its linkages to other components of the study such as measurement. To answer the previous questions, first extract the concepts and conceptual definitions from the written text in the introduction, the literature review, or the discussion of the framework. Then you must judge the adequacy of the definitions and the linkages of concepts to variables and their measurement.

RESEARCH EXAMPLE Extracting Concepts and Conceptual Definitions from a Published Quantitative Study

The following framework was extracted from a study by Schmelzer, Case, Chappell, and Wright (2000) entitled "Colonic cleansing, fluid absorption, and discomfort following tap water and soapsuds enemas." The study was published in *Applied Nursing Research*. Concepts have been circled and conceptual definitions have been underlined to show you how to identify and mark them in published studies. In physiological studies, some concepts may not be defined because their meanings are commonly held within the discipline. These are referred to as primitive concepts.

The ideal enema solution would effectively cleanse the colon with minimal side effects. The following sections describe the colonic cleansing mechanism and the dangers of excessive fluid absorption, rectal mucosal damage, and discomfort.

Colonic Cleansing

Enemas cleanse the colon by stimulating propulsion and secretion. Three major factors influence an enema's ability to stimulate defecation; enema volume, the presence of chemical irritants, and the osmolarity or tonicity of the solution (Wood, 1994). The instillation of a large fluid volume into the intestinal lumen stimulates propulsion; chemical irritants stimulate both propulsion and secretion to rapidly empty the colon (Chang, Sitrin, & Black, 1996). Hypertonic solutions such as sodium phosphate enemas stimulate defecation by drawing fluid from the body into the lumen of the colon through osmosis and by directly irritating rectal mucosa. To promote fluid absorption from the colon, hypotonic solutions are thought to slow propulsion (Chang et al., 1996; Wood, 1994). Because tap water, a hypotonic solution, does not irritate colonic mucosa (Niv, 1990), its effect must be the result of volume alone. Soapsuds solutions are also hypotonic, but both a large volume and chemical irritation stimulate defecation.

Few studies have addressed optimal enema volume and individual tolerance. Nursing texts recommend volumes ranging from 0.5 to 1 liter (Craven & Hirnle, 1996; Sorensen & Luckmann, 1986), but up to 2 liters have been given (Hageman & Goei, 1993). Because the adult rectal capacity is about 400 ml (Doughty & Jackson, 1993), larger volumes (500 to 2000 ml) would reach the sigmoid colon and beyond resulting in stretching of bowel lumen

Fluid Absorption

Fluid absorption is one of the colon's major functions. Of the approximately 9 L of fluid that enter the colon daily, about 8.8 L is absorbed by the epithelial cells lining the lumen of the colon (Chang et al., 1996). Osmosis promotes absorption when luminal contents are hypotonic to plasma. Tap water enemas were used to rehydrate patients before intravenous access was available (Harmer & Henderson, 1944), but repeated tap water enemas can cause hyponatremia and fluid overload (Chertow & Brady, 1994).

The amount of fluid absorbed from stools is related to the length of time it is in contact with the colon's epithelial cells (Chang et al., 1996). After the enema is instilled, nurses report telling patients to resist defecating as long as possible (Schmelzer & Wright, 1996), and nursing textbooks suggest that longer retention produces better results (Craven & Hirnle, 1996; Sorensen & Luckmann, 1986). This practice, however, would seem to promote greater water absorption, decrease the available volume to stimulate defecation, and increase the risk of fluid overload.

Mucosal Irritation

When endocrine cells and sensory neurons detect chemical changes from foreign antigens, toxins or chemicals, they initiate a secretory response to dilute the irritant and powerful propulsive forces to eject it from the body (Wood, 1994). This response may be useful if the irritation is mild enough to stimulate defecation without damaging the mucosal cells; however, excessive irritation can damage mucosal cells and the resulting inflammation could dramatically increase secretion and propulsion (Chang et al., 1996).

Although tap water is not an irritation (Niv, 1990), soapsuds enemas have been associated with severe mucosal irritation and colitis (Kim, Cho, & Levinsohn, 1980; Orchard & Lawson, 1986; Toffler & Barry, 1972). Despite these reports, soapsuds enemas are still frequently used to treat constipation (Schmelzer & Wright, 1993; 1996).

"Extraneous Variables

The size of the enema returns can be influenced by certain factors including age, gender, and the time since the last bowel movement...."

Margin annotations: concept; concept; concept; concept; conceptual definition of defecation; concept; concept; concept; concept; concept; conceptual definition of osmolarity; concept; conceptual definition of hypertonic; concept; concept; conceptual definition of fluid absorption; concept; concept; conceptual definition of chemical irritate; conceptual definition of stimulates propulsion; conceptual definition of secretory response

Statements

Statements express claims that are important to the theory. An **existence statement** declares that a given concept exists or that a given relationship between concepts occurs. For example, an existence statement might claim that a condition referred to as *stress* exists and that there is a relationship between the concept of stress and the concept of health. A **relational statement** clarifies the type of relationship that exists between or among concepts. For example, one relational statement might propose that high levels of stress are related to declining levels of health. Another relational statement might propose that exercise is related to weight.

It is the statements of a theory that are tested through research, not the theory itself. Testing a theory involves determining the truth of each relational statement in the theory. However, a single study might test only one relational statement. As more studies examine a single relational statement, increasing evidence of the truth or falsity of that statement is confirmed. Many studies are required to validate all the statements in a theory.

In theories, **propositions** (relational statements) can be expressed at various levels of abstraction. The statements found in conceptual models (general propositions) are at a high level of abstraction. Statements found in theories (specific propositions) are at a moderate level of abstraction. Hypotheses are at a low level of abstraction and are specific. As statements are expressed in a less abstract way, they become more narrow in scope (Fawcett & Downs, 1992), as shown below.

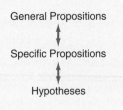

Statements at varying levels of abstraction that express relationships between or among the same conceptual ideas can be arranged in hierarchical form, from general to specific. This should allow the reader to see the logical links among the various levels of abstraction.

📖 RESEARCH EXAMPLE   Statements in the Study

Roy and Roberts (1981) developed statement sets related to Roy's nursing model that could be used in frameworks for research, as shown in the following excerpts.

General Proposition

The magnitude of the internal and external stimuli will positively influence the magnitude of the physiological response of an intact system.

Specific Proposition

The amount of mobility in the form of exercising positively influences the level of muscle integrity.

Hypothesis

If the nurse helps the patient maintain muscle tone through proper exercising, the patient will experience fewer problems associated with immobility. (Roy & Roberts, 1981, p. 90)

CRITIQUE GUIDELINES   Statements in the Study

In critiquing a published study, use critical reasoning to identify the statements expressed as propositions and hypotheses. The following questions may help you identify and critique these statements:

1. What statements are expressed within the publication?
2. Are all of the study concepts included within the statements?
3. Are the statements expressed as both propositions and hypotheses (or research questions)?
4. Are one or more statements being tested by the study design?

Extracting Statements from a Published Study

In some studies, the statements are implied, rather than clearly stated. Sometimes they are located within the "Introduction" or "Literature Review," rather than within a clearly expressed framework. If the statements are implied and not clearly stated, use critical reasoning to extract them from the text and express them as statements. To begin, search the "Introduction," the "Background and Significance," the "Literature Review," and the "Framework" for sentences that seem to express relationships between concepts included in the study. Next, write down a single sentence that seems to be a relational statement and express it graphically. For example, the statement "Exercise is related to weight" could be expressed as follows:

Exercise ⟷ Weight

The next statement can be identified as a relational statement and should be written down and expressed graphically. Continue this step until you have graphically expressed all of the statements related to the selected concepts. If the linkages among your graphic expressions are examined, the theoretical ideas embedded in the text will gradually become clearer.

RESEARCH EXAMPLE   Extracting Statements

A study by Schmelzer and colleagues (2000) illustrates the extraction of statements from text in a published study (see p. 178). It should be noted that all of the concepts previously identified are included in these statements. General propositions are underlined in red, specific propositions are underlined in green, and hypotheses are underlined with a double rule. When marking text in an article, you may use a variety of colored highlighters to differentiate these various types of statements. You may also want to write notes in the margins.

Background

The ideal enema solution would effectively cleanse the colon with minimal side effects. The following sections describe the colonic cleansing mechanism and the dangers of excessive fluid absorption, rectal mucosal damage, and discomfort.

Colonic Cleansing

general proposition —— Enemas cleanse the colon by stimulating propulsion and secretion. Three major factors influence an enema's ability to stimulate defecation: enema volume, the presence of chemical irritants, and the osmolarity or tonicity of the solution (Wood, 1994). The instillation of a large fluid volume into the intestinal lumen stimulates propulsion; chemical irritants stimulate both propulsion and secretion to rapidly empty the colon (Chang, Sitrin, & Black, 1996). Hypertonic solutions, such as sodium *specific proposition* —— phosphate enemas, stimulate defecation by drawing fluid from the body into the lumen of the colon through osmosis and by directly irritating rectal mucosa. To promote fluid absorption from the colon, hypotonic solutions are thought to slow propulsion (Chang et al., 1996; Wood, 1994). Because tap *specific proposition* —— water, a hypotonic solution, does not irritate colonic mucosa (Niv, 1990), its effect must be the result of volume alone. Soapsuds solutions are also hypotonic, but both a large volume and chemical irritation stimulate defecation.

(right margin: specific proposition, specific proposition, specific proposition*)*

Few studies have addressed optimal enema volume and individual tolerance. Nursing texts recommend volumes ranging from 0.5 to 1.0 liter (Craven & Hirnle, 1996; Sorensen & Luckmann, 1986), but up to 2 liters have been given (Hageman & Goei, 1993). Because the adult rectal capacity is about 400 ml (Doughty & Jackson, 1993), larger volumes (500 to 2000 ml) would reach the sigmoid colon and beyond.

Fluid Absorption

Fluid absorption is one of the colon's major functions. Of the approximately 9 liters of fluid that enter the colon daily, about 8.8 liters is absorbed by the epithelial cells lining the lumen of the colon (Chang et al., 1996). Osmosis promotes absorption when luminal contents are hypotonic to plasma. —— *general proposition*
Tap water enemas were used to rehydrate patients before intravenous access was available (Harmer & Henderson, 1944), but repeated tap water enemas can cause hyponatremia and fluid overload (Chertow & Brady, 1994).

specific proposition —— The amount of fluid absorbed from stools is related to the length of time it is in contact with the colon's epithelial cells (Chang et al., 1996). After the enema is instilled, nurses report telling patients to resist defecating as long as possible (Schmelzer & Wright, 1996), and nursing textbooks suggest that longer retention produces better results (Craven & Hirnle, 1996; Sorensen & Luckmann, 1986). This practice, however, would seem to promote greater water absorption, decrease the available volume to stimulate defecation, and increase the risk of fluid overload.

Mucosal Irritation

specific proposition —— When endocrine cells and sensory neurons detect chemical changes from foreign antigens, toxins or chemicals, they initiate a secretory response to dilute the irritant and powerful propulsive forces to eject it from the body (Wood, 1994). This response may be useful if the irritation is mild enough to stimulate defecation without damaging the mucosal cells; however, excessive irritation can damage mucosal cells and the resulting inflammation could dramatically increase secretion and propulsion (Chang et al., 1996).

Although tap water is not an irritation (Niv, 1990), soapsuds enemas have been associated with severe mucosal irritation and colitis (Kim, Cho, & Levinsohn, 1980; Orchard & Lawson, 1986; Toffler & Barry, 1972). Despite these reports, soapsuds enemas are still frequently used to treat constipation (Schmelzer & Wright, 1993; 1996).

Extraneous Variables

specific proposition —— The size of the enema returns can be influenced by certain factors including age, gender, and the time since the last bowel movement.... Renal function, serum albumin, and overall hydration status influence an individual's response to a large fluid load. Serum blood urea nitrogen (BUN) and creatinine reflect renal function, and hematocrit and sodium levels provide information about hydration status.

Conceptual Map

One strategy for expressing a theory is a **conceptual map** that graphically shows the inter-relationships of the concepts and statements (Artinian, 1982; Fawcett & Downs, 1992; Moody, 1989; Newman, 1979; Silva, 1981). A conceptual map is developed to explain which concepts contribute to or partially cause an outcome. The map should be supported by references from the literature. A conceptual map summarizes and integrates what is known about a phenomenon more succinctly and clearly than does a literary explanation, thus allowing a grasp of the "wholeness" of a phenomenon.

A conceptual map includes all of the major concepts in a theory or framework. These concepts are linked by arrows expressing the proposed linkages between concepts. Each linkage shown by an arrow is a graphic illustration of a relational statement (proposition) of the theory.

RESEARCH EXAMPLE   Conceptual Map

Mapping is useful in identifying gaps in the logic of the theory and reveals inconsistencies, incompleteness, and errors (Artinian, 1982). Schmelzer, and colleagues (2000) did not provide a conceptual map with their framework. The statements extracted from their published study were used to construct the map in Figure 6-1. The findings of their study are provided next.

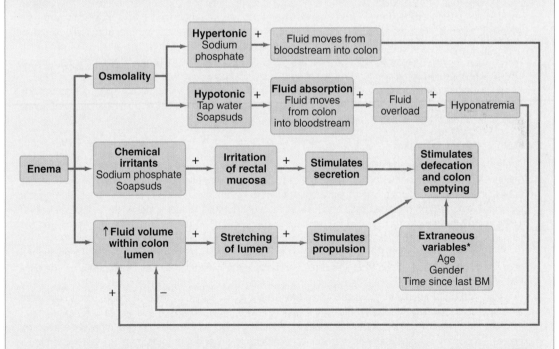

Figure 6-1. Conceptual map constructed from statements extracted from study. BM, bowel movement. *Effect might be explained by variations in colon muscle tone. (Data from Schmelzer, M., Case, P., Chappell, S. M., & Wright, K. B. [2000]. Colonic cleansing, fluid absorption, and discomfort following tap water and soapsuds enemas. *Applied Nursing Research, 13*[2], 83–91.)

(continues)

RESEARCH EXAMPLE *(continued)*

Soapsuds enemas produced significantly larger net outputs than tap water, had similar absorption rates, and were equally well tolerated. Seventeen of the 25 subjects in the study had negative net outputs. This means that more liquid was inserted than was expelled. These findings raise two questions. First, why were soapsuds enemas well tolerated in this study? Several sources condemn soapsuds enemas, citing damage to rectal mucosa. Responses to the questionnaire indicate subjects tolerated the soapsuds enemas as well as the tap water enemas and had few complaints of discomfort. Second, why did so many in both treatment groups have negative net outputs?

Soapsuds Enema Tolerance

Gastroenterologists have noted irritation when viewing rectal mucosa immediately after soapsuds enemas (Davila & Willenbucher, 1998). Mucosal irritation has also been noted following Fleet's Phospho-Soda enemas and bisacodyl suppositories (Saunders, Haggitt, Kimmey, & Silverstein, 1990), both popular preparations.

Although mild irritation might be acceptable, three cases of severe rectal mucosal damage are cited by those condemning soapsuds enemas (Davila & Willenbucher, 1998): two cases were young men who gave themselves enemas containing a variety of household detergents (Toffler & Barry, 1972; Kim, Cho, & Levinsohn, 1980); the third was a hospitalized patient who was given daily soapsuds enemas for 5 consecutive days (Orchard & Lawson, 1986). In all three cases, excessive amounts of the soapsuds enemas were given.

No one has attempted to test various types and concentrations of soap to determine the optimal solution. In a 1944 article condemning soapsuds enemas, Hicks recognized that a major problem with soapsuds enemas was the lack of a standard preparation. He surveyed several metropolitan Canadian hospitals and found haphazard practices for soapsuds enemas at all but one. The situation is not much better today. Nursing textbooks recommend anywhere from 5 mL per 1000 mL of water (Kozier, Erb, & Olivari, 1991), but these recommendations have no scientific basis.

No one has studied the severity and duration of the irritation or the effects of varying concentrations and preparations of soap. Research that includes macroscopic and microscopic examination of the rectal mucosa is needed to establish the safety of soapsuds solutions.

Negative Net Outputs

The researchers were surprised by the number of enema returns that were smaller than the amount of solution instilled. The mean net output following the simulated tap water enemas was −175.3 g, and all but one subject in the tap water group had negative outputs. Although the mean net output of the soapsuds enema group was 10.5 g, 6 of the 13 subjects also had negative net outputs. What happened to the fluid left behind in the colon? If absorption accounted for the decreased output, PEG concentrations in the enema returns should have been greater than 2 (2.01 and 2.09 g/L).

The mean percentage of PEG recovery was 68% following the tap water enema and 72% following the soapsuds enema. Because the PEG was diluted and only partially recovered in the enema returns, the original enema solution must have been diluted by liquid and stool already in the colon and only partially excreted. Also, all enema returns were collected for 1 hour following the enema, adequate time to eliminate all enema solution. Thus, the fluid remaining in the colon was probably absorbed into the body over time.

The large volume of tap water stimulated defecation, though not enough to completely empty the bowel. Because the soapsuds enema produced significantly larger net outputs than tap water enemas, it must be a stronger defecation stimulus. (pp. 89–90)

Frameworks for Physiological Studies

Until recently, physiological studies tended to lack a clearly defined framework. Some physiological researchers discounted the importance of the theoretical dimension of research. This was due in part to the emphasis in nursing on psychosocial theories. In addition, some researchers tended to discount biological knowledge. The theoretical basis for physiological studies is derived from physics, physiology, genetics and pathophysiology and may not be considered theory by some researchers. However, it is Scientific Theory. The knowledge in these areas is well tested through research, and theoretical relationships often are referred to as laws and principles. The theoretical relationships may be considered facts rather than theories. However, propositions can be developed and tested using these laws and principles and then applied to nursing problems.

Developing a framework to clearly express the logic on which the study is based is helpful both to the researcher and to readers of the published study. The critique of a physiological framework is no different from that of other frameworks. However, concepts and conceptual definitions in physiological frameworks may be less abstract than concepts and conceptual definitions in many psychosocial studies. Concepts in physiological studies might be such terms as cardiac output, dyspnea, wound healing, blood pressure, tissue hypoxia, metabolism, and functional status.

Schmelzer and colleagues' (2000) study described in the preceding Research Example box is an example of a physiologic study framework.

Frameworks Based on Middle Range Theories

Most frameworks for nursing studies are based on middle range theories. These studies test the validity of the middle range theory and also examine the parameters within which the middle range theory can be applied. Some middle range theories that were developed outside of nursing are now being used as the basis for frameworks in nursing studies. Other middle range theories were developed within nursing to explain nursing phenomena. These theories also should be tested before being applied to nursing practice.

RESEARCH EXAMPLE Framework Based on Middle Range Theory

Wilson (2005) used Pender's Health Promotion Model (Pender, Murdaugh, & Parsons (2001), a middle range theory, as a basis for her study of *health-promoting behaviors of sheltered homeless women.*

The purpose of this study was to describe sociodemographic and personal characteristics, health practices, and health-promoting behaviors in a population of sheltered homeless women in a specific Midwest geographical region to increase awareness, understanding, and provide further insight into the complex area of homelessness and health.

The theoretical framework for this study was based upon Pender's revised Health Promotion Model. The Health Promotion Model (HPM) provides a framework to examine influences on participation in health-promoting behaviors and provides direction for effective interventions. The HPM illustrates that each person is a multidimensional holistic individual who continually interacts with both interpersonal and physical environments and emphasizes the active role of the individual in the achievement of an improved healthy state.

(continues)

RESEARCH EXAMPLE *(continued)*

The 3 major constructs of the HPM (individual characteristics and experiences, behavior-specific cognition and affect, and behavioral outcomes) were used to select specific study variables as conceptualized within the model. Health-promoting behaviors, the outcome of the HPM, were examined in this population and relationships among study variables explored. (p. 51)

The Health Promoting Lifestyle Profile II scale was administered to 137 homeless women and gathered data on a number of descriptive variables (e.g., age, ethnicity, employment status, length of time homeless, cause of homelessness).

CRITIQUE

The study measured all of the major concepts in Pender's Health Promotion Model. The sample, which included subjects from 5 shelters for women, was of sufficient size (137 homeless women) to provide a reasonable test of Pender's relationships. Pender's model was useful in identifying the inadequacies in health services for homeless women. The author recommends that the model be used provide a framework for the provision of health services to homeless women.

FINDINGS

The homeless women who participated in the study had high rates of unemployment, high numbers of co-morbid conditions, and high housing instability. Although these women had good access to health care, they had limited access to health promotion and prevention services. When offered, the homeless women participated in a variety of health-promoting activities.

IMPLICATIONS FOR PRACTICE

Pender's HPM (Health Promotion Model) is of great value to guide health care interventions for sheltered homeless women and should be used to assess current influences and provide a framework for services directed at increasing their health. Individual characteristics and past experiences are important to assess in order to provide in-depth understanding of the individual. Immediate competing demands have direct effects on the participation of health-promoting behaviors, and, for the homeless, include issues such as availability of childcare. Additionally, basic needs (shelter, food, safety) can be viewed as competing demands as these take priority status and must be adequately addressed before health promotion needs can become a focus. Half of the women reported that they had been staying with friends and/or family members being "doubled-up" on a temporary basis before seeking shelter services, validating the research of others. Housing instability, coupled with the added stress on families who host others and on those who are homeless, suggests that the homeless, prior to seeking shelter services (when "doubled-up"), have unstable support systems validating the critical importance of establishment and maintenance of strong social and emotional support networks. Shelter staff and services can have both positive and negative effects on the practice of health behaviors; an adequate knowledge base of the importance of health-promoting behaviors and recognition of its value can have positive influences on homeless residents to practice health behaviors. Additionally, if participation in health-promoting behaviors is rewarded, residents may also value these behaviors and recognize them as benefits to action, as depicted in the HPM.

Situational influences are of critical importance as a motivator of action for health-promoting behaviors as depicted by Pender. If opportunities to engage in health-promoting behaviors are not readily available (planned exercise programs, availability of exercise equipment, knowledge about nutritional components, educational offerings related to personal health responsibilities, etc), it is unlikely that homeless women will participate. The decision of one to participate in health-promoting behaviors does not come from one single factor but from the interaction of many. . .

Health care providers are challenged to find innovative methods to decrease health disparities that are prevalent in this vulnerable population. Healthy People 2010 (U.S. Department of Health and Human Services, 2000) focuses on the health of all Americans, including vulnerable and underserved populations. This critical document provides direction for elimination of socioeconomic disparities in health and includes primary level strategies aimed at accessible health promotion and disease prevention care and services. Improved access to care is one critical method to address these disparities, but increased understanding of the nature and extent of health disparities that exist among vulnerable populations must be targeted so effectual program and policy development can occur directed toward those at greatest risk for adverse health outcomes. . . Creation and establishment of collaborative partnerships designed to implement effective interventions and programs that will enhance the health and well-being of homeless women is of vital importance. Development of outreach services to homeless shelters as well as community sites that serve the impoverished (food banks, churches, low-income housing, community centers) is strongly warranted. Shelter-based interventions are needed that address holistic care for physical, psychological, spiritual, and social resources and not just housing, food, safety, and specific disease concerns. Interventions that support participation in health-promoting behaviors must be accessible, affordable, and appropriate to the needs and lifestyles of being homeless. Culturally appropriate interventions and programs that develop resiliency and strengthening of personal resources are needed to positively impact the health of this unique at-risk group. Social justice must become the guiding force so that all persons, regardless of socioeconomic status will have opportunities for a healthier life. (pp. 60-62)

Frameworks Derived from Qualitative Studies

Middle range theories are developed in some qualitative studies as an outcome of the study. These theories can then be used as a basis for clinical practice and/or as a framework in other qualitative or quantitative studies.

RESEARCH EXAMPLE Framework Derived from a Qualitative Study

Rich and Grey (2005) conducted a study of young black males who were victims of violence. The researchers sought to understand the participants' experience of violence. Although a number of studies have been conducted in this area and have identified risk factors for violence, these researchers were interested in understanding how these risk factors worked together to precipitate violence. The framework that served as a basis for their work was that of Elijah Anderson (1999), an ethnographic researcher who described a "code of the street"—a set of informal rules governing interpersonal public behavior, including violence. The researchers interviewed 47 participants who had experienced violence (being shot, stabbed, or physically assaulted by another person) within 1 to 2 weeks of the interview. Twenty-three participated in a second interview. Rich and Grey provide a conceptual map of their findings (Figure 6-2) which may be useful as a framework for further research.

(continues)

RESEARCH EXAMPLE *(continued)*

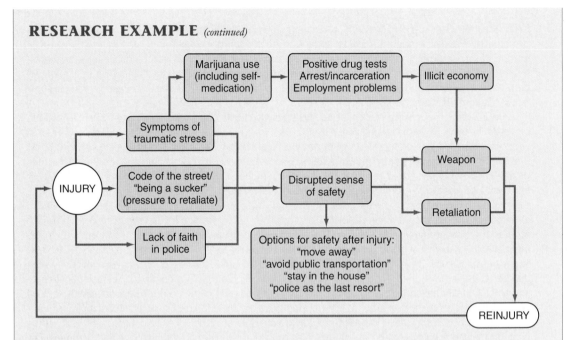

Figure 6-2. Model illustrating pathways to recurrence. (Redrawn from Rich, J. A., & Grey, C. M. [2005]. Pathways to recurrent trauma among young Black men: Traumatic stress, substance use, and the "Code of the Street." *American Journal of Public Health, 95*[5], 816–824.

CRITIQUE

The description of the gathering of data and reduction and analysis of data suggests a well-planned study. The sample size (47) was unusually large for a qualitative study and indicates the investment of the researchers in their topic. The study includes a mix of qualitative and quantitative methods, including a scale to assess posttraumatic stress disorder. The researchers used a grounded theory approach to qualitative analysis.

FINDINGS

The participants believed that if they did not retaliate against an assailant, they were at greater risk for future injuries

Respect means receiving the deference one deserves.

When someone "disrespects" you physically, emotionally, or materially, you must respond aggressively to regain respect.

Being a sucker is when someone says or does something harmful and the affected person does not retaliate.

Tolerating disrespect damages the affected person's identity, as well as increasing the risk of further victimization.

The participants have no confidence in the police or the judicial system to protect them.

These researchers' findings generally are consistent with those of Anderson (1999).

IMPLICATIONS FOR PRACTICE

Rich and Grey's model "suggests points of intervention to break the cycle of recurrent violence. The code of the street—especially the meaning of respect and 'being a sucker'—should be acknowledged and incorporated in violence prevention strategies targeting young Black men. Alternate ways of establishing a sense of safety, strength, self-esteem, and masculinity, if made available to these young men, might reduce their drive for retaliation as a response to disrespect. Educational programs that allow undereducated men to complete high school and begin college, in addition to job training programs that prepare men for meaningful work, could provide an alternative way to establish an identity."

"Efforts to improve relationships between the police and young Black male victims might address fears of racial profiling and lead to victims cooperating with the police to apprehend their assailants. . ."

"Health care providers should work to ensure that victims are safe when they are released from the hospital, particularly if they could be targeted as key witnesses or are at high risk for retaliation. The Department of Justice, according to which there are currently fewer than 12 hospital centers in the country that offer comprehensive services to victims of gun violence, has advocated for hospital-based interventions targeting victims of non-fatal violence."

"Diagnosis and treatment of symptoms of trauma could remove one of the forces driving perceptions of vulnerability. In our experience, few victims are routinely referred for mental health services after their assault. Lack of insurance coverage and lack of culturally competent mental health services make it difficult for those who are in distress to find treatment. Effective treatment of symptoms could potentially interrupt a cascade toward weapon carrying, substance abuse, and further alienation from stabilizing institutions such as employment, education, and health care." (Rich & Grey, 2005, pp. 822-823)

Frameworks Including Conceptual Nursing Models

Building a body of knowledge related to a particular conceptual model requires an organized program of research. This program of research is referred to as a research tradition. A group of scholars dedicated to conducting research related to the model develop theories compatible with the model, including propositions for testing. An organized plan for testing these propositions is agreed on. Researchers conducting studies consistent with a particular research tradition often maintain a network of communication regarding their work. In some cases annual conferences focused on the model are held to share research findings, explore theoretical ideas, and maintain network contacts. Conceptual models of nursing do not have well-established research traditions (Fawcett, 1989). However, research traditions are being developed for some nursing models.

One example of a nursing model with an emerging research tradition is Orem's (2001) Model of Self-Care. This model focuses on the domain of nursing practice and on what nurses actually do when they practice nursing. Orem proposes that people generally know how to take care of themselves (self-care). If they are dependent in some way (e.g., by being very young, aged, or handicapped), family members usually take on this responsibility (dependent care). When people are ill or have some pathologic condition (e.g., diabetes or a colostomy), they or their family members often acquire special skills to provide that care (therapeutic self-care). A person's capacity to provide self-care is referred to as self-care agency. A self-care deficit occurs when self-care demand exceeds self-care agency. These ideas are expressed graphically in Figure 6-3.

(continues)

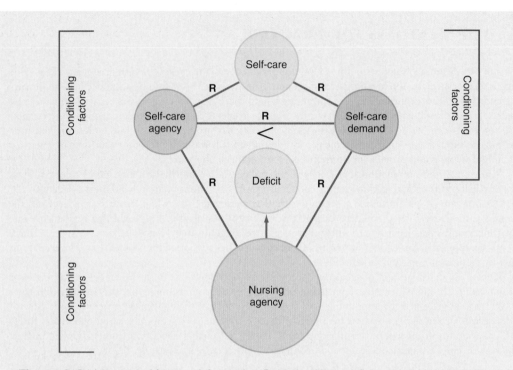

Figure 6-3. A conceptual framework for nursing. R, relationship; <, deficit relationship, current or projected. (From Orem, D. E. [1995]. *Nursing: Concepts of practice* [5th ed.]. St. Louis: Mosby. Used with permission.)

Nursing care is provided only when there is a deficit in the self-care or dependent care that the person and the family provides (self-care deficit). In this case the nurse (or nurses) develops a nursing system to provide the needed care. This system involves prescribing, designing, and providing the needed care. The goal of nursing care is to facilitate resumption of self-care by the person or family members, or both. Three types of nursing systems are recognized in this model: wholly compensatory, partly compensatory, and supportive-educative. Selection of one of these systems is based on the capacity of the person to perform self-care.

The notion of self-care as an important construct for nursing has drawn nurse researchers to Orem's work. Multiple studies have examined self-care in a variety of nursing situations. Instruments consistent with Orem's model have been developed to measure some of her concepts. Orem developed three theories related to her model: the Theory of Self-Care Deficits, the Theory of Self-Care, and the Theory of Nursing Systems (also referred to as the General Theory of Nursing). However, few propositions emerging from Orem's theories have been tested.

For a number of years, Dodd and colleagues have been conducting studies based on Orem's model.* Many of these studies have been funded through the National Institutes of Health (NIH). This is an important example of the carefully planned programs of research that are necessary to validate the usefulness of a nursing theory in guiding nursing practice.

---

*Dibble, Padilla, Dodd, & Miaskowski, 1998; Dodd, 1982a,b, 1983a,b, 1984a,b,c, 1987a,b, 1988a,b, 1991, 1996; 1997; 1999; 2000; Dodd, et al., 1986-1990; Dodd et al., 1988-1992; Dodd & Dibble, 1993; Dodd, Dibble, Miaskowski, et al., 2001; Dodd, Dibble, & Thomas, 1992a,b; Dodd, Janson, Facione, et al., 2001; Dodd, Larson, & Dibble, 1996; Dodd, Miaskowski, Dibble, et al., 2000; Dodd, Miaskowski, & Paul, 2001; Dodd & Mood, 1981; Dodd, Thomas, & Dibble, 1991; Dodd, West, Tripathy, et al., 2000; Facione & Dodd, 1995; Facione, Dodd, Holzemer, & Meleis, 1997; Jansen, Miaskowski, Dodd, & Dowling, 2005; Larson, Dodd, & Aksamit, 1998; Larson, Miaskowski, MacPhail, et al., 1998; Lovely, Miaskowski, & Dodd, 1999; Mandrell, Ruccione, Dodd, et al., 2000; Messias, Yeager, Dibble, & Dodd, 1997; Miaskowski, 2000; Musci & Dodd, 1990; Piper, Dibble, Dodd, Weiss, Slaughter, & Paul, 1998; Schumacher, Koresawa, West, Dodd, Paul, Tripathy, et al., 2005.

RESEARCH EXAMPLE   Frameworks Including Conceptual Nursing Models

In 1996, Dodd et al. conducted a study funded by the National Cancer Institute to test the effectiveness of a nurse-initiated systematic oral hygiene teaching program to prevent chemotherapy-induced oral mucositis in patients. In previous studies Dodd and colleagues (1986-1990; 1988-1992), had found that nursing management of mucositis in patients receiving chemotherapy for cancer was in disarray. Because most patients are receiving chemotherapy as outpatients, it is not possible to monitor closely the condition of a patient's mouth.

> Many patients were told that they might experience oral problems because of their chemotherapy, but they were not instructed in any type of preventive mouth care. Therefore, most patients who experienced mouth problems initially tried to self-manage using a trial-and-error approach. When patients sought assistance from their physicians or nurses, they were offered a variety of remedies with instructions to swish and spit. Many patients indicated that this approach was not only ineffective, it actually increased their discomfort and mouth problems. (Dodd et al., 1996, p. 922)

Basing her claims on Orem's Theory of Self-Care Agency, Dodd proposed that a nurse-initiated systematic oral hygiene teaching program, (PRO-SELF: Mouth Aware [PSMA] Program) that is offered before the development of mucositis, would enhance the patient's self-care agency and result in a decrease in the incidence and severity of mucositis (Figure 6-4). The Oral Assessment Guide (Eilers, Berger, & Peterson, 1988) was used to guide clinician ratings of chemotherapy-related changes in the oral mucosa. The study developed to validate this proposition also tested the effectiveness of two mouthwashes used in the mouth care protocol: chlorhexidine and a placebo control (sterile water). The findings of the study validated Orem's concept of self-care agency.

> The PSMA program provided patients with the knowledge and skills needed to perform the systematic oral hygiene protocol. Evidence exists that the patients used the PSMA program as instructed. Data from this study suggest that the use of a systematic oral hygiene program prescribed in the PSMA program may have reduced the incidence of chemotherapy-induced mucositis from an *a priori* estimate of 44% to less than 26%. (p. 926)

(continues)

RESEARCH EXAMPLE (continued)

Mouth Care

Each day you MUST:
1. **Look** at your whole mouth, including your lips and tongue *every morning* before brushing, flossing, and rinsing. **Check** for problems listed below.
2. **Brush** your teeth for 90 seconds *twice a day*—after breakfast and before bedtime.
3. **Floss** your teeth at least *once a day.*
4. **Rinse** your mouth with one capful of the medicated mouthwash for 30 seconds *twice a day*—after breakfast and before bedtime. Swish thoroughly and spit out.
5. **Do NOT eat or drink ANYTHING, including WATER, FOR 30 MINUTES** after using the medicated mouthwash.
6. **Avoid** smoking, alcoholic beverages, and spicy foods.

Mouth Problems to Check for Daily
*If you have any of the following **problems,*** you must call your nurse AS SOON AS POSSIBLE.
1. **Sores** in your mouth
2. **White spots** in your mouth
3. **Pain** in your mouth
4. **Difficulty** eating or drinking
5. Unusual amount of **bleeding**
   Nurse's name _____
   Phone number _____

*Specific instructions for denture wearer were provided.

Figure 6-4. PRO-SELF Mouth Aware Prevention Program for Non-Denture Wearers. (From Dodd, M. J. et al. [1996]. Randomized clinical trial of chlorhexidine versus placebo for prevention of oral mucositis in patients receiving chemotherapy. *Oncology Nursing Forum, 23*[6], 921. Used with permission.)

No significant difference was found in the effectiveness of the two mouthwashes used in the study. Thus, Dodd and colleagues recommend the use of water in implementing the PSMA program. This study was selected for the 1996 Oncology Nursing Society (ONS)/Schering Corporation Excellence in Cancer Nursing Research Award.

CRITIQUE GUIDELINES   Conceptual Model–Theory Frameworks

Critiquing a framework that includes both a conceptual model and a theory is more complex than critiquing a framework based only on a theory. Identify the constructs and their definitions, as well as the concepts and their definitions. Also, identify both general and specific propositions and link them to the hypotheses or research questions.

Including a conceptual model as well as a theory in a framework is a relatively new idea in nursing. Therefore, few published studies have frameworks that include a conceptual model, a theory, and a conceptual map illustrating the linkage between the model and the theory. The map for such a framework must include both the conceptual model and a testable theory.

KEY CONCEPTS

- Research is based on theory.
- Researchers use theories to organize what is known about a phenomenon.
- A conceptual model, similar to a theory but more abstract, broadly explains phenomena of interest, expresses assumptions, and reflects a philosophical stance.
- A framework is a brief explanation of a theory or those portions of a theory to be tested in a study.
- Every study has a framework, although some frameworks are poorly expressed.
- The framework must identify and define the concepts and the relational statements being tested.
- Testing a theory involves determining the truth of each relational statement in the theory.
- Critiquing a framework requires the identification and evaluation of the concepts, their definitions, and the statements linking the concepts.
- An organized program of research is important for building a body of knowledge related to the phenomena explained by a particular conceptual model.

TIPS FOR FURTHER STUDY

- Are you having difficulty identifying frameworks in research reports? Try the "Exercises in Critique" in your *Study Guide*, Chapter 6.
- If you are having problems distinguishing the different types of nursing theories, complete the Open-Book Quiz on http://evolve.elsevier.com/Burns/understanding/.
- Are you still trying to understand how theories can guide nursing practice? See "Going Beyond" in your *Study Guide*, Chapter 6.

REFERENCES

Acton, G. J. (1997). Affiliated-individuation as a mediator of stress and burden in caregivers of adults with dementia. *Journal of Holistic Nursing, 15*(4), 336–357.

Ajzen, I. (1991). The theory of planned behavior. *Organizational Behaviour and Human Decision Processes, 50*(2), 179–211.

Algase, D.L., Beck, C.K., Ianowski, A., Whall, A., Benert, S., Richards, R., & Beattie, E. (1996). Need-driven dementia-compromised behavior. An alternative view of disruptive behavior. *American Journal of Alzheimer's Disease, 11*(6), 10, 12–19.

Anderson, E. (1999). *Code of the street: Decency, violence and the moral life of the inner city.* New York: Norton.

Antonovsky, A. (1987). *Unraveling the mystery of health: How people manage stress and stay well.* San Francisco: Jossey-Bass.

Artinian, B. (1982). Conceptual mapping. Development of the strategy. *Western Journal of Nursing Research, 4*(4), 379–393.

August-Brady, M. (2000). Prevention as intervention. *Journal of Advanced Nursing, 31*(6), 1304–1308.

Backman, K. (2003). Middle-range theory development in nursing science: Self-care of home-dwelling elderly [Finnish]. *Holtotiede, 15*(3), 115–130.

Bandura, A. (1982). Self-efficacy mechanism in human agency. *American Psychologist, 37*(2), 122–147.

Bandura, A. (1986). *Social foundations of thought and action: A social cognitive theory.* Englewood Cliffs, NJ: Prentice-Hall.

Bandura, A. (1989). Regulation of cognitive processes through perceived self-efficacy, *Developmental Psychology, 25*(5), 729–735.

Bandura, A. (1997). *Self-efficacy: The exercise of control.* New York: W. H. Freeman.

Beck, C. T. (1993). Teetering on the edge: A substantive theory of postpartum depression. *Nursing Research, 42*(1), 42–48.

Becker, M. H. (1976). *Health belief model and personal health behavior.* Thorofare, New Jersey; Slack.

Bowlby, J. (1969). *Attachment and loss,* vol. 1: *Attachment.* London: Hogarth Press.

Bowlby, J. (1973). *Attachment and loss,* vol. 2: *Separation.* New York: Basic Books.

Brooks, E. M., & Thomas, S. (1997). The perception and judgment of senior baccalaureate student nurses in clinical decision making. *Advances in Nursing Science, 19*(3), 50–69.

Burke, S. O., Kauffmann, E., Costello, E. A., & Dillon, M. C. (1991). Hazardous secrets and reluctly taking charge: Parenting a child with repeated hospitalizations. *Image—The Journal of Nursing Scholarship 23*(1), 39–45.

Cargile, A., Giles, H., & Clement, R. (1995). Language, conflict, and ethnolinguistic identity theory. In J. B. Gittler (Ed.) *Research in human social conflict 1* (pp. 189–208). Philadelphia, PA: Elsevier.

Casalenuovo, G. A. (2002). *Fatigue in diabetes mellitus: Testing a middle range theory of well-being derived from Neuman's theory of optimal client system stability and the Neuman Systems Model.* Doctoral dissertation, University of Tennessee.

Champion, V. L. (1985). Use of the health belief model in determining frequency of breast self-examination. *Research in Nursing &Health, 8*(4), 373–379.

Chang, E., Sitrin, M., & Black, D. (1996). *Gastrointestinal, hepatobiliary, and nutritional physiology.* Philadelphia: Lippincott-Raven.

Chapman, K. J., & Pepler, C. (1998). Coping, hope and anticipatory grief in family members with palliative home care. *Cancer Nursing, 21*(4), 226–234.

Chenitz, W. C. (1983). Entry into a nursing home as status passage: A theory to guide nursing practice. *Geriatric Nursing, 4*(2), 92–97.

Chertow, G. M., & Brady, H. R. (1994). Hyponatremia from tap-water enema [Letter]. *Lancet, 344*(8924), 748.

Colling, K. B., & Buettner, L. L. (2002). Simple pleasures: Interventions from the need-driven dementia-compromised behavior model. *Journal of Gerontological Nursing, 28*(10), 16–20.

Cox, C. L. (1982). An interaction model of client behavior: Theoretical prescription for nursing. *Advances in Nursing Science, 5*(1), 41–56.

Craven, R., & Hirnle, C. (1996). *Fundamentals of nursing: human health and function* (2nd ed., pp. 1249–1253). Philadelphia: Lippincott.

Crist, J. (2002). Middle-range theory of critical analysis of disparity: Adapting the Andersen Use Model. 35th Annual Communicating Nursing Research Conference/16 Annual WIN Assembly. Health Disparities: Meeting the Challenge. Held April 18–20, 2002, Palm Springs, California.

Davila, A., & Willenbucher, R. (1998). Other diseases of the colon and rectum. In M. Feldman, B. F. Schorschmidt, & M. Sleisenger (Eds.), *Sleisenger and Fordran's Gastrointestinal and Liver Disease/Pathology/Diagnosis/Management* (p. 1994), Philadelphia, PA: W. B. Saunders.

Deane, K. A., & Degner, L. F. (1998). Information needs, uncertainty, and anxiety in women who had a breast biopsy with benign outcome. *Cancer Nursing, 21*(2), 117–126.

Dethloff, S. B. (2004). Case study. A family decision to discontinue dialysis treatment for a parent: An advanced practice nurse (APN) guided process. *Nephrology Nursing Journal, 31*(4), 443–444.

Dibble, S. L., Padilla, G. V., Dodd, M. J., & Miaskowski, C. (1998). Gender differences in the dimensions of quality of life. *Oncology Nursing Forum, 25*(3), 577–583.

Dodd, M. (1984c). Measuring informational intervention for chemotherapy knowledge and self-care behavior. *Research in Nursing & Health, 7*(1), 43–50.

Dodd, M. J. (1982a). Cancer patients' knowledge of chemotherapy: Assessment and informational interventions. *Oncology Nursing Forum, 9*(3), 39–44.

Dodd, M. J. (1982b). Assessing patient self-care for side effects of cancer chemotherapy Part I. *Cancer Nursing, 5*(6), 447–451.

Dodd, M. J. (1983a). Assessing patient self-care for side effects of cancer chemotherapy Part II. *Cancer Nursing, 5*(6), 63–67.

Dodd, M. J. (1983b). Self-care for side effects of cancer chemotherapy: An assessment of nursing interventions Part II. *Cancer Nursing, 6*(1), 63–67.

Dodd, M. J. (1984a). Patterns of self-care in cancer patients receiving radiation therapy. *Oncology Nursing Forum, 11*(3), 23–27.

Dodd, M. J. (1984b). Self-care for patients with breast cancer to prevent side effects of chemotherapy: A concern for public health nursing. *Public Health Nursing, 1*(4), 202–209.

Dodd, M. (1984c). Measuring informational intervention for chemotherapy knowledge and self-care behavior. *Research in Nursing & Health, 7*(1), 43–50.

Dodd, M. J. (1987a). *Managing side effects of chemotherapy and radiation therapy: A guide for nurses and patients.* Norwich, CT: Appleton & Lange.

Dodd, M. J. (1987b). Efficacy of proactive information on self-care in radiation therapy patients. *Heart & Lung: The Journal of Acute and Critical Care, 16*(5), 538–544.

Dodd, M. J. (1988a). Efficacy of proactive information on self-care in chemotherapy patients. *Patient Education and Counseling, 11*(3), 215–225.

Dodd, M. J. (1988b). Patterns of self-care in patients with breast cancer. *Western Journal of Nursing Research, 10*(1), 7–24.

Dodd, M. J. (1991). *Managing the side effects of chemotherapy and radiation: A guide for patients and their families* (2nd ed.). Englewood Cliffs, NJ: Prentice-Hall.

Dodd, M. J. (1996). *Managing the side effects of chemotherapy and radiation therapy: A guide for patients and their families* (3rd ed.). San Francisco: University of California, School of Nursing Press.

Dodd, M. J. (1997). Self care: Ready or not! *Oncology Nursing Forum, 24*(6), 983–990.

Dodd, M. J. (1999). Self-care: Not as simple as we hoped. 32nd Annual Communicating Nursing Research Conference/13th Annual WIN Assembly, Nursing Research: For the Health of Our Nation, held April 22–24, 1999, at the Bahia Hotel, San Diego. *Communicating Nursing Research, 32*, 43–46.

Dodd, M. J. et al. (1986–1990). *Coping and self-care of cancer families: Nurse prospectus* (Final report). Funded by the National Institutes of Health, R01 CA 1440.

Dodd, M. J. et al. (1988–1992). *Self-care interventions to decrease chemotherapy morbidity* (Final report). Funded by the National Institutes of Health and the National Cancer Institute, R01 CA 48312.

Dodd, M. J. et al. (1992). *Self-care intervention to decrease chemotherapy morbidity.* Invited paper presented at the Seventeenth Annual Congress of the Oncology Nursing Society, San Diego, CA.

Dodd, M. J., & Dibble, S. L. (1993). Predictors of self-care: A test of Orem model. *Oncology Nursing Forum, 20*(6), 895–901.

Dodd, M. J., & Mood, D. W. (1981). Chemotherapy: Helping patients to know the drugs they are receiving and their possible side effects. *Cancer Nursing, 4*(4), 311–318.

Dodd, M. J., Dibble, S. L., & Thomas, M. L. (1992a). Outpatient chemotherapy: Patients and family members concerns and coping strategies. *Journal of Public Health Nursing, 9*(1), 37–44.

Dodd, M. J., Dibble, S., Miaskowski, C., Paul, S., Cho, M., MacPhail, L., et al. (2001). A comparison of the affective state and quality of life of chemotherapy patients who do and do not develop chemotherapy-induced oral mucositis. *Journal of Pain and Symptom Management, 21*(6), 498–505.

Dodd, M. J., Janson, S., Facione, N., Faucett, J., Froelicher, E. S., Humphries, J., et al. (2001). Advancing the science of symptom management. *Journal of Advanced Nursing, 33*(5), 668–676.

Dodd, M. J., Larson, P. J., Dibble, S. L., Miaskowski, C., Greenspan, D., MacFail, E., et al. (1996). Randomized clinical trial of chlorhexidine versus placebo for prevention of oral mucositis in patients receiving chemotherapy. *Oncology Nursing Forum, 23*(6), 921–927.

Dodd, M. J., Miaskowski, C., & Paul, S. M. (2001). Symptom clusters and their effect on the functional status of patients with cancer. *Oncology Nursing Forum, 28*(3), 465–470.

Dodd, M. J., Miaskowski, C., Dibble, S. L., Paul, S. M., MacPhail, L., Greenspan, D., et al. (2000). Factors influencing oral mucositis in patients receiving chemotherapy. *Cancer Practice: A Multidisciplinary Journal of Cancer Care, 8*(6), 291–297.

Dodd, M. J., Thomas, M. L., & Dibble, S. L. (1991). Self-care for patients experiencing cancer chemotherapy side effects: A concern for home care nurses. *Home Healthcare Nurse, 9*(6), 21–26.

Dodd, M., West, C., Tripathy, D., Miaskowski, C., Paul, S., & Koo, P. (2000). A RCT of the effectiveness of the PRO-SELF Pain Control Program. 33rd Annual Communicating Nursing Research Conference/14th Annual WIN Assembly: Building on a Legacy of Excellence in Nursing Research, April 13–15, 2000, Denver, Colorado. *Communicating Nursing Research, 33,* 242.

Dorsey, C. J., & Murdaugh, C. L. (2003). The theory of self-care management for vulnerable populations. *Journal of Theory Construction & Testing, 7*(2), 43–49.

Doughty, D. B., & Jackson, D. B. (1993). *Gastrointestinal disorders.* St. Louis: Mosby.

Duff, D. L. (2002). *Negotiating uncertainty following a severe traumatic brain injury: Family impact and influence.* Doctoral dissertation. University of Calgary.

Dunn, K. S. (2001). *Adaptation to chronic pain: Religious and non-religious coping in Judeo-Christian elders.* Doctoral dissertation, Wayne State University, Detroit.

Dunn, K. S. (2004). Toward a middle-range theory of adaptation to chronic pain. *Nursing Science Quarterly, 17*(1), 78–84.

Dunn, K. S. (2005). Testing a middle-range theoretical model of adaptation to chronic pain. *Nursing Science Quarterly, 18*(2), 146–156.

Eakes, G. G., Burke, M. L., & Hainsworth, M. A. (1998). Middle-range theory of chronic sorrow. *Image—The Journal of Nursing Scholarship, 30*(2), 179–184.

Eilers, J., Berger, A. M., & Peterson, M. C. (1988). Development, testing, and application of the oral assessment guide. *Oncology Nursing Forum, 15*(3), 325–330.

Engebretson, J., & Littleton, L. Y. (2001). Cultural negotiation: A constructivist-based model for nursing practice. *Nursing Outlook, 49*(5), 223–230.

Facione, N. C., Dodd, M. H., Holzemer, W., & Meleis, A. I. (1997). Helpseeking for self-discovered breast symptoms: Implications for early detection. *Cancer Practice: A Multidisciplinary Journal of Cancer Care, 5*(4), 220–227.

Facione, N., & Dodd, M. J. (1995). Women narratives of help seeking for breast cancer. *Cancer Practice, 3*(4), 219–225.

Fairfax, J. (2002). *Theory of quality of life of stroke survivors.* Doctoral dissertation. Wayne State University, Detroit.

Fawcett, J. (1989). *Analysis and evaluation of conceptual models of nursing* (2nd ed.). Philadelphia: F.A. Davis.

Fawcett, J. H., & Downs, F. (1992). *The relationship of theory and research* (2nd ed.). Norwalk, CT: Appleton-Century-Crofts.

Fessenden, C. C. (2002). *Adoption of testicular self-examination.* Doctoral dissertation. Wayne State University, Detroit.

Gift, A. G. (1992). Dyspnea. *Nursing Clinics of North America, 25*(4), 955–965.

Good, M. & Moore, S. M. (1996). Clinical practice guidelines as a new source of middle range theory: Focus on acute pain. *Nursing Outlook, 44*(2), 74–79.

Good, M. A. (1998). A middle range theory of acute pain management: Use in research. *Nursing Outlook, 46*(3), 120–124.

Hageman, M. J., & Goei, R. (1993). Cleansing enema prior to double-contrast barium enema examination: Is it necessary? *Radiology, 187*(1), 109–112.

Harmer, B., & Henderson, V. (1944). *Textbook of the principles and practice of nursing* (p. 663). New York: Macmillan.

Hicks, E. S. (1944). Observations regarding enemas. *Canadian Medical Association, 51,* 358–359.

Hildebrandt, E. (1994). Building community participation in health care: A model and example from South Africa. *Journal of Nursing Scholarship, 28*(2) 155–159.

Hitchcock, J. M., & Wilson, H. S. (1992). Personal risking: lesbian self-disclosure of sexual orientation to professional health care providers. *Nursing Research, 41*(3), 178–183.

Hrabe, D. P. (2001). *Relationship development among chronically ill women in a computer-mediated environment.* Doctoral dissertation, University of Arizona.

Huth, M. M., & Moore, S. M. (1998). Prescriptive theory of acute pain management in infants and children. *Journal of the Society of Pediatric Nurses, 3*(1), 23–32.

Jansen, C. E., Miaskowski, C., Dodd, M. L., & Dowling, G. (2005). Chemotherapy-induced cognitive impairment in women with breast cancer: a critique of the literature. *Oncology Nursing Forum, 32*(2): 329–342.

Jenerette, C. M. (2004). *Testing the theory of self-care management for vulnerable populations in a sample of adults with sickle cell disease.* Doctoral dissertation. University of South Carolina,

Jezewski, M. A. (1995). Evolution of a grounded theory: Conflict resolution through culture brokering. *Advances in Nursing Science, 17*(3), 14–30.

Jirovec, M. M., Jenkins, J., Isenberg, M., & Baiardi, J. (1999). Urine control theory derived from Roy's

conceptual framework. *Nursing Science Quarterly, 12*(3), 251–255.

Kim, J., Dodd, M. L., West, C., Paul, S., Facione, N., Schumacher, K., et al. (2004). The PRO-SELF Pain Control Program improves patients' knowledge of cancer pain management. *Oncology Nursing Forum, 31*(6), 1137–1143.

Kim, S. K., Cho, C., & Levinsohn, E. M. (1980). Caustic colitis due to detergent enema. *American Journal of Roentgenology, 134*(2), 397–398.

Kinney, C. K. (1990). Facilitating growth and development: A paradigm case for modeling and role-modeling. *Issues in Mental Health Nursing, 11*(4), 375–395.

Klaus, M. H., & Kennell, J. H. (1976). *Maternal-infant bonding: The impact of early separation or loss on family development.* St. Louis: Mosby.

Kolcaba, K. (1994). A theory of comfort for nursing. *Journal of Advanced Nursing, 19*(6), 1178–1184.

Kozier, B., Erb, G., & Olivari, R. (1991). *Fundamentals of nursing: Concepts, process and practice* (4th ed.). (p. 1169). Redwood City, CA: Addison-Wesley.

Kreulen, G. J. (1994). Self-care, utilization, cost, quality and health status outcomes of a psychobehavioral nursing intervention: Women experiencing treatment for breast cancer. University of Arizona. Unpublished dissertation.

Kylma, J., & Vehvilainen-Julkunen, K. (1997). Hope in nursing research: A meta-analysis of the ontological and epistemological foundations of research on hope. *Journal of Advanced Nursing, 25*(2), 364–371.

Larson P. J., Dodd M. J., & Aksamit I. (1998). A symptom-management program for patients undergoing cancer treatment: The Pro-Self Program. *Journal of Cancer Education, 13*(4), 248–252.

Larson, P. J., Miaskowski, C., MacPhail, L., Dodd, M. J., Greenspan, D., et al. (1998). The PRO-SELF Mouth Aware program: An effective approach for reducing chemotherapy-induced mucositis. *Cancer Nursing, 21*(4), 263–268.

Lazarus, R., & Folkman, S. (1984). *Stress, appraisal, and coping.* New York: Springer.

Lenz, E. R., Pugh. C., Milligan, R. A., Gift, A. G., & Suppe, F. (1997). The middle-range theory of unpleasant symptoms: An update. *Advances in Nursing Science, 19*(3), 14–27.

Leventhal, H., Benyamini, Y., Brownee, S., Diefenbach, M., Levelthan, E., Patrick-Miller, L., et al. (1997). Illness representations: Theoretical foundation. In: Petrie, K. J. and Weinman, J. (2003). *Percentions of Health and Illness,* pp. 19–46. Singapore: Harwood Academic Publishers.

Levesque, L., Ricard, N., Ducharme, F., Duquette, A., & Bonin, J. (1998). Empirical verification of a theoretical model derived from the Roy Adaptation Model: Findings from five studies. *Nursing Science Quarterly, 11*(1), 31–39.

Liehr, P., & Smith, M. J. (1999). Middle range theory: Spinning research and practice to create knowledge for the new millennium. *Advances in Nursing Science, 21*(4), 81–91.

Lindsey, A. M., Larson, P. J., Dodd, M. J., Brecht, M., & Packer, A. (1994). Comorbidity, nutritional intake, social support, weight, and functional status over time in older cancer patients receiving radiotherapy. *Cancer Nursing, 17*(2), 113-124.

Lovely, M. P., Miaskowski, C., & Dodd, M. (1999). Relationship between fatigue and quality of life in patients with glioblastoma multiformae. *Oncology Nursing Forum, 26*(5), 921–925.

Luce, G. (1970). *Biological rhythms in psychiatry and medicine.* Washington, DC: U.S. Public Health Service.

Mahlungulu, S. N., & Uys, L. R. (2004). Spirituality in nursing: An analysis of the concept. *Curationis: South African Journal of Nursing, 27*(2), 15–26.

Mandrell, B. N., Ruccione, K, Dodd, M. L., Moore, J., Nelson, A. E., et al. (2000). Consensus statements: Applying the concept of self-care to pediatric oncology patients. *Seminars in Oncology Nursing, 16*(4), 315–316.

Marsh, V., Beard, M. T., & Bailey, C. (2002). Multitrait-multimethod matrix in scientific inquiry. *Journal of Theory Construction & Testing, 6*(1), 94–97.

McCubbin, H. I., & Patterson, J. M. (1983). The family stress process: the double ABCX model of adjustment and adaptation. *Marriage and Family Review, 6*(7), 7–37.

Mefford, L. C. (2004). A theory of health promotion for preterm infants based on Levine's conservation model of nursing. *Nursing Science Quarterly, 17*(3), 260–266.

Meleis, A. I., Sawyer, L. M., Im, E., Hilfinger/Messias, D. K., & Schumacher, K. (2000). Experiencing transitions: An emerging middle-range theory. *Advances in Nursing Science, 23*(1), 12–28.

Mercer, R. T. (1986). *First time motherhood: Experiences from teens to forties.* New York: Springer.

Messias, D. K. H., Yeager, K. A., Dibble, S. L., & Dodd, M. J. (1997). Patients' perspectives of fatigue while undergoing chemotherapy. *Oncology Nursing Forum, 24*(1), 43–48.

Miaskowski, C. J. (2000). Improving pain management: An ongoing journey. *Oncology Nursing Forum, 27*(6), 938–944.

Miaskowski, C., Dodd, M. L., West, C., Schumacher, K., Paul, S. M., Tripathy, D., et al. (2004). Randomized clinical trial of the effectiveness of a self-care intervention to improve cancer pain management. *Journal of Clinical Oncology, 22*(9), 1713–1720.

Miaskowski, C., Mack, K. A., Dodd, M. L., West, C., Paul, S. M., Tripathy, D., et al. (2002). Oncology outpatients with pain from bone metastasis require more than around-the-clock dosing of analgesics to achieve adequate pain control. *Journal of Pain, 3*(1), 12–20.

Mishel, M. H. (1988). Uncertainty in illness. *The Journal of Nursing Scholarship, 20*(4), 225–232.

Mishel, M. H. (1990). Reconceptualization of the uncertainty in illness theory. *The Journal of Nursing Scholarship, 22*(4), 256–262.

Moody, L. E. (1989). Building a conceptual map to guide research. *Florida Nursing Review, 4*(1), 1.

Morse, J. M., & Doberneck, B. (1995). Delineating the concept of hope. *Image—The Journal of Nursing Scholarship, 27*(4), 277–285.

Morse, J. M., & Johnson, H. K. (1991). *The Illness Experience: Dimensions of Suffering.* Newbury Park, CA: Sage.

Morse, J. M., Solberg, S. M., Neander, W. L., Bottorff, J. L., & Johnson, J. L. (1990). Concepts of caring and caring as a concept. *Advances in Nursing Science, 13*(1), 1–14.

Musci, I., & Dodd, M. (1990). Predicting self-care with patients and family members affective states and family functioning. *Oncology Nursing Forum, 17*(3), 394–400.

Myers, J. S. (2002). *Low-income immigrant parents and their children's health care: A problem-solving process.* Doctoral dissertation, George Mason University.

Newman, M. A. (1979). *Theory development in nursing.* Philadelphia: F. A. Davis.

Niv, Y. (1990). Enema preparation for proctosigmoidoscopy does not cause mucosal changes (Letter to the editor). *Southern Medical Journal, 79*(11), 1459–1460.

Olson, J., & Hanchett, E. (1997). Nurse expressed empathy, patient outcomes, and development of a middle-range theory. *The Journal of Nursing Scholarship, 29*(1), 71–76.

Orchard, J., & Lawson, R. (1986). Severe colitis induced by soap enemas. *Southern Medical Journal, 79*(11), 1459–1460.

Orem, D. E. (1995). *Nursing: Concepts of practice* (5th ed.). St. Louis: Mosby.

Orem, D. E. (2001). *Nursing: Concepts of practice* (6th ed.). St. Louis: Mosby.

Patterson, G. R. (1982). *Coercive family process.* Eugene, OR: Castoglia.

Pender, N. J. (1987). *Health promotion in nursing practice.* Norwalk, CT: Saunders.

Pender, N. J., Murdaugh, C. L., & Parsons, M. A. (2001). *Health promotion in nursing practice* (4th edition). Upper Saddle River, NJ: Prentice Hall.

Peterson, S. J., & Bredow, T. S. (2004). *Middle range theories: Application to nursing research.* Philadelphia, PA: Lippincott, Williams, & Wilkins.

Phillips, L. R., & Rempusheski, V. F. (1986). Caring for the frail elderly at home: Toward a theoretical explanation of the dynamics of poor quality family caregiving. *Advances in Nursing Science, 8*(4), 62–84.

Piper, B. F., Dibble, S. L., Dodd, M. J., Weiss, M. C., Slaughter, R. E., & Paul, S. M. (1998). The revised Piper Fatigue Scale: Psychometric evaluation in women with breast cancer. *Oncology Nursing Forum, 25*(4), 677–684.

Polk, L. V. (1997). Toward a middle-range theory of resilience. *Advances in Nursing Science, 19*(3), 1–13.

Powell-Cope, G. M. (1994). Family caregivers of people with AIDS: Negotiating partnerships with professional health care providers. *Nursing Research, 43*(6), 324–330.

Prochaska, J. O., & Velicer, W. F. (1997). The transtheoretical model of health behavior change. *American Journal of Health Promotion, 12*(1), 38–48.

Purnell, L. (2005). The Purnell Model for cultural competence. *The Journal for Multicultural Nursing & Health, 11*(2), 7–15.

Quinn, A. A. (1991). A theoretical model of the peri-menopausal process. *Journal of Nurse-Midwifery, 36*(1), 25–29.

Ray, M. (1989). The theory of bureaucratic caring for nursing practice in the organizational culture. *Nursing Administration Quarterly, 13*(2), 31–42.

Reed, P. (1991). Toward a nursing theory of self-transcendence: Deductive reformulation using developmental theories. *Advances in Nursing Science, 13*(4), 64–77.

Rich, J. A., & Grey, C. M. (2005). Pathways to recurrent trauma among young Black men: Traumatic stress, substance use, and the "Code of the Street." *American Journal of Public Health, 95*(5), 816–824.

Rogers, M. E., Malinski, V. M., & Barrett, E. A. M. (1994). *Martha E. Rogers: Her life and her work*. Philadelphia: F. A. Davis.

Roy, C., & Andrews, H. A. (1999). *Roy adaptation model*. Norwalk, CT: Appleton & Lange.

Roy, C., & Roberts, S. L. (1981). *Theory construction in nursing: An adaptation model*. Englewood Cliffs, NJ: Prentice-Hall.

Ruland, C. M., & Moore, S. M. (1998). Theory construction based on standards of care: A proposed theory of the peaceful end of life. *Nursing Outlook, 46*(4), 169–175.

Rumpt, J. (2002). Searching the essence of physiotherapy: A comparison of the Multi-dimensional-Load and Tolerance Model and the Movement Continuum Theory [Dutch]. *Nederlands Tijdschrift Voor Fysiotherapie, 112*(1), 9–16.

Sanford, R. C. (2000). Caring through relation and dialogue: A nursing perspective for patient education. *Advances in Nursing Science, 22*(3), 1–15.

Saunders, D. R., Haggitt, R. C., Kimmey, M. B., & Silverstein, F. E. (1990). Morphological consequences of bisacodyl on normal human rectal mucosa: Effects of a prostaglandin E_1 analog on mucosal injury. *Gastrointestinal Endoscopy, 36*(2), 101–104.

Schmelzer, M., & Wright, K. (1993). Say nope to soap, *American Journal of Nursing, 93*(3), 21.

Schmelzer, M., & Wright, K. (1996). Enema administration techniques used by experienced registered nurses. *Gastroenterology Nursing, 19*(5), 171–175.

Schmelzer, M., Case, P., Chappell, S. M., & Wright, K. B. (2000). Colonic cleansing, fluid absorption, and discomfort following tap water and soapsuds enemas. *Applied Nursing Research, 13*(2), 83–91.

Schumacher, K. L., Koresawa, S., West, C., Dodd, M. L., Paul, S. M., Tripathy, D., et al. (2002). The usefulness of a daily pain management diary for outpatients of cancer-related pain. *Oncology Nursing Forum, 29*(9), 1304-1313.

Schumacher, K. L., Koresawa, S., West, C., Dodd, M., Paul, S. M., Tripathy, D., et al. (2005). Focus on Research Methods: Qualitative research contribution to a randomized clinical trial. *Research in Nursing & Health, 28*(3), 268-280.

Schumacher, K. L., Koresawa, S., West, C., Hawkins, C., Johnson, C., Wais, E., et al. (2002). Putting cancer pain management regimens into practice at home. *Journal of Pain and Symptom Management, 23*(5), 369-382.

Schumacher, K. L., West, C., Dodd, M. L., Paul, S. M., Tripathy, D., Koo, P., et al. (2002). Pain management autobiographies and reluctance to use opioids for cancer pain management. *Cancer Nursing, 25*(2), 125-133.

Selye, H. (1976). *The stress of life*. New York: McGraw-Hill.

Silva, M. C. (1981). Selection of a theoretical framework. In S. D. Krampitz & N. Pavlovich (Eds.). *Readings for nursing research* (pp. 17–28). St. Louis: Mosby.

Smith, C. E., Pace, K., Kochinda, C., Kleinbeck, S., Koehler, J., & Popkess-Vawter, S. (2002). Caregiver effectiveness model evolution to a midrange theory of home care: A process for critique and replication. *Advances in Nursing Science, 25*(1), 50–64.

Smith, M. J., & Liehr, P. R. (2003). *Middle range theory for nursing*. New York, NY: Springer.

Sorensen, K., & Luckmann, J. (1986). *Basic nursing: A physiologic approach* (2nd ed., pp. 839–842). Philadelphia: Saunders.

Stark, P. L. & McGovern, J. P. (1992). *The meaning of suffering*. NLN Publications, Merck, pp. 25–42. (15–2461)

Swanson, E. A., Jensen, D. P., Specht, J., Johnson, M. L., & Maas, M. (1997). Caregiving: Concept analysis and outcomes. *Scholarly Inquiry for Nursing Practice: An International Journal, 11*(1), 65–79.

Swanson, K. M. (1991). Empirical development of a middle range theory of caring. *Nursing Research, 40*(3), 161–166.

Swanson, K. M. (1993). Nursing as informed caring for the well-being of others. *The Journal of Nursing Scholarship, 25*(4), 352–357.

Thomas, S. P. (1991). Toward a new conceptualization of women's anger. *Issues in Mental Health Nursing, 12*(1), 31–49.

Thompson, J. E., Oakley, D., Burke, M., Jay, S., & Conklin, M. (1989). Theory building in nurse-midwifery: The care process. *Journal of Nurse-Midwifery, 34*(4), 120–130.

Toffler, R. B., & Barry, J. M. (1972). Colonic mucosal slough following detergent enemas. *American Journal of Gastroenterology, 58*(6), 638–640.

Tollett, J. H., & Thomas, S. P. (1995). A theory-based nursing intervention to instill hope in homeless veterans. *Advances in Nursing Science, 18*(2), 76–90.

Tsai, P. (2003). A middle-range theory of caregiver stress. *Nursing Science Quarterly, 16*(2), 137–145.

Tsai, P., Tak, S., Moore, C., & Palencia, I. (2003). Testing a theory of chronic pain. *Journal of Advanced Nursing, 43*(2), 158–169.

U.S. Department of Health and Human Services (2000). *Healthy People 2010*. Washington, D.C: Author. For sale by the U.S. Government Printing Office.

University of California, San Francisco School of Nursing Symptom Management Group. (1994). A model for symptom management. *Image—The Journal of Nursing Scholarship, 26*(4), 272–276.

Walker, L. O. (1992). *Parent-infant nursing science: Paradigms, phenomena, methods*. Philadelphia: F.A. Davis.

Watson, J. (1985). *Nursing: Human science and human care. A theory of nursing*. Norwalk, CT: Appleton & Lange.

Whittemore, R., & Roy, C. (2002). Adapting to diabetes mellitus: A theory synthesis. *Nursing Science Quarterly, 15*(4), 311–317.

Williams, A. E. (2004). *Ethnic disparities in orthopaedic trauma*. Doctoral dissertation, University of Colorado Health Sciences Center, Denver.

Wilson, I. B., & Cleary, P. D. (1995). Linking clinical variables and health-related quality of life: A conceptual model of patient outcomes. *Journal of the American Medical Association, 273*(1), 59–65.

Wilson, M. (2005). Health-promoting behaviors of sheltered homeless women. *Family & Community Health, 28*(1), 51–63.

Wood, J. (1994). Physiology of the enteric nervous system. In L. R. Johnson (Ed.), *Physiology of the gastrointestinal tract* (3rd ed., pp. 423–482). New York: Raven Press.

Wuest, J. (2001). Precarious ordering: Toward a formal theory of woman's caring. *Health Care for Women International, 22*(1/2), 167–193.

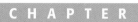

Examining Ethics in
Nursing Research

Chapter Overview

Learning Outcomes

After completing this chapter, you should be able to:

1. Identify the historical events influencing the development of ethical codes and regulations for research.

2. Identify the ethical principles that are important in conducting research on human subjects.

3. Describe the human rights that require protection in research.

4. Critique the informed consent and institutional review processes in published studies.

5. Examine the benefit-risk ratio of published studies.

6. Describe the types of possible scientific misconduct in the conduct, reporting, and publication of health care research.

Key Terms

STUDY TOOLS

Be sure to visit http:/elsevier.com/evolve/Burns/understanding for additional examples and self-tests.
Also, a review of this chapter's concepts and practice exercises can be found in Chapter 7 of the Study
Guide for *Understanding Nursing Research: Building an Evidence-Based Practice*, 4th edition.

What is unethical research? Are unethical studies that violate subjects' rights or involve scientific misconduct conducted today? It would be nice to believe that unethical studies are a thing of the past. However, this is not the case. Some recent studies in nursing and other disciplines do include evidence of scientific misconduct with the violation of subjects' rights and the publication of inaccurate scientific information (Njie & Thomas, 2001).

Misconduct can occur during the conduct, reporting, and publication of studies. Scientific misconduct in research includes such fraudulent practices as fabrication, falsification, or forging of data; dishonest manipulation of the study design or methods with protocol violations; misrepresentation of findings; and plagiarism (Rankin & Esteves, 1997). Scientific misconduct is a major problem, and greater than half of the top 50 research institutions in the United States have been investigated for fraud. Thus, the ethical aspects of published studies and of research conducted in clinical agencies should be critiqued. Most published studies include ethical information about subject selection and the data collection process in the "Methods" section of the report. Institutional review boards (IRBs) in universities and clinical agencies have been organized to examine the ethical aspects of studies before they are conducted.

To provide a background for examining ethical aspects of studies, this chapter describes the ethical codes and regulations that currently guide the conduct of biomedical and behavioral research. A new regulation entitled the Health Insurance Portability and Accountability Act (HIPAA) was enacted in 2003 to protect the privacy of people's health information. The HIPAA regulations have important implications for researchers conducting studies in health care. This chapter provides an overview of this act and the other regulations that have been developed to promote ethical conduct of research (Olsen, 2003). The elements of ethical research detailed in this chapter are (1) protecting human rights, (2) understanding informed consent, (3) understanding institutional review of research, and (4) balancing the benefits and risks in a study. Critique guidelines are provided for examining the ethical aspects of published studies and research proposed for conduct in clinical agencies. The chapter concludes with a discussion of two timely ethical issues: scientific misconduct and the use of animals in research.

Historical Events Influencing the Development of Ethical Codes and Regulations

Since the 1940s four experimental projects have been highly publicized for their unethical treatment of human subjects: the Nazi medical experiments, the Tuskegee Syphilis Study, the Willowbrook Study, and the Jewish Chronic Disease Hospital Study (Berger, 1990; Levine, 1986). Although these were biomedical studies and the primary investigators were physicians, the evidence suggests that nurses understood the nature of the research, identified potential research subjects, delivered treatments to the subjects, and served as data collectors. These unethical studies demonstrate the importance of ethical conduct for nurses while they are reviewing, participating in, or conducting nursing or biomedical research (Havens, 2004). These studies also influenced the formulation of ethical codes and regulations that currently direct the conduct of research.

Nazi Medical Experiments

From 1933 to 1945 the Third Reich in Europe performed atrocious unethical medical activities. The programs of the Nazi regime included sterilization, euthanasia, and medical experimentation for the purpose of producing a population of "racially pure" Germans who were destined to rule the world. The medical experiments were conducted on prisoners of war and persons considered to be racially valueless, such as Jews, who were confined in concentration camps. The experiments involved exposing subjects to high altitudes, freezing temperatures, malaria, poisons, spotted fever (typhus), or untested drugs and performing surgical procedures, usually without any form of anesthesia for the subjects. Extensive examination of the records from some of these studies indicated that they were poorly conceived and conducted. Thus, little if any useful scientific knowledge was generated by this research (Berger, 1990; Steinfels & Levine, 1976).

The Nazi experiments violated numerous rights of the research subjects. The selection of subjects for these studies was racially based and unfair, and the subjects had no choice: they were prisoners who were forced to participate. As a result of these experiments, subjects frequently were killed, or they sustained permanent physical, mental, and social damage (Levine, 1986).

Nuremberg Code

Those involved in the Nazi experiments were brought to trial before the Nuremberg Tribunals, and their unethical research received international attention. The mistreatment of human subjects in these studies led to the development of the Nuremberg Code in 1949; this code is presented in Table 7-1. The code includes guidelines that should help you evaluate

Table 7-1	The Nuremberg Code

1. The voluntary consent of the human subject is absolutely essential....
2. The experiment should be such as to yield fruitful results for the good of society, unprocurable by other methods or means of study, and not random and unnecessary in nature.
3. The experiment should be so designed and based on the results of animal experimentation and a knowledge of the natural history of the disease or other problem under study that the anticipated results will justify the performance of the experiment.
4. The experiment should be so conducted as to avoid all unnecessary physical and mental suffering and injury.
5. No experiment should be conducted where there is an *a priori* reason to believe that death or disabling injury will occur, except, perhaps, in those experiments where the experimental physicians also serve as subjects.
6. The degree of risk to be taken should never exceed that determined by the humanitarian importance of the problem to be solved by the experiment.
7. Proper preparations should be made and adequate facilities provided to protect the experimental subject against even remote possibilities of injury, disability, or death.
8. The experiment should be conducted only by scientifically qualified persons. The highest degree of skill and care should be required through all stages of the experiment of those who conduct or engage in the experiment.
9. During the course of the experiment the human subject should be at liberty to bring the experiment to an end if he has reached the physical or mental state where continuation of the experiment seems to him to be impossible.
10. During the course of the experiment the scientist in charge must be prepared to terminate the experiment at any stage, if he has probable cause to believe, in the exercise of the good faith, superior skill and careful judgment required of him that a continuation of the experiment is likely to result in injury, disability, or death to the experimental subject....

From Nuremberg Code (1986). In R. J. Levine (Ed.), *Ethics and regulation of clinical research* (2nd ed., pp. 425–426). Baltimore and Munich: Urban & Schwarzenberg.

the consent process, the protection of subjects from harm, and the balance of benefits and risks in a study (Nuremberg Code, 1986).

Declaration of Helsinki

The Nuremberg Code provided the basis for the development of the Declaration of Helsinki, which was adopted in 1964 and revised in 1975, 1983, 1989, 1996, and 2000 by the World Medical Association. A major focus of the initial document was the differentiation of therapeutic research from nontherapeutic research. **Therapeutic research** provides patients with an opportunity to receive an experimental treatment that might have beneficial results. **Nontherapeutic research** is conducted to generate knowledge for a discipline; the results of the study might benefit future patients but probably will not benefit those acting as research subjects. The Declaration of Helsinki includes the following ethical principles: (1) the investigator should protect the life, health, privacy, and dignity of human subjects; (2) the investigator should exercise greater care to protect subjects from harm in nontherapeutic research; and (3) the investigator should conduct research only when the importance of the objective outweighs the inherent risks and burdens to the subjects. (The ethical principles of the Declaration of Helsinki can be reviewed online at http://www.wma.net/e/policy/b3.htm.) Most institutions conducting clinical research adopted the Nuremberg Code and Declaration of Helsinki; however, episodes of scientific misconduct related to mistreatment of subjects continued to occur in biomedical and behavioral research (Levine, 1986).

Tuskegee Syphilis Study

In 1932, the U.S. Public Health Service initiated a study of syphilis in African American men in the small rural town of Tuskegee, Alabama (Levine, 1986; Rothman, 1982). The study, which continued for 40 years, was conducted to determine the natural course of syphilis in African American men. Many of the subjects who consented to participate in the study were not informed about the purpose and procedures of the research. Some were unaware that they were subjects in a study. By 1936 it was apparent that the men with syphilis had developed more complications than those observed in the men in the control group. Ten years later the death rate among those with syphilis was twice as high as it was for the control group. The subjects were examined periodically but were not treated for syphilis, even when penicillin was determined to be an effective treatment for the disease in the 1940s. Information about an effective treatment for syphilis was withheld from the subjects, and deliberate steps were taken to deprive them of treatment (Brandt, 1978).

Published reports of the Tuskegee Syphilis Study started appearing in 1936, and additional papers were published every 4 to 6 years. No effort was made to stop the study; in fact, in 1969 the Centers for Disease Control and Prevention (then called the Center for Disease Control) decided that the study should continue. In 1972, an account of the study in the *Washington Star* sparked public outrage; only then did the Department of Health, Education, and Welfare (DHEW) stop the study. The study was investigated and found to be ethically unjustified (Brandt, 1978).

Willowbrook Study

From the mid-1950s to the early 1970s, Dr. Saul Krugman conducted research on hepatitis at Willowbrook, an institution for the mentally retarded in Staten Island, New York (Rothman, 1982). The subjects were children who were deliberately infected with the hepatitis virus. During the 20-year study, Willowbrook closed its doors to new inmates because of overcrowded conditions. However, the research ward continued to admit new inmates, and parents had to give permission for their child to be in the study to gain admission to the institution (Levine, 1986).

From the late 1950s to the early 1970s, Krugman's research team published several articles describing the study protocol and findings. In 1966, Beecher cited the Willowbrook Study in *The New England Journal of Medicine* as an example of unethical research. The investigators defended injecting the children with the hepatitis virus because they believed most of the children would acquire the infection on admission to the institution. They also stressed the benefits the subjects received, which were a cleaner environment, better supervision, and a higher nurse-patient ratio on the research ward (Rothman, 1982). Despite the controversy, this unethical study continued until the early 1970s.

Jewish Chronic Disease Hospital Study

Another highly publicized unethical study was conducted at the Jewish Chronic Disease Hospital in New York in the 1960s. The purpose of this study was to determine patients' rejection responses to live cancer cells. Twenty-two patients were injected with a suspension containing live cancer cells that had been generated from human cancer tissue (Levine, 1986).

Because these patients were not informed that they were taking part in research or that the injections they received were live cancer cells, their rights were not protected. In addition, the study was never presented for review to the research committee of the Jewish Chronic Disease Hospital, and the physicians caring for the patients were unaware that the study was being conducted. The physician directing the research was an employee of the Sloan-Kettering Institute for Cancer Research, and there was no indication that this institution had conducted a review of the research project (Hershey & Miller, 1976). This unethical study was conducted without the informed consent of the subjects and without institutional review and had the potential to injure, disable, or cause the death of the human subjects. The study was stopped immediately and steps were taken to ensure proper care for the patients exposed to the cancer cells and the review of all future research to be conducted in this agency.

Department of Health, Education, and Welfare 1973 Regulations for the Protection of Human Research Subjects

The continued conduct of harmful, unethical research from the 1960s to the 1970s made additional controls necessary. In 1973, the DHEW published its first set of regulations for the protection of human research subjects. These regulations also provided protection for persons having limited capacity to consent, such as people who are ill, mentally impaired, or dying (Levine, 1986). According to the DHEW regulations, all research involving human subjects had to undergo full institutional review, which increased the protection of human subjects. However, reviewing all studies without regard for the degree of risk involved greatly increased the time for study approval and reduced the number of studies conducted.

National Commission for the Protection of Human Subjects of Biomedical and Behavioral Research

Because the issue of protecting human subjects in research was not resolved by the DHEW regulations, the National Commission for the Protection of Human Subjects of Biomedical and Behavioral Research (1978) was formed. This commission was established by the National Research Act (Public Law 93-348), which was passed in 1974. The commission identified three **ethical principles** that are relevant to the conduct of research involving human subjects: respect for persons, beneficence, and justice. The **principle of respect for persons** indicates that people should be treated as autonomous agents with the right to self-determination and the freedom to participate or not participate in research. Those persons with diminished autonomy, such as children, people who are terminally or mentally ill, and prisoners, are entitled to additional protection. The **principle of beneficence** encourages the researcher to do good and "above all, do no harm." The **principle of justice** states that human subjects should be treated fairly in terms of the benefits and the risks of research. Before it was dissolved in 1978, the commission developed ethical research guidelines based on these three principles and made recommendations to the U.S. Department of Health and Human Services (DHHS) in the *Belmont Report*. (Information on this report and the three ethical principles—respect for persons, beneficence, and justice—can be obtained online at http://ohsr.od.nih.gov/guidelines/belmont.html.)

Current Federal Regulations for the Protection of Human Subjects

In response to the commission's recommendations, the DHHS developed a set of federal regulations for the protection of human research subjects in 1981, and these regulations were revised in 1983, 1991, and 2001 (U.S. DHHS, 1981, 1983, 1991, 2001, 2005). The 2005 regulations are part of the *Code of Federal Regulations* (CFR), Title 45 Part 46 Protection of Human Subjects. These regulations provide direction for (1) protection of human subjects in research, with additional protection for pregnant women, human fetuses, neonates, children, and prisoners; (2) documentation of informed consent; and (3) implementation of the IRB process (access these regulations online at http://ohsr.od.nih.gov/guidelines/45cfr46.html).

Most of the biomedical and behavioral research conducted in the United States is governed by the DHHS Protection of Human Subjects Regulations (U.S. DHHS, 2005) and/or the U.S. Food and Drug Administration (FDA, 2002; online at http://www.fda.gov/oc/gcp/). The FDA, within the DHHS, manages the CFR Title 21 Food and Drugs, Part 50 Protection of Human Subjects and Part 56 Institutional Review Boards. The FDA has additional human subject protection regulations that apply to clinical investigations involving products regulated by the FDA under the Federal Food, Drug, and Cosmetic Act and research that supports applications for research or marketing permits for these products. Thus, these regulations apply to studies of drugs for humans, medical devices for human use, biological products for human use, human dietary supplements, and electronic products (FDA, 2002; online at http://vm.cfsan.fda.gov/~lrd/cfr50.html). The physician and nurse researchers conducting clinical trials to generate new drugs and refine existing drug treatments must comply with these FDA regulations. Table 7-2 clarifies the focus of the U.S. DHHS and FDA Protection of Human Subjects Regulations.

The U.S. DHHS and FDA regulations provide guidelines for the protection of subjects in federally and privately funded research to ensure their privacy and the confidentiality of the information obtained through research. With the mechanisms for the electronic access and transfer of individuals' information, however, the public became concerned about the potential abuses of the health information of persons in all circumstances, including research projects. Thus, a new federal regulation—the Health Insurance Portability and Accountability Act (HIPAA), or Public Law 104-191—was enacted on August 21, 1996, and implemented on April 14, 2003, to protect people's private health information (U.S. DHHS, 2003). (HIPAA regulations can be accessed online at http://www.hhs.gov/ocr/hipaa/finalreg.html.) Table 7-2 clarifies the focus of HIPAA regulations as compared with the DHHS and FDA regulations (U.S. DHHS, 2004, August 4b).

The DHHS developed regulations entitled the *Standards for Privacy of Individually Identifiable Health Information*, and compliance with these regulations is known as the Privacy Rule (U.S. DHHS, 2003, 45 CFR Parts 160 and 164). The HIPAA Privacy Rule established a category entitled protective health information (PHI), which allows covered entities, such as health plans, health care clearinghouses, and health care providers that transmit health information, to use or disclose PHI to others only in certain situations. These situations are discussed later in this chapter.

The HIPAA Privacy Rule has an impact not only on the health care environment but also on the research conducted in this environment. A person must provide his or her signed permission, or authorization, before that person's PHI can be used or disclosed for research purposes. Researchers must modify their current studies and develop their new research

Table 7-2　Clarification of the Focus of Federal Regulations and Impact on Research

Area of Distinction	HIPAA Privacy Rule	DHHS Protection of Human Subjects Regulations Title 45 CFR Part 46	FDA Protection of Human Subjects Regulations Title 21 CFR Parts 50 & 56
Overall objective	Establish a federal floor of privacy protections for most individually identifiable health information by establishing conditions for its use and disclosure by certain health care providers, health plans, and health care clearinghouses	To protect the rights and welfare of human subjects involved in research conducted or supported by DHHS. Not specifically a privacy regulation	To protect the rights, safety, and welfare of subjects involved in clinical investigations regulated by the FDA. Not specifically a privacy regulation
Applicability	Applies to HIPAA-defined covered entities, regardless of the source of funding	Applies to human subjects' research conducted or supported by DHHS and research with private funding	Applies to research involving products regulated by the FDA. Federal support is not necessary for FDA regulations to be applicable. When research subject to FDA jurisdiction is federally funded, both the DHHS Protection of Human Subjects Regulations and FDA Protection of Human Subjects Regulations apply

From U.S. Department of Health and Human Services. (2004, August 4b). How do other privacy protections interact with the privacy rule? HIPAA Privacy Rule: Information for Researchers. Retrieved December 3, 2005, from http://privacyruleandresearch.nih.gov/pr_05.asp

DHHS, Department of Health and Human Services; FDA, Food and Drug Administration; HIPAA, Health Insurance Portability and Accountability Act.

projects to comply with the HIPAA Privacy Rule. The DHHS developed a website entitled "HIPAA Privacy Rule: Information for Researchers" to address the impact of this rule on the informed consent and IRB processes in research and to answer common questions about HIPAA (available at http://privacyruleandresearch.nih.gov/) (U.S. DHHD, 2004, August 4c). Because this is a relatively new law, the exact impact it will have on the protection of people's privacy and on the conduct of research is yet to be determined (Frank-Stromborg, 2004; Olsen, 2003; Stone, 2003).

Protecting Human Rights

What are human rights? How are these rights protected during research? **Human rights** are claims and demands that have been justified in the eyes of an individual or by the consensus of a group of people. Nurses who critique published studies, review research for conduct in their agencies, or assist with data collection for a study have an ethical responsibility to determine whether the rights of the research subjects are protected. The human rights that require protection in research are the rights to (1) self-determination, (2) privacy, (3) anonymity and confidentiality, (4) fair treatment, and (5) protection from discomfort and harm (American Nurses Association, 2001; American Psychological Association, 2002).

Right to Self-Determination

The right to self-determination is based on the ethical principle of respect for persons, and it indicates that humans are capable of controlling their own destiny. Thus, humans should be treated as autonomous agents, who have the freedom to conduct their lives as they choose without external controls. Subjects are treated as autonomous agents in a study if the researcher has (1) informed them about the study, (2) allowed them to choose whether to participate, and (3) allowed them to withdraw from the study at any time without penalty (Levine, 1986).

Violation of the Right to Self-Determination

A subject's right to self-determination can be violated through the use of coercion, covert data collection, and deception. Coercion occurs when one person intentionally presents an overt threat of harm or an excessive reward to another to obtain compliance. Some subjects are coerced to participate in research because they fear harm or discomfort if they do not participate. For example, some patients feel that their medical and nursing care will be negatively affected if they do not agree to be research subjects. Other subjects are coerced to participate in studies because they believe that they cannot refuse the excessive rewards offered, such as large sums of money, special privileges, or jobs (Emanuel, 2004; U.S. DHHS, 2005).

With covert data collection, subjects are unaware that research data are being collected (Reynolds, 1979). For example, in the Jewish Chronic Disease Hospital Study, most of the patients and their physicians were unaware of the study. The subjects were informed that they were receiving an injection of cells, but the word "cancer" was omitted (Beecher, 1966).

The use of deception (the actual misinforming of subjects for research purposes) (Kelman, 1967) also can violate a subject's right to self-determination. A classic example of deception is seen in the Milgram (1963) study, in which the subjects thought they were administering electric shocks to another person, but the person was really a professional actor who pretended to feel the shocks. If deception is used in a study, the research report should indicate how the subjects were deceived and that the subjects were informed of the actual research activities and the findings at the end of the study.

Persons with Diminished Autonomy

Persons have diminished autonomy when they are vulnerable and less advantaged because of legal or mental incompetence, terminal illness, or confinement to an institution (Levine, 1986; U.S. DHHS, 2005). These persons require additional protection of their right to self-determination because of their decreased ability or inability to give informed consent. In addition, these persons are vulnerable to coercion and deception. The research report should include justification for the use of subjects with diminished autonomy, and the need for justification increases as the subjects' risks and vulnerability increase.

Legal and Mental Limitations of Those Consenting to Research

Minors (neonates and children), pregnant women and fetuses, mentally impaired persons, and unconscious patients are legally and/or mentally unable to give informed consent. These individuals often lack the ability to comprehend information about a study and/or to make decisions about participating in or withdrawing from the study. These persons have a range of vulnerability from minimal to absolute. The use of persons with diminished autonomy as research subjects is more acceptable if the following are true: (1) the research is therapeutic, that is, the subjects might benefit from the experimental process; (2) the researcher is willing to use both vulnerable and nonvulnerable people as subjects; (3) the risk is minimized in the study; and (4) the consent process is strictly followed to ensure the rights of the prospective subjects (U.S. DHHS, 2005).

Neonates

A neonate is defined as a newborn and is identified as either viable or nonviable on delivery. Viable neonates are able to survive after delivery, if given the benefit of available medical therapy, and can independently maintain a heartbeat and respiration. "A nonviable neonate means that a newborn after delivery, although living, is not viable" (U.S. DHHS, 2001, 45 CFR Section 46.202). Neonates are extremely vulnerable and require extra protection to determine their involvement in research. However, viable neonates, neonates of uncertain viability, and nonviable neonates may be involved in research if the following conditions are met: (1) the study is scientifically appropriate and the preclinical and clinical studies have been conducted and provide data for assessing the potential risks to the neonates; (2) the study provides important biomedical knowledge, which cannot be obtained by other means, and will not add risk to the neonate; (3) the research holds out the prospect of enhancing the probability of survival of the neonate; (4) both parents are fully informed about the research during the consent process; and (5) researchers will have no part in determining the viability of a neonate. In addition, for "nonviable neonates, the vital functions of the neonate should not be artificially maintained because of the research and the research should not terminate the heartbeat or respiration of the neonate" (U.S. DHHS, 2001, 45 CFR Section 46.205).

RESEARCH EXAMPLE **Ethical Conduct of Research with Neonates**

Holditch-Davis, Brandon, and Schwartz (2003) conducted a study in preterm infants to increase understanding of infant behaviors related to sleeping and waking, their characteristics, and illness severity. The ethical aspects of the study were described as follows:

. . .[T]he study was approved by the institutional committee for protection of human subjects [IRB]. Infants were enrolled as soon as their medical conditions were no longer critical if an additional hospital stay of at least 1 week was anticipated and informed consent was obtained from the parents... (p. 310).

All other infants, including those with intraventricular hemorrhage, were eligible so that the sample would be representative of preterm infants in intensive care units (p. 309).

(continues)

CRITIQUE

Holditch-Davis, et al. (2003) obtained IRB approval for their study and parental informed consent. They also attempted to ensure that the neonates' conditions were stable to decrease the risks related to the study. They included a variety of neonates with different types of illnesses to increase the representativeness of the sample. All of these activities promoted the ethical conduct of this study according to the DHHS regulations (U.S. DHHS, 2001).

IMPLICATIONS FOR PRACTICE

The development of infant behaviors occurred over the preterm period. The behaviors included yawn, sigh, negative facial expression, startle/jerk, jitter, large body movements, mouth movements, and hiccups. The sighs and hiccups usually decreased over time. Additional research is needed before clinically useful interpretations of infant behaviors can be made. Studies need to focus on the occurrence of infant behaviors in sleeping and waking and how the behaviors are affected by different stimuli, illness severity, and age.

Children

The laws defining the minor status of a child are statutory and vary from state to state. Often a child's competence to give consent is operationalized by age, with incompetence being irrefutable up to age 7 (Broome, 1999; Thompson, 1987). However, by age 7 children can think in terms of concrete operations and can provide meaningful assent to participation as research subjects. With advancing age and maturity the child can play a stronger role in the consent process.

The DHHS regulations require "soliciting the assent of the children (when capable) and the permission of their parents or guardians. Assent means a child's affirmative agreement to participate in research…. Permission means the agreement of parent(s) or guardian to the participation of their child or ward in research" (U.S. DHHS, 1983, Section 46.402). The decision about using children as research subjects also is influenced by the therapeutic nature of the research and the risks versus benefits. Thompson (1987) developed a guide for obtaining informed consent based on the child's level of competence, the therapeutic nature of the research, and the risks versus benefits (see Table 7-3). Broome (1999) developed an example assent form that is presented in Table 7-4. During a study, the child needs to be given an option to ask questions and to withdraw from the study if he or she desires.

There is an increased need for ethical research using children as subjects. Researchers are being urged to conduct clinical trials with children to determine the effectiveness of selected pharmacological and nonpharmacological treatments for various age groups (Rosato, 2000).

Pregnant Women and Fetuses

Pregnant women require additional protection in research because of the presence of the fetus. Federal regulations define pregnancy as encompassing the period of time from

Table 7-3	Guide to Obtaining Informed Consent, Based on the Relationship between a Child's Level of Competence, the Therapeutic Nature of the Research, and Risk versus Benefits*

	Nontherapeutic		Therapeutic	
	MMR-LB	MR-LB	MR-HB	MMR-HB
Child, incompetent (generally 0-7 yr)				
Parents' consent	Necessary	Necessary	Sufficient*	Sufficient
Child's assent	Optional†	Optional†	Optional	Optional
Child, relatively competent (7 yr and older)				
Parents' consent	Necessary	Necessary	Sufficient‡	Recommended
Child's assent	Necessary	Necessary	Sufficient§	Sufficient

MMR, more than minimal risk; *MR*, minimal risk; *LB*, low benefit; *HB*, high benefit.
*A parent's refusal can be superseded by the principle that a parent has no power to forbid the saving of a child's life.
†Children making a "deliberate objection" would be precluded from participation by most researchers.
‡In cases not involving the privacy rights of a "mature minor."
§In cases involving the privacy rights of a "mature minor."

Table 7-4	Sample Assent Form for Children Ages 6 to 12 Years: Pain Interventions for Children with Cancer

Oral Explanation
I am a nurse who would like to know if relaxation, special ways of breathing, and using your mind to think pleasant things help children like you to feel less afraid and feel less hurt when the doctor has to do a bone marrow aspiration or spinal tap. Today, and the next five times you and your parent come to the clinic, I would like for you to answer some questions about the things in the clinic that scare you. I would also like you to tell me about how much pain you felt during the bone marrow or spinal tap. In addition, I would like to videotape (take pictures of) you and your mom and/or dad during the tests. The second time you visit the clinic I would like to meet with you and teach you special ways to relax, breathe, and use your mind to imagine pleasant things. You can use the special imagining and breathing then during your visits to the clinic. I would ask you and your parents to practice the things I teach you at home between your visits to the clinic. At any time you could change your mind and not be in the study anymore.

To child:
1. I want to learn special ways to relax, breathe, and imagine.
2. I want to answer questions about things children may be afraid of when they come to the clinic.
3. I want to tell you how much pain I feel during the tests I have.
4. I will let you videotape me while the doctor does the tests (bone marrow and spinal taps).

If the child says YES, have him/her put an "X" here:

If the child says NO, have him/her put an "X" here:

Date:

Child's signature:

From Broome, M. E. (1999). Consent (assent) for research with pediatric patients. *Seminars in Oncology Nursing, 15*(2), 101.

implantation until delivery. "A woman is assumed to be pregnant if she exhibits any of the pertinent presumptive signs of pregnancy, such as missed menses, until the results of a pregnancy test are negative or until delivery" (U.S. DHHS, 2005, 45 CFR section 46.202). Research conducted with pregnant women should have the potential to directly benefit the woman or the fetus. If the investigation is thought to provide a direct benefit just to the fetus, then the consent of the pregnant woman and the father needs to be obtained. Studies with "pregnant women should include no inducements to terminate the pregnancy and the researcher should have no part in any decision to terminate a pregnancy" (U.S. DHHS, 2005, 45 CFR Section 46.204).

Persons with Mental Illness or Cognitive Impairment

Certain persons, because of mental illness, cognitive impairment, or a comatose state, are incompetent and incapable of giving informed consent. Persons are said to be incompetent if, in the judgment of a qualified clinician, they have those attributes that ordinarily provide the grounds for designating incompetence (Levine, 1986). Incompetence can be temporary (e.g., with inebriation), permanent (e.g., with advanced senile dementia), or subjective or transitory (e.g., with behavior or symptoms of psychosis). If a person is judged incompetent and incapable of giving consent, the researcher must seek approval from the prospective subject and his or her legally authorized representative. A legally authorized representative is a person or another body authorized under applicable law to consent on behalf of a prospective subject to the subject's participation in the research procedure(s) (U.S. DHHS, 2005).

Terminally Ill Subjects

Participating in research may carry increased risks with minimal or no benefits for terminally ill subjects. In addition, the dying subject's condition potentially may affect the study results, leading the researcher to misinterpret the findings. For example, cancer patients have become an overstudied population. It is not unusual that the majority of procedures performed on cancer patients is a result of research protocols that include blood work, bone marrow scans, lumbar punctures, and biopsies (Strauman & Cotanch, 1988). These biomedical research treatments can easily compromise the care of these patients, which poses ethical dilemmas for clinical nurses. More nurses will be responsible for ensuring adherence to ethical standards in research as they participate in institutional review of research and serve as patient advocates in the clinical setting (Havens, 2004; Njie & Thomas, 2001).

Persons Confined to Institutions

Prisoners are people who are confined to institutions and are designated as having diminished autonomy by federal law (U.S. DHHS, 2005). Prison inmates may feel coerced to participate in research because they fear harm or desire the benefits of early release, special treatment, or monetary gain.

Hospitalized patients are a vulnerable population but are not designated as having diminished autonomy by law. However, patients are vulnerable because they are ill and are confined in settings that are controlled by health care personnel. Some hospitalized patients feel obligated to be research subjects because they want to assist a particular nurse or physician with his or her research. Others feel coerced to participate because they fear that their care will be adversely affected if they refuse. Thus, researchers should be cautious about protecting the rights of patients in health care agencies who participate in research.

CRITIQUE GUIDELINES Self-Determination

When critiquing studies, evaluate the subjects' capacity for self-determination and assess whether the rights of subjects with diminished autonomy were protected. Ask questions such as the following:

1. Did the subjects have diminished autonomy because of legal or mental incompetence, terminal illness, or confinement to an institution?
2. If they did, were special precautions taken in obtaining consent from these subjects and their parents or guardians?

Right to Privacy

Privacy is the freedom people have to determine the time, extent, and general circumstances under which their private information will be shared with or withheld from others. Private information includes that concerning a person's attitudes, beliefs, behaviors, opinions, and records. The research subject's privacy is protected if the subject is informed, consents to participate in a study, and voluntarily shares private information with a researcher. An **invasion of privacy** occurs when private information is shared without a person's knowledge or against his or her will. The invasion of subjects' right to privacy brought about the Privacy Act of 1974. As a result of this act, people now have the right to provide or prevent access of others to their records (Levine, 1986). A research report often will indicate that the subjects' privacy was protected and may include the details of how this was accomplished.

The HIPAA Privacy Rule expanded the protection of a person's privacy—specifically, his or her protected, individually identifiable health information—and described the ways in which covered entities can use or disclose this information. **Covered entities** are health care providers, health plans, employers, and health care clearinghouses (public or private entities that process or facilitate the processing of health information). **Individually identifiable health information** (IIHI) means

> ...any information, including demographic information collected from an individual that is created or received by health care provider, health plan, or healthcare clearinghouse; and related to past, present, or future physical or mental health or condition of an individual, the provision of health care to an individual, or the past, present, or future payment for the provision of health care to an individual, and identifies the individual; or with respect to which there is a reasonable basis to believe that the information can be used to identify the individual. (U.S. DHHS, 2003, 45 CFR, Section 160.103)

According to the HIPAA Privacy Rule, the IIHI is protected health information (PHI) that is transmitted by electronic media, maintained in electronic media, or transmitted or maintained in any other form or medium. Thus, the HIPAA privacy regulations affect nursing research in the following areas:

1. Accessing data from a covered entity, such as reviewing a patient's medical record in clinics or hospitals;
2. Developing health information, such as the data developed when an intervention is implemented in a study to improve a subject's health; and
3. Disclosing data from a study to a colleague in another institution, such as sharing data from a study to facilitative development of an instrument or scale (Frank-Stromborg, 2004; Olsen, 2003).

The DHHS developed guidelines to assist researchers, health care organizations, and health care providers determine when they can use and disclose IIHI. IIHI can be used or disclosed to a researcher in the following situations:

- The protected health information (PHI) has been de-identified under the HIPAA Privacy Rule.
- The data are part of a limited data set and a data use agreement with the researcher(s) is in place.
- The person who is a potential subject for a study provides authorization for the researcher to use and disclose his or her PHI.
- A waiver or alteration of the authorization requirement is obtained from an IRB or privacy board. (U.S. DHHS, 2004, August 4a)

The first two items are discussed in this section of the text. The authorization process is discussed in the section "Understanding Informed Consent," and the waiver or alteration of authorization requirement is covered in the section "Understanding Institutional Review."

De-Identifying Protected Health Information under the Privacy Rule

Covered entities, such as health care providers and agencies, can allow researchers access to health information if the information has been de-identified. De-identifying health data involves removing the 18 elements that could be used to identify a specific person or that person's relatives, employer, or household members. The 18 identifying elements are

- Names.
- All geographic subdivisions smaller than a state, including street address, city, county, precinct, ZIP Code, and their equivalent geographical codes, except for the initial three digits of a ZIP Code if, according to the current publicly available data from the Bureau of the Census.
- The geographic unit formed by combining all ZIP Codes with the same three initial digits contains more than 20,000 people.
- The initial three digits of a ZIP Code for all such geographic units containing 20,000 or fewer people are changed to 000.
- All elements of dates (except year) for dates directly related to an individual, including birth date, admission date, discharge date, date of death; and all ages over 89 and all elements of dates (including year) indicative of such age, except that such ages and elements may be aggregated into a single category of age 90 or older.

- Telephone numbers.
- Facsimile numbers.
- Electronic mail addresses.
- Social security numbers.
- Medical record numbers.
- Health plan beneficiary numbers.
- Account numbers.
- Certificate/license numbers.
- Vehicle identifiers and serial numbers, including license plate numbers.
- Device identifiers and serial numbers.
- Web universal resource locators (URLs).
- Internet protocol (IP) address numbers.
- Biometric identifiers, including fingerprints and voiceprints.
- Full-face photographic images and any comparable images.
- Any other unique identifying number, characteristic, or code, unless otherwise permitted by the Privacy Rule for re-identification. (U.S. DHHS, 2004, August, 4a; online at http://privacyruleandresearch.nih.gov/pr_08.asp)

A person's health information also can be de-identified using statistical methods. However, the covered entity and the researcher must ensure that the individual subject cannot be identified, or that there is a very small risk that the subject could be identified from the information used. The statistical method used for de-identification of the health data must be documented, and the study must certify that the 18 elements for identification have been removed or revised to prevent identification of a specific person. This certification information must be kept for a period of 6 years by the researcher.

Limited Data Set and Data Use Agreement

Covered entities—health care provider, health plan, and health care clearinghouse—may use and disclose a limited data set to a researcher for a study without an individual subject's authorization or an IRB waiver. However, a limited data set is considered PHI, and the covered entity and the researcher need to have a data use agreement. The **data use agreement** limits how the data set may be used and how it will be protected. The HIPAA Privacy Rule requires that the following information be included in a data use agreement:

- Specifies the permitted uses and disclosures of the limited data set.
- Identifies the researcher who is permitted to use or receive the limited data set.
- Stipulates that the recipient (researcher) will:
  - ◆ Not use or disclose the information other than permitted by the agreement.
  - ◆ Use appropriate safeguards to prevent the use or disclosure of the information, except as provided for in the agreement.
  - ◆ Hold any other person (co-researchers, statisticians, or data collectors) to the standards, restrictions, and conditions stated in the data use agreement with respect to the health information.
  - ◆ Not identify the information or contact the individuals whose data are in the limited data set. (U.S. DHHS, 2004, August 4a; online at http://privacyruleandresearch.nih.gov/pr_08.asp)

Right to Anonymity and Confidentiality

On the basis of the right to privacy, the research subject has the right to anonymity and the right to assume that the data collected will be kept confidential. Complete **anonymity** exists when the subject's identity cannot be linked, even by the researcher, with his or her individual responses (American Nurses Association, 2001).

In most studies, researchers know the identity of their subjects, and they promise the subjects that their identity will be kept anonymous from others and that the research data will be kept confidential. **Confidentiality** is the researcher's management of private information shared by a subject. The researcher must refrain from sharing that information without the authorization of the subject. Confidentiality is grounded in the following premises:

> (1) Individuals can share personal information to the extent they wish and are entitled to have secrets; (2) one can choose with whom to share personal information; (3) those accepting information in confidence have an obligation to maintain confidentiality; and (4) professionals, such as researchers, have a duty to maintain confidentiality that goes beyond ordinary loyalty. (Levine, 1986, p. 164)

A **breach of confidentiality** can occur when a researcher, by accident or direct action, allows an unauthorized person to gain access to the raw data of a study. Confidentiality also can be breached in reporting or publishing a study if a subject's identity is accidentally revealed, violating the subject's right to anonymity (Ramos, 1989). Breach of confidentiality is of special concern in qualitative studies that have few subjects and involve the reporting of long quotes made by the subjects. Such long quotes often can reveal the identity of a subject to others, resulting in a breach of confidentiality (Munhall, 2001a; Sandelowski, 1994). Breaches of confidentiality that can be especially harmful to subjects include those regarding religious preferences; sexual practices; income; racial prejudices; drug use; child abuse; and personal attributes such as intelligence, honesty, and courage. Thus, the research report needs to be examined for evidence that subject confidentiality was maintained during data collection and analysis. In addition, the research findings should be reported so that a subject or group of subjects cannot be identified by their responses.

RESEARCH EXAMPLE Protection of Research Subjects' Rights

Barber, Grubbs, and Cottrell (2005) conducted a study of the self-perception of children diagnosed with attention deficit/hyperactivity disorder (ADHD). These researchers addressed how they conducted research with children, who have diminished autonomy; protected their privacy; and maintained the confidentiality of the research data.

Children aged 8-12 years who came for an appointment at a local pediatric office or local health agency with an ADHD clinic along with their parent or guardian were approached and asked to participate voluntarily in a short question-and-answer session with the researcher. A copy of the data collection tool was offered to the parent or guardian. Parents of the potential study participants were asked to read a parent information letter and give written informed consent [parent or guardian consent]. The procedure was explained to each child, and he or she was allowed to ask any question or express any concern regarding participation. Consent to participate was gained in the presence of each child's parent or guardian. Complete confidentiality was guaranteed [confidentiality]. Each child gave written assent by signing a form indicating that they were voluntarily taking part in the study [child assent]. After consent was obtained, each child was led to a private location away from others [privacy]. The parent or guardian was asked to remain close by.... The children were encouraged to answer truthfully and to voice any questions or concern. They were also assured that nobody other than the researcher would know their answers [confidentiality].... Parents or guardians were informed that overall results of the study would be made available to the practitioner and provided upon request. (Barber et al., 2005, p. 239)

CRITIQUE

Barber and colleagues (2005) clearly described their process of obtaining informed consent and protecting the rights of their research subjects. They documented that the children, who were minors and incompetent to give consent, were provided with a detailed explanation of the research and given the opportunity to assent to participate in the study in front of their parents or guardian. Researchers asked the parents and guardians, who also were provided an explanation of the study verbally and in writing, to give their informed consent for their child to participate in the study. The data for the study were collected in a private location that ensured privacy for the child but with the parent remaining close if needed. Confidentiality of the research data was ensured twice in the study example, and the analysis of the data produced "overall results," so individual subjects and their data could not be identified.

IMPLICATIONS FOR PRACTICE

Barber et al. (2005) found that children with ADHD had negative self-perceptions and lower self-esteem than that of their peers. Over the years, the cumulative effects on self-esteem and self-perception may have significant life consequences for these children. The researchers recommended focusing on fostering self-esteem and positive self-perception in children with ADHD through support groups and behavioral training.

Right to Fair Treatment

The right to fair treatment is based on the ethical principle of justice. According to this principle, people must be treated fairly and receive what they are due or owed. The research report needs to indicate that the selection of subjects and their treatment during the study were fair.

Fair Selection and Treatment of Subjects

In the past, injustice in subject selection resulted from social, cultural, racial, and sexual biases in society. For many years, research was conducted on categories of people who were thought to be especially suitable as research subjects, such as persons living in poverty, charity patients, prisoners, slaves, peasants, dying persons, and others who were considered undesirable (Reynolds, 1979). Researchers often treated these subjects carelessly and had little regard for the harm and discomfort they experienced. The Nazi medical experiments, the Tuskegee Syphilis Study, the Willowbrook Study, and the Jewish Chronic Disease Hospital Study all exemplify unfair subject selection.

Another concern with subject selection is that some researchers select subjects because they like them and want them to receive the specific benefits of a study. Other researchers have been swayed by power or money to make certain patients subjects so these patients can receive potentially beneficial treatments. Random selection of subjects can eliminate some of the researcher's biases that may influence subject selection.

Each study must include a specific researcher-subject agreement regarding the researcher's role and the subject's participation in a study (American Psychological Association, 2002). While conducting the study, the researcher must treat the subjects fairly and respect that agreement. For example, the activities or procedures that the subject is to perform should not be changed without the subject's consent. The benefits promised to the subjects should be provided. In addition, subjects who participate in studies should receive equal benefits regardless of age, race, or socioeconomic level.

The research report needs to indicate that the selection and treatment of the subjects were fair. Subjects must have been selected for reasons directly related to the problem being studied and not for their easy availability, compromised position, manipulability, or friendship with the researcher (National Commission for the Protection of Human Subjects of Biomedical and Behavioral Research, 1978). In addition, the "Procedures" section of the research report must indicate fair and equal treatment of the subjects during data collection.

The Barber et al. (2005) study of the self-perception of children with ADHD, presented earlier in this chapter, demonstrated fair selection and treatment of subjects. The children selected for the study were those who came for an appointment at a local pediatric office or ADHD clinic and they were asked if they would like to participate. This indicates that the children and their parents or guardians were in the office or clinic of their own free will and that they had the right to participate or not in the study. During the study, the children's privacy was protected and confidentiality of the research data was maintained. In addition, "the children and their parents were given the chance to ask any questions or voice any concern regarding participation in the study" (Barber et al., 2005, p. 239). These steps by the researchers indicate the fair treatment of the subjects and their parents and guardians during the study.

Right to Protection from Discomfort and Harm

The right to protection from discomfort and harm from a study is based on the ethical principle of beneficence, which states that one should do good and, above all, do no harm. According to this principle, members of society must take an active role in preventing discomfort and harm and promoting good in the world around them. In research, **discomfort and harm** can be physical, emotional, social, or economic, or any combination of these four (Weijer, 2000). Reynolds (1972) identified five categories of studies based on levels of discomfort and harm: no anticipated effects, temporary discomfort, unusual levels of temporary discomfort, risk of permanent damage, and certainty of permanent damage.

No Anticipated Effects

In some studies, no positive or negative effects are expected for the subjects. For example, studies that involve reviewing patients' records, students' files, pathology reports, or other documents have no anticipated effects on the research subjects. In this type of study, the researcher does not interact directly with the subjects; however, there is still a potential risk of invading a subject's privacy. With the HIPAA regulations, a subject's IIHI must be protected during data collection and analysis and in publication of the final report (U.S. DHHS, 2003).

Temporary Discomfort

Studies that cause temporary discomfort are described as minimal-risk studies, in which the discomfort is similar to what the subject would encounter in his or her daily life and is temporary, ending with termination of the experiment (U.S. DHHS, 2005). Many nursing studies require the completion of questionnaires or participation in interviews, which usually involve minimal risk or are a mere inconvenience for the subjects. The physical discomfort may include fatigue, headache, or muscle tension. The emotional and social risks may include anxiety or embarrassment associated with answering certain questions. The economic risks may include the time commitment for the study or travel costs to the study site.

Most clinical nursing studies examining the effect of a treatment involve minimal risk. For example, a study may involve examining the effects of exercise on the blood glucose levels of diabetic subjects. For the study, the subjects are asked to test their blood glucose level one extra time per day. Discomfort occurs when the blood is obtained, and there is a potential risk of physical changes that may occur with exercise. The subjects also may feel anxiety and fear associated with the additional blood testing, and the testing may be an added expense. The diabetic subjects in this study will encounter similar discomforts in their daily lives, however, and the discomfort will cease with the termination of the study.

Unusual Levels of Temporary Discomfort

In studies that involve unusual levels of temporary discomfort, subjects frequently have discomfort both during the study and after it has been completed. For example, subjects may have prolonged muscle weakness, joint pain, and dizziness after participating in a study that required them to be confined to bed for 10 days to determine the effects of immobility. Studies that require subjects to experience failure, extreme fear, or threats to their identity or to act in unnatural ways involve unusual levels of temporary discomfort. In some qualitative studies, subjects are asked questions that open old wounds or involve reliving traumatic events (Ford & Reuter, 1990). For example, asking subjects to describe their rape experience could precipitate feelings of extreme anger, fear, sadness, or any combination of these emotions. In such studies, investigators need to indicate in the research report that they were vigilant in assessing the subjects' discomfort and referred them as necessary for appropriate professional intervention.

Risk of Permanent Damage

In some studies, the possibility exists for subjects to sustain permanent damage; this is more common in biomedical research than in nursing research. For example, new drugs and surgical procedures being tested in medical studies have the potential to cause subjects permanent physical damage. Some topics investigated by nurses have the potential to permanently damage subjects emotionally and socially. Studies examining sensitive information, such as sexual behavior, child abuse, AIDS or human immunodeficiency virus status, or drug use, can be very risky for subjects. These studies have the potential to cause permanent damage to a subject's personality or reputation. There also are potential economic risks, such as those resulting from a decrease in job performance or loss of employment.

Certainty of Permanent Damage

In some research, such as the Nazi medical experiments and the Tuskegee Syphilis Study, the subjects experienced permanent damage. Conducting research that will permanently damage subjects is highly questionable, regardless of the benefits that will be gained. Frequently the benefits gained from such a study are experienced not by the research subjects but by others in society. Studies causing permanent damage to subjects violate the fifth principle of the Nuremberg Code (see Table 7-1).

Understanding Informed Consent

What is informed consent? How is informed consent obtained from research subjects? "Informing" is the transmission of essential ideas and content from the investigator to the prospective subject. "Consent" is the prospective subject's agreement to participate in a study as a subject. Every prospective subject, to the degree that he or she is capable, should have the opportunity to choose whether to participate in research (FDA, 1998a; U.S. DHHS, 2005). **Informed consent** includes four elements: (1) disclosure of essential study information to the subject, (2) comprehension of this information by the subject, (3) competence of the subject to give consent, and (4) voluntary consent of the subject to participate in the study.

Essential Information for Consent

Informed consent requires the researcher to disclose specific information to all prospective subjects. The following information is identified as essential for obtaining informed consent from research subjects (FDA, 1998a; U.S. DHHS, 2005):

1. *Introduction of research activities.* The initial information presented to prospective subjects clearly indicates that a study is to be conducted and that they are being asked to participate as subjects.
2. *Statement of the research purpose.* The researcher states the immediate purpose of the research and any long-range goals related to the study.
3. *Selection of research subjects.* The researcher explains to prospective subjects why they were selected to participate in the study.

4. *Explanation of procedures.* Prospective subjects receive a complete description of the procedures to be followed and identification of any procedures that are experimental in the study (U.S. DHHS, 2001, Section 46.116a).

5. *Description of risks and discomforts.* Prospective subjects are informed of any reasonably foreseeable risks or discomforts (physical, emotional, social, and economic) that might result from the study.

6. *Description of benefits.* The investigator describes any benefits to the subjects or to other people or future patients that may reasonably be expected from the research, including any financial advantages or other rewards for participating in the study.

7. *Disclosure of alternatives.* The investigator discloses the appropriate alternative procedures or courses of treatment, if any, that might be advantageous to the subjects (FDA, 1998a; U.S. DHHS, 2005). For example, the researchers of the Tuskegee Syphilis Study should have informed the subjects with syphilis that penicillin was an effective treatment for the disease.

8. *Assurance of anonymity and confidentiality.* Prospective subjects should know the extent to which their responses and records will be kept confidential. Subjects are promised that their identity will remain anonymous in reports and publications of the study.

9. *Offer to answer questions.* The researcher offers to answer any questions the prospective subjects may have.

10. *Voluntary participation.* Consent form includes a statement that participation is voluntary and that refusal to participate will involve no penalty or loss of benefits to which the subject is otherwise entitled.

11. *Option to withdraw.* Subjects are informed that they may discontinue participation (withdraw from a study) at any time without penalty or loss of benefits (U.S. DHHS, 1991, Section 46.116a).

12. *Consent to incomplete disclosure.* In some studies, subjects are not completely informed of the study purpose because that knowledge would alter their actions. However, prospective subjects must be told when certain information is being withheld deliberately.

A **consent form** is a written document that includes the elements of informed consent required by the DHHS Regulations (U.S. DHHS, 2005) and FDA Regulations (1998a). In addition, a consent form may include other information required by the institution where the study is to be conducted or by the agency funding the study. An example of a consent form is presented in Figure 7-1; the **boldface** terms indicate the essential consent information.

Comprehension of Consent Information

Informed consent implies not only that the researcher has imparted information to the subjects but also that the prospective subjects have comprehended that information. The researcher must take the time to teach the subjects about the study. The amount of information to be taught depends on the subjects' knowledge of research and the specific research topic. The benefits and risks of a study need to be discussed in detail, with examples that the potential subject can understand. Nurses often serve as patient advocates in clinical agencies and need to assess whether patients involved in research understand the purpose and the potential risks and benefits of their participation in a study (Burns & Grove, 2005).

Study title: The Needs of Family Members of Critically Ill Adults
Investigator: Linda L. Norris, R.N.

Ms. Norris is a registered nurse studying the emotional and social needs of family members of patients in the Intensive Care Units **(research purpose)**. Although the study will not benefit you directly, it will provide information that might enable nurses to identify family members' needs and to assist family members with those needs **(potential benefits)**.

The study and its procedures have been approved by the appropriate people and review boards at The University of Texas at Arlington and X hospital **(IRB approval)**. The study procedures might cause fatigue for you or your family **(potential risks)**. The procedures include: (1) responding to a questionnaire about the needs of family members of critically ill patients and (2) completing a demographic data sheet **(explanation of procedures)**. Participation in this study will take approximately 20 minutes **(time commitment)**. You are free to ask any questions about the study or about being a subject and you may call Ms. Norris at (999) 999-9999 (work) or (999) 999-9999 (home) if you have further questions **(offer to answer questions)**.

Your participation in this study is voluntary; you are under no obligation to participate **(alternative option and voluntary consent)**. You have the right to withdraw at any time and the care of your family member and your relationship with the health care team will not be affected **(option to withdraw)**.

The study data will be coded so they will not be linked to your name. Your identity will not be revealed while the study is being conducted or when the study is reported or published. All study data will be collected by Ms. Norris, stored in a secure place, and not shared with any other person without your permission **(assurance of anonymity and confidentiality)**.

I have read this consent form and voluntarily consent to participate in this study.

(If Appropriate)

_____   _____
Subject's Signature   Date   Legal Representative   Date

I have explained this study to the above subject and to have sought his/her understanding for informed consent.

_____
Investigator's Signature   Date

Figure 7-1. Sample consent form.

Competence to Give Consent

Autonomous persons, who are capable of understanding the benefits and risks of a proposed study, are competent to give consent. Persons with diminished autonomy due to legal or mental incompetence, terminal illness, or confinement to an institution frequently are not legally competent to consent to participate in research (see the earlier section "Right to Self-Determination"). Frequently, the researcher determines the competence of the subject (Douglas & Larson, 1986). In the research report the investigator often will indicate the competence of the subjects and the process that was used for obtaining informed consent.

Voluntary Consent

Voluntary consent means that the prospective subject has decided to take part in a study of his or her own volition without coercion or any undue influence (Douglas & Larson, 1986). Voluntary consent is obtained after the prospective subject has been given the essential information about the study and has demonstrated comprehension of this information. All of these elements of informed consent need to be documented in a consent form.

Documentation of Informed Consent

The documentation of informed consent depends on (1) the level of risk involved in the study and (2) the discretion of the researcher and those reviewing the study for institutional approval. Most studies require a written consent form, although in some studies, the requirement for written consent is waived. Nurses may be asked to identify subjects for studies, obtain consent forms for studies, collect study data, or participate in an IRB to review the ethics of a study. Thus, they need to be aware of the process for documenting consent in research.

Written Consent Waived

The requirements for written consent may be waived in research that "presents no more than minimal risk of harm to subjects and involves no procedures for which written consent is normally required outside of the research context" (U.S. DHHS, 2001, 45 CFR Section 46.117c). For example, researchers using questionnaires to collect relatively harmless data do not need to obtain a signed consent form from the subjects. The subject's completion of the questionnaire may serve as consent. The top of the questionnaire might contain a statement such as "Your completion of this questionnaire indicates your consent to participate in this study."

Written consent also is waived in a situation in which "the only record linking the subject and the research would be the consent document and the principal risk would be potential harm resulting from a breach of confidentiality. Each subject will be asked whether the subject wants documentation linking the subject with the research, and the subject's wishes will govern" (U.S. DHHS, 2001, 45 CFR Section 46.117c). Thus, in this situation, subjects are given the option to sign or not sign a consent form that links them to the research. The four elements of consent—disclosure, comprehension, competency, and voluntariness—are essential in all studies, whether written consent is waived or required.

Written Consent Documents

The short form consent document includes the following statement: "The elements of informed consent required by Section 46.116 [see the section "Information Essential for Consent"] have been presented orally to the subject or the subject's legally authorized representative" (U.S. DHHS, 2001, 45 CFR Section 46.117a). The researcher must develop a written summary of what is to be said to the subject in the oral presentation, and the summary must be approved by an IRB. When the oral presentation is made to the subject or to the subject's representative, a witness is required. The subject or the representative must sign the short form consent document. "The witness shall sign both the short form and a copy of the summary, and the person actually obtaining consent shall sign a copy of the summary" (U.S. DHHS, 2001, 45 CFR Section 46.117a). Copies of the summary and short form are given to the subject and the witness; the original documents are retained by the researcher. The researcher must keep these documents for 3 years. The short form written consent documents typically are used in studies that present minimal or moderate risk to the subjects.

The formal written consent document includes the elements of informed consent required by the DHHS (U.S. DHHS, 2005) and FDA (1998a) regulations (see the previous section "Information Essential for Consent"). In addition, a consent form may include other information required by the institution where the study is to be conducted or by the agency funding the study. A sample consent form is presented in Figure 7-1, p. 217, with descriptors of the essential consent information. The consent form can be read by the subject or read to the subject by the researcher; however, it is wise also to explain the study to the subject. The form is signed by the subject and is witnessed by the investigator or research assistant collecting the data. This type of consent can be used for any type of study, from minimal risk to high risk. All persons signing the consent form—including the subject, researcher, and any witnesses—must receive a copy of it. The original consent form is kept by the researcher for a period of 3 years.

Studies that involve subjects with diminished autonomy require a written consent form. If these prospective subjects have some comprehension of the study and agree to participate as subjects, they must sign the consent form. However, the form also must be signed by the subject's legally authorized representative. The representative indicates his or her relationship with the subject under the signature (see Figure 7-1). Sometimes nurses are asked to sign a consent form as a witness for a biomedical study. They must know the study purpose and procedures and the subject's comprehension of the study before signing the form.

HIPAA Privacy Rule: Authorization for Research Uses and Disclosure

The HIPAA Privacy Rule provides people, as research subjects, the right to authorize covered entities (health care provider, health plan, and health care clearinghouse) to use or disclose their PHI for research purposes. This authorization is regulated by the HIPAA and is in addition to the informed consent that is regulated by the DHHS (U.S. DHHS, 2005, CFR 45 Part 46) and the FDA (1998a, CFR 21 Part 50). The authorization focuses on the privacy risks and states how, why, and to whom the PHI will be shared. The authorization "Core Elements" can be found online at http://privacyruleandresearch.nih.gov/authorization.asp (U.S. DHHS, 2004, July 1). The authorization information can be included as part of the consent form, but it probably is best to have two separate forms (U.S. DHHS, 2003, April 17; Olsen, 2003). The DHHS has developed a sample authorization form, which is presented in Figure 7-2.

AUTHORIZATION TO USE OR DISCLOSE (RELEASE) HEALTH INFORMATION
THAT IDENTIFIES YOU FOR A RESEARCH STUDY

REQUIRED ELEMENTS:

If you sign this document, you give permission to [name or other identification of specific health care provider(s) or description of classes of persons, e.g., all doctors, all health care providers] at [name of covered entity or entities] to use or disclose (release) your health information that identifies you for the research study described below:
[Provide a description of the research study, such as the title and purpose of the research.]

The health information that we may use or disclose (release) for this research includes
[complete as appropriate]:
[Provide a description of information to be used or disclosed for the research project. This description may include, for example, all information in a medical record, results of physical examinations, medical history, lab tests, or certain health information indicating or relating to a particular condition.]
The health information listed above may be used by and/or disclosed (released) to:
[Name or class of persons involved in the research; i.e., researchers and their staff**]

[Name of covered entity] is required by law to protect your health information. By signing this document, you authorize [name of covered entity] to use and/or disclose (release) your health information for this research. Those persons who receive your health information may not be required by Federal privacy laws (such as the Privacy Rule) to protect it and may share your information with others without your permission, if permitted by laws governing them.

Please note that [include the appropriate statement]:
- You do not have to sign this Authorization, but if you do not, you may not receive research-related treatment. **(When the research involves treatment and is conducted by the covered entity or when the covered entity provides health care solely for the purpose of creating protected health information to disclose to a researcher)**

- [Name of covered entity] may not condition (withhold or refuse) treating you on whether you sign this Authorization. **(When the research does not involve research-related treatment by the covered entity or when the covered entity is not providing health care solely for the purpose of creating protected health information to disclose to a researcher)**

Please note that [include the appropriate statement]:
- You may change your mind and revoke (take back) this Authorization at any time, except to the extent that [name of covered entity(ies)] has already acted based on this Authorization. To revoke this Authorization, you must write to: [name of the covered entity(ies) and contact information]. **(Where the research study is conducted by an entity other than the covered entity)**

- You may change your mind and revoke (take back) this Authorization at any time. Even if you revoke this Authorization, [name or class of persons at the covered entity involved in the research] may still use or disclose health information they already have obtained about you as necessary to maintain the integrity or reliability of the current research. To revoke this Authorization, you must write to: [name of the covered entity(ies) and contact information]. **(Where the research study is conducted by the covered entity)**

_____   _____
Signature of participant or participant's   Date
personal representative

_____   _____
Printed name of participant or participant's   If applicable, a description of the personal
personal representative   representative's authority to sign for the participant

** Where a covered entity conducts the research study, the Authorization must list ALL names or other identification, or ALL classes, of persons who will have access through the covered entity to the protected health information (PHI) for the research study (e.g., research collaborators, sponsors, and others who will have access to data that includes PHI). Examples may include, but are not limited to the following:

- Data coordinating centers that will receive and process PHI;
- Sponsors who want access to PHI or who will actualy own the research data; and/or
- Institutional Review Boards or Data Safety and Monitoring Boards.

If the research study is conducted by an entity other than the covered entity, the authorization need only list the name or other identification of the outside researcher (or class of researchers) and any other entity to whom the covered entity is expected to make the disclosure.

Figure 7-2. The Authorization to Use or Disclose (Release) Health Information That Identifies You for a Research Study. (From U.S. Department of Health and Human Services. (2004, July 1). Information for covered entities and researchers on authorizations for research uses or disclosures of protected health information. HIPAA Privacy Rule: Information for Researchers. Available at http://privacyruleand research.nih.gov/authorization.asp)

RESEARCH EXAMPLE Informed Consent

Research reports often discuss the consent process and identify some of the essential consent information that was provided to the potential subjects. Some mention of the consent process for that study is required, but the depth of the discussion will vary according to the research purpose and the types of subjects included in the study. Yeh, Chang, and Chang (2005) conducted a study of the perceived quality of life of children with cancer using the children's self-reports and parent-proxy reports; thus, both children and parents were subjects in the study. The following excerpt documents the process for obtaining informed consent from these subjects.

> The hospital's established procedures for protecting confidentiality were strictly followed. Eligible parents were approached by one of three trained data collectors who are registered nurses. The parents received verbal and written explanations of the study and procedures and were asked about their willingness to participate in our study along with their sick children. After parental consent and child assent were obtained, participants were scheduled for face-to-face interviews that took place at the hospital ward or at the outpatient clinics for baseline assessment.... Any information on the questionnaires identifying participants was removed immediately upon receipt of the packet and all materials were stored in a locked place. (Yeh et al., 2005, p. 356)

CRITIQUE

Yeh and colleagues (2005) clearly identified the informed consent process in their research report. The researchers indicated that the study subjects (children and parents) were provided verbal and written information about the study and the parents were asked to sign a consent form and the children were asked to assent to the study. The researchers also strictly followed confidentiality procedures of the agency and removed any specific information identifying individual participants from the data collected. The data were securely stored so that only the researchers had access to the data for analysis. On the basis of the research report, Yeh et al. followed the DHHS (U.S. DHHS, 2005) and HIPAA (U.S. DHHS, 2004, July 1) guidelines for the consent process.

IMPLICATIONS FOR PRACTICE

Yeh et al. (2005) found that the parents consistently reported better quality of life for their children than was perceived by the child. This study provides initial understanding of parents' and children's perceptions of quality of life and how these perceptions might vary. Further research is needed to determine changes in the perceived quality of life over time through acceptance of diagnosis, treatment, and after treatment by both children and parents. A better understanding of the perceived quality of life is needed before interventions can be developed to support the child and parents in dealing with a cancer diagnosis.

Understanding Institutional Review

In institutional review, a study is examined for ethical concerns by a committee of the researcher's peers. The first federal policy statement on protection of human subjects by institutional review was issued by the PHS in 1966. The statement required that research involving human subjects must be reviewed by a committee of peers or associates to confirm that (1) the rights and welfare of the persons involved were protected, (2) the appropriate methods were used to secure informed consent, and (3) the potential benefits of the investigation were greater than the risks (Levine, 1986).

In 1974, DHEW passed the National Research Act, which required that all research involving human subjects undergo institutional review. The DHHS reviewed and revised these guidelines in 1981, 1983, 1991, 2001, and 2005 (45 CFR Sections 46.107–46.115; online at http://ohsr.od.nih.gov/guidelines/45cfr46.html). The FDA (1998b, 21 CFR Sections 56.103–56.124; online at http://www.fda.gov/oc/ohrt/irbs/appendixc.html) also has very similar guidelines for institutional review of research. The regulations describe the membership, functions, and operations of the body responsible for institutional review. An **institutional review board (IRB)** is a committee that reviews research to ensure that the investigator is conducting the research ethically. Universities, hospital, corporations, and many managed care centers have IRBs to promote the conduct of ethical research and to protect the rights of prospective subjects at their institutions.

Each IRB has at least five members of varying backgrounds (cultural, economic, educational, gender, racial) to promote complete, scholarly, and fair review of research that is commonly conducted in an institution. If an institution regularly reviews studies with vulnerable subjects, such as children, neonates, pregnant women, prisoners, and the mentally disabled, the IRB needs to include one or more members with knowledge about and experience in working with these subjects. The members must have sufficient experience and expertise to review a variety of studies, including quantitative, qualitative, and outcomes research (Munhall, 2001b). The IRB members must not have a conflicting interest related to a study conducted in an institution. Any member having a conflict of interest with a research project being reviewed must excuse himself or herself from the review process, except to provide information requested by the IRB. The IRB also must include one member whose primary concern is nonscientific, such as an ethicist, lawyer, or minister. At least one of the IRB members must be someone who is not affiliated with the institution (FDA, 1998b; U.S. DHHS, 2005). The IRBs in hospitals often are composed of physicians, nurses, lawyers, scientists, clergy, and community lay persons.

Levels of Reviews Conducted by Institutional Review Boards

The functions and operations of an IRB involve the review of research at three different levels: (1) exempt from review, (2) expedited review, and (3) complete review. The level of the review required for each study is decided by the IRB chairperson and/or committee, but not by the researcher. Studies usually are **exempt from review** if they pose no apparent risks for the research subjects. The studies that typically are considered exempt from review by the federal regulations are identified in Table 7-5. Nursing studies that carry no foreseeable risks or that involve procedures posing a mere inconvenience for subjects usually are identified as exempt from review by the chairperson of the IRB committee.

Studies that carry some risks, which are viewed as minimal, qualify for an **expedited review**. "**Minimal risk** means that the probability of and magnitude of harm or discomfort anticipated in the research are not greater in and of themselves than those ordinarily encountered in daily life or during the performance of routine physical or psychological examinations or tests" (U.S. DHHS, 2005, 45 CFR Section 46.102i). Expedited review procedures also can be used to review minor changes in previously approved research. Under expedited review procedures, the review may be carried out by the IRB chairperson or by one or more

Table 7-5	Research Qualifying for Exemption from Review

Unless otherwise required by department or agency heads, research activities in which the only involvement of human subjects will be in one or more of the following categories are exempt from review.

(1) Research conducted in established or commonly accepted educational settings, involving normal educational practices, such as (i) research on regular and special education instructional strategies, or (ii) research on the effectiveness of or the comparison among instructional techniques, curricula, or classroom management methods.

(2) Research involving the use of educational tests (cognitive, diagnostic, aptitude, achievement), survey procedures, interview procedures or observation of public behavior, unless: (i) information obtained is recorded in such a manner that human subjects can be identified, directly or through identifiers linked to the subjects; and (ii) any disclosure of the human subjects' responses outside the research could reasonably place the subjects at risk of criminal or civil liability or be damaging to the subjects' financial standing, employability, or reputation.

(3) Research involving the use of educational tests (cognitive, diagnostic, aptitude, achievement), survey procedures, interview procedures, or observation of public behavior that is not exempt under paragraph (b)(2) of this section, if: (i) the human subjects are elected or appointed public officials or candidates for public office; or (ii) Federal statute(s) require(s) without exception that the confidentiality of the personally identifiable information will be maintained throughout the research and thereafter.

(4) Research involving the collection or study of existing data, documents, records, pathological specimens, or diagnostic specimens, if these sources are publicly available or if the information is recorded by the investigator in such a manner that subjects cannot be identified, directly or through identifiers linked to the subjects.

(5) Research and demonstration projects which are conducted by or subject to the approval of Department or Agency heads, and which are designed to study, evaluate, or otherwise examine: (i) Public benefit or service programs; (ii) procedures for obtaining benefits or services under those programs; (iii) possible changes in or alternatives to those programs or procedures; or (iv) possible changes in methods or levels of payment for benefits or services under those programs.

(6) Taste and food quality evaluation and consumer acceptance studies, (i) if wholesome foods without additives are consumed or (ii) if a food is consumed that contains a food ingredient at or below the level and for a use found to be safe, or agricultural chemical or environmental contaminant at or below the level found to be safe, by the Food and Drug Administration or approved by the Environmental Protection Agency or the Food Safety and Inspection Service of the U.S. Department of Agriculture.

From U.S. Department of Health and Human Services. (2001, November 13). Protection of human subjects. *Code of Federal Regulations*, Title 45, Part 46. Retrieved January 10, 2004, from http://ohrp.osophs.dhhs.gov/humansubjects/guidance/45cfr46.htm

experienced reviewers designated by the chairperson from among members of the IRB. In reviewing the research, the reviewers may exercise all of the authorities of the IRB except disapproval of the research. A research activity may be disapproved only after a complete review of the IRB (FDA, 1998b; U.S. DHHS, 2005). Table 7-6 identifies research that usually qualifies for expedited review.

A study that carries greater than minimal risks must receive a **complete review** by an IRB. To obtain IRB approval, researchers must ensure that

(1) risks to subjects are minimized, (2) risks to subjects are reasonable in relation to anticipated benefits, (3) selection of subjects is equitable, (4) informed consent will be sought from each prospective subject or the subject's legally authorized representative, (5) informed consent will be appropriately documented, (6) the research plan makes adequate provision for monitoring data collection for subjects' safety, and (7) adequate provisions are made to protect the privacy of subjects and to maintain the confidentiality of data. (FDA, 1998b, 21 CFR 56.111; U.S. DHHS, 2005, 45 CFR Section 46.111)

Table 7-6	Research Qualifying for Expedited Institutional Review Board Review

Expedited review (by committee chairpersons or designated members) for the following research involving no more than minimal risk is authorized:

1. Collection of hair and nail clippings, in a nondisfiguring manner; deciduous teeth and permanent teeth if patient care indicates a need for extraction.
2. Collection of excreta and external secretions including sweat, uncannulated saliva, placenta removed at delivery, and amniotic fluid at the time of rupture of the membrane before or during labor.
3. Recording of data from subjects 18 years of age or older using noninvasive procedures routinely employed in clinical practice. This includes the use of physical sensors that are applied either to the surface of the body or at a distance and do not involve input of matter or significant amounts of energy into the subject or an invasion of the subject's privacy. It also includes such procedures as weighing, testing sensory acuity, electrocardiography, electroencephalography, thermography, detection of naturally occurring radioactivity, diagnostic echography, and electroretinography. It does not include exposure to electromagnetic radiation outside the visible range (for example, x-rays, microwaves).
4. Collection of blood samples by venipuncture, in amounts not exceeding 450 ml in an 8-week period and no more than two times per week, from subjects 18 years of age or older and who are in good health and not pregnant.
5. Collection of both supragingival and subgingival dental plaque and calculus, provided the procedure is not more invasive than routine prophylactic scaling of the teeth and the process is accomplished in accordance with accepted prophylactic techniques.
6. Voice recordings made for research purposes such as investigations of speech defects.
7. Moderate exercise by healthy volunteers.
8. The study of existing data, documents, records, pathological specimens, or diagnostic specimens.
9. Research on individual or group behavior or characteristics of individuals, such as studies of perception, cognition, game theory, or test development, where the investigator does not manipulate subjects' behavior and research will not involve stress to subjects.
10. Research on drugs or devices for which an investigational new drug exemption or an investigational device exemption is not required.

From U.S. Department of Health and Human Services. (2001, November 13). Protection of human subjects. *Code of Federal Regulations*, Title 45, Part 46. (Additional regulations that apply to research involving fetuses, pregnant women, human in vitro fertilization, and prisoners are available online at http://ohrp.osophs.dhhs.gov/humansubjects/guidance/45cfr46.htm.)

RESEARCH EXAMPLE Institutional Review Board Approval in a Study

Published studies often indicate that a research project was approved by an IRB. For example, Steele and Porche (2005) conducted their study to test the Theory of Planned Behavior to predict the intentions of rural women in Southeastern Louisiana to obtain a mammogram. The researchers described the following approval process for their study.

The institutional review board [IRB] at Louisiana State University Health Sciences Center approved the study. Upon obtaining written permission to collect data within the agencies, participants were recruited by posting flyers in rural churches, health clinics, hospitals, senior centers, and school employee lunchrooms. Women who accessed the rural community-based organization during the study period, attended briefing sessions, and met the eligibility requirements were asked to participate [subject selection]. The researcher discussed the purpose of the study with each participant, answered any questions, and allowed time for them to review and sign the consent form [informed consent]. . . A financial incentive of a $10 gift certificate was given to all participants who completed the questionnaire. (Steele & Porche, 2005, p. 335)

(continues)

CRITIQUE

Steele and Porche (2005) presented the essential content that documents the ethics of a study. The study was presented to IRB committees and approved for conduct in a rural town in Louisiana. The subjects were fairly selected because fliers were placed in numerous sites and participants who met the eligibility criteria were invited to participate. So subjects had a choice to participate or not in the study. Steele and Porche followed the elements of informed consent because they provided subjects with an explanation of the study and allowed questions before the subjects signed a written consent form. The subjects were offered a very small financial incentive of a $10 gift certificate to encourage their participation. The incentive was not large enough for people to feel that they had to participate just to receive the money.

IMPLICATIONS FOR PRACTICE

The study provided support for the use of the Theory of Planned Behavior to predict the likelihood of women in a rural town to obtain a mammogram. The perceived behavior control was the strongest predictor of mammography intention. However, more research is needed to explain the women's attitudes toward mammography and their motivation to get a mammogram. This additional knowledge is needed before an intervention can be developed to increase mammography intention and use (Steele & Porche, 2005).

Influence of HIPAA Privacy Rule on Institutional Review Boards

Under the HIPAA Privacy Rule, an IRB or institutional established privacy board can act on requests for a waiver or an alteration of the authorization requirement for a research project. If an IRB and privacy board both exist in an agency, the approval of only one board is required, and it probably will be the IRB for research projects. Researchers can choose to obtain a signed authorization form from potential subjects or can ask for a waiver or an alteration of the authorization requirement. An altered authorization requirement occurs when an IRB approves a request that some but not all of the required 18 elements be removed from health information that is to be used in research. The researcher also can request a partial or complete waiver of the authorization requirement from the IRB. The partial waiver involves the researcher's obtaining PHI to contact and recruit potential subjects for a study. An IRB can give a researcher a complete waiver of authorization in studies in which the informed consent requirements also might be waived (U.S. DHHS, 2004, July 8). (The HIPAA regulations related to IRBs can be found online at http://privacyruleandresearch.nih.gov/irband-privacyrule.asp.)

The HIPAA Privacy Rule does not change the IRB membership and functions that are designated under the DHHS and FDA Protection of Human Subjects Regulations. For clarification, the responsibilities of the IRB/privacy board for HIPAA (U.S. DHHS, 2004, July 8) and the responsibilities of the IRB under the DHHS (U.S. DHHS, 2005) and FDA (1998a, 1998b) are outlined in Table 7-7.

Table 7-7	Comparison of IRB/Privacy Board Responsibilities for HIPAA, DHHS, and FDAC

Area of Distinction	HIPAA Privacy Rule	DHHS Protection of Human Subjects Regulations Title 45 CFR Part 46	FDA Protection of Human Subjects Regulations Title 21 CFR Parts 50 & 56
Permissions for research	Authorization	Informed consent and authorization	Informed consent and authorization
IRB/privacy board responsibilities	Requires the covered entity to obtain authorization for research use or disclosure of PHI unless a regulatory permission applies. Because of this, the IRB or privacy board would see only requests to waive or alter the authorization requirement. In exercising Privacy Rule authority, the IRB or privacy board does not review the authorization form.	Requires the covered entity to obtain authorization for research use or disclosure of PHI unless a regulatory permission applies. Because of this, the IRB or privacy board would only see requests to waive or alter the authorization requirement. In exercising Privacy Rule authority, the IRB or privacy board does not review the authorization form.	The IRB must ensure that informed consent will be sought from, and documented for, each prospective subject or the subject's legally authorized representative, in accordance with, and to the extent required by, FDA regulations. If specified criteria are met, the requirements for either obtaining informed consent or documenting informed consent may be waived. The IRB must review and approve the authorization form if it is combined with the informed consent document. Privacy boards have no authority under the FDA Protection of Human Subjects Regulations.

U.S. Department of Health and Human Services. (2004, August 4a). How can covered entities use and disclose protected health information for research and comply with the Privacy Rule? HIPAA Privacy Rule: Information for Researchers. Retrieved online December 3, 2005, from http://privacyruleandresearch.nih.gov/pr_08.asp

DHHS, Department of Health and Human Services; FDA, Food and Drug Administration; HIPAA, Health Insurance Portability and Accountability Act; IRB, institutional review board; PHI, protected health information.

Examining the Benefit-Risk Ratio of a Study

Nurses who serve on an IRB for their agencies, serve as patient advocate when research is conducted in their agencies, or are asked to collect data for a study should examine the balance of benefits and risks in studies. To determine this balance, or **benefit-risk ratio**, the benefits and risks associated with the sampling method, consent process, procedures, and potential outcomes of the study are assessed (see Figure 7-3). Informed consent must be obtained from subjects, and selection and treatment of subjects during the study must be fair. An important outcome of research is the development and refinement of knowledge. The type of knowledge that might be obtained from the study and who will be influenced by the knowledge also must be identified.

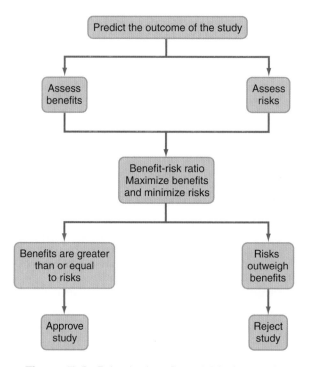

Figure 7-3. Balancing benefits and risks for a study.

The type of research conducted—therapeutic or nontherapeutic—affects the potential benefits for the subjects. In therapeutic research, subjects might benefit from the study procedures in areas such as skin care, range of motion, touch, and other nursing interventions. The benefits might include improved physical condition, which could facilitate emotional and social benefits. Some researchers have noted that participation in descriptive research has encouraged subjects to process and disclose thoughts regarding life-altering events, and that these actions have been beneficial to the subjects' health and well-being. Nontherapeutic nursing research does not benefit subjects directly, but it is important because it generates and refines nursing knowledge for future patients, the nursing profession, and society (King, 2000). All research subjects benefit by having an increased understanding of the research process and knowing the findings from a particular study.

Examining the benefit-risk ratio also involves assessing the type, degree, and number of risks that subjects might encounter while participating in a study. The risks involved depend on the purpose of the study and the procedures used to conduct the study. Risks can be physical, emotional, social, or economic and can range in level from no anticipated risk or mere inconvenience to certain risk of permanent damage (see the earlier section "Right to Protection from Discomfort and Harm") (Levine, 1986; Reynolds, 1972). If the risks outweigh the benefits, the study probably is unethical and should not be conducted. If the benefits outweigh the risks, the study probably is ethical and has the potential to add to nursing's knowledge base (see Figure 7-3).

RESEARCH EXAMPLE   Benefit-Risk Ratio

The benefit-risk ratio can be analyzed for a study that focused on the effects of an exercise and diet program on the subjects' serum lipid values and cardiovascular risk level (Bruce, 1991; Bruce & Grove, 1994). The serum lipid levels examined were serum cholesterol, low-density lipoprotein (LDL), and high-density lipoprotein (HDL). The subjects voluntarily agreed to participate in the study and signed a consent form. All subjects were treated fairly during subject selection and data collection. The potential benefits to the participants included (1) increased knowledge about exercise and diet, (2) increased knowledge about serum lipid values and cardiovascular risk level at the start of the program and 1 year later, (3) improved levels of serum lipids, (4) lowered cardiovascular risk level, and (5) improved exercise and diet habits. The risks included the discomfort of having blood drawn twice and the time spent participating in the study. These discomforts were temporary; they ended with the termination of the study. In addition, the discomforts did not exceed what the subjects would experience in their daily lives. The amount of time that the subjects spent participating in the study was minimized through efficient organization and precise scheduling of research activities.

Assessment of the benefit-risk ratio suggests that the benefits are greater in number and importance than the risks; the risks are temporary and can be minimized by the researcher. The researcher received approvals from the university and clinical agency IRBs and also obtained informed consent from each subject. The informed consent process involved the following: (1) providing each subject with essential information about the study, both orally and in writing; (2) giving each subject the choice of whether to participate in the study; and (3) having each subject read and sign a consent form. Thus, this study was ethical and provided benefits both to the subjects and their families and for the development of nursing knowledge regarding the effects of exercise and diet on serum lipid levels and cardiovascular risk level.

If you were a member of the IRB that reviewed this study, you and the other committee members probably would recommend approving the study for implementation in your agency. Because the risks of the study are minimal, the review process probably would be expedited. If you were a patient advocate, you would examine the risks and benefits, determine whether the study had received IRB approval, and examine the appropriateness of the informed consent process. Because the study meets ethical guidelines, you probably would encourage patients to be subjects in this study so that they might receive the identified benefits. You probably also would be willing to identify potential subjects or collect data for the researcher.

CRITIQUE GUIDELINES   The Ethics of a Study

The ethical aspects of a study include having the research project approved by the IRB for the setting and obtaining informed consent from the subjects. This information needs to be included in published studies. In addition, the conduct of research must meet the DHHS (U.S. DHHS, 2005), FDA (2002), and HIPAA (U.S. DHHS, 2003) regulations for the conduct of ethical research with human subjects. Consider the following questions when critiquing the ethical aspects of a study.

1. Was the benefit-risk ratio of the study acceptable? What was the level of risk of the study: no anticipated effects, temporary discomfort, unusual levels of temporary discomfort, risk

(continues)

CRITIQUE GUIDELINES *(continued)*

of permanent damage, or certainty of permanent damage? Was this level of risk reasonable for the study based on the potential benefit of the knowledge generated? Did the benefits outweigh the risks?

2. Was the study approved by the appropriate IRB?
3. Was informed consent obtained from the subjects? Was the information that was essential for consent provided? Were the subjects capable of comprehending the information? Did the researcher take any action to ensure that the subjects comprehended the consent information? Were the subjects competent to give consent? If the subjects were not competent to give consent, who acted as their legally authorized representatives? Did it seem that the subjects participated voluntarily in the study?
4. Were the rights of the subjects protected during sampling, data collection, and data analysis? Was privacy provided during data collection? Were the subjects' identities kept anonymous? Were the research data kept confidential? Were the data analyzed and the findings presented in a way to ensure the anonymity of the subjects in the research report?
5. Were the U.S. DHHS (2005), FDA (2002), and HIPAA (U.S. DHHS, 2003) regulations followed in the development and implementation of the study?

Understanding Scientific Misconduct

The goal of research is to generate sound scientific knowledge, which is possible only through the honest conduct, reporting, and publication of quality research. However, during the last 20 years an increasing number of fraudulent studies have been published in prestigious scientific journals. In the late 1980s, scientific misconduct was deemed a serious problem and was investigated by the DHHS (1989). In 1989, two new federal agencies were organized for reporting and investigating scientific misconduct. The Office of Scientific Integrity Review (OSIR) was established to manage scientific misconduct by grant recipients. The Office of Scientific Integrity (OSI) supervises the implementation of the rules and regulations related to scientific misconduct and manages any investigations (Hawley & Jeffers, 1992, U.S. DHHS, 1989). The investigations by the OSIR and the OSI revealed a variety of fraudulent behaviors. In some instances, the fraudulent studies were never conducted, and the researchers fabricated the data and study results. In other cases, the findings were consciously distorted.

An example of scientific misconduct was evident in the publications of Dr. Robert Slutsky, a heart specialist at the University of California, San Diego, School of Medicine. He resigned in 1986 when confronted with inconsistencies in his research publications. His publications contained "statistical anomalies that raised the question of data fabrication" (Friedman, 1990, p. 1416). In 6 years, Slutsky published 161 articles, and during one period he was completing an article every 10 days. Eighteen of the articles were found to be fraudulent and now have retraction notations, and 60 articles were questionable (Friedman, 1990).

Dr. Stephen Breuning, a psychologist at the University of Pittsburgh, engaged in deceptive and misleading practices in reporting his research on retarded children. He used his fraudulent research to obtain more than $300,000 in federal grants. In 1988 he was criminally charged with research fraud. He pleaded guilty, was fined $20,000, and faced up to 10 years in prison (Chop & Silva, 1991).

Role of the Office of Research Integrity in Promoting the Conduct of Ethical Research

Currently, the Office of Research Integrity (ORI) promotes the integrity of biomedical and behavioral research in about 4,000 institutions worldwide (ORI, 2005b; online at http://ori.dhhs.gov/). The ORI protects the integrity of the PHS's extramural and intramural research programs. The extramural program provides funding to research institutions, and the intramural program provides funding for research conducted within the federal government. The current functions of the ORI are as follows:

- Develop and promulgate policies, procedures, rules, and regulations aimed at preventing, monitoring, and imposing administrative actions concerning misconduct and protecting whistle blowers from retaliation
- Administer an assurance program
- Review completed investigations conducted by applicants or awardees' institutions
- Provide on-site technical assistance to institutions during inquiries and investigations when requested
- Review institutional findings and recommend administrative actions to the Assistant Secretary of Health, who makes the final decisions regarding misconduct, subject to appeal
- Present misconduct findings in administrative hearings before the DHHS Departmental Appeals Board (DAB)
- Promote scientific integrity through a variety of educational programs and activities (ORI, 2005a)

Over the last 10 years, the ORI has had a major role in the investigation of allegations of misconduct in research within several institutions.

Misconduct or *misconduct in science* means fabrication, falsification, plagiarism, or other practices that seriously deviate from those that are commonly accepted within the scientific community for proposing, conducting, or reporting research. It does not include honest error or honest differences in interpretations or judgments of data. (ORI, 2005a)

Fabrication is the making up of results and recording or reporting them. **Falsification** is manipulating research materials, equipment, or processes, or changing or omitting data or results, such that the research is not accurately represented in the research record. **Plagiarism** is the appropriation of another person's ideas, processes, results, or words without giving appropriate credit, including those obtained through confidential review of others' research proposals and manuscripts (ORI, 2005a).

The DHHS regulations implemented by the ORI classifies research misconduct as (1) an act that involves a significant departure from the acceptable practice of the scientific community for maintaining the integrity of the research record; (2) an act that was committed intentionally; and (3) an allegation that can be proved by a preponderance of evidence. From 1993 to 1997, the ORI received about 1000 allegations of scientific misconduct that resulted in 150 investigations, with 76 findings of scientific misconduct and 74 findings of no misconduct. The most common sites for the investigations were medical schools (68%), hospitals

(11%), and research institutes (10%). The persons charged with misconduct were primarily males who held a PhD or MD degree and were mostly associate professors, professors, and postdoctoral fellows. The administrative actions taken against the 76 respondents found to have committed scientific misconduct included disbarment from receiving federal funding for periods ranging from 18 months to 8 years; prohibition from PHS advisory service; and other actions requiring supervised research, certification of data, certification of sources, and correction or retraction of articles (ORI, 2005b). Each year the ORI provides a summary of its investigations and actions (which can be accessed online at http://ori.dhhs.gov).

Examining the Use of Animals in Research

The use of animals as research subjects is a controversial issue of growing concern to nurse researchers (Burns & Grove, 2005). A small but increasing number of nurse scientists are conducting physiological studies that require the use of animals. Many scientists, especially physicians, believe the current animal rights movement could threaten the future of health research. Animal rights groups are active in antiresearch campaigns and are backed by massive resources, with a treasury that was estimated at $50 million in 1988 (Pardes, West, & Pincus, 1991). Some of these groups are trying to raise the consciousness of researchers and society to ensure that animals are used wisely in the conduct of research and are treated humanely.

Two important questions should be addressed: (1) Should animals be used as subjects in research? (2) If animals are used in research, what mechanisms ensure that they are treated humanely? The type of research project influences the selection of subjects. Animals are just one of a variety of subjects used in research; others include human beings, plants, and computer data sets. If possible, most researchers use nonanimal subjects because this approach generally is less expensive. If the studies are low risk, which most nursing studies are, human beings frequently are used as subjects. However, some studies require the use of animals to answer the research question. Approximately 17 to 22 million animals are used in research each year, and 90% of them are rodents. The combined percentage of dogs and cats used in research is only 1% to 2% (Goodwin & Morrison, 2000).

Because animals are deemed valuable subjects for selected research projects, what mechanisms ensure that animals are treated humanely? At least five separate types of regulations exist to protect research animals from mistreatment. The federal government, state governments, independent accreditation organizations, professional societies, and individual institutions work to ensure that research animals are used only when necessary and only under humane conditions. At the federal level, animal research is conducted according to the guidelines of the Public Health Service (PHS) Policy on Humane Care and Use of Laboratory Animals, which was adopted in 1986 and reprinted essentially unchanged in 1996 (National Institutes of Health [NIH], 2003). The PHS Policy on Humane Care and Use of Laboratory Animals defines *animal* as any live, vertebrate animal that is used or intended to be used in research, research training, experimentation, or biological testing or for a related purpose. Any institution proposing research involving animals must have a written Animal Welfare Assurance statement acceptable to the PHS that documents compliance with the PHS policy. All assurances are evaluated by the NIH's OPRR to determine the adequacy of the institution's proposed program for the care and use of animals in PHS-conducted or -supported activities (NIH, 2003).

Compliance with the PHS policy has promoted the humane care and treatment of animals in research. In addition, over 700 institutions conducting health-related research have sought accreditation by the American Association for Accreditation of Laboratory Animal Care (AAALAC), which was developed to ensure the humane treatment of animals in research (Goodwin & Morrison, 2000). In conducting research, the subjects should be carefully selected; and if animals are used as subjects, they should be humanely treated.

KEY CONCEPTS

- Four experimental projects have been highly publicized for their unethical treatment of human subjects: (1) the Nazi medical experiments, (2) the Tuskegee Syphilis Study, (3) the Willowbrook Study, and (4) the Jewish Chronic Disease Hospital Study.
- Two historical documents, the Nuremberg Code and the Declaration of Helsinki, have had a strong impact on the conduct of research.
- The DHHS (1981, 1983, 1991, 2001, 2005) and the FDA (1998a, 1998b, 2002) passed regulations to promote ethical conduct in research, including (1) general requirements for informed consent and (2) guidelines for IRB review of research.
- The HIPAA was enacted in 2003 to protect the privacy of people's health information.
- The human rights that require protection in research are (1) self-determination, (2) privacy, (3) anonymity and confidentiality, (4) fair treatment, and (5) protection from discomfort and harm.
- Informed consent involves (1) transmission of essential study information to the potential subject, (2) comprehension of that information by the potential subject, (3) competence of the potential subject to give consent, and (4) voluntary consent by the potential subject to participate in the study.
- An institutional review board consists of a committee of peers who examine studies for ethical concerns with three levels of review: exempt, expedited, and complete.
- To balance the benefits and risks of a study, the type, degree, and number of risks are examined, and the potential benefits are identified.
- Scientific misconduct is a serious ethical problem of the last few decades, with the conducting, reporting, and publication of fraudulent research.

TIPS FOR FURTHER STUDY

- Review the studies in the *Study Guide* and identify the steps that were taken to protect the rights of the subjects. Were the studies reviewed by institutional review board (IRB)? Did the subjects sign consent forms?
- Apply the Benefit/Risk Ratio to a study in the *Study Guide*. Was the study conducted ethically? Provide a rationale for your decision.
- Obtain a study from the *Journal of Pediatric Nursing* and describe how the children's rights are protected in the study. Do children have diminished autonomy in research? Provide a rationale for your response.
- Read about the Health Insurance Portability and Accountability Act (HIPAA) and the conduct of research online at http://privacyruleandresearch.nih.gov. How has this act affected the conduct of research?
- Contact the IRB chair in a clinical agency. Ask them about the role of the IRB in the conduct of research in the agency.

REFERENCES

American Nurses Association. (2001). *Code of ethics for nurses with interpretive statements*. Washington, DC: Author. Copy available for viewing only at http://www.nursingworld.org/ethics/ecode.htm

American Psychological Association. (2002). *Ethical principles of psychologists and code of conduct*. Washington, DC: Author.

Barber, S., Grubbs, L., & Cottrell, B. (2005). Self-perception in children with attention deficit/hyperactivity disorder. *Journal of Pediatric Nursing, 20*(4), 235–245.

Beecher, H. K. (1966). Ethics and clinical research. *The New England Journal of Medicine, 274*(24), 1354–1360.

Berger, R. L. (1990). Nazi science: The Dachau hypothermia experiments. *The New England Journal of Medicine, 322*(20), 1435–1440.

Brandt, A. M. (1978). Racism and research: The case of the Tuskegee syphilis study. *Hastings Center Report, 8*(6), 21–29.

Broome, M. E. (1999). Consent (assent) for research with pediatric patients. *Seminars in Oncology Nursing, 15*(2), 96–103.

Bruce, S. L. (1991). *The effect of a coronary artery risk evaluation program on the serum lipid values of a selected military population*. Unpublished master's thesis, University of Texas at Arlington.

Bruce, S. L., & Grove, S. K. (1994). The effect of a coronary artery risk evaluation program on serum lipid values and cardiovascular risk levels. *Applied Nursing Research, 7*(2), 67–74.

Burns, N., & Grove, S. K. (2005). *The practice of nursing research: Conduct, critique, and utilization* (5th ed.). Philadelphia: Saunders.

Chop, R. M., & Silva, M. C. (1991). Scientific fraud: Definitions, policies, and implications for nursing research. *Journal of Professional Nursing, 7*(3), 166–171.

Douglas, S., & Larson, E. (1986). There's more to informed consent than information. *Focus on Critical Care, 13*(2), 43–47.

Emanuel, E. J. (2004). Ending concerns about undue inducement. *The Journal of Law, Medicine & Ethics: A Journal of the American Society of Law, Medicine & Ethics, 32*(1), 100–105.

Food and Drug Administration. (1998a). A guide to informed consent. *Code of Federal Regulations*, Title 21 Part 50. Retrieved December 2, 2005, from http://www.fda.gov/oc/ohrt/irbs/informedconsent.html

Food and Drug Administration. (1998b). Institutional review boards. *Code of Federal Regulations*, Title 21 Part 56. Retrieved December 2, 2005, from http://www.fda.gov/oc/ohrt/irbs/appendixc.html

Food and Drug Administration. (2002, April 1). Protection of human subjects. *Code of Federal Regulations*, Title 21 Part 50. Retrieved December 2, 2005, from http://www.access.gpo.gov/nara/cfr/waisidx_02/21cfr50_02.html

Ford, J. S., & Reuter, L. I. (1990). Ethical dilemmas associated with small samples. *Journal of Advanced Nursing, 15*(2), 187–191.

Frank-Stromborg, M. (2004). They're real and they're here: The new federally regulated privacy rules under HIPAA. *Dermatology Nursing, 16*(1), 13–25.

Friedman, P. J. (1990). Correcting the literature following fraudulent publication. *Journal of the American Medical Association, 263*(10), 1416–1419.

Goodwin, F. K., & Morrison, A. R. (2000). Science and self-doubt. *Reason, 32*(5), 22–28.

Havens, G. A. (2004). Ethical implications for the professional nurse of research involving human subjects. *Journal of Vascular Nursing, 22*(1), 19–23.

Hawley, D. J., & Jeffers, J. M. (1992). Scientific misconduct as a dilemma for nursing. *Image—The Journal of Nursing Scholarship, 24*(1), 51–55.

Hershey, N., & Miller, R. D. (1976). *Human experimentation and the law*. Germantown, MD: Aspen.

Holditch-Davis, D., Brandon, D. H., & Schwartz, T. (2003). Development of behaviors in preterm infants: Relation to sleeping and waking. *Nursing Research, 52*(5), 307–317.

Kelman, H. C. (1967). Human use of human subjects: The problem of deception in social psychological experiments. *Psychological Bulletin, 67*(1), 1–11.

King, N. M. (2000). Defining and describing benefit appropriately in clinical trials. *The Journal of Law, Medicine & Ethics: A Journal of the American Society of Law, Medicine & Ethics, 28*(4), 332–343.

Levine, R. J. (1986). *Ethics and regulation of clinical research* (2nd ed.). Baltimore and Munich: Urban & Schwarzenberg.

Milgram, S. (1963). Behavioral study of obedience. *Journal of Abnormal and Social Psychology, 67*(4), 371–378.

Munhall, P. L. (2001a). Ethical considerations in qualitative research. In P. L. Munhall (Ed.), *Nursing research: A qualitative perspective* (3rd ed., pp. 537–549). Sudbury, MA: Jones & Bartlett.

Munhall, P. L. (2001b). Institutional review of qualitative research proposals: A task of no small consequence. In P. L. Munhall (Ed.), *Nursing research: A qualitative perspective* (3rd ed., pp. 551–563). Sudbury, MA: Jones & Barlett.

National Commission for the Protection of Human Subjects of Biomedical and Behavioral Research. (1978). *Belmont report: Ethical principles and guidelines for research involving human subjects*. DHEW Publication No. (05) 78–0012. Washington, DC: U.S. Government Printing Office.

National Institutes of Health. (2003). Office of Laboratory Animal Welfare: Public Health Service policy on humane care and use of laboratory animals. Retrieved December 3, 2005, from http://grants.nih.gov/grants/olaw/olaw.htm

Njie, V. P., & Thomas, A. C. (2001). Quality issues in clinical research and the implications on health policy (QICRHP). *Journal of Professional Nursing, 17*(5), 233–242.

Nuremberg Code. (1986). In R. J. Levine (Ed.), *Ethics and regulation of clinical research* (2nd ed., pp. 425–426). Baltimore and Munich: Urban & Schwarzenberg.

Office of Research Integrity. (2005a). Handling misconduct. Retrieved December 3, 2005 from http://ori.dhhs.gov/misconduct

Office of Research Integrity. (2005b). About the Office of Research Integrity. Retrieved December 3, 2005, from http://ori.dhhs.gov/

Olsen, D. P. (2003). Methods: HIPAA privacy regulations and nursing research. *Nursing Research, 52*(5), 344–348.

Pardes, H., West, A., & Pincus, H. A. (1991). Physicians and the animal-rights movement. *The New England Journal of Medicine, 324*(23), 1640–1643.

Ramos, M. C. (1989). Some ethical implications of qualitative research. *Research in Nursing & Health, 12*(1), 57–63.

Rankin, M., & Esteves, M. D. (1997). Perceptions of scientific misconduct in nursing. *Nursing Research, 46*(5), 270–276.

Reynolds, P. D. (1972). On the protection of human subjects and social science. *International Social Science Journal, 24*(4), 693–719.

Reynolds, P. D. (1979). *Ethical dilemmas and social science research.* San Francisco: Jossey-Bass.

Rosato, J. (2000). The ethics of clinical trials: A child's view. *The Journal of Law, Medicine & Ethics: A Journal of the American Society of Law, Medicine & Ethics, 28*(4), 362–378.

Rothman, D. J. (1982). Were Tuskegee and Willowbrook "studies in nature"? *Hastings Center Report, 12*(2), 5–7.

Sandelowski, M. (1994). Focus on qualitative methods: The use of quotes in qualitative research. *Research in Nursing & Health, 17*(6), 479–482.

Steele, S. K., & Porche, D. J. (2005). Testing the theory of planned behavior to predict mammography intention. *Nursing Research, 54*(5), 332–338.

Stone, P. W. (2003). Ask an expert: HIPAA in 2003 and its meaning for nurse researchers. *Applied Nursing Research, 16*(4), 291–293.

Steinfels, P., & Levine, C. (1976). Biomedical ethics and the shadow of Nazism. *Hastings Center Report, 6*(4), 1–20.

Strauman, J. J., & Cotanch, P. H. (1988). Oncology nurse research issues: Over-studied populations. *Oncology Nursing Forum, 15*(5), 665–667.

Thompson, P. J. (1987). Protection of the rights of children as subjects for research. *Journal of Pediatric Nursing, 2*(6), 392–399.

U.S. Department of Health and Human Services. (1981, January 26). Final regulations amending basic HHS policy for the protection of human research subjects. *Code of Federal Regulations,* Title 45 Part 46.

U.S. Department of Health and Human Services. (1983, March 8). Protection of human subjects. *Code of Federal Regulations,* Title 45 Part 46.

U.S. Department of Health and Human Services. (1989). Final rule: Responsibilities of awardee and applicant institutions for dealing with and reporting possible misconduct in science. *Federal Register, 54,* 32446–32451.

U.S. Department of Health and Human Services. (1991, June 18). Protection of human subjects. *Code of Federal Regulations,* Title 45 Part 46.

U.S. Department of Health and Human Services. (2001, November 13). Protection of human subjects. *Code of Federal Regulations,* Title 45 Part 46.

U.S. Department of Health and Human Services. (2003, April 17). Standards for privacy of individually identifiable health information; final rule. *Code of Federal Regulations,* Title 45 Public Welfare, Parts 160 and 164. Retrieved December 2, 2005, from http://www.hhs.gov/ocr/hipaa/finalreg.html

U.S. Department of Health and Human Services. (2004, July 1). Information for covered entities and researchers on authorizations for research uses or disclosures of protected health information. HIPAA Privacy Rule: Information for Researchers. Retrieved December 2, 2005, from http://privacyruleandresearch.nih.gov/authorization.asp

U.S. Department of Health and Human Services. (2004, July 8). Institutional review boards and the HIPAA Privacy Rule. HIPAA Privacy Rule: Information for Researchers. Retrieved December 2, 2005 from http://privacyruleandresearch.nih.gov/irbandprivacyrule.asp

U.S. Department of Health and Human Services. (2004, August 4a). How can covered entities use and disclose protected health information for research and comply with the Privacy Rule? HIPAA Privacy Rule: Information for Researchers. Retrieved December 3, 2005, from http://privacyruleandresearch.nih.gov/pr_08.asp

U.S. Department of Health and Human Services. (2004, August 4b). How do other privacy protections interact with the privacy rule? HIPAA Privacy Rule: Information for Researchers. Retrieved December 3, 2005, from http://privacyruleandresearch.nih.gov/pr_05.asp

U.S. Department of Health and Human Services. (2004, August 4c). HIPAA Privacy Rule: Information for Researchers. Retrieved December 3, 2005, from http://privacyruleandresearch.nih.gov

U.S. Department of Health and Human Services. (2005, June 23). Protection of human subjects. *Code of Federal Regulations,* Title 45 Part 46. Retrieved December 2, 2005, from http://ohsr.od.nih.gov/guidelines/45cfr46.html

Weijer, C. (2000). The ethical analysis of risk. *The Journal of Law, Medicine & Ethics: A Journal of the American Society of Law, Medicine & Ethics, 28*(4), 344–361.

Yeh, C., Chang, C., & Chang, P. (2005). Evaluating quality of life in children with cancer using children's self-reports and parent-proxy reports. *Nursing Research, 54*(5), 354–362.

Clarifying Research Designs

Learning Outcomes

After completing this chapter, you should be able to:

1. Identify the designs of published studies.
2. Critique the quality of designs of quantitative nursing studies.
3. Select studies sufficiently well designed to provide evidence on which practice can be based.
4. Model designs of published studies.

Key Terms

STUDY TOOLS

Be sure to visit http://evolve.elsevier.com/Burns/understanding for additional examples and self-tests. Also, a review of this chapter's concepts and practice exercises can be found in Chapter 8 of the Study Guide for *Understanding Nursing Research: Building an Evidence-Based Practice*, 4th edition.

A **research design** is a blueprint for conducting a study. The purpose of a design is to maximize control over factors that can interfere with the validity of the findings. Just as the blueprint for a house must be individualized to the specific house being built, so must the design be made specific to a study. The control provided by the design increases the probability that the study results will accurately reflect reality.

To critique studies, you must learn how to identify the study design and evaluate threats to validity resulting from design flaws. Validity is important because studies must be well designed to contribute to evidence-based practice. Designs that provide evidence that nursing interventions are effective in achieving desired outcomes are particularly important.

As background information necessary to identify and critique designs of published studies, this chapter includes the concepts important to design, identifies some designs commonly used in nursing studies, and describes the elements of a good design. The chapter also includes content related to defining experimental interventions, mapping designs, and identifying replication studies.

Concepts Important to Design

Many terms used in discussing research design have special meanings within this context. Understanding the meanings of these concepts is critical to understanding the purpose of a specific design. Some of the major concepts used in research design are causality, multicausality, probability, bias, control, manipulation, and validity.

Causality

Causality basically says that things have causes, and causes lead to effects. Not all studies examine cause and effect. Studies may describe specific variables, or examine relationships among the variables. In a critique, you must determine whether the purpose of the study is to examine causality, examine relationships among variables, or describe variables. You may be able to determine whether the purpose of a study is to examine causality by reading the purpose statement and the propositions within the framework. For example, the purpose of a causal study may be to examine the effect of a specific preoperative educational program on length of hospital stay. The proposition may state that preoperative teaching results in a decreased hospitalization period. Preoperative teaching is not the only factor affecting length of hospital stay. Other important factors include the diagnosis, type of surgery, patient's age, initial physical condition of the patient, and complications that occurred after surgery. However, from the perspective of causality, it is important to design the study so that the effect of a single cause—in this case, a preoperative education program—can be examined apart from the other factors affecting length of hospital stay.

Multicausality

Very few phenomena in nursing can be clearly pinned down to a single cause and a single effect. A number of interrelating variables can be involved in producing a particular effect. Thus, studies developed from a multicausal perspective will include more variables than those using a strict causal orientation. The presence of multiple causes for an effect is referred to as **multicausality**. For example, diagnosis, patient age, patient condition, and complications after surgery all will be involved in causing the length of hospital stay. Because of the complexity of causal relationships, a theory is unlikely to identify every element involved in causing a particular phenomenon. However, the greater the proportion of causal factors that can be identified and examined in a single study, the clearer the understanding will be of the overall phenomenon. This greater understanding is expected to increase the ability to predict and control the effect.

Probability

Probability addresses relative rather than absolute causality. A cause may not produce a specific effect each time that particular cause occurs. Thus, researchers recognize that a particular cause *probably* will result in a specific effect. Using a probability orientation, researchers design studies to examine the probability that a given effect will occur under a defined set of circumstances. The circumstances may be variations in multiple variables.

For example, while assessing the effect of multiple variables on length of hospitalization, the researcher may choose to examine the probability of a given length of hospital stay under a variety of specific sets of circumstances. One specific set of circumstances may be that the patient had 15 minutes of preoperative teaching, underwent a specific type of surgery, was a certain age, had a particular level of health before surgery, and experienced a specific complication. The probability of a given length of hospital stay could be expected to vary as the set of circumstances varied. When examining probability, the researcher finds that hypotheses are complex, with multiple variables.

Bias

The term **bias** means a slant or deviation from the true or expected. Bias in a study distorts the findings from what the results would have been without the bias. Because studies are conducted to determine the real and the true, researchers place great value on identifying and removing sources of bias in their study or controlling their effects on the study findings. Designs are developed to reduce the possibility and effects of bias. Any component of a study that deviates or causes a deviation from a true measurement of the study variables contributes to distorted findings. Many factors related to research can be biased; these include attitudes or motivations of the researcher (conscious or unconscious), the components of the environment in which the study is conducted, selection of the individual subjects, composition of the sample, the groups formed, the measurement tools, the data collection process, the data, and the statistics.

For example, some of the subjects for the study might be taken from a unit of the hospital in which the patients are participating in another study involving high-quality nursing care; or one nurse, selecting patients for the study, might assign the patients who are most interested in the study to the experimental group. Each of these situations introduces bias to the study.

An important focus in critiquing a study is to identify possible sources of bias. This requires careful examination of the researcher's report of the study methods, including strategies for obtaining subjects and performing measurements. However, not all biases can be identified from the published report of a study. The article may not provide sufficient detail about the methods to detect all of the biases.

Control

One method of reducing bias is to increase the amount of control in the design. Control means having the power to direct or manipulate factors to achieve a desired outcome. For example, in a study of preoperative teaching, subjects may be randomly selected and then randomly assigned to the experimental or control group. The researcher may control the duration of preoperative teaching sessions, the content taught, the method of teaching, and the teacher. The time that the teaching occurred in relation to surgery also may be controlled, as well as the environment in which it occurred. Measurement of the length of hospital stay may be controlled by ensuring that the number of days or hours was calculated exactly in the same way for each subject. Limiting the characteristics of subjects, such as diagnosis, age, type of surgery, and incidence of complications, is a form of control. Control is particularly important in experimental and quasi-experimental studies. The greater the researcher's control over the study situation, the more credible (or valid) the study findings. The purpose of research designs is to maximize control of elements in the study situation.

Manipulation

Manipulation is a form of control used most commonly in experimental or quasi-experimental research. Controlling the treatment or intervention is the most commonly used manipulation. For example, in a study of the effects of preoperative teaching, the situation might be manipulated so that one group of subjects received preoperative teaching and another did not. In a study on oral care, the frequency of care might be manipulated.

When experimental designs are used to explore causal relationships in nursing research, the nurse must be free to manipulate the variables under study. If the freedom to manipulate a variable (e.g., the type, amount, or frequency of pain control measures) is under someone else's control (e.g., a physician or the staff nurses), a bias is introduced into the study. Thus, the treatment each subject receives may differ. The researcher will then be, so to speak, comparing apples and oranges. In descriptive and correlational studies, little or no effort is made to manipulate factors in the circumstances of the study. Instead, the purpose is to examine the situation as it exists. As a result of the subjective nature of observation, the possibility that bias will influence findings is greater in these kinds of studies.

CRITIQUE GUIDELINES Study Design

When critiquing a study, ask the following questions:

1. Which elements were controlled? What elements could have been controlled to improve the study design?
2. What was the feasibility of controlling particular elements of the study? What was the effect of *not* controlling certain elements on the validity of the study findings?
3. Which elements of the design were manipulated and how they were manipulated?
4. How adequate was the manipulation? What elements should have been manipulated to improve the validity of the findings?
5. What type of design was used in the study? Descriptive studies have little if any control of elements or manipulation. In moving from correlational designs to quasi-experimental and then experimental designs, the amount of control or manipulation increases.

Designs for Nursing Studies

A variety of study designs are used in nursing research; the four types most commonly used are descriptive, correlational, quasi-experimental, and experimental. Descriptive and correlational studies examine variables in natural environments and do not include treatments provided by the researcher. Quasi-experimental and experimental studies are designed to examine cause and effect. These studies are conducted to examine differences in dependent variables that are thought to be caused by independent variables (treatments). This section briefly describes the four types of designs and provides specific examples of each. More detail on specific designs is available in other sources (Burns & Grove, 2005).

The algorithm shown in Figure 8-1 may be used to determine the type of study design for a published study. The algorithm includes a series of yes or no responses to specific questions about the design. The algorithm starts with the question "Is there a treatment?" The answer leads to the next question, with the four types of design being identified in the algorithm. Then a second algorithm provided for each type of design can be used to identify the specific design used in the study.

Descriptive Design

The descriptive study is designed to gain more information about characteristics within a particular field of study. Its purpose is to provide a picture of a situation as it naturally happens. A descriptive design may be used to develop theories, identify problems with current practice, justify current practice, make judgments, or determine what other practitioners in similar situations are doing. No manipulation of variables is involved in a descriptive design. In many aspects of nursing, a clearer picture of the phenomenon is needed before causality can be examined. Protection against bias is achieved through (1) conceptual and operational definitions of variables, (2) sample selection and size, (3) valid and reliable instruments, and (4) data collection procedures that partially control the environment. Descriptive

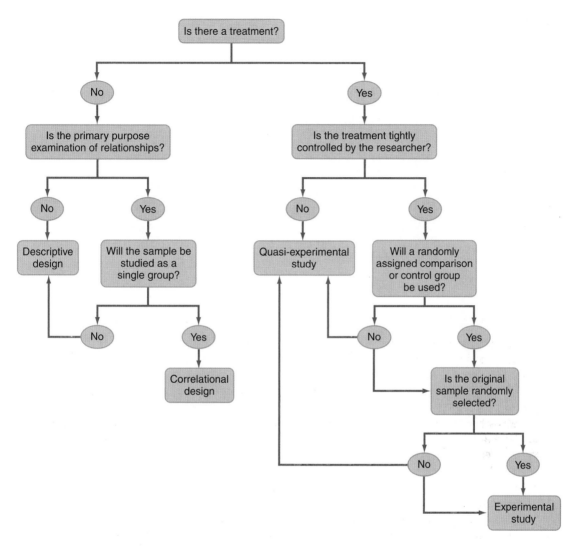

Figure 8-1. Algorithm for determining the type of study design.

studies differ in level of complexity. Some contain only two variables; others may include multiple variables.

Use the algorithm shown in Figure 8-2 to determine the type of descriptive design used in a published study.

Typical Descriptive Design

The most commonly used design in the category of descriptive studies is presented in Figure 8-3. The design is used to examine characteristics of a single sample. The **descriptive**

design includes identifying a phenomenon of interest, identifying the variables within the phenomenon, developing conceptual and operational definitions of the variables, and describing the variables. The description of the variables leads to an interpretation of the theoretical meaning of the findings and the development of hypotheses.

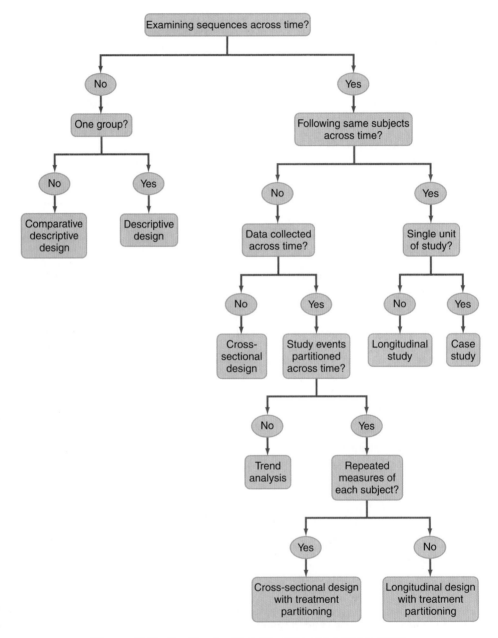

Figure 8-2. Algorithm for determining type of descriptive design.

CLARIFICATION ──────▶ MEASUREMENT ──────▶ DESCRIPTION ──────▶ INTERPRETATION

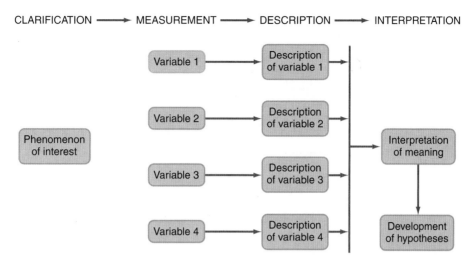

Figure 8-3. Typical descriptive design.

RESEARCH EXAMPLE   Typical Descriptive Design

An example of a descriptive design is the study by O'Leary-Kelley, Puntillo, Barr, Stotts, and Douglas (2005) describing the nutritional adequacy of enteral feeding for patients receiving mechanical ventilation. The investigators studied a convenience sample of 60 hospitalized subjects and used the Harris-Benedict equation (HBE) to calculate energy requirements for the sample. Energy provided by the enteral feedings and reason and duration of interruptions in feedings were recorded for 3 consecutive days.

The variables described were (1) energy requirements of each subject, (2) energy provided by the enteral feedings of each subject, (3) reasons for interruptions of feeding for each subject, and (4) duration of interruptions of feeding for each subject. Two other variables were calculated from the preceding four variables: (5) the percent of each subject's energy requirement provided by the feedings and (6) the percent of each subject's energy requirement not provided because of each identified cause of interruption. Examining these variables, the authors concluded that "more than two thirds of ICU patients treated with mechanical ventilation received less than 90% of their nutritional requirements…. [H]alf of these patients received less than 50% of their required energy during the 3-day study period" (p. 226).

CRITIQUE

This well-thought-out descriptive study controlled the following elements: (1) all subjects were hospitalized and receiving mechanical ventilation; (2) all subjects were being fed enterally; (3) energy requirements of patients were measured using the same measurement method; (4) energy provided by feeding of each patient was measured consistently; (5) reasons for interruptions were recorded; and (6) the duration of interruptions of feeding was recorded.

Elements that could have been altered (controlled) to improve the study design include using a larger sample size, limiting the age of subjects, requiring that the same enteral feeding be provided to each subject, limiting the sample to subjects with the same severity of illness, and measuring the nutritional adequacy for subjects at the beginning of the study. The nutritional adequacy for subjects could have been

(continues)

CRITIQUE *(continued)*

measured at the beginning of the study, or the subjects could have been limited to patients with a given level of nutritional adequacy. The sample could have been limited to subjects with a specific health problem resulting in mechanical ventilation. However, limiting these variables in a study designed to examine the overall problem in patients receiving enteral feedings would not have given the overall picture of this serious problem in patient care. Manipulation is not appropriate in a descriptive study.

In addition, controlling these elements would not have been feasible for the following reasons. The study was conducted in a single intensive care unit. Patients had various physicians ordering feedings. Patients were admitted for various health conditions, were of various ages, and had differing severity of illness. Controlling these elements would have required using multiple intensive care units over a period of several years. The cost of control of these elements in both money and time would be great. Thus, the feasibility of increasing control is low. The effects of not controlling these elements on the validity of the study findings are not serious. The study provides an initial broad examination that clarifies a clinical problem. This provides a clearer picture of the phenomenon of concern, revealing the seriousness of the problem.

IMPLICATIONS FOR PRACTICE

Because the problem seems to occur across a variety of types of patients, it serves as a warning sign clinically that there is a need for greater efforts to reduce interruptions of feeding: "Most critically ill patients receiving mechanical ventilation who are fed enterally do not receive their energy requirements, primarily because of frequent interruptions in enteral feedings" (p. 222). Meeting energy requirements is essential to recovery. Protein is needed for maintenance and repair of body tissues. Without adequate nutrition, the immune system and other body defenses cannot function adequately. Nurses caring for critically ill patients receiving parenteral nutrition must protect their patients' welfare and facilitate healing by ensuring that their patients receive sufficient feedings to meet their energy requirements. Results provide information that can be used in future experimental studies designed to test the effectiveness of interventions to reduce interruptions or increase the energy provided by the feedings. An accumulated body of knowledge from such studies can be used as an evidence base to guide nursing practice.

The study authors also provide recommendations for measurement of energy requirements in both clinical practice and research. In a subset of 25 of their subjects, energy requirements were determined by both the HBE, which has been the accepted standard for determining energy requirements for critically ill patients, and indirect calorimetry. However, the authors conclude that "the accuracy of the HBE is limited in ventilator-dependent patients, patients who are either morbidly obese or severely malnourished and underweight, transplant patients, and patients with marked fluid overload, ascites, extensive limb amputations, or paraplegia" (p. 223). They recommend the use of indirect calorimetry as a more accurate approach to estimating energy requirements in critically ill patients. Indirect calorimetry calculates energy expenditure indirectly by measuring pulmonary gas exchange.

Comparative Descriptive Design

The **comparative descriptive design** (Figure 8-4) is used to describe variables and to examine differences in variables in two or more groups that occur naturally in a setting. The results obtained from these analyses are frequently not generalized to a population.

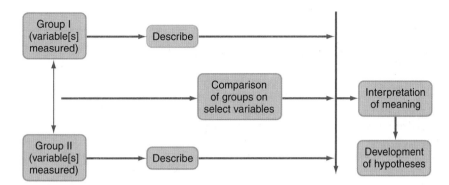

Figure 8-4. Comparative descriptive design.

RESEARCH EXAMPLE   Comparative Descriptive Design

Johnson's (2005) study comparing health-promoting lifestyle behaviors of African American men and women is an example of the comparative descriptive design. The purpose of the study was to expand the body of knowledge in the complex area of homelessness and health. The sample comprised 223 African Americans living in the southeast United States. Pender's Health Promotion Model was used as the theoretical framework. The Health Promoting Lifestyle Profile (HPLP), based on Pender's model, was used to measure the health behaviors. Because men and women have been shown in studies to differ in their health behaviors, African American men and women were compared to determine if there were differences and the extent of any such differences in health behaviors of homeless men and women. The study found no statistically significant gender differences in the HPLP total scores. No differences based on income, education, or marital status were found. However, significant differences were found between men and women in their scores for interpersonal relationship support, health responsibility, and nutrition, with women having higher scores than men. In addition to addressing the major questions of the study, the study author provided considerably detailed and specific findings, which is common in descriptive studies. Some of the findings are as follows:

Homeless African American women had a higher level of employment than that of homeless white women.

Women in the sample had a higher level of education than African American homeless women in previous studies. However, critical social supports often were missing.

Although previous studies found limited access to health care, the present study found adequate access to acute health care services. However, it is not clear that health promotion and primary disease prevention services are available.

Common physical problems found at a higher rate included hypertension, respiratory conditions, and diabetes.

CRITIQUE

The elements that were controlled in the study were (1) identity of subjects as homeless African American men and women and (2) use of the same measure to determine health behaviors of subjects. Elements that could have been controlled to improve the study design were the length of time each subject was

(continues)

CRITIQUE *(continued)*

homeless, availability of health care, and the nature of available health care. However, controlling these study elements is not feasible. Manipulation is not appropriate in descriptive studies.

The findings are valid and provide a glimpse of health problems and health behaviors of the homeless population in this nation. Results of the study also were compared with those of previous studies of the same population. The study results provide a broad array of information to add to the knowledge base of nursing. Examination of this study and the author's literature review suggest that the body of knowledge needed to provide evidence-based practice related to homeless health care is currently inadequate. Additional studies are needed, with more controls. Interventions for the homeless population that have demonstrated outcomes of improved health behaviors also are needed. Approaches to providing health services related to health promotion that are acceptable to the homeless population need to be developed and tested.

IMPLICATIONS FOR PRACTICE

This study indicates that although (at least in the Southeast, where the study was conducted) available health care is available to the homeless for acute health problems, health promotion and disease prevention activities are needed. Also needed is facilitation of social support for the homeless in a way acceptable to this population. A likely assumption is that homeless people are not interested in health promotion and disease prevention. Accordingly, nurses need to be creative in developing health promotion and disease prevention strategies that enable and motivate homeless people to become involved in promoting their own health and preventing diseases that are prevalent among the homeless. The general population needs to understand that communicable diseases that begin in society's most vulnerable can spread to threaten all members of society. Economically, the health of the entire workforce of a nation predicts the welfare of that nation. To the extent that homeless people are left to their own devices, without the resources they need, the nation as a whole suffers. Nurses are mandated by society to provide care not only to individuals and families but also to communities and to populations. Providing comprehensive care to the homeless will require working with the homeless to develop creative—and effective—solutions.

Case Study Design

The **case study design** involves an intensive exploration of a single unit of study, such as a person, a very small number of subjects, or a family, group, community, or institution. Although the number of subjects tends to be small, the number of variables in a case study usually is large. In fact, it is important to examine all variables that may have an impact on the situation being studied.

Case studies were commonly used in nursing 40-50 years ago but appear in the literature less frequently today. Well-designed case studies are a good source of descriptive information and can be used as evidence to support or invalidate theories. Information from a variety of sources can be collected on each concept of interest using different data collection methods. Case studies may use physiologic measures and/or valid psychosocial measures. This strategy can greatly expand the understanding of the phenomenon under study. Case studies also are useful for demonstrating the effectiveness of a therapeutic technique. In fact, the reporting of a case study can be the vehicle by which the technique is introduced to other practitioners. The case study design also has potential for revealing important findings that can generate new hypotheses for testing. Thus, the case study can lead to the design of large sample studies to examine factors identified by the case study.

The case study design depends on the circumstances of the case but usually includes an element of time. The researcher typically explores the subject's history and previous behavior patterns in detail. As the case study proceeds, the researcher may become aware of components important to the focus of the study that were not originally included in the study. Both quantitative and qualitative elements are likely to be incorporated into the case study design.

RESEARCH EXAMPLE Case Study Design

An example of a case study design is presented in Ulster and Antle's (2005) article "In the darkness there can be light: A family's adaptation to a child's blindness." The following is the abstract from that study:

Blindness or significant visual impairment can be very difficult for families to cope with. In this article, the authors present an in-depth case study of a family's journey through diagnosis and treatment for retinoblastoma (RB), a rare form of childhood eye cancer affecting the retina. As a part of the analysis of this family's experience, the authors examine assumptions about children's abilities to cope and predominant notions of quality of life through the experiences of one child, Alex, and his family.... In spite of signs of psychological trauma, Alex demonstrated a remarkable adaptive ability and had more insights about his experiences than anticipated. Similarly, following a period of considerable worry for their child's health and his ability to adjust to blindness, the parents, too, feel their family has a good quality of life. (Ulster & Antle, 2005, p. 209)

CRITIQUE

In this case study, no elements were controlled. Control is inappropriate in case studies. Validity is limited to the subject of the study. Manipulation is not appropriate. The clarification of the process of care provides insights useful for practice, as well as for developing frameworks and designing studies to extend the findings to larger samples and test interventions for providing care in similar situations.

IMPLICATIONS FOR PRACTICE

This case study provides the reader with an experience of caring for a child who has suddenly become blind, and with a perspective on the experience of his parents as their child is treated for cancer and becomes blind. The caring nurse can be as traumatized by the experience as are the child and the parents. Using description, the study author introduces approaches to nursing care that facilitate coping by the parents and the child. The nurse-reader can learn to apply similar caring approaches in similar situations. Contribution to evidence-based practice must wait for additional studies designed by nurse researchers who are perhaps inspired by studies such as this one.

Correlational Design

The purpose of a **correlational design** is to examine relationships between or among two or more variables in a single group. This examination can occur at any of several levels: descriptive correlational, in which the researcher can seek to describe a relationship; predictive correlational, in which the researcher can predict relationships among variables; or the model testing design, in which all of the relationships proposed by a theory are tested simultaneously.

In correlational designs, a large range in the variable scores is necessary to determine the existence of a relationship. Thus, the sample should reflect the full range of scores possible on the variables being measured. Some subjects should have very high scores and others very low scores, and the scores of the rest should be distributed throughout the possible range. Because of the need for a wide variation on scores, correlational studies generally require large sample sizes. Subjects are not divided into groups, because group differences are not examined.

To determine the type of correlational design used in a published study, use the algorithm shown in Figure 8-5. More detail on specific correlational designs referred to in this algorithm is available elsewhere (Burns & Grove, 2005).

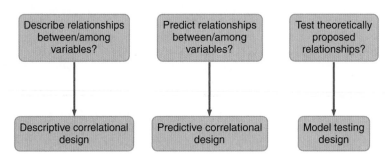

Figure 8-5. Algorithm for determining type of correlational design.

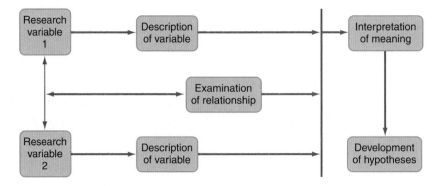

Figure 8-6. Descriptive correlational design.

Descriptive Correlational Design

The purpose of a **descriptive correlational design** is to describe variables and examine relationships among these variables. Using this design will facilitate the identification of many interrelationships in a situation (Figure 8-6). The study may examine variables in a situation that has already occurred or is currently occurring. Researchers make no attempt to control or manipulate the situation. As with descriptive studies, variables must be clearly identified and defined.

RESEARCH EXAMPLE   Descriptive Correlational Design

An example of a descriptive correlational design is Rew, Taylor-Seehafer, Thomas, and Yockey's (2001) study titled "Correlates of Resilience in Homeless Adolescents."

Purposes. To (a) describe reasons adolescents give for their homelessness, (b) explore relationships among resilience and selected risk and protective factors, (c) identify differences in risk and protective factors by gender and sexual orientation, and (d) determine best predictors of resilience. (p. 33)

Design. Descriptive and exploratory correlational design was used to collect and analyze data from a convenience sample of 59 homeless adolescents who sought health and social services from a community street-outreach project in central Texas in 1998. (p. 33)

Methods. Paper and pencil survey consisting of valid measures (Resilience Scale, UCLA-Revised Loneliness Scale, Beck Hopelessness Scale, Social Connectedness Scale, and Death-Related Attitude Schedule) was administered in a street-outreach setting.

Findings. Nearly half the sample (47%) reported a history of sexual abuse and 36% self-identified as gay, lesbian, or bisexual in orientation. Over half (51%) were thrown out of their homes by their parents, 37% left home because their parents disapproved of their alcohol or drug use, and nearly one-third left home because parents sexually abused them. Lack of resilience was significantly related to hopelessness, loneliness, life-threatening behaviors, and connectedness, but not to gender or sexual orientation. Hopelessness and connectedness explained 50% of the variance in resilience.

Participants who perceived themselves as resilient, although disconnected from other people, were less lonely, less hopeless, and engaged in fewer life-threatening behaviors than were those who perceived themselves as not being resilient. They survived by adapting to street life and by becoming overly self-reliant. (p. 33)

CRITIQUE

The study sample is limited to adolescents who were homeless and sought health care at a specific clinic. Measures were valid and reliable scales. Increasing the sample size by extending the time for data collection would have improved the study design. It is not clear how many potential subjects declined to participate because of the number of scales to be completed. This would affect validity of the study, because adolescents who declined to participate may be different from those who agreed. Were those who were resilient more likely to participate than those who were not? Were those who sought care at a clinic different from those who did not? What percent of the estimated number of homeless adolescents in the

(continues)

CRITIQUE *(continued)*

city was represented in the study findings? A descriptive correlational design allows the examination of multiple variables in the study but does not have the depth of description of a case study. However, the authors are able to examine a broad circle of information about a relatively unknown population to contribute to the nursing body of knowledge. Manipulation is inappropriate with this type of design.

IMPLICATIONS FOR PRACTICE

Rew and colleagues' (2001) study has provided answers to questions many people have asked: Why do adolescents leave home, how do they live, where do they live, what do they do, how do they survive? Few nurses encounter these young people, much less try to provide care to them. These children are elusive and live on the margins of society where ordinary folk do not go. They are different in many ways from the African American adult homeless population described earlier in this chapter (Johnson, 2005). How can they be reached? Is it possible to move some of them back into the mainstream of society? What can nurses do to help them? These findings may be useful in understanding them and in planning interventions to promote health and well-being in this vulnerable population. The understanding gained from the study needs to be used to develop interventions designed to provide effective means of providing care to homeless adolescents. Such interventions must be tested through well-designed studies in order to provide evidence-based knowledge that can be used to guide practice.

Predictive Correlational Design

The purpose of a predictive correlational design is to predict the value of one variable based on values obtained for another variable(s). Prediction is one approach to examining causal relationships between variables. Because causal phenomena are being examined, the terms *dependent* and *independent* are used to describe the variables. One variable is classified as the dependent variable, and all other variables are independent variables. A predictive design (Figure 8-7) study attempts to predict the level of the dependent variable from the independent variables. The independent variables that are most effective in prediction are highly correlated with the dependent variable but not highly correlated with other independent variables used in the study. Predictive correlational designs require the development of a theory-based mathematical hypothesis proposing variables expected to effectively predict the dependent variable. Researchers then use regression analysis to test the hypothesis.

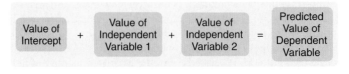

Figure 8-7. Predictive design.

RESEARCH EXAMPLE   Predictive Correlational Design

Dormire and Yarandi (2001) conducted a predictive correlational study of predictors of risk for adolescent childbearing (pp. 81–86):

Purpose. The purpose of this study was to develop a predictive model that identifies young women at risk for adolescent motherhood (p. 81).

Variables. Variables in this study were self-esteem, perceptions of childbearing, race, social status, and relationships with family members and friends. (p. 81)

Sample. Stratified sample of 357 adolescents was drawn from public health units and public schools in six randomly selected counties in North Central Florida. (p. 81)

Instruments. Four research instruments in addition to a demographic instrument were used to obtain data: 1) Hollingshead Four Factor Index of Social Status (Hollingshead, 1975), 2) Parental Bonding Instrument (Parker, Tupling & Brown, 1979), 3) Rosenberg Self-Esteem Scale (Rosenberg, 1965), and 4) Parenting Perceptions Instrument (PPI) (Dormire, 1992). (p. 83)

Procedure. Those girls who consented to participate in the study first completed a demographic questionnaire that included the questions appropriate for calculation of social status. The demographic questionnaire included data regarding variables that are part of the social context (i.e., number of friends pregnant, years of education, and mother's age at first pregnancy), because other researchers have identified these factors as related to adolescent childbearing. While these factors were not the major focus of the research, they were conceptually a fit and provided additional social context data. (p. 83) Following this the three scales were administered.

Analysis. A stepwise logistic regression was used to investigate the combined effects of these variables for identification of risk for adolescent motherhood. (p. 81)

Findings. In this [sic] data, the greatest likelihood of childbearing (97.66%) is represented by an [sic] 14-year-old African American adolescent who did not know her dad, lived in an unskilled laborer household, felt positively about being a mother at her current age, knew three friends who were pregnant, and had two friends who were mothers. The power of this combination of variables is evident in comparing probability for a 14-year-old with all of the same variable levels; her probability of motherhood is 80.6%. This comparison indicates that, although age is an important variable in adolescent motherhood, the social factors of the model presented in this research are critical to identifying those adolescents at greatest risk. (p. 84)

Conversely, calculation of the probabilities for adolescents with differing social status characteristics finds reduction of motherhood probability. An 18-year-old adolescent who is White, lives in a home with a parent in a professional occupation, knows her father, does not want to be a mother at her current age, and has no friends either pregnant or parenting has only a 12.5% probability of motherhood. The 14-year-old with these same characteristics has a 1.4% probability. (p. 84)

CRITIQUE

The elements that were controlled in the design were age, valid measurement scales, and a large stratified sample. The design could have been improved by determining the number of adolescents who actually became mothers during adolescence. This determination was possible but would have required following the subjects over a period of several years, with a considerable expenditure of time and available funds. Unfortunately, without this information, the study requires an assumption that the level of risk is closely related to actual occurrence of motherhood during adolescence, which is not tested in this study. Manipulation is not used in this type of design.

(continues)

IMPLICATIONS FOR PRACTICE

With instruments that are readily available to practitioners, nurses can evaluate these variables and determine the risk of adolescent motherhood to individuals. Several of the variables significant to risk assessment can be obtained through interview alone…. Subsequent nursing interventions can be directed toward prevention to those at greatest risk. Nurses in any clinical setting can refer adolescents identified to be at risk for early pregnancy to prevention programs available in their communities. (p. 86) Prediction of adolescent pregnancy can contribute to evidence-based practice. However, evidence-based practice requires longitudinal studies that demonstrate the effectiveness of the predictions. A further contribution to evidence-based practice requires the testing of interventions that are demonstrated to reduce the risk of adolescent pregnancies.

Model Testing Design

Some studies are designed specifically to test the accuracy of a hypothesized causal model (middle range theory). The **model testing design** requires that all variables relevant to the model be measured. A large, heterogeneous sample is required. Investigators identify all of the paths expressing relationships between concepts and develop a conceptual map (Figure 8-8). The analysis determines whether the data are consistent with the model.

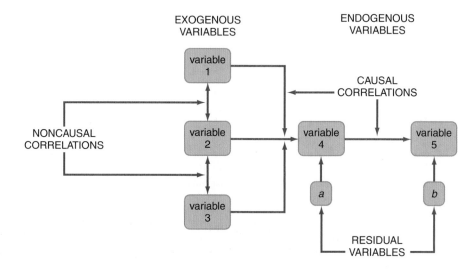

Figure 8-8. Model-testing design.

RESEARCH EXAMPLE Model Testing Design

Rempel and Fong (2005) used a model testing design to test the ability of the Reasons Model to predict the breastfeeding intentions of 317 first-time mothers before and after breastfeeding experience:

> The Reasons Model proposes that three levels of reasons for (pro) and against (con) adherence to health-related advice predict intentions: evidence-based (Level I); self-consequential (Level II); and affective, schema-related (Level III) reasons. (p. 443)

Measures included the Breastfeeding Reasons Questionnaire, Breastfeeding intentions, and Postpartum Questionnaires. Subjects were followed from the third trimester to 12 months postpartum, with contacts at birth, 1 month, 2 months, 4 months, 6 months, 9 months, and 12 months so long as breastfeeding was continuing. Those who began breastfeeding and then stopped before the 12th month were contacted one time after discontinuation to assess actual breastfeeding duration and reasons for weaning.

Map of Model

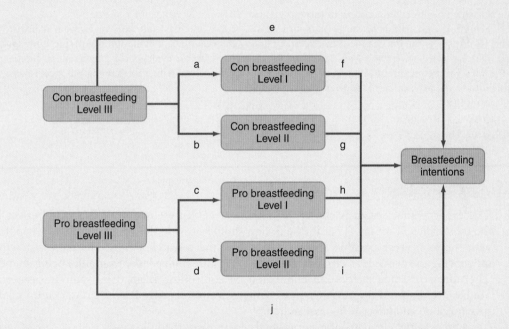

Path analytic model: Reasons predicting breastfeeding intentions.

Findings

Path analyses showed that the Reasons Model was able to predict breastfeeding intentions. Level III reasons most strongly predicted prenatal and early postpartum intentions. Level II con breastfeeding reasons predicted later postpartum intentions. Breastfeeding intentions significantly predicted behavior. The ability to predict future behavior is an important guide to nursing practice and contributes to evidence-based practice.

(continues)

CRITIQUE

In this study, researchers controlled the following elements: sample size, valid and reliable scales, and longitudinal follow-up of subjects, testing of the Reasons Model, and demonstrating a measured link between intention to breastfeed and breastfeeding behavior. This is a strong design and needs no further controls. Manipulation is not appropriate in this design.

IMPLICATIONS FOR PRACTICE

It is important to know the reasons people give for their behavior. These reasons reflect their feelings and their values. If a nurse is recommending a particular behavior, such as breastfeeding, a mother's acceptance of that recommendation must fit with her personal values and self-understanding. By understanding this, the nurse "will be in a much better position to assist individuals to make and maintain choices that will promote their own health and the health of those they love" (Rempel & Fong, 2005, p. 463).

Theoretical explanation of the pathways of cause for the preferred outcome of long-term breastfeeding is critical to the development of effective nursing interventions. The design of nursing interventions must be based on strong, well-tested theories and have strong evidence of effectiveness. Studies incorporating these principles will help to generate evidence-based guidelines for nursing practice, related in this case to the promotion of long-term breastfeeding.

Testing Causality

The experimental design is chosen to obtain a true representation of cause and effect by the most efficient means. That is, the design should provide the greatest amount of control with the least error possible. To examine cause, the researcher must eliminate all factors influencing the dependent variable other than the cause (independent variable) being studied. The effects of some factors are eliminated by controlling them (e.g., sampling criteria). Studies are designed to prevent other elements from intruding into the observation of the specific cause and effect being researched.

The essential elements of experimental research are the following:

- Random assignment of subjects to groups
- Precisely defined independent variable
- Researcher-controlled manipulation of the independent variable
- Researcher control of the experimental situation and setting, including a control or comparison group
- Clearly identified sampling criteria
- Carefully measured dependent variables
- Controlled environment for conduct of study

Quasi-Experimental Design

Use of a quasi-experimental design facilitates the search for knowledge and examination of causality in situations in which complete control is not possible. This type of design was developed to control as many threats to validity as possible in a situation in which some of the components of true experimental design are lacking. A nonequivalent comparison group, one in which the control group is not selected by random means, commonly is used in quasi-experimental studies.

In most quasi-experimental studies, experimental and comparison subjects are selected from the same pool of potential subjects. Occasionally, with this type of design, comparison and treatment groups may evolve naturally. For example, groups may include subjects who choose a treatment as the experimental group and subjects who choose not to receive a treatment as the comparison group. These groups cannot be considered equivalent, however, because the subjects in the control group usually differ in important ways from those in the treatment group.

Quasi-experimental study designs vary widely. The most frequently used design in social science research is the untreated comparison group design with pretest and posttest (Figure 8-9). With this design, the researcher has a group of subjects who receive the experimental treatment (or intervention) and a comparison group of subjects who receive no treatment (or, in some cases, the standard care provided in the circumstances under study).

Another commonly used design is the posttest-only design with a comparison group (Figure 8-10). This design is used in situations in which a pretest is not possible. For example, if the researcher is examining differences in the amount of pain that a subject feels during a painful procedure, and a nursing intervention is used to reduce pain for subjects in the experimental group, it might not be possible (or meaningful) to pretest the amount of pain

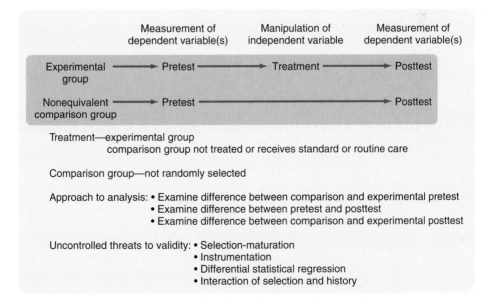

Figure 8-9. Pretest and posttest design with a comparison group.

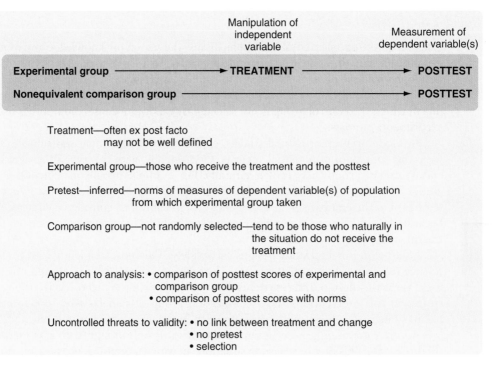

Figure 8-10. Posttest-only design with a comparison group.

before the procedure. This design incorporates a number of threats to validity because of the lack of a pretest and thus is sometimes referred to as a pre-experimental design.

Use the algorithm shown in Figure 8-11 to determine the type of quasi-experimental study design used in a published study. More details about specific designs identified in this algorithm are available in other sources (Burns & Grove, 2005).

RESEARCH EXAMPLE   Quasi-Experimental Pretest-Posttest Design with Control Group

Velsor-Friedrich, Pigott, and Srof (2005) conducted a quasi-experimental study using a pretest-posttest design with a control group. The study was funded by the National Institute of Nursing Research. Following is their abstract:

INTRODUCTION

Asthma is the most prevalent chronic illness, affecting more than 7 million children younger than 17 years. Asthma has become a leading public health concern because of the dramatic rise in the incidence of this disease during the past 15 years, particularly in minority populations. This study tested a two-part intervention on selected psychosocial and health outcomes of 8- to 13-year-old inner city minority students with asthma. (p. 163)

(continues)

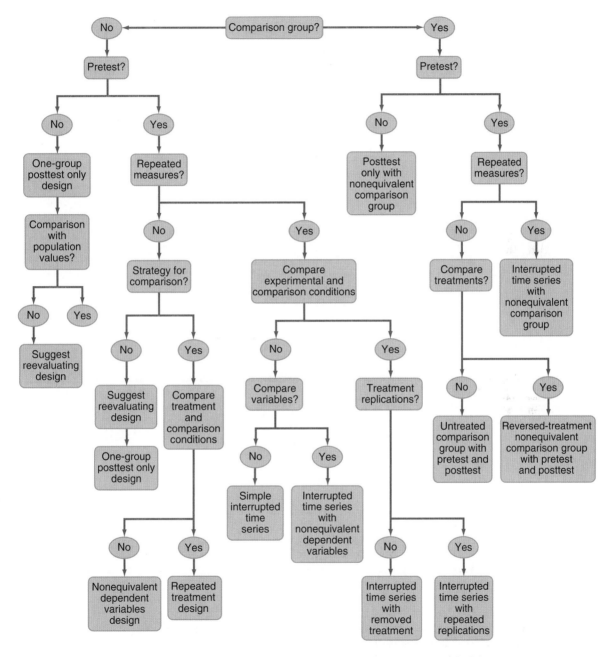

Figure 8-11. Algorithm for determining type of quasi-experimental design.

RESEARCH EXAMPLE *(continued)*

The framework for the study was Orem's (2001) Self-Care Deficit Theory. Variables included the self-care abilities of self-esteem; asthma self-efficacy; asthma knowledge; and knowledge, skill, and motivation for self-care.

In the 2 weeks prior to the initiation of the intervention, baseline information was collected regarding the student's asthma health using an asthma diary. (p. 165)

The intervention in this study was composed of student participation in the asthma education program, Open Airways, followed by 5 monthly visits with the nurse practitioner [NP] in the school-based clinic. The Open Airways Asthma Education Program was developed at Columbia University in conjunction with the American Lung Association. The purposes of the Open Airways Program are to: (a) empower children with asthma by teaching them how to prevent asthma episodes and emergencies; and (b) to help schools control asthma by creating partnerships in asthma care with school personnel, school nurses, physicians, and families (American Lung Association, 2004; U.S. Department of Health & Human Services, 1984). The program consists of six, 45-minute sessions offered once per week in which small groups of children learn new asthma management skills. The session topics include: (a) basic information about asthma; (b) how to recognize and respond to asthma symptoms; (c) using asthma medication and deciding when to seek help; (d) how to keep physically active; (e) identifying and controlling triggers to minimize asthma symptoms; and (f) handling programs related to asthma and school. The curriculum incorporates an interactive teaching approach utilizing group discussion, stories, games, and role-play to promote children's active involvement in the learning process. The program focuses on the child's independent actions as self-managers, emphasizing the child's responsibility for recognizing asthma symptoms and initiating a plan of action (American Lung Association; U.S. Department of Health & Human Services, 2000). The curriculum reflects recommendations for asthma management that are consistent with the NAEPP (National Asthma Education and Prevention Program Guidelines, 1997; 2002). (p. 166)

The second part of the intervention consisted of 5 monthly visits with the NP at the school-based health clinic. These follow-up visits were initiated after the students completed the asthma educational program. During the visits, the NP assessed the student's asthma health, including auscultation of breath sounds, assessment of current medication use and availability, and history of symptoms, visits to the emergency department, and hospitalizations. Students were asked to demonstrate skills such as flow meter techniques. The NP included age-appropriate asthma education information (from the Open Airways curriculum) as deemed necessary to reinforce and/or increase asthma knowledge. The NP at each of the four schools was given a packet of asthma information to review with the children if needed. Adjustments to asthma management plans were made as determined by the NP. (p. 166)

PROCEDURE

An asthma screening survey developed in a previous study (Velsor-Friedrich, Pigott, & Louloudes, 2004) was used to determine which children in the four schools had asthma. The survey was given to every child in each of the four Midwestern elementary schools. A letter, written by the principal of each school, asked parents to complete the survey and return it to the school the next day. As an incentive, the classrooms with the highest returns received a pizza lunch party. The returned surveys were reviewed and a list was compiled of children who had been diagnosed with asthma by a physician or who had demonstrated asthma-related symptoms and frequent asthma-related emergency department visits or hospital admissions. The return rate of completed surveys ranged from 25% to 27% per each school. The diagnosis of asthma or the presence of asthma-related symptoms was reported in approximately 22% of the returned surveys. (p. 166)

Parents of children identified with asthma were sent a letter explaining the study and were asked to complete the consent and child assent forms if they were interested in having their child participate in the study. From the four schools, 83 signed consent-assents were returned. Of those, 73 met the inclusion criteria guidelines and those children were enrolled in the study. After a year, at the conclusion of the study, the sample included 52 students with 21 (28%) lost to attrition. Reasons for attrition included 18 students who moved to another area or transferred to another school. Therefore, only three students dropped out of the study. (p. 166)

There were 52 children in the sample, with 28 children in the treatment group and 24 children in the comparison group. It is not clear from the published study how assignments to group were made. Although the comparison group received no treatment during the study, the asthma educational program was provided to the comparison group at the conclusion of the study.

The first hypothesis is supported in part. School-aged children with asthma showed significant improvements in self-care ability following participation in a school-based asthma intervention. The significant findings on the self-care measures suggest that the Open Airways curriculum plus the NP follow-up with individualized asthma management plans is an effective course of action for improving students' asthma knowledge, self-efficacy, general self-care practices and asthma self-care practices. (p. 169)

Despite significant findings related to self-care practice, the hypothesized improvement in health outcomes was not supported. There were no significant differences between the treatment and control groups on measures of peak expiratory flow rate (PEFR), symptom frequency, rescue medication use, urgent doctor visits, or school absenteeism. (p. 169)

CRITIQUE

The elements that were controlled in this study were the ages of the children, the method of seeking subjects, and the carefully developed treatment. The year-long follow-up evaluation of the children allows careful examination of children's response to the educational program and the NP interventions. The tracking of self-care measures used by the children also was a strength. Elements that could have been controlled to improve the study design include clarifying the method used for assignment to groups and increasing the percentage of the population sampled, but the feasibility of the latter is not great. Parents of children in this age group, regardless of economic status or ethnicity, often are not given notes sent home, and the parents tend not to ask or to examine material brought home by children. Those who do read the note often will not respond. Follow-up notes or letters in the mail will increase samples somewhat, but response is still limited. This is a problem with most studies of children's health behaviors that use schools as a source of subjects.

Children in the treatment group did increase self-care measures; however, the use of the self-care measures did not result in an improvement in outcome measures such as PEFR, frequency of symptoms, rescue medication use, urgent doctor visits, and school absenteeism. Thus, the study did not demonstrate the effectiveness of the intervention. It also did not demonstrate that using the selected self-care measures improves health status. This may be due to the small sample size. Testing an intervention such as this one usually requires a sample size of at least 200 who complete the study. It may be, however, that the treatment is not strong enough to cause a change in outcomes, or that the treatment just does not work. Determining which of these is the case will require more studies, larger samples, and further development of the intervention.

(continues)

> ### IMPLICATIONS FOR PRACTICE
>
> "The study supports the ongoing benefit of school-based asthma programming for improved asthma self-care practice among African American inner-city school-aged children. Comprehensive school-based programs combining Open Airways and NP-facilitated asthma management plans should be built on a structure that provides for health care continuity. However, the multiple factors influencing asthma episodes, coupled with the rising asthma morbidity despite adherence to NAEPP guidelines, requires a coordinated multilevel public health-focused effort. The school-based approach should be part of a larger community based program that works to enhance familial health practices concerning asthma self-care. Models for parental involvement demonstrate the benefits of home based assessment and intervention. Training of health workers to provide follow-through care in the home can help to decrease barriers. Well-planned asthma-specific assessments can lead to individualization of care." (p. 170)
>
> The study also provides an evidence base for nursing practice. However, the evidence base needs to be strengthened with large sample clinical trials that prove the effectiveness of the intervention in improving health status, as well as self-care activities. The authors prescribe the elements that need to be added to the intervention to bring about the desired outcome.

Experimental Designs

A variety of **experimental designs**, some relatively simple and others very complex, have been developed for a variety of studies focused on examining causality. In some cases, researchers may combine characteristics of more than one design to meet the needs of their study. Names of designs vary from one text to another. When reading and critiquing a published study, determine the author's name for the design (some authors do not name the design used) and read the description of the design to determine the type of design used in the study.

Use the algorithm shown in Figure 8-12 to determine the type of experimental study design used in a published study. More details about specific designs referred to in Figure 8-12 are available in other texts (Burns & Grove, 2005).

Pretest-Posttest Design

The most common experimental design used in nursing studies is the pretest-posttest design. This design is shown in Figure 8-13, except that the experimental study is more tightly controlled. Multiple groups (both experimental and control) can be used to great advantage in this design. For example, one control group can receive no treatment, whereas another control group receives a placebo treatment. Each one of multiple experimental groups can receive a variation of the treatment, such as a different frequency, intensity, or duration of nursing care measures. These additions greatly increase the generalizability of study findings.

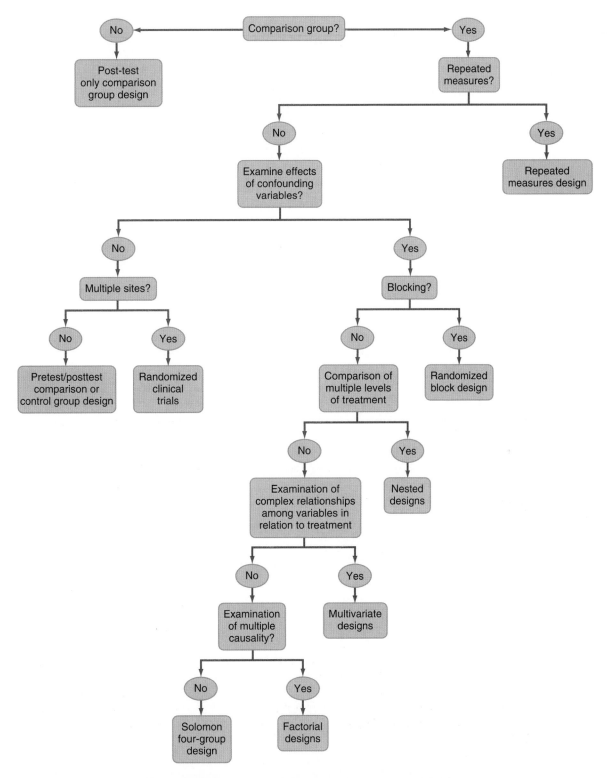

Figure 8-12. Algorithm for determining type of experimental design.

	Measurement of dependent variable(s)	Manipulation of independent variable	Measurement of dependent variable(s)
Randomized experimental group	Pretest ──────────→	Treatment ──────────→	Posttest
Randomized comparison or control group	Pretest ──────────────────────────────→		Posttest

Treatment: Under control of researcher

Approach to analysis: • Comparison of pretest and posttest scores
 • Comparison of comparison and experimental groups
 • Comparison of pretest/posttest differences between samples

Uncontrolled threats to validity: • Testing
 • Instrumentation
 • Mortality
 • Restricted generalizability as control increases

Figure 8-13. The classic experimental design: Pretest-posttest control group design.

RESEARCH EXAMPLE Experimental Pretest-Posttest Design

Williams and Schreier (2005) conducted a study of the role of education in managing fatigue, anxiety, and sleep disorders in women undergoing chemotherapy for breast cancer. The study was funded by the Pitt County Chapter of the American Cancer Society (ACS), an Oncology Nursing Society (ONS) Foundation grant supported by GlaxoSmithKline, the Leo Jenkins Cancer Center, and the ACS Institutional Research Grant.

The settings were at a tertiary medical center in the Southeastern United States and a satellite cancer treatment clinic. The medical center serves a 29-county rural area with a diverse population. A considerable number of patients are African American, poor, and with low education levels. Seventy-one subjects who were newly diagnosed with breast cancer were included in the study. All received intravenous chemotherapy regimes that included CYTOXAN cyclophosphamide (Methrotrexate), ADRUCH Flurouracil (CMF) or ADRIAMYCIN (Doxorubicin Hydrochloride Injection, USP), and cyclophosphamide (AC). All subjects were 18 years of age or older; English speaking; capable of hearing normal conversations; oriented to time, place, and person; and living in a community setting. All subjects had a Karnofsky Performance Scale rating greater than 70% and were not undergoing any therapy other than chemotherapy. Patients were randomly assigned to the treatment or control group.

A 20-min audiotape that consisted of education about exercise and relaxation to manage anxiety, fatigue, and sleep problems was developed for the study. The transcript for the tape was developed based on prior research studies that documented the most effective SCBs [self-care behaviors] for anxiety.... The transcript for the tape was written at the fifth-grade level to ensure that patients with low literacy would comprehend the material. The computerized Flesch Readability Scale was used to determine the reading level of the transcript. A mock audiotape was made and reviewed for clarity and inclusiveness by three professional nurses and three formerly treated patients with breast cancer. A professional female reader recorded the tape in a sound studio where background music was added. A printed self-care diary (SCD) of SCBs that mirrored the audiotape was also written at or below a fifth-grade level as determined by the Flesch Readability Scale and given to the women in the experimental group.

The SCD in this study included frequently experienced SEs [side effects] of anxiety, fatigue, and sleep disturbance and the SCBs for these SEs. The printed SCD given to women in the experimental group contained information that was consistent with the SCD interview questions. Subjects were asked to indicate whether they had experienced a specific SE or event and to rate the severity of the event on a scale ranging from 1 *(not severe)* to 5 *(extremely severe)*. The incidence and severity of SEs were obtained by summing and averaging. (p. 139)

The State-Trait Anxiety Inventory [STAI] was used to measure anxiety. All subjects were interviewed by the same interviewer three times by telephone before the first treatment, 1 month later, and 3 months later. The interviewers were graduate-level nursing students. At the first interview, all women completed demographic data and the trait and state anxiety scales were administered. All the women completed a pretest on their knowledge of SCBs. At the end of 1 month, all participants completed the SCD (1st SCD) and the state anxiety scale of the STAI. At the end of 3 months, all participants were interviewed using the SCD (2nd SCD) and the state anxiety scale of the STAI and completed a posttest on knowledge of chemotherapy SEs.

Overall, women who received education demonstrated more SCBs, a wider range of SBCs, increased use of SCBs over time, and less anxiety. Nursing time for education in busy clinics is minimal. Patient anxiety in the clinic environment interferes with learning. Audiotapes are an effective tool for use at home, providing for teaching and reinforcement of patient education. (p. 138)

CRITIQUE

Williams and Schreier (2005) controlled the following subject variables in the design of this study: new diagnosis of breast cancer, similar chemotherapy protocols and no other treatments, English as native language, normal ability to communicate, age of 18 years or older, and residence in a community setting, confirmation of orientation, and a Karnofsky score higher than 70%. Thus, the subjects were as similar as possible. The treatment audiotape had undergone considerable refinement before use in the study. Because the tape was recorded, the treatment was exactly the same for each subject. The researchers gave a printed self-care diary to each subject in the experimental group to record the symptoms experienced and the self-care strategies the subject used to reduce symptoms. The symptoms being studied were the same for each subject. All subjects were interviewed by telephone on a preset schedule. Interviewers asked the exact same questions for each subject. All of the interviewers were graduate-level nursing students. Thus, Williams and Schreier controlled everything possible to control in the study.

IMPLICATIONS FOR PRACTICE

It is well known that patients undergoing chemotherapy experience numerous SEs from treatment. Severity of SEs can lead to patients' failure to complete their therapy, and certain SEs can lead to complications that might require hospitalization. Often, the significance and severity of SEs exceed patients' ability to adequately care for themselves without assistance from nurses and other care providers. Patients who are undergoing outpatient chemotherapy require active interventions to lessen anxiety and relieve treatment-related SEs. Teaching women how to manage the SEs of treatment has been shown to decrease their symptom distress. Nurses have a major role in managing SEs and assisting patients in managing SEs. They can provide the education needed to assist patients in performing effective self-care. (p. 142)

This study provides a strong contribution to the evidence base needed to provide high-quality care to patients undergoing chemotherapy.

Randomized Clinical Trial

The **randomized clinical trial** has been used in medicine since 1945. However, until recently it has not been used in nursing. The clinical trial uses large numbers of subjects to test the effects of a treatment and compare the results with those of a control group that has not received the treatment (or that has received a traditional treatment). Subjects are drawn from a reference population, using clearly defined criteria, and then are randomly assigned to treatment or control groups. Baseline states must be comparable in all groups included in the study. The same treatment is given and is consistently applied, and outcomes are measured consistently. Care is taken to ensure that randomization procedures are rigidly adhered to in a study. Because of the need to have large samples and to be able to generalize to a variety of clinical settings and patients, the study may be carried out simultaneously in multiple geographic locations coordinated by the primary researcher. Use of this design has the potential to greatly improve the scientific base for nursing practice (Fetter et al., 1989; Tyzenhouse, 1981). Burns and Grove (2005) have defined the criteria that must be met for a nursing study to be defined as a clinical trial.

RESEARCH EXAMPLE   Randomized Clinical Trial

Kim, Dodd, West, Paul, Facione, Schumacher, et al. (2004) conducted a clinical trial of the PRO-SELF Pain Control Program. The study was supported by a grant from the National Cancer Institute (CA 64734). Unrestricted grants from Janssen Pharmaceutica and Purdue Pharma LP provided additional support.

Two hundred twelve outpatients with cancer were recruited from a university-based cancer center, two community-based oncology practices, one outpatient radiation therapy center, one health maintenance organization, one veteran's administration facility, and one military hospital, all in northern California. The study was approved by the Committee on Human Research at the University of California, San Francisco, and at each of the study sites. Only those patients (n = 174) who completed the study were included in the analysis. Some patients (n = 38) did not complete the entire study for a variety of reasons, including increased severity of illness, intervening cancer treatments that required hospitalization, and death. No differences were found in any of the demographic, disease, or baseline pain characteristics among patients who did and did not complete the study. (p. 1132)

The participants were adult (>18 years old) outpatients with cancer who were able to read, write, and understand English. All participants had a Karnofsky Performance Status (KPS) score of 50 or more, an average pain score of 2.5 or more on a 0–10 numeric rating scale (based on an average of seven days' baseline ratings of pain intensity), and radiographic evidence of bone metastasis. (p. 1132)

INSTRUMENTS

Patients completed a demographic questionnaire, the KPS (Karnofsky Pain Scale) rating scale (Karnofsky & Burchenal, 1949), and the PES (Pain Experience Scale) (Ferrell, Rhiner, & Rivera, 1993). In addition, patients' medical records were reviewed for disease and treatment information. (p. 1139)

The demographic questionnaire obtained information about age, gender, marital status, living arrangements, education level, ethnicity, and employment status. Baseline information about patients' pain was obtained using a numeric rating scale ranging from 0 (no pain) to ten (excruciating pain) for pain now and average, worst, and least pain. In addition, patients were asked to rate the number of hours per day and days per week that they experienced pain that interfered with their mood or activities. (p. 1139)

The KPS rating scale measures patients' ability to accomplish normal activities of daily living and their need for caregivers' assistance (Karnofsky & Burchenal, 1949). The KPS scale used in this study consisted of eight items for ranking functional status. They ranged from 30 (i.e., disability requiring hospitalization) to 100 (i.e., adequate health status with no complaints and no evidence of disease). Reliability and validity of the KPS scores on each item indicate a more correct response (i.e., more agreement or more disagreement with the statement (Ferrell, et al., 1993). Reliability and validity of the KPS have been established. (Karnofsky, 1977).

The PES contains 13 visual analog scales that measure an individual's knowledge about cancer pain and its management as well as an individual's perception of the pain experience (Ferrell, et al, 1993). The knowledge portion of the PES contains nine items that address knowledge about addiction, physical dependence, frequency of drug administration, scheduling of drug administration, and side effects associated with opioid analgesics. Each item is rated using a 10-mm visual analog scale anchored on the left with the work "disagree" and on the right with the word "agree." Patients were asked to mark an "X" on the line to indicate their level of agreement with each item. Some items were reverse coded so that each item was score[d] to reflect the degree of correctness. A total PES knowledge score was determined by summing the scores for each of the individual items and then converting that score to a 100% scale. The reliability and validity of the PES are well established. Higher scores on each item indicate a more correct response (i.e., more agreement or more disagreement with the statement). (Ferrell, et al.,1993)

DATA COLLECTION PROCEDURE

Patients were approached by a recruitment nurse who explained the study procedures and obtained informed consent. Patients completed the demographic questionnaire and KPS rating at the time of enrollment and were randomized into the PRO-SELF© or standard care group. At weeks 1, 3, and 6, a research nurse assigned solely to the PRO-SELF© or standard care groups visited patients in their homes. The same nurse conducted telephone interviews at weeks 2, 4, and 5. (Ferrell, et al., 1993, p. 1139)

During the week 1 visit, both groups of patients completed the PES (Ferrell, et al., 1993) to assess their knowledge about cancer pain and its management. The patients' responses to the PES questionnaire became the basis for the educational session with patients in the PRO-SELF© group. This session was tailored to meet individual learning needs. In addition, patients in the PRO-SELF© group were given written instructions regarding pain and side-effect management, taught how to use a weekly pillbox, and taught how to use a script to assist them in communicating with their physicians about unrelieved pain. During the subsequent home visits and follow-up phone calls, the educational content of the PRO-SELF© program was reinforced and patients were coached about how to modify their pain management plan to improve outcomes (see West et al. (2003) for a complete description of the PRO-SELF© program). The PES was readministered to both groups of patients at the final home visit to evaluate the effectiveness of the PRO-SELF© Pain Control Program. (p. 1139)

CRITIQUE

Kim and colleagues (2002) conducted this study in seven settings, thus controlling the setting as a cause of the effects being examined. The measurement instruments all were well known, valid methods of measurement. The researchers selected subjects on the basis of their fit with the defined criteria for the sample and then randomly assigned subjects to experimental or control group. Research nurses were assigned to either the experimental group or the control group, to avoid accidental exposure of the control group to elements of the intervention. A schedule of home visits and phone calls ensured consistency in research nurse activities. Thus, the study had a high level of control designed to provide a high degree of validity of the study findings. The research nurses consistently administered the intervention to all subjects in the experimental group. The study was implemented by nurses highly experienced in conducting research in this field of study.

(continues)

IMPLICATIONS FOR PRACTICE

The findings from this study demonstrate that the PES can be used as the basis for patient education in cancer pain management. Oncology nurses can use patients' responses to items on a survey such as the PES to individualize their teaching and spend more time on the identified knowledge deficits. This individualized approach to education about pain management may save staff time and improve patient outcomes. However, even with five weeks of education, patients did not achieve scores of 100% on the PES. (p. 1142)

Defining Experimental Interventions

In quasi-experimental and experimental studies, investigators develop an intervention that is expected to result in differences in posttest measures between the treatment and control or comparison groups. This intervention may be physiologic, psychosocial, educational, or a combination of these. The specific steps or components of the intervention need to be carefully planned, and a rationale is given for providing the intervention in a particular way. The intervention is described in detail in the published study. Labels for interventions such as "preoperative teaching" are to be avoided because they do not contribute to comprehension of the exact nature of the intervention. Readers may be easily led astray by such labels—each person has his or her own expectations of what should occur during preoperative teaching. Nursing is currently developing classifications of nursing interventions. It is hoped that these classifications will be useful to the researcher in clarifying the intervention provided. The goal of the intervention being investigated is to maximize the differences between the control and the experimental groups. Thus, it is important to choose the best intervention that can be provided under the circumstances of the study.

Although control and comparison groups traditionally have received no intervention, adherence to this expectation is not possible in many nursing studies. For example, it would be unethical not to provide preoperative teaching to a patient. Furthermore, in many studies it is possible that just spending time with a patient or having a patient participate in activities that he or she considers beneficial may in itself cause an effect. Therefore, the study often includes a control or comparison group intervention. This intervention usually is the standard care the patient would receive if a study were not being conducted. The researcher must describe in detail the standard care that the control or comparison group receives so that the study can be adequately critiqued. Because the quality of this standard care is likely to vary considerably among subjects, variance in the control or comparison group is likely to be high. The risk of a Type II error is greater than when the control or comparison group receives no treatment.

CRITIQUE GUIDELINES Interventions

When critiquing the interventions in a study, ask the following questions:

1. Was the experimental intervention described in detail?
2. Was justification from the literature provided for development of the experimental intervention?
3. Was the experimental intervention the best that could be provided given current knowledge?
4. Was a protocol developed to ensure consistent or reliable implementation of the treatment with each subject throughout the study? (See Burns & Grove [2005] for discussion of intervention protocols.)
5. Did the study report indicate who implemented the treatment? If more than one person implemented the treatment, were they trained to ensure consistency in the delivery of the treatment?
6. Was any control or comparison group intervention described?
7. Was an intervention theory provided to explain why the intervention causes the outcomes and exactly how the intervention produced the desired effects?

Intervention research methods are presented in the textbook by Burns and Grove (2005, Chapter 13, "Intervention Research").

RESEARCH EXAMPLE Interventions

Peden, Rayens, Hall, and Grant (2005) describe the intervention used in their study "Testing an intervention to reduce negative thinking, depressive symptoms, and chronic stressors in low-income single mothers." This research was funded by Grant RO1 NR0506-01 awarded to Drs. Peden, Hall, and Rayens by the National Institute of Nursing Research, National Institutes of Health.

Those single mothers assigned to receive the cognitive-behavioral intervention participated in six 1-hour or four 90-minute group sessions that targeted identification of negative thinking and its effects on feelings and depressive behaviors. The intervention is based on the premise that women who are at risk for depression have modifiable risk factors. The modifiable risk factor targeted is negative thinking. Cognitive-behavioral strategies are designed to teach people that through self-control they can alter their thoughts, feelings, and behaviors. Cognitive-behavioral strategies are focused on teaching skills to regulate thoughts and moods. An important aspect of skill teaching is practice of the skills between sessions. The primary technique was developed by Meichenbaum (1977). Through practice, specifically the use of audiotapes, people learn to interrupt negative thinking. Once the negative thinking is interrupted, a more positive thought is inserted. These positive thoughts are referred to as affirmations. Participants listen daily to affirmations audiotaped in their own voice, and they place written affirmations in their work and home environments. This use of other visual cues is another mechanism for incorporating positive thoughts into their thinking style. (pp. 270-271)

The intervention was designed using specific content from Verona Gordon's *Insight* (1991) program, *The Depression Workbook* (Copeland, 1992), and Dr. Peden's own clinical practice with depressed women. Affirmations and direct actions were adapted from the Insight program, with permission. *The Depression Workbook* included information on thought stopping, affirmations, and distorted thinking styles. Depressed women benefit from group treatment (Gordon & Tobin, 1991; Van Servellen & Dull, 1981) because it allows

(continues)

RESEARCH EXAMPLE *(continued)*

contact with peers with similar problems, reduces isolation, promotes change, and is cost-effective. To ensure fidelity in implementing the intervention, a script was written for each session. Upon assignment to the intervention group, each participant received a notebook containing handouts on the weekly topics, a schedule for each session, and homework assignments. Group size varied from four to eight participants. The intervention is educational and was offered by a master's-educated psychiatric nurse with experience in leading client groups. Each group leader was trained by the PI in intervention delivery. A more complete description of the weekly sessions is available (Peden et al., 2001). (p. 271)

CRITIQUE

The researchers did not describe the intervention in sufficient detail to enable the nurse-reader to provide the intervention. Nurses interested in using the intervention will need to contact the researcher. The literature provided justification for development of the experimental intervention. The experimental intervention merged findings from previous practice and research and thus has validity as the best that could be provided as indicated by the current literature. Using a script ensured consistent or reliable implementation of the treatment with each subject throughout the study. The intervention was provided by a master's-educated psychiatric nurse with experience in leading client groups. Each group leader was trained specifically to provide the intervention by the primary investigator. No control group intervention was described.

IMPLICATIONS FOR PRACTICE

The intervention had been tested previously in a randomized, controlled prevention trial conducted with 136 low-income single mothers with children between the ages of 2 and 6 years. "The findings in this study support the recommendations of the National Institute of Mental Health Psychosocial Intervention Development Workgroup (Hollon et al., 2002) to design interventions to prevent the onset of clinical depression in at-risk populations. Single mothers with small children are at risk for depression. The intervention was effective in decreasing depressive symptoms, and this beneficial effect lasted 6 months after the intervention. Negative thinking and chronic stressors also decreased significantly…. This research indicates the mental health benefits of altering negative thinking through an easy-to-administer and cost-effective nursing intervention. It also provides further support for the use of affirmations as a way to improve mood in at-risk people. Such an intervention might have little direct effect on changing the chronic stressors faced by this vulnerable population; however, nurses can provide strategies to improve the way single mothers perceive the chronic stressors they face. Additional clinical implications include depression screening as a routine practice for all mothers, with particular attention to women experiencing multiple stressors. Referral to mental health professionals for further evaluation and treatment can decrease the incidence of depression in this vulnerable population" (Peden, et al, 2005, p. 273).

This study contributes an evidence-based intervention that can be applied to at-risk populations to address a serious problem in nursing practice.

"Depression is a costly problem. It not only interferes with the health of mothers but also has the potential to negatively affect the mental health of their children. Early recognition and treatment of depressive symptoms can improve the mental health of low-income, single-mother families. Interventions focused on reducing negative thinking are one key to preventing clinical depression in low-income, single mothers" (Peden, et al, 2005, p. 273).

Mapping the Design

In quasi-experimental and experimental studies, investigators can map the design to clarify the points at which measurements are taken and treatments are provided for various groups in the study. Generally, the symbol O is used for an observation or a measurement. Several measurements or observations may be indicated by this symbol. The symbol T is used for a treatment. For example, in a study with two groups, experimental and control, in which subjects received a pretest and a posttest (pretest-posttest control group design), the design can be mapped as follows.

	Pretest	**Treatment**	**Posttest**
Experimental group	O_1	T	O_2
Control or comparison group	O_1		O_2

This design map could be used for a quasi-experimental or an experimental study. In the quasi-experimental study, the control group is called the "comparison" (or "nonequivalent") group. Experimental design subjects are randomly selected and then randomly assigned to groups.

If the study includes several posttests at monthly intervals, the design can be mapped as follows:

			Posttests			
	Pretest	**Treatment**	**1 mo**	**2 mo**	**3 mo**	**4 mo**
Experimental group	O_1	T	O_2	O_3	O_4	O_5
Control or comparison group	O_1		O_2	O_3	O_4	O_5

Researchers can express variations in the design map for more than two groups, by adding more rows, for repeated treatments, by placing the "T" at each place the treatment is administered, or for multiple treatments. Multiple treatments may be labeled T_1, T_2, T_3, and so on.

Role of Replication Studies in Evidence-Based Practice

Replication studies involve reproducing or repeating a study to determine whether similar findings will be obtained (Taunton, 1989). The intent of replication is to determine whether the findings from the original study hold up despite minor changes in the research conditions. If the findings generated through replication are consistent with the original study findings, these findings are more credible and have the potential to be used in practice.

Replication is essential for knowledge development for several reasons: (1) replication establishes the credibility of the findings, (2) it extends the generalizability of the findings over a range of instances and contexts, (3) it provides support for theory development, and (4) it decreases the acceptance of erroneous results (Beck, 1994). Thus, replication studies are essential to generate knowledge that can be used in practice.

Beck (1994) conducted a computerized and manual review of the nursing literature from 1983 through 1992 and found only 49 replication studies. Possibly, the number of replication studies is limited because replication is viewed by some as less scholarly or less important than original research. However, the lack of replication studies severely limits the development of a scientific knowledge base for nursing (Beck, 1994; Martin, 1995). Thus, replication of studies is an important priority for nursing because it will greatly influence the generation of nursing knowledge that can be synthesized for use in practice (Burns & Grove, 2005).

KEY CONCEPTS

- A research design is a blueprint for conducting a study that maximizes control over factors that could interfere with the validity of the findings.
- Elements central to the study design include the presence or absence of a treatment, number of groups in the sample, number and timing of measurements to be performed, method of sampling, time frame for data collection, planned comparisons, and control of extraneous variables.
- Four common types of quantitative designs are used in nursing: descriptive, correlational, quasi-experimental, and experimental.
- The three essential elements of experimental research are (1) the random assignment of subjects to groups; (2) the researcher's manipulation of the independent variable; and (3) the researcher's control of the experimental situation and setting, including a control or comparison group.
- The purpose of design is to maximize the possibility of obtaining valid answers to research questions or hypotheses. A good design provides the subjects, the setting, and the protocol within which these comparisons can be clearly examined.
- Critiquing a design involves examining the study environment, sample, treatment, and measurement.

TIPS FOR FURTHER STUDY

- Are you having difficulty identifying the design of a published study? Work through "Making Connections" in your *Study Guide*.
- For help in evaluating the quality of a design, try answering the questions in Chapter 8 of the Companion CD-ROM.
- To prepare for developing a design model of a published study, practice "Mapping the Design" in your *Study Guide*.
- To clarify the concept of validity, work through the "Matching Questions" in the Open-Book Quiz at http://evolve.elsevier.com/Burns/understanding/.
- Test your understanding of causality with Chapter 8 of the Companion CD-ROM.

REFERENCES

American Lung Association. (2004). *Open airways*. Retrieved March 3, 2004, from http://www.lungs.org/

Beck, C. T. (1994). Replication strategies for nursing research. *Image—The Journal of Nursing Scholarship, 26*(3), 191–194.

Burns, N., & Grove, S. K. (2005). *The practice of nursing research: Conduct, critique and utilization* (5th ed.). Philadelphia: Saunders.

Copeland, M. E. (1992). *The depression workbook: A guide for living with depression and manic depression*. Oakland, CA: New Harbinger.

Dormire, S. L. (1992). *Human agency perspectives in adolescent motherhood: Self-esteem and socio-cultural variables*. Unpublished doctoral dissertation. University of Florida Gainsville.

Dormire, S. L., & Yarandi, H. (2001). Predictors of risk for adolescent childbearing. *Applied Nursing Research*, *14*(2), 81–86.

Ferrell, B. R., Rhiner, M., & Rivera, L. M. (1993). Development and evaluation of the family pain questionnaire. *Journal of Psychosocial Oncology*, *10*(4), 21–35.

Fetter, M. S., et al. (1989). Randomized clinical trials: Issues for researchers. *Nursing Research*, *38*(2), 117–120.

Gordon, V. C., & Tobin, M. (1991). *Insight: A cognitive enhancement program for women*. Available from Verona Gordon, University of Minnesota, Minneapolis, MN.

Hollingshead, A. (1975). *Four factor index of social status*. New Haven: Yale University Press.

Hollon, S., Munoz, R. F., Barlow, D., Beardslee, W., Bell, C., Bernal, G., et al. (2002). Psychosocial intervention development for the prevention and treatment of depression: Promoting innovation and increasing access. *Biological Psychiatry*, *52*(6), 610–630.

Johnson, R. L. (2005). Gender differences in health-promoting lifestyles of African Americans. *Public Health Nursing*, *22*(2), 130–137.

Karnofsky, D. (1977). Performance scales. In G. T. Kennealey & M. S. Mitchell (Eds.), *Factors that influence the therapeutic response in cancer* (pp. 191–205). New York: Plenum Press.

Karnofsky, D., & Burchenal, J. (1949). The clinical evaluation of chemotherapeutic agents in cancer. In C. M. Macleod (Ed.). *Evaluation of chemotherapeutic agents* (pp. 199–205). New York: Columbia University Press.

Kim, J., Dodd, M., West, C., Paul, S., Facione, N., Schumacher, K., et al.. (2004). The PRO-SELF© Pain Control Program improves patients' knowledge of cancer pain management. *Oncology Nursing Forum*, *31*(6), 1137–1143.

Martin, P. A. (1995). More replication studies needed. *Applied Nursing Research*, *8*(2), 102–103.

Meichenbaum, D. (1977). *Cognitive-behavior modification: An integrative approach*. New York: Plenum Press.

National Asthma Education and Prevention Program. (1997). Practical guide for the diagnosis and management of asthma: Expert panel 2 report. NIH Publication No. 97–4053. Washington, DC. U.S. GPO.

National Asthma Education and Prevention Program. (2002). Expert panel report. Guidelines for the diagnosis and management of asthma. Update on Selected Topics. NIH Publication No. 02–5075. Washington, DC. U.S. GPO.

O'Leary-Kelley, C. M., Puntillo, K. A., Barr, J., Stotts, N., & Douglas, M. K. (2005). Nutritional adequacy in patients receiving mechanical ventilation who are fed enterally. *American Journal of Critical Care*, *14*(3), 222–231.

Orem, D. E. (2001). *Nursing concepts of practice*, 6th Ed. Philadelphia, PA: Mosby.

Parker, G., Tupling, H., & Brown, L. B. (1979). A parental bonding instrument. *British Journal of Medical Psychology*, *52*, 1–10.

Peden, A. R., Rayens, M. K., Hall, L. A., & Beebe, L. H. (2001). Preventing depression in high-risk college women: A report of an 18-month follow-up. *Journal of American College Health*, *49*(6), 299–306.

Peden, A. R., Rayens, M. K., Hall, L. A., & Grant, E. (2005). Testing an intervention to reduce negative thinking, depressive symptoms, and chronic stressors in low-income single mothers. *The Journal of Nursing Scholarship*, *37*(3), 268–274.

Rempel, L. A. & Fong, G. T. (2005). Why breastfeed? A longitudinal test of the Reasons Model among first-time mothers. *Psychology and Health*, *20*(4), 443–466.

Rew, L., Taylor-Seehafer, M., Thomas, N. Y., & Yockey, R. D. (2001). Correlates of resilience in homeless adolescents. *The Journal of Nursing Scholarship*, *33*(1), 33–40.

Rosenberg, M. (1965). *Society and the adolescent self-image*. Princeton, NJ: Princeton University Press.

Taunton, R. L. (1989). Replication: Key to research application. *Dimensions of Critical Care Nursing*, *8*(3), 156-158.

Tyzenhouse, P. S. (1981). Technical notes: The nursing clinical trial. *Western Journal of Nursing Research*, *3*(1), 102–109.

U.S. Department of Health and Human Services. (1984). Open airways self-management program. NIH publication No. 84–2365. U.S. Department of Health and Human Services. Rockville, MD: National Heart, Lung and Blood Institute. U.S. GPO.

U.S. Department of Health and Human Services. (2000). *Healthy people 2010*. Washington, DC: Author. For sale by the U.S. Government Printing Office, Superintendent of Documents. U.S. GPO.

Ulster, A. A. & Antle, B. J. (2005). In the darkness there can be light: A family's adaptation to a child's blindness. *Journal of Visual Impairment & Blindness*, *99*(4), 209–218.

Van Servellen, G. M., & Dull, L. V. (1981). Group psychotherapy for depressed women: A model. *Journal of Psychosocial Nursing and Mental Health Services*, *19*(8), 25–31.

Velsor-Friedrich, B., Pigott, T., & Louloudes, A. (2004). The effects of a school-based intervention on the self-care and health of African-American inner-city children with asthma. *Journal of Pediatric Nursing*, *19*(4), 247–256.

Velsor-Friedrich, B., Pigott, T., & Srof, B. (2005). A practitioner-based asthma intervention program with African American inner-city school children. *Journal of Pediatric Health Care*, *19*(3), 163–171.

West, C. M., Dodd, M. J., Paul, S. M., Schumacher, K., Tripathy, D., Koo, P., et al. (2003). The PRO-SELF© Pain Control Program—an effective approach for cancer pain management. *Oncology Nursing Forum*, *31*(6), 65–73.

Williams, S. A., & Schreier, A. M. (2005). The role of education in managing fatigue, anxiety, and sleep disorders in women undergoing chemotherapy for breast cancer. *Applied Nursing Research*, *18*(3), 138–147.

Outcomes Research

Chapter Overview

Learning Outcomes

After completing this chapter, you should be able to:

1. Discriminate between traditional quantitative research and outcomes research
2. Explain the theoretical basis of outcomes research.
3. Explain the importance of outcomes research.
4. Identify nursing-sensitive patient outcomes.
5. Describe some of the unique methodologies of outcomes research.

Key Terms

STUDY TOOLS

Be sure to visit http://evolve.elsevier.com/Burns/understanding for additional examples and self-tests. Also, a review of this chapter's concepts and practice exercises can be found in Chapter 9 of the Study Guide for *Understanding Nursing Research: Building an Evidence-Based Practice*, 4th edition.

Outcomes research focuses on the end results of patient care. In order to explain the end results, nurse researchers also must understand the processes used to provide patient care. The strategies used in outcomes research are, to some extent, a departure from the accepted scientific methodology for health care research, and they incorporate evaluation methods, epidemiology, and economic theory. The findings of outcome studies continue to have a powerful impact on the provision of health care and the development of health policy.

The momentum propelling outcomes research comes not from scholars but from policy makers, insurers, and the public. These groups increasingly demand that providers justify interventions and systems of care in terms of improved patient lives and that costs of care be considered in the evaluation of treatment outcomes (Hinshaw, 1992). A major shift has occurred in published nursing studies, with the number of studies using traditional quantitative or qualitative methods being dwarfed by the number of outcomes studies. A large number of nursing and multidisciplinary journals focused on outcomes research have been initiated. A listing of these journals is presented in Table 9-1.

This chapter provides an explanation of the theoretical basis of outcomes research, a brief history of the emerging endeavors to examine outcomes, the importance of outcomes research designed to examine nursing practice, and methodologies used in outcomes research.

The Theoretical Basis of Outcomes Research

The theory on which outcomes research is based emerged from evaluation research. The theorist Avedis Donabedian (1976, 1978, 1980, 1982, 1987) proposed a theory of quality health care and the process of evaluating it.

Donabedian's Theory of Quality Health Care

Quality is the overriding construct of Donabedian's Theory of Quality Health Care, although he never defines this concept (Mark, 1995). The cube shown in Figure 9-1 helps explain the elements of quality health care. The three dimensions of the cube are health, subjects of care, and providers of care. The concept health has many aspects; three are shown on the cube: physical-physiological function, psychological function, and social function. Donabedian (1987, p. 4) proposes that "the manner in which we conceive of health and of our responsibility for it, makes a fundamental difference to the concept of quality and, as a result, to the methods that we use to assess and assure the quality of care."

Loegering, Reiter, and Gambone (1994) modified Donabedian's levels to include the patient, family, and community as providers of care as well as recipients of care. They suggest that access to care is one dimension of the provision of care by the community. Figure 9-2 illustrates their modifications.

Table 9-1	Nursing and Multidisciplinary Journals Focused on Outcomes Research

Best Practice
Clinical Effectiveness in Nursing
Effective Health Care
Evidence-Based Mental Health
Evidence-Based Practice
Health Education Research
Health Promotion Practice
Health Technology Assessment
International Journal of Health Care Quality Assurance Incorporating Leadership in Health Services
Journal of Care Management
Journal of Clinical Ethics
Journal of Clinical Outcomes Management
Journal for Health Care Quality
Journal of Health Services and Research Policy
Journal of Integrated Care Pathways
Journal of Nursing Care Quality
Journal of Nursing Quality Assurance
Journal of Quality in Clinical Practice
Journal of Rehabilitation Outcomes Measurement
Nursing and Health Policy Review
Outcomes Management
Outcomes Management for Nursing Practice
Patient Satisfaction Management
Quality in Health Care
Quality in Primary Care
Quality and Safety in Health Care
Quality Management in Health Care

Donabedian (1987) identifies three objects of evaluation in appraising quality: structure, process, and outcome. A complete quality assessment program requires the simultaneous use of all three concepts and an examination of the relationships among the three. However, researchers have had little success in accomplishing this theoretical goal. Studies designed to examine all three concepts would require sufficiently large samples of various structures, each with the various processes being compared and large samples of subjects who have experienced the outcomes of those processes. The funding and the cooperation necessary to accomplish this goal are not yet available.

Evaluating Outcomes

The goal of outcomes research, the evaluation of outcomes as defined by Donabedian, is not as simplistic as it might immediately appear. Donabedian's theory requires that identified outcomes be clearly linked with the process that caused the outcome. To accomplish this linking, the researcher must define the process and justify the causal links with the selected outcomes. The identification of desirable outcomes requires dialogue between the subjects of care and the providers of care. Although the providers of care may delineate what is

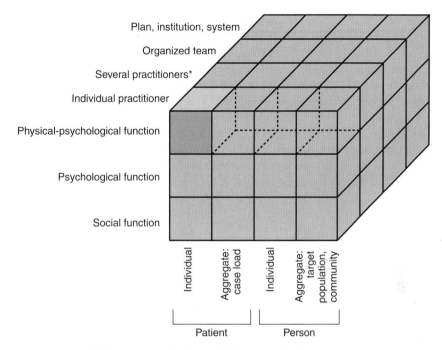

Figure 9-1. Level and scope of concern as factors in the definition of quality. (From Donabedian, A. [1987]. Some basic issues in evaluating the quality of health care. In L. T. Rinke [Ed.], *Outcome measures in home care* [Vol. 1, pp. 3–28]. New York: National League for Nursing.)

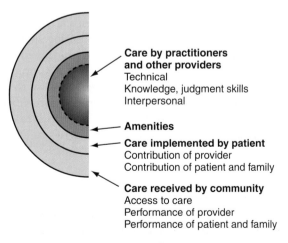

Care by practitioners and other providers
Technical
Knowledge, judgment skills
Interpersonal

Amenities

Care implemented by patient
Contribution of provider
Contribution of patient and family

Care received by community
Access to care
Performance of provider
Performance of patient and family

Figure 9-2. Various levels at which the quality of health care can be assessed. (From Donabedian, A. [1988]. The quality of care: How can it be assessed? *Journal of the American Medical Association, 260*[12], 1744. Copyright 1988, American Medical Association.)

achievable, the subjects of care must clarify what is desirable. The outcomes also must be relevant to the goals of the health care professionals, the health care system of which the professionals are a part, and society.

Outcomes are time dependent. Some outcomes may not be apparent for a long period after the process that is purported to cause them, whereas others may be apparent immediately. Some outcomes are temporary and others are permanent. Thus, the selection of an appropriate time frame for determining the selected outcomes must be established.

A final obstacle to outcomes evaluation is one of attribution. This requires assigning the place and degree of responsibility for the outcomes observed. A specific outcome often is influenced by a multiplicity of factors. Lewis (1995) points out that health care represents only one dimension of a complex situation. Patient factors, such as compliance, predisposition to disease, age, propensity to use resources, high-risk behaviors (e.g., smoking), and lifestyle, also must be taken into account. Environmental factors such as air quality, public policies related to smoking, and occupational hazards also must be included. Responsibility for outcomes may be distributed among providers, patients, employers, insurers, and the community.

As yet, little scientific basis has been established for judging the precise relationship between each of these factors and the selected outcome. Many of the influencing factors may be outside the jurisdiction or influence of the health care system or of the providers within it. One solution to this problem of identifying relevant outcomes is to define a set of closely related outcomes specific to the condition for which care is being provided. Critical pathways and care maps may be useful in defining at least related outcomes. However, related outcomes do not provide the degree of evidence of examining the desired outcomes.

Evaluating Process

The process of clinical management has been, for most health care professionals, an art rather than a science. Understanding the process sufficiently to study it must begin with much careful reflection, dialogue, and observation. Clinical management has multiple components, many of which have not yet been clearly defined or tested. Bergmark and Oscarsson (1991, pp. 139–140) suggest the following questions as important to consider in evaluating process: (1) "What constitutes the 'therapeutic agent'?" (2) "Do practitioners actually do what they say they do?" (3) "Do practitioners always know what they do?" Current outcomes studies are using process variables that are easy to identify. Answers to questions such as those posed by Bergmark and Oscarsson are more difficult to define and initially will require observation, interviews, and the use of qualitative research methodologies.

Three components of process of particular interest to Donabedian are standards of care, practice styles, and costs of care.

Standards of Care

A **standard of care** is a norm by which quality of care is judged. Clinical guidelines, critical paths, and care maps define standards of care. According to Donabedian (1987), a practitioner has legitimate responsibility to apply available knowledge in the management of a dysfunctional state. This management consists of (1) the identification or diagnosis of the dysfunction, (2) the decision whether to intervene, (3) the choice of intervention objectives, (4) the choice of methods and techniques to achieve the objectives, and (5) the skillful execution of the selected techniques.

Donabedian (1987) recommends the development of criteria to be used as a basis for judging the quality of care. These criteria may take the form of clinical guidelines or care maps based on previous validation of the contribution of the care to outcomes. The clinical guidelines published by the Agency for Healthcare Research and Quality (AHRQ) establish norms on which the validity of clinical management can be judged. However, the core of the problem, from Donabedian's perspective, is clinical judgment. Analysis of the process of making diagnoses and therapeutic decisions is critical to the evaluation of the quality of care. The emergence of decision trees and algorithms is a response to Donabedian's concerns and provides a means of evaluating the adequacy of clinical judgments.

Practice Styles

The style of practice is another dimension of the process of care that influences quality; however, it is problematic to judge what constitutes "goodness" in style and to provide justification for the decisions. Moreover, diverse styles of interpersonal relationships are possible. Most studies examining practice styles are conducted with physicians as subjects. A few studies of practice styles of nurses, however, are beginning to appear in the literature (Bircumshaw & Chapman, 1988; Fullerton, Hollenbach, & Wingard, 1996).

Costs of Care

A third dimension of the examination of quality of care is cost. Maintaining a specified level of quality of care necessarily has cost consequences. Providing more and better care is likely to increase costs but also is likely to produce savings. Economic benefits can be obtained by preventing illness, preventing complications, maintaining a higher quality of life, or prolonging productive life.

A related issue is who bears the costs of care. Some measures purported to reduce costs have instead simply shifted costs to another party. For example, in certain instances a hospital can reduce its costs by discharging a particular type of patient early, but total costs will increase if the necessary community-based health care raises costs above those incurred by keeping the patient hospitalized longer. In this case, the third-party provider may experience higher costs. In many cases, the costs are shifted from the health care system to the family as out-of-pocket costs. Studies examining changes in costs of care must consider *total* costs.

Evaluating Structure

Structures of care are the elements of organization and administration that guide the processes of care. The first step in evaluating structure is to identify and describe the elements of the structure. Various administration and management theories may be used to identify the elements of structure to be studied. Examples of such elements are leadership, tolerance of innovativeness, organizational hierarchy, decision-making processes, distribution of power, financial management, and administrative decision-making processes.

The second step is to evaluate the impact of various structure elements on the process of care and on outcomes. This evaluation requires comparing different structures that provide the same processes of care. In the evaluation of structures, the unit of measure is the structure. The evaluation requires access to a sufficiently large sample of like structures with similar processes and outcomes, which can then be compared with a sample of another structure providing the same processes and outcomes. For example, a researcher may decide to compare various structures providing primary health care, such as the private physician office, the health maintenance organization (HMO), the rural health clinic, the community-oriented primary care clinic, and the nurse-managed center. Another researcher may wish to examine surgical care provided within the structures of a private outpatient surgical clinic, a private hospital, a county hospital, and a teaching hospital associated with a health science center. In each of these studies, the focus will be the impact of structure on processes of care and outcomes of care. See Figures 9-3 through 9-6 for examples of frameworks for outcomes studies with this focus.

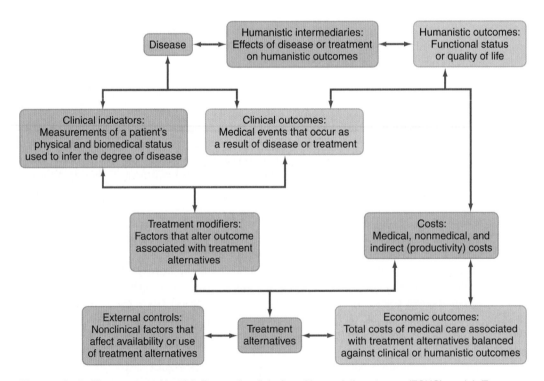

Figure 9-3. The conceptual model: Economic, clinical, and humanistic outcome (ECHO) model. (From Kozma, C. M., Reeder, C. E., & Schulz, R. M. [1993]. Economic, clinical, and humanistic outcomes: A planning model for pharmacoeconomic research. *Clinical Therapeutics, 15*[6], 1125.)

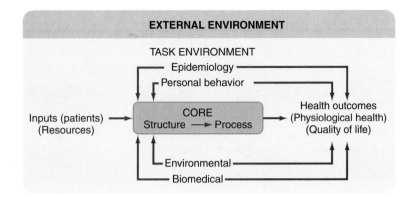

Figure 9-4. A systems perspective of health services research. (From Anderson, R. M., Davidson, P. L., & Ganz, P. A. [1994]. Symbiotic relationships of quality of life, health services research and other health research. *Quality of Life Research, 3*[5], 367.)

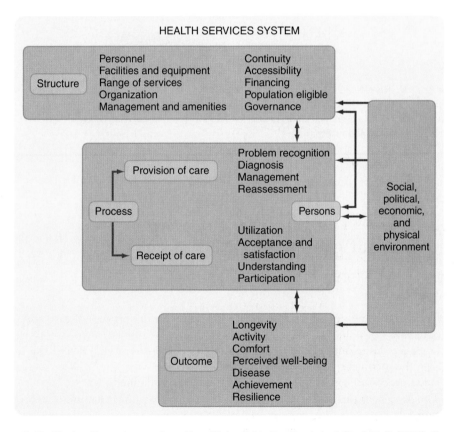

Figure 9-5. The health services system. (From Vivier, P. M., Bernier, J. A., & Starfield, B. [1994]. Current approaches to measuring health outcomes in pediatric research. *Current Opinions in Pediatrics, 6*[5], 531.)

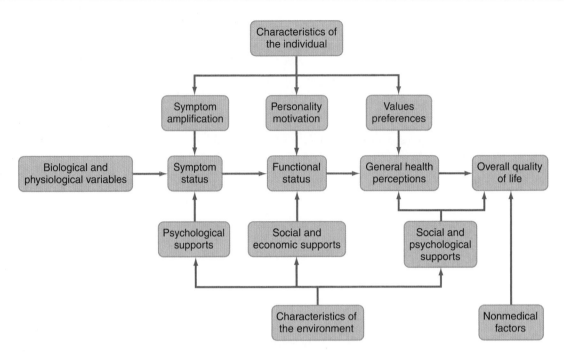

Figure 9-6. Relationships among measures of patient outcome in a health-related quality-of-life conceptual model. (From Wilson, I. B., & Cleary, P. D. [1995]. Linking clinical variables with health-related quality of life: A conceptual model of patient outcomes. *Journal of the American Medical Association, 273*[1], 60. Copyright 1995, the American Medical Association.)

CRITIQUE GUIDELINES Structure of Care

When critiquing an outcomes research study, consider structure of care. Then ask yourself the following questions:

1. Do the outcome variables show a clear link between the process of care and the identified outcome?
2. Does the desirability of the selected outcome reflect the preference of the patient, rather than the provider?
3. Is the process of care leading to the outcome clearly defined?
4. The process of care is driven by the structure of care. Is the structure of care defined in the study?
5. The practice style of providers is a major factor in the process of care. Is the practice style defined?

The Agency for Health Services Research

Nurses participated in the initial federal involvement in the quality of health care. In 1959, two National Institutes of Health Study Sections, the Hospital and Medical Facilities Study Section and the Nursing Study Section, met to discuss concerns about the adequacy and appropriateness of medical care, patient care, and hospital and medical facilities. As a result of their dialogue, a Health Services Research Study Section was initiated. This study section eventually became the Agency for Health Services Research (AHSR). With small amounts of funding from Congress, the AHSR continued to study the effectiveness of health services, primarily supporting the research of economists, epidemiologists, and health policy analysts (White, 1993). Two projects that were to have the greatest impact were small area analyses and the Medical Outcomes Study (MOS).

Small Area Analyses

In the 1970s, an epidemiologist named Wennberg began a series of studies examining small area variations in medical practice across towns and counties. He found a wide variation in the tonsillectomy rate from one town to another in the New England area that could not be explained by differences such as health status, insurance, and demographics. These findings were replicated for a variety of medical procedures. Investigators began a search for the underlying causes of such variation and their implications for health status (O'Connor, Plume, & Wennberg, 1993; Wennberg, Barry, Fowler, & Mulley, 1993). Studies also revealed that many procedures, such as coronary artery bypass, were being performed on patients who did not have appropriate clinical indications for such surgery (Power, Tunis, & Wagner, 1994).

The Medical Outcomes Study

The Medical Outcomes Study (MOS) was the first large-scale study to examine factors influencing patient outcomes. The study was designed to identify elements of physician care associated with favorable patient outcomes. The conceptual framework for the MOS is shown in Figure 9-7. Variations in use of resources and in physician technical and inter-personal styles were examined (Greenfield et al., 1992; Kelly, Huber, Johnson, McCloskey, & Maas, 1994; Riesenberg & Glass, 1989; Stewart et al., 1989). Kelly and colleagues noted, however, that the MOS failed to control for the effects of nursing interventions, staffing patterns, and nursing practice delivery models on medical outcomes. Coordination of care, counseling, and referrals—activities more commonly performed by nurses than by physicians—were considered in the MOS to be components of medical practice.

The Agency for Health Care Policy and Research

The Agency for Health Care Policy and Research (AHCPR), created in 1989 by Congress, replaced the AHSR. The congressional mandate for the AHCPR was

> ...to carry out research, demonstrations, guideline development, training, and dissemination activities with respect to health care services and systems of information regarding the following

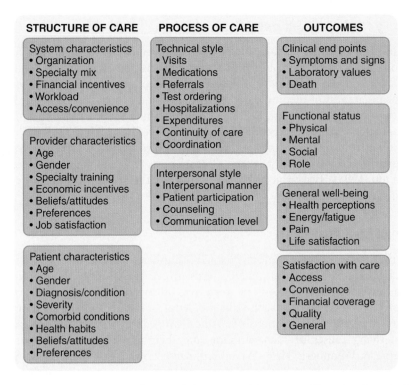

Figure 9-7. The Medical Outcomes Study (MOS) conceptual framework. (From American Medical Association. [1989]. *Journal of the American Medical Association, 262,* 925–930. Copyrighted 1989, American Medical Association.)

areas: the effectiveness, efficiency, quality, and outcomes of health services; clinical practice, including primary care; health care technologies, facilities, and equipment; health care costs, productivity, and market forces; health promotion and disease prevention; health statistics and epidemiology; and medical liability. (Gray, 1992, p. 40)

A National Advisory Council for Health Care Policy, Research, and Evaluation also was established by Congress. The Council was required to include (1) health care researchers; (2) health care professionals (specifically including nurses); (3) professionals from the fields of business, law, ethics, economics, and public policy; and (4) persons representing the interests of consumers. The budget for the AHCPR increased to $1.9 million in 1988, $5.9 million in 1989, and $37.5 million in 1990.

The AHCPR initiated several major research efforts to examine medical outcomes. Two of the most significant, described next, are the Medical Treatment Effectiveness Program (MEDTEP) and a component of MEDTEP referred to as Patient Outcomes Research Teams (PORTs) (Greene, Bondy, & Maklan, 1994).

The Medical Treatment Effectiveness Program

MEDTEP was established by Congress in 1989 to be implemented by the AHCPR. The purpose of the program was to improve the effectiveness and appropriateness of medical practice. The term medical was used by Congress when the program was mandated. However, it was broadly interpreted to include health care in general and nursing care in particular—an important consideration from the perspective of the nursing profession. The program was charged to develop and disseminate scientific information about the effects of health care services and procedures on patients' survival, health status, functional capacity, and quality of life, a remarkable shift from the narrow focus of traditional medical research. MEDTEP funded three research areas: (1) patient outcomes research, (2) database development, and (3) research on effective methods of disseminating the information gathered. In 1993, the program implemented studies to examine the effects of pharmaceuticals on patient outcomes and provided $19 million to establish Research Centers on Minority Populations (Clinton, 1993).

Patient Outcomes Research Team Projects

In 1994, Congress mandated patient outcomes research team projects (PORTs), that is, large-scale, multifaceted, and multidisciplinary projects to "identify and analyze the outcomes and costs of current alternative practice patterns in order to determine the best treatment strategy and to develop and test methods for reducing inappropriate variations" (U.S. Congress, 1994, p. 67). The PORTs were required to "conduct literature reviews and syntheses; analyze practice variations and associated patient outcomes, using available data augmented by primary data collection where desired; disseminate research findings; and evaluate the effects of dissemination" (U.S. Congress, 1994, p. 67). Questions typically addressed by PORTs include the following:

> Do patients benefit from the care provided?
> What treatments work best?
> Has the patient's functional status improved?
> From whose viewpoint has the patient's outcome been evaluated?
> Are health care resources well spent? (Tanenbaum, 1994; Wood, 1990)

A major task of PORTs was to disseminate their findings and change the practice of health care providers to improve patient outcomes. A framework for dissemination was developed that identified the audiences for disseminated products, the media involved, and the strategies that foster assimilation and adoption of information (Goldberg, Cummings, Steinberg, Ricci, Shannon, Soumerai, et al., 1994).

A Cost of Care Workgroup, consisting of a representative from each PORT, was convened in 1994 with the following four goals: (1) to determine the best methods for estimating the cost of certain conditions using claims data, (2) to evaluate methods for estimating the cost of care using billing information and patient interview data, (3) to examine methods for determining the indirect cost of care, and (4) to evaluate methods for comparing the cost of care internationally (Lave et al., 1994).

In 1992, the National Center for Nursing Research (NCNR) sponsored a Conference on Patient Outcomes Research: Examining the Effectiveness of Nursing Practice. In the keynote speech, Hinshaw, then director of the NCNR, made the following suggestions:

> From a nursing perspective, particular clinical conditions need to be identified that are more specific to nursing's focus on prevention, health promotion, symptom management, and the amelioration of the effects of acute and chronic illnesses. We are all familiar with clinical conditions that are central to our practice, such as skin integrity, pain, urinary incontinence, nausea and vomiting, nutritional deficits, confusion, restricted mobility, depression, fatigue, and illness-related stress. It will be particularly important in our research programs that we begin to both define and refine the patient outcomes specific to interventions focused on such clinical conditions. (Hinshaw, 1992, p. 9)

Examining the impact of nursing on overall hospital outcomes requires inclusion of nursing data in the large databases used to analyze outcomes. The cost of adding new variables to these databases is high. Nursing professionals are competing with the voices of others who wish to add their own relevant variables. However, with the force of the American Nurses Association (ANA), the voice of the profession is being heard.

The NCNR, now the National Institute for Nursing Research (NINR), developed a partnership with the AHCPR to fund outcomes studies of importance to nursing. Calls for proposals jointly supported by the AHCPR and the NINR are announced each year. (These calls for proposals can be found on the NINR home page on the World Wide Web: http://ninr.nih.gov/ninr/.)

With a growing budget and strong political support, proponents of the AHCPR were becoming a powerful force demanding change in health care, because of the demand for health care reform that existed throughout the government and among the public. The role of the AHCPR, however, was the focus of considerable controversy. For example, a subset of spinal orthopedic surgeons strongly opposed the guidelines for the treatment of back pain. From 1994-1998, this group of physicians assailed members of Congress with visits, letters, and telephone calls. The AHCPR was under attack by powerful forces and was in danger of being eliminated or of having its budget greatly reduced. In fact, for the 1997 fiscal year budget, Congress cut AHCPR funding by $35 million, thereby ending the funding of MEDTEP and new PORTs. The following year, however, Congressional members recognized that the opposition to the agency had been based on special interests and that the contested PORT findings were valid (Deyo, Psaty, Simon, Wagner, & Omenn, 1997; Fardon, Garfin, & Saal, 1997).

The intimidation of agencies and researchers by special-interest groups has serious implications for both scientists and society. Fardon, Garfin, and Saal, in a letter to *The New England Journal of Medicine* (1997), express concern about this problem.

> Harassment of researchers and funding agencies is a substantial disincentive to pursuing certain research on medical care or health risks. In effect, special-interest groups with money and power want to define acceptable questions and shape the range of acceptable answers. Eliminating public, peer-reviewed funding would slow the production of objective knowledge, force investigators to seek funding that may not be free of conflict of interest, and leave patients, physicians, and insurers without essential scientific evidence. University faculty members are governed by financial conflict-of-interest rules intended to prevent them from conducting research in which they or their relatives might have a financial stake. Thus, the elimination of public research support and the intimidation of independent investigators are inimical to larger social interests. Professional societies, universities, and the government need to weigh in quickly and heavily against strategies and specific cases of intimidation and vengeful budget cuts…. Inquiry may be warranted concerning the extent to which special-interest groups block or delay the publication

of unwanted findings. Journals may need to make a special effort to avoid relying on otherwise highly qualified reviewers and editorialists who have financial conflicts of interests, especially consultants to firms whose products receive negative evaluations. Journals may also need to set up defenses against potential threats of withholding advertising.... When funding agencies come under attack from groups with narrow interests, prompt and unambiguous responses from universities and professional organizations are needed. Self-interested attacks must be pointed out to politicians, who may otherwise be unable to distinguish self-interested parties from disinterested ones (Deyo et al., 1997, pp. 1315-1316).

The AHCPR operated without authorization from 1995 until December 6, 1999, receiving operating funds through congressional appropriations. The reauthorization act changed the name of the AHCPR to the Agency for Healthcare Research and Quality (AHRQ). The AHRQ is designated as a scientific research agency. The term *policy* was removed from the agency name, to avoid the perception that this body determined federal health care policies and regulations. The word *quality* was added to the agency's name, establishing the AHRQ as the lead federal agency on quality of care research, with a new responsibility to coordinate all federal quality improvement efforts and health services research. The new legislation eliminated the requirement that the AHRQ develop clinical practice guidelines. However, the AHRQ still supports these efforts through Evidence-Based Practice Centers and the dissemination of evidence-based guidelines through its National Guideline Clearinghouse. The new legislation defines the AHRQ's mission as follows:

> Meet the information needs of its customers—patients and clinicians, health system leaders, and policymakers—so that they can make more informed healthcare decisions.
> Build the evidence base for what works and doesn't work in healthcare and develop the information, tools, and strategies that decisionmakers can use to make good decisions and provide high-quality healthcare based on evidence.
> Develop scientific knowledge in these areas but will not mandate guidelines or standards for measuring quality. (One Hundred Sixth Congress of the United States, 1999, pp. 2–3)

The proposed budget for the AHRQ in fiscal year 2004 was $279 million.

The United States is not the only country making demands for improvements in quality of care and reductions in costs. Many countries around the world are experiencing similar concerns and addressing them in relation to their particular government structure. Thus, the movement into outcomes research and the application of the approaches described in this chapter constitute a worldwide phenomenon.

Reviews of Evidence from Existing Knowledge

The extensive review of published and unpublished work related to a particular health care problem was taken over by a number of organizations located in various countries. The most well known of these is the Cochrane Collaboration located in England. The Cochrane Collection is available on the Internet and through some search engines such as CINAHL. Such reviews may conclude that available knowledge is insufficient for the development of clinical guidelines, or they may propose clinical guidelines and/or a protocol developed from the material reviewed. Reviews are evaluated regularly, and a judgment is made about the need to update the review. The date of the initial review and all updates are provided.

Clinical Guideline Panels

Clinical guideline panels are developed to incorporate available evidence on health outcomes into sets of recommendations concerning appropriate management strategies for patients with the studied conditions. Any professional group may gather a group to develop guidelines on a particular topic. Some groups seek funding for the project, whereas others, such as professional organizations, conduct the work as an aspect of the organizational work. Medical schools and nursing schools have submitted guidelines as have medical and nursing organizations and volunteer agencies such as the American Cancer Society. Guidelines developed across the world are included. Some guidelines are evidence-based, whereas others are not. The evidence-based guidelines have considerably more validity. (Current guidelines can be obtained from the National Guideline Clearinghouse of AHRQ at the following Internet address: http:/www.guideline.gov/.)

Outcomes Research and Nursing Practice

Outcome studies provide rich opportunities to build a stronger scientific underpinning for nursing practice (Rettig, 1991): "Nursing needs to be able to explain the impact of care provided by its practitioners through measures of outcomes of patient care that reflect nursing practice" (Moritz, 1991, p. 113).

The American Nurses Association's "Nursing's Safety & Quality Initiative"

In the late 1980s and early 1990s, hospitals were confronted with managed care requirements to reduce costs. To accomplish this goal, hospitals across the country reduced their nursing staff and replaced them with unlicensed personnel having very little training for their assignments. Managed care dictated earlier patient discharges, resulting in patient loads that were sicker and required complex care. Nurses repeatedly complained that patient care was inadequate and that patients were experiencing complications and dying needlessly because of the inadequate staffing of RNs. However, nursing had little concrete evidence of these statements. Many nurses left nursing practice or changed to community areas of nursing practice. The RNs remaining in hospital practice tended to be new graduates who were placed in positions of responsibility without adequate experience. Assignment loads became increasingly difficult. Nurses tended to leave the hospital after 2 years, and more new graduates replaced them. A shortage of nurses, already in place, was exacerbated by this situation. Recruitment of new students became increasingly difficult as greater numbers of news items discussed the problems.

In 1994 the ANA, in collaboration with the American Academy of Nursing Expert Panel on Quality Health Care (Mitchell, Ferketich, & Jennings, 1998), launched an initiative to identify indicators of quality nursing practice, and to collect and analyze data using these indicators across the United States. The goal was to identify or develop nursing-sensitive quality measures. Donobedian's theory was used as the framework for the project. The committee conducted an extensive literature review, expert panel discussions, and focus group interviews to identify 21 nursing care indicators relevant to nursing care quality in acute care. On the basis of Donobedian's theory or established evidence of a strong link to nursing care quality, the committee then reduced the list of indicators to 10. The 10 indicators currently being collected and 4 others undergoing pilot testing are listed in Table 9-2.

Table 9-2	American Nurses Association Acute Care Nursing-Sensitive Quality Indicators

Patient falls

Patient falls with injury

Pressure ulcers—% of patients with documented ulcer (stage I–IV on day of prevalence study. Also have Hospital-acquired ulcer—% of patients with documented ulcer (stage I–IV) on day of prevalence study

Nurse satisfaction

Nursing Hours Per Patient Day (HPPD)—RN, LPN/LVN, UAP—number of productive hours worked by nursing staff with direct patient care responsibilities

Staff mix—the total number of productive hours worked by each skill mix category (RN, LPN, UAP)/total staff hours

Type of unit (critical care, step down, medical, surgical and combined)

Number of staffed beds designated by the hospital

Agency staff—total number of productive hours worked by contract staff

Urban vs. rural category

New Indicators Undergoing Pilot Testing

Pediatric pain

Peripheral intravenous infiltration

Restraint use

Patient aggression

LPN, licensed practical nurse; LVN, licensed vocational nurse; RN, registered nurse; UAP, unlicensed assistive personnel.

From American Nurses Association–National Center for Nursing Quality. Retrieved on XXX 00, 200X, from http://nursingworld.org/quality/prtdatabase.htm

If nursing care could be compared among hospitals, nursing would have the evidence to justify claims of patient harms from the changes in RN staffing. ANA entered a new area of research and asked questions that had not previously been studied. No one knew what indicators were sensitive to the nursing care provided to patients or what relationships existed between nursing inputs and patient outcomes. They had to persuade hospitals to participate in the study at a time when hospitals had a severe case of "data paranoia" (fear of providing data to anyone outside the hospital because of how third parties might interpret the data). Every hospital had a different way of measuring the indicators selected by ANA. Persuading them to change to a standardized measure of the indicators for consistency across hospitals was a major endeavor (Jennings, Loan, DePaul, Brosch, & Hildreth, 2001; Rowell, 2001). Nurse researchers and cooperating hospitals instituted the mechanisms required for data collection and began multiple pilot studies. These pilot studies identified multiple obstacles to the project. They learned that not only must the indicators be measured consistently, but that data collection must be standardized. As studies continued, indicators were amplified and continue to be tested. As this testing continues, further alterations in the indicators occur (Anonymous, 1997; Campbell-Heider, Krainovich-Miller, King, Sedhom, & Malinski, 1998; Jennings et al., 2001).

The ANA proposes that all hospitals collect and report on the 10 nursing-sensitive quality indicators. The ANA is working to ensure that these indicators are included in data collected by accrediting organizations and by the federal government, and that the data be shared with key groups. The ANA also is encouraging state nurses' associations to lobby state legislatures to include the nursing-sensitive quality indicators into regulations or state law.

In 1998, the ANA provided funding to develop a national database to house data collected using nursing-sensitive quality indicators. This database, named The National Database of Nursing Quality Indicators (NDNQI), is a program of the National Center for

Nursing Quality, funded by the ANA. The database is housed at the University of Kansas Medical Center Research Institute (KUMCRI) and of the University of Kansas School of Nursing. In 2001, data from nursing-sensitive quality indicators were being collected from more than 120 hospitals in 24 states across the United States. By 2005, that number had increased to 767 hospitals in the 50 states and the District of Columbia. The National Center for Nursing Quality analyzes the data quarterly and provides feedback reports to all participating hospitals. Confidential benchmarking reports are provided to allow hospitals to compare their results with those of other hospitals (Rowell, 2001).

In 1997, the ANA appointed members of an Advisory Committee on Community-Based Non-Acute Care Indicators to identify the first core set of indictors for non-acute care settings. Some of the members had helped develop the Acute Care Indicators, giving the committee some continuity of the work. The committee began by selecting a theoretical base for its work: Evans and Stoddart's (1990) determinants of health model and also Donabedian's model of quality. As its work progressed, the committee chose to synthesize a model to guide the identification and testing of indicators (Figure 9-8). The committee followed the acute care group's process in selecting the indicators. A hired contractor conducted the literature review, while the committee conducted focus groups and interviews with key stakeholders such as consumers of care, registered nurses, policy makers, regulators, payers, facility administrators, and purchasers. Owing to budget constraints, the ANA limited development to 10 indicators (see Table 9-3). The committee requests that all nurses and nursing organizations join with the ANA to continue to expand this work (Head, Maas, & Johnson, 2003; Sawyer et al., 2002). (For current information on the ANA's Safety & Quality Initiative, visit the following website: http://nursingworld.org/quality.)

A number of studies on the effects of nursing staff mix on patient outcomes have been published recently (Blegen, Goode, & Reed, 1998; Buerhaus & Needleman, 2000; Cho, Ketefian, Barkauskas, & Smith, 2003; Hall, Doran, Baker, Pink, Sidani, O'Brien, et al., 2001; Houser, 2000; Needleman, Buerhaus, Mattke, Steward, & Zelevinsky, 2002a, 2002b). These studies are finding a significant effect of staffing mix on patient outcomes.

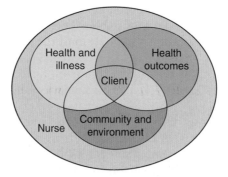

Figure 9-8. Model used to guide identification and testing of community-based non-acute care indicators by the American Nurses Association (ANA) Advisory Committee (1997). (In Sawyer, L.M., Berkowitz, B., Larrabee, J.H., Marino, B.L., Martin, K.S., et al: Expanding American Nurses Association Nursing Quality Indicators to community-based practices. *Outcomes Management*, 6(2), p. 53.)

Table 9-3	Nursing-Sensitive Quality Indicators for Community-Based Non-Acute Care Indicators

- Pain management (symptom severity)—The treatment and prevention of pain and discomfort. Effectiveness is related to level of functioning and activities of daily living and includes measures of frequency, intensity and duration of pain symptoms.
- Consistency of communication (strength of therapeutic alliance)—Consistent RN/advanced practice registered nurses (APRN) provider identified in the data/record.
- Staff mix (utilization of services)—Total number of direct care hours or total number of encounters provided by RN or APRN staff who have client care responsibilities (per episode/encounter/case as appropriate to the setting) and (RNs, LPNs, UAPs caring for clients)—The percent of registered nursing care hours as a total of all nursing care hours; secondary measure—percent of APRNs.
- Client satisfaction—The degree to which the care received met client expectations regarding nursing care, pain management, patient education and overall care.
- Prevention of tobacco use (risk reduction)—The number of clients attending educational sessions per year provided and/or coordinated by RNs about the risks of tobacco use (includes: coordination of educational sessions/programs either with individuals or groups).
- Cardiovascular prevention (risk reduction)—The number of clients attending educational sessions per year provided and/or coordinated by RNs about risks of cardiovascular disease.
- Care giver activity (protective factors)—The existence or frequency of primary care giver involvement.
- Identification of primary care giver (protective factors)
- ADL/IADL (level of function)—The degree to which the normal physical or entire action of a system occurs (physical or psychological).
- Psychosocial interaction (level of function)—The degree to which the normal action of a system occurs.

ADL/IADL, activities of daily living/instrumental activities of daily living; LPN, licensed practical nurse; LVN, licensed vocational nurse; RN, registered nurse; UAP, unlicensed assistive personnel.

From American Nurses Association. Retrieved on April 1, 2006, from http://nursingworld.org/readroom. Go to nursing-sensitive indicators for community-based nonacute care settings.

The most significant of these studies, conducted by Needleman et al. (2002a, 2002b), used discharge and staffing data from 799 hospitals in 11 states to estimate nurse staffing levels for RNs, LPN/LVNs, and aides, as well as the frequency of a wide range of complications developed by patients during their hospital stay. The data cover 6 million patients discharged from hospitals in 1997. These investigators found that low levels of RN staffing among a hospital's nurses were associated with higher rates of serious complications such as pneumonia, upper gastrointestinal bleeding, shock, and cardiac arrest, including deaths among patients with these three complications, as well as sepsis or deep vein thrombosis. These complications occurred 3% to 9% more often than in hospitals with lower levels of RN staffing.

Sochalski (2001), after a review of studies on staff mix, cautions that

...missing from these studies is a more thorough explanation of *how* nurse staffing affects patient outcomes. That is, does increasing staffing levels and/or skill mix, under any circumstances, yield better outcomes, or are the effects of staffing titrated by other features in the practice environment that influence nursing's ability to deliver the quality of care that results in better patient outcomes? Trying to establish minimum staffing ratios in the absence of clear information on just how staffing levels affect outcomes may result in ratios that overestimate or underestimate what is really needed to improve patient care. Furthermore, if the effect of staffing on patient outcomes can only be fully achieved in the presence of other features in the practice environment, then it will be the presence or absence of these features and not solely staffing levels that will produce the desired patient results. Without a clear understanding of the circumstances under which staffing affects outcomes, we lack the capacity to improve patient outcomes if efforts are directed only at changing staffing levels. (p. 11)

Standing, Anthony, and Hertz (2001) conducted a triangulated study of outcomes after delegation to unlicensed assistive personnel (UAP), funded by the National Council of State Boards of Nursing. This report describes the qualitative analysis of interviews of RNs who described a delegation with a positive outcome and a delegation with a negative outcome. Negative outcomes after delegation ranged from family or client upsets, to fractures or other injuries, to death. In some cases, the UAP performed activities that had not been delegated to them. Negative outcomes were most frequently due to the UAP's not receiving or following directions, or not adhering to established policy. Positive outcomes included enhanced client well-being as indicated by increased socialization and other measures, prevention of poor client outcomes, and enhanced unit functioning.

Nursing-Sensitive Patient Outcomes

Donobedian states that a clear link must be established between an outcome and the process that resulted in the outcome. Thus, selecting a nursing-sensitive outcome requires a clear explanation of the process that led to that outcome. The process that needs to be defined is likely to be a complex combination of nursing acts, acts of other professionals, organizational acts, and patient characteristics and behaviors. Nursing acts are not clearly defined and are inconsistent across nurses and institutions. Few studies have attempted to describe a particular nursing process, much less link it to outcomes.

Stetler, Morsi, and Burns (2000) have worked to develop a comprehensive, in-depth profile of nursing-sensitive outcomes of hospital nursing care at the unit level and to use the information in routine quality monitoring. They used a prevention framework based on the work of Stetler and DeZell (1989). The framework describes the nurse's role in preventing complications in a nosocomial hospital environment; treatment consequences; a patient's health status, disease state, or evolving condition; and the patient's inability to care for themselves safely. From a safety perspective, the framework classifies outcomes as positive or negative. Outcomes are further classified in terms of preventability, impact, severity, and a holistic view of patient safety. Positive behaviors protect or rescue patients from potential or actual negative events. These actions are categorized as (1) detection/reporting, (2) detection/prevention, and (3) facilitation of resolution/prevention.

Other work has included development of a model of nursing effectiveness to use in studies of patient outcomes.

Irvine, Sidani, and Hall (1998) have developed The Nursing Role Effectiveness Model (Figure 9-9) to guide the examination and explanation of the links between nursing processes and patient outcomes. The model is based on Donabedian's theory of quality care. Roles are defined as

...positions in organizations that have attached to them a set of expected behaviors. Professional roles are complex because they consist of components that are based on normative expectations concerning standards of practice that have been established by external regulatory bodies and secondly, on normative expectations that have evolved over time that are unique to the organization. (p. 59)

The Nursing Role Effectiveness Model has three major components: structure, the nurses' role, and patient/health outcomes. Structure has three subcomponents: nurse, organizational, and patient. Nurse variables that influence quality of nursing care include factors such as experience level, knowledge, and skill level. Organizational components that can affect quality of nursing care include staff mix, workload, and assignment patterns. Patient characteristics that can affect quality of care include health status, severity, and morbidity. Nurses' role has three subcomponents: nurses' independent role, nurses' dependent role, and nurses' interdependent role. Independent role functions include assessment, diagnosis, nurse initiated interventions, and follow-up care. The patient/health outcomes of the independent role are clinical/symptom control, freedom from complications, functional status/self-care, knowledge of disease and its treatment, satisfaction and costs. The dependent role functions include execution of medical orders and physician-initiated treatments. It is the dependent role functions that can lead to patient/health outcomes of adverse events. Interdependent role functions include communication, case management, coordination of care, and continuity/monitoring and reporting. The interdependent role results in team functioning and affects the patient/health outcomes of the independent role.

The Propositions of The Nursing Role Effectiveness Model were stated as follows (Irvine, Sidani, & Hall, 1998):

Nursing's capacity to engage effectively in the independent, dependent, and interdependent role functions is influenced by individual nurse variables, patient variables, and organizational structure variables. (p. 61)

Nurses' interdependent role function depends upon the nurse's ability to communicate and articulate her/his opinion to other members of the health care team. (p. 61)

Nurse, patient, and system structural variables have a direct effect on clinical, functional, satisfaction, and cost outcomes. (p. 61)

Nurses' independent role function can have a direct effect on clinical, functional, satisfaction, and cost outcomes. (p. 61)

Medication errors and other adverse events associated with nurses' dependent role function can ultimately affect all categories of patient outcome. (p. 62)

Nursing's interdependent role function can affect the quality of interprofessional communication and coordination. The nature of inter-professional communication and coordination can influence other important patient outcomes and costs such as risk-adjusted length of stay, risk-adjusted mortality rates, excess home care costs following discharge, unplanned visits to the physician or emergency department, and unplanned re-hospitalization. (p. 62)

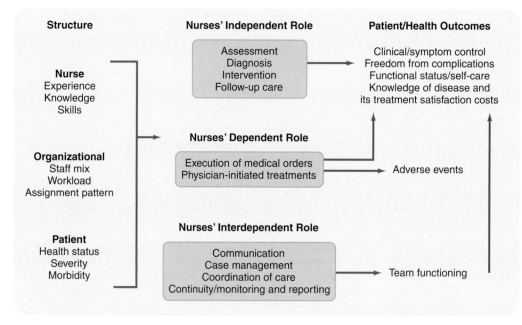

Figure 9-9. The Nursing Role Effectiveness Model. (From Irvine, D., Sidani, S., & Hall, L. M. [1998]. Linking outcomes to nurses' roles in health care. *Nursing Economics, 16*[2], 59.)

Sidani and Irvine (1999) subsequently modified The Nursing Role Effectiveness Model to evaluate the nurse practitioner role in acute care settings, providing a guide for nurse practitioners interested in studying their roles. These investigators selected variables relevant to acute care nurse practitioner (ACNP) practice to operationalize the components of the model, and proposed relationships among the elements of the three components. Using this framework, the research group examined the organizational factors influencing nurse practitioners' role implementation in acute care settings (Irvine et al., 2000). They also conducted a study examining the practice patterns of ACNPs (Sidani et al., 2000). Practice patterns of ACNPs also have been examined by Rosenfeld, McEvoy, and Glassman (2003). Organizational changes resulting from implementing the APN's role in acute care were studied by Cummings, Fraser, and Tarlier (2003).

In 2002, Doran, Sidani, Keatings, and Doidge conducted an empirical test of The Nursing Role Effectiveness Model. These investigators found that The Nursing Role Effectiveness Model was effective in guiding the evaluation of outcomes of nursing care. They noted that "for the most part the hypothesized relationships among the variables were supported. However, further work is needed to develop an understanding of how nurses engage in their coordinating role functions and how we can measure these role activities" (p. 30).

Advanced-Practice Nursing Outcomes Research

Advanced-practice nurses (APNs) and their organizations have been slow to move into research measuring outcomes of their practice. Early studies examined broad variables that allow comparisons with other practitioners. Nurse-sensitive outcomes that document effectiveness of specific interventions have yet to be identified, however (Kleinpell-Nowell & Weiner, 1999). Computerized electronic patient records make the study of clinical practice considerably easier, but the use of these electronic records varies widely among APNs. APNs are very familiar with Current Procedural Terminology (CPT) codes and International Classification of Diseases-9 (ICD-9) codes. However, most are unfamiliar with standardized nursing languages, such as Nursing Outcomes Classification (NOC) and Nursing Interventions Classification (NIC), which tend to be used in electronic databases. Still, a few studies of APN practice are beginning to appear in the literature.

RESEARCH EXAMPLE Advanced-Practice Nursing Outcomes Research

Barton, Gilbert, Erickson, Baramee, Sowers, and Robertson (2003) used the Omaha System, a nursing-sensitive database, to describe and document faculty practice at the University of Colorado Health Science Center. This system includes all of the nursing elements (diagnosis, intervention, outcome) and has been tested through 11 years of federally funded research. Barton et al. used Teleform software, developed by Cardiff (Vista, California) to collect data. This allowed data to be scanned, faxed, or entered using the Internet. Although the study focused on use of the system and reported only preliminary results, the project demonstrated an effective way to examine the clinical practice of APNs.

Ingersoll, McIntosh, and Williams (2000) conducted a study asking APNs what measures they recommended for use in measuring their effect on patient outcomes. Indicators listed were rated by a second group of APNs on validity, sensitivity, feasibility, utility, and cost. The highest-ranked indicators were satisfaction with care delivery, symptom resolution/reduction, perception of being well cared for, compliance/adherence with treatment plan, knowledge of patients and families, trust of care provider, collaboration among care providers, frequency and type of procedures ordered, and quality of life.

Donohue (2003) conducted a qualitative study examining nurse practitioner–client interaction in a women's health clinic to determine what the women's expectations were of the nurse practitioner visit and what was actually received. Clients indicated that they expected and received services, health information, trust, self-disclosure, support, affirmation, time, acceptance, and respect.

Practice-Based Research Networks

A practice-based research network (PBRN) is a group of practices focused on patient care that are affiliated in order to analyze their clinical practices in communities. Such networks have consisted of primary care physicians for a number of years, but no networks of advanced-practice registered nurses (APRNs) (i.e., APNs) have yet been established. Thus, questions about APRNs have not been studied. Little is known about APRNs or their practice patterns. Developing a PBRN of primary care APRNs will let researchers address questions about whether care by APRNs is different from care provided by other disciplines. In 2000, the AHRQ awarded a grant to Yale University School of Nursing in collaboration with five other schools of nursing to develop a PBRN of APRNs providing primary care. The name of the network is APRNet (Advanced Practice Registered Nurses' Research Network). Its purpose is to "conduct and facilitate practice-based research relevant to APRN primary care practice; develop culturally competent, evidence-based practice models for APRNs; and translate research findings into primary care practice" (McCloskey, Grey, Deshefy-Longhi, & Grey, 2003, p. 39). Initial data gathering has been primarily descriptive and examines the characteristics of practitioners participating in the network. A series of studies is planned to determine how APRN practices operate, how APRN services are determined and billed, and what clinical outcomes are obtained

Methodologies for Outcomes Studies

A research tradition for the outcomes model is still emerging. A research tradition defines an acceptable research methodology. The lack of an established set of methods should encourage greater creativity in seeking new strategies for studying the phenomena of concern. Small single studies using untried methods may be useful. Research teams need to develop research programs with a planned sequence of studies focused on a particular outcome concern. The PORTs defined a research process for conducting programs of funded outcomes studies. These programs are complex and may consist of multiple studies using a variety of research strategies whose findings must be merged before conclusions are reached.

Although starting a research program as extensive as a PORT would be unrealistic without the level of funding the PORTs received, ideas for developing the methodology of outcomes research programs on a smaller scale may emerge from an examination of these plans. For example, measurement methods used in PORTs are available for smaller studies. The following steps were constructed combining PORT plans proposed by Freund, Dittus, Fitzgerald, and Heck, (1990), Sledge (1993), and Turk and Rudy (1994).

1. Perform a critical review of the published literature or a meta-analysis.
2. Conduct large database analyses on the basis of the results of the critical literature review.
3. Identify outcomes measures for use in the study, and evaluate their sensitivity to change.
4. Identify variables that might affect the outcomes.
5. Achieve consensus on definitions for all variables to be used in the research program.
6. Develop assessment instruments or techniques.
7. Conduct patient surveys or focus groups to gain information on outcomes, such as level of functional status and perceived pain, and on how these outcomes may improve or regress over time.
8. Determine patterns of care (who provides care at what points of time for what purposes?).
9. Perform a cohort analysis: Monitor a cohort of patients, some of whom will receive one treatment and others of whom will not receive the treatment, to assess changes in outcomes over time. Use a telephone survey at selected intervals to gather information. Evaluate the proportion of patients who improve, as well as the group mean differences.
10. Determine, through follow-up studies, differences in patient selection or interventions that are associated with different outcomes. Evaluate the durability of change by conducting sufficiently long follow-up. Determine the percentage of patients dropping out of groups receiving different treatments and, when possible, determine their reasons for dropping out.

11. Determine the clinical significance of improvement, as well as the statistical significance.
12. Determine the cost-benefit ratio and cost-effectiveness of the treatments under evaluation.
13. Use decision analyses to synthesize information about patients' outcomes and preferences for various types of outcomes.
14. Disseminate information to both patients and health care providers about which persons would and which would not benefit from the procedure.
15. Conduct a clinical trial to evaluate the effects of the intervention.
16. Incorporate findings into treatment guidelines.
17. Modify provider and patient behavior so that proven, effective treatment is given to persons who are most likely to benefit.

The PORTs recognized the need to allow diversity in research strategies, measures, and analyses to facilitate methodological advances (Fowler, Cleary, Magaziner, Patrick, & Benjamin, 1994). Creative flexibility often is necessary to develop ways to answer new questions. Finding ways to determine the impact of a condition on a person's life is difficult. Interpreting results also can be problematic, because clinical significance is considered as important as statistical significance. This issue requires a judgment by the research team about what constitutes clinical significance in that particular area of study.

This section describes some of the sampling issues, research strategies, measurements, and statistical approaches being used by researchers in outcomes studies. The descriptions provided are not sufficient to guide the researcher in using the approaches described but rather provide a broad overview of a variety of methods being used. For additional information, refer to the citations for each topic. Outcomes studies cross a variety of disciplines; thus, the emerging methodology is being enriched by a cross-pollination of ideas, some of which are new to nursing research.

Samples and Sampling

The preferred sampling methods differ in outcomes studies; random sampling is not considered desirable and is seldom used. Heterogeneous, rather than homogeneous, samples are obtained. Traditional researchers use sampling criteria that restrict the subjects to decrease possible biases and variance and to increase the possibility of identifying a statistically significant difference. Outcomes researchers, however, seek large heterogeneous samples that reflect, as much as possible, all patients who would receive care in the real world. Outcomes samples must include, for example, patients with various comorbid conditions and patients with various levels of health. In addition, persons who do not receive treatment for their condition should be identified. Evaluating the representativeness of such samples is problematic. Similarly, locating untreated patients and including them in follow-up studies constitute other challenges. Outcomes researchers must devise ways to overcome these challenges.

Traditional researchers and statisticians argue that when patients are not selected randomly, biases and confounding variables are more likely to occur. Further, they argue, this issue is a particular problem when the sample size is small. In nonexperimental studies, variation is likely to be greater, resulting in a higher risk of a Type II error. Traditional analysts consider nonrandomized studies to be based on observational data and therefore lacking in credibility (Orchard, 1994). Using this argument, traditionalists claim that the findings of most outcomes studies are not valid and should not be used as a basis to establish guidelines for clinical practice or to build a body of knowledge.

Slade, Kuipers, and Priebe (2002) suggest that

> …research questions are designed so that they can be answered by Randomized Controlled Trials (RCTs). Specifically, the use of RCTs involves the identification of an intervention which is given to patients in the experimental group, but not the control group. This encourages the asking of particular types of research questions, typically of the form "Does intervention X work for disorder Y?" However, one might argue that the RCT methodology limits the questions that can be asked, and hence can restrict the potential findings from research. Furthermore, if different questions were being asked, the RCTs would not always be the best methodology to employ…. The question "Which patients with condition Y does intervention X work for?" may prove to have more clinical relevance, and answering this question may involve asking the question "How does intervention X work?", a question which cannot be answered just by using RCTs. (pp. 12–13)

Large Databases as Sample Sources

One source of samples used for outcomes studies is large databases. Two broad categories of databases emerge from patient care encounters: clinical databases and administrative databases, as illustrated in Figure 9-10. Providers such as hospitals, HMOs, and health care professionals create clinical databases. The clinical data are generated either as a result of routine documentation of care or in relation to a research protocol. Some databases are data registries that have been developed to gather data related to a particular disease, such as cancer (Lee & Goldman, 1989). With the use of a clinical database, it is possible to link observations made by many practitioners over long periods. Links can be made between the process of care and outcomes (Mitchell et al, 1994; Moses, 1995).

Insurance companies, government agencies, and others not directly involved in providing patient care create administrative databases. These databases have standardized sets of data for enormous numbers of patients and providers (Deyo et al., 1994; McDonald & Hui,

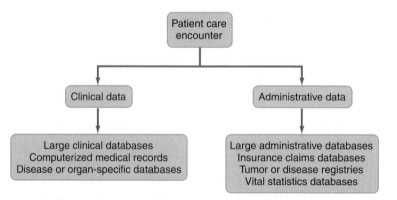

Figure 9-10. Types of databases emanating from patient care encounters. (From Lange, L. L., & Jacox, A. [1993]. Using large databases in nursing and health policy research. *Journal of Professional Nursing, 9*[4], 204.)

1991). An example is the Medicare database managed by the Health Care Financing Administration (HCFA). These large administrative databases can be used to determine the incidence or prevalence of disease, geographic variations in medical care utilization, characteristics of medical care, outcomes of care, and complementarity with clinical trials. Wray and colleagues (1995) caution, however, that analyses should be restricted to outcomes specific to a particular subgroup of patients, rather than one adverse outcome of all disease states.

Problems with the quality of data in the large databases are well recognized. The data have been gathered and entered by hundreds of people in a variety of settings. Few quality checks on the data are performed, and within the same data sets, records may have different lengths and structures. Missing data are common. Sampling and measurement errors are inherent in all large databases. Sampling error is a result of the way in which cases are selected for inclusion in the database; measurement error emerges from problems related to the operational definition of concepts. Thus, reliability and validity of the data are concerns (Davis, 1990; Lange & Jacox, 1993).

Large databases are used in outcomes studies to examine patient care outcomes. The outcomes that can be examined are limited to those recorded in the database and thus tend to be rather general. Existing databases can be used for analyses such as assessment of nursing care delivery models, variation in nursing practices, or evaluation of patients' risk of hospital-acquired infection, hospital-acquired pressure ulcer, or falls. Lange and Jacox (1993) identify the following important health policy questions related to nursing that should be examined through the use of large databases:

1. What is standard nursing practice in various settings?
2. What is the relationship between variations in nursing practice and patient outcomes?
3. What are the effects of different nursing staff mixes on patient outcomes and costs?
4. What are the total costs for episodes of treatment of specific conditions, and what part of those are attributable to nursing care?
5. Who is being reimbursed for nursing care delivery? (Lange & Jacox, p. 207)

To examine these questions, nurses must develop the statistical and methodological skills needed for working with large databases. Large databases contain patient and institutional information from huge numbers of patients. They exist in computer-readable form, require special statistical methods and computer techniques, and can be used by researchers who were not involved in the creation of the database.

Regrettably, nursing data are noticeably missing from these large databases and hence from funded health policy studies using them. A nursing minimum data set has been repeatedly recommended for inclusion in these databases (Werley, Devine, Zorn, Ryan, & Westra, 1991; Werley & Lang, 1988; Zielstorff, Hudgings, Grobe, & the National Commission on Nursing Implementation Project Task Force on Nursing Information Systems, 1993). This minimum data set would comprise a set of variables necessary and sufficient to describe an episode of illness or the care given by a provider. The ANA has mandated the formation of a Steering Committee on Databases to Support Clinical Nursing Practice. The following nursing classification schemes are being used in national databases:

- The North American Nursing Diagnosis Association (NANDA) classification
- The Omaha System: Applications for Community Health Nursing classification
- The Home Health Care Classification
- The Nursing Interventions Classification (NIC)

- The Nursing Outcomes Classification (NOC)
- Temple (1990) expressed the following concerns regarding the use of large data sets, rather than controlled trials, to assess effectiveness of treatments:

> We have traveled this route before with uncontrolled observations. It has always been hoped, and has often been asserted, that uncontrolled databases can be adjusted in some way that will allow valid comparisons of treatments. I know of no systematic attempt to document this. Outcomes researchers counter these criticisms by pointing out that experimental studies lack external validity and are not useful for application in clinical settings. They claim that the findings of clinical trials are not being used by clinicians because they are not representative of the patients seeking care. (p. 211)

Research Strategies for Outcomes Studies

Outcomes research programs usually consist of studies with a mix of strategies carried out sequentially. Although these strategies could be referred to as designs, for some the term design as used in Chapter 8 is inconsistent with the use of the term here. Research strategies for outcomes studies have emerged from a variety of disciplines, and innovative new strategies continue to appear in the literature. Strategies for outcomes studies tend to allow less control than is possible with traditional research designs and cannot be as easily categorized. The numerous research strategies for outcomes studies described next are only a sampling from the literature:

- Consensus knowledge building
- Practice pattern profiling
- Prospective cohort studies
- Retrospective cohort studies
- Population-based studies
- Clinical decision analysis
- Study of the effectiveness of interdisciplinary teams
- Geographical analyses
- Economic studies
- Ethical studies
- Defining and testing of interventions

Consensus Knowledge Building

Consensus knowledge building usually is performed by a multidisciplinary group representing a variety of constituencies. Initially, an extensive international search of the literature on the topic of concern, including unpublished studies, studies in progress, dissertations, and theses, is conducted. Several separate reviews may be performed, focusing on specific questions about the outcomes of care, diagnosis, prevention, or prognosis. Because meta-analytic methods often cannot be applied to the literature pertinent to PORTs, systematic approaches to critique and synthesis have been developed to identify relevant studies and gather and analyze data abstracted from the studies (Powe et al., 1994).

The results are dispersed to researchers and clinical experts in the field, who are asked to carefully examine the material and then participate in a consensus conference. The consensus conference yields clinical guidelines, which are published and widely distributed to clinicians. The clinical guidelines also are used as practice norms to study process and outcomes in that field. Gaps in the knowledge base are identified and research priorities determined by the consensus group.

Preliminary steps in this process may include conducting extensive integrative reviews and seeking consensus from a multidisciplinary research team and locally available clinicians. A review can be accomplished by establishing a website and conducting dialogue with experts via the Internet. The review may then be published in Sigma Theta Tau's online journal, *Knowledge Synthesis in Nursing*, and then dialogue related to the review may be conducted over the Internet. The Delphi method also has been used to seek consensus (Vermeulen, Ratko, Erstad, Brecher, & Matuszewski, 1995).

Practice Pattern Profiling

Practice pattern profiling is an epidemiological technique that focuses on patterns of care, rather than on individual occurrences of care. Large database analysis is used to identify a provider's pattern of practice and compare it with that of similar providers or with an accepted standard of practice. The technique has been used to determine overutilization and underutilization of services, to determine costs associated with a particular provider's care, to uncover problems related to efficiency and quality of care, and to assess provider performance. The provider being profiled may be an individual practitioner, a group of practitioners, or a health care organization such as a hospital or an HMO.

The provider's pattern is expressed as a rate aggregated over time for a defined population of patients under the provider's care. For example, the analysis may examine the number of sigmoidoscopy claims filed per 100 Medicare patients seen by the provider in a given year. Other analyses may examine (1) whether diabetic patients have had at least one annual serum glucose test and have received an ophthalmology examination or (2) the frequency of flu shots, Papanicolaou smears, and mammograms for various target populations (Lasker, Shapiro, & Tucker, 1992; McNeil, Pedersen, & Gatsonis, 1992).

Profiling can be used when the data contain hierarchical groupings. For example, patients may be grouped by nurse, nurses by unit, and units by larger organizations. The analysis uses regression equations to examine the relationship of an outcome to the characteristics of the various groupings. To be effective, the analysis must include data on the different sources of variability that might contribute to a given outcome.

The structure of the analysis reflects the structure of the data. Patient characteristics, for example, may include data on disease severity, comorbidity, emergent status, behavioral characteristics, socioeconomic status, and demographics. Nurse characteristics may consist of level of education, specialty status, years of practice, age, gender, and certifications. Unit characteristics may comprise number of beds, nursing management style used on the unit, ratio of patients to nurses, and the proportion of staff who are registered nurses (RNs) (McNeil et al., 1992).

Profiles are designed to generate some type of action, such as demonstrating that a provider's rates are too high or too low compared with the norm. By examining aggregate patterns of practice, profiling can be used to evaluate the care provided by different organizations or received by different populations of patients. Critical pathways or care maps can then be used to determine the proportion of patients whose data diverged from the pathway for a particular nurse, group of nurses, or group of nursing units. Profiling can be used for quality improvement, assessment of provider performance, and utilization review.

Methods of improving outcomes are not addressed by profiling, although this process can identify problem areas. It can be used to determine how and by whom performance should be changed to improve outcomes. Profiling also can identify outliers (persons with extreme scores or values), allowing more detailed examination of the reasons for the disparity of data.

The databases currently being used for profiling are not ideal, because they were developed for other purposes. Outcomes that can be examined are limited to broad outcomes, such as morbidity and mortality rates, complication rate, readmission rate, and frequency of utilization of various services (Lasker et al., 1992; McNeil et al., 1992). Table 9-4 lists examples of the large database measures that might be used in profiling.

Table 9-4	Examples of Large Database Measures Used in Profiling		
Quality of Care Issue	Measures	Example(s)	Criteria
Access	Proportion of population receiving care during the year, classified by age and sex	% of children under age 2 seen for at least one well-care visit	National
		% of children seen in emergency rooms for any reason, for trauma, and for medical problems	Trends
Preventive	Portion of population in specific age and sex groups receiving recommended tests or procedures	% of children by group having recommended immunizations in previous year	National recommendation
		% of women age 50 and over having mammography in past year	National recommendation
		% of deliveries with prenatal care beginning in first trimester	National recommendation
Diagnosis	% of population diagnosed (and under care) for specific chronic conditions by age and sex	% of adults diagnosed at one or more visits as having essential hypertension by age and sex	Epidemiologic data on prevalence of hypertension
Treatment	*Medications* Average number of new prescriptions per person per year	Average number of new prescriptions for antibiotics per person per year	Trends and comparison data
	Surgery Rate of surgical procedures per year: total, inpatient, and ambulatory (if applicable)	Cesarean section rate for all deliveries	Trends and comparison data
Outcomes	Hospital readmissions within 3 months of discharge	% of readmissions for some condition	Comparison data and trends
		% of readmission identifying a complication	

Reproduced in part from Steinwachs, D. M., Weiner, J. P., & Shapiro, S. (1989). Management information systems and quality. In N. Goldfield & D. B. Nash (Eds.), *Providing quality care: The challenge to clinicians* (pp. 160–180). Philadelphia: American College of Physicians.

Prospective Cohort Studies

A **prospective cohort study** is an epidemiological study in which a group of people are identified who are at risk for experiencing a particular event. Sample sizes for these studies often must be very large, particularly if only a small portion of the at-risk group will experience the event. The entire group is followed over time to determine the point at which the event occurs, variables associated with the event, and outcomes for persons who experienced the event compared with those who did not.

The Harvard Nurses Health Study, which is still being conducted, is an example of a prospective cohort study. This study recruited 100,000 nurses to determine the long-term consequences of the use of birth control pills. Nurses are sent a questionnaire every 2 years to gather data about their health and health behaviors. The study has been in progress for more than 20 years. Multiple studies using the large data set yielded by this Harvard study have been reported in the literature. Prospective cohort nursing studies could be conducted on a smaller scale on other populations, such as patients identified as being at high risk for the development of pressure ulcers.

Retrospective Cohort Studies

A **retrospective cohort study** is an epidemiological study in which a group of people are identified who have experienced a particular event. This is a common research technique used to study occupational exposure to chemicals. Events of interest to nursing that can be studied in this manner include a procedure, an episode of care, a nursing intervention, and a diagnosis. For example, nurses may use a retrospective cohort study to follow a cohort of women who have received a mastectomy for breast cancer or of patients in whom a urinary bladder catheter was placed during and after surgery. The cohort is evaluated after the event to determine the occurrence of changes in health status, usually identified as the development of a particular disease or death. Nurses also may be interested in the pattern of recovery after an event or, in the case of catheterization, the incidence of bladder infections in the months after surgery.

On the basis of the study findings, epidemiologists calculate the relative risk of the identified change in health for the group. For example, if death is the occurrence of interest, the expected number of deaths is determined. The observed number of deaths divided by the expected number of deaths and multiplied by 100 yields a **standardized mortality ratio (SMR),** which is regarded as a measure of the relative risk for the persons in the studied group to die of a particular condition. For example, in nursing studies, patients may be evaluated at specific intervals after discharge from a health care facility (Swaen & Meijers, 1988).

In retrospective studies, researchers commonly ask patients to recall information relevant to their previous health status. This information often is used to determine the amount of change occurring before and after an intervention. However, because recall can easily be distorted, and researchers thereby misled, retrospective studies should be used with caution. Herrmann (1995) identified three sources of distortion in recall, as follows: (1) the question posed to the subject may be conceived or expressed incorrectly, (2) the recall process may be in error, and (3) the research design used to measure recall can result in the recalled event's appearing to be different from what actually occurred. Herrmann (1995, p. AS90) also identified four bases of recall:

Direct recall: the subject "accesses the memory without having to think or search memory" resulting in correct information.

Indirect recall: the subject "accesses the memory after thinking or searching memory," resulting in correct information.

Limited recall: "access to the memory does not occur but information that suggests the contents of the memory is accessed," resulting in an educated guess.

No recall: "neither the memory nor information relevant to the memory may be accessed," resulting in a wild guess.

Population-Based Studies

Population-based studies also are important in outcomes research. Conditions must be studied in the context of the community, rather than of the medical system. To avoid selection bias with this method, all cases of a condition occurring in the defined population are included, rather than only patients treated at a particular health care facility. Efforts may be made to include people with the condition who have not received treatment.

Community-based norms of tests and survey instruments obtained in this manner provide a clearer picture of the range of values than does evaluation of the limited spectrum of patients seen in specialty clinics. Estimates of instrument sensitivity and specificity are more accurate. This method is useful in elucidating the natural history of a condition or in identifying the long-term risks and benefits of a particular intervention (Guess, Jacobsen, Girman, Oesterling, Chute, Panser, et al., 1995).

Clinical Decision Analysis

Clinical decision analysis is a systematic method of describing clinical problems, identifying possible diagnostic and management courses of action, assessing the probability and value of various outcomes, and then calculating the optimal course of action. Decision analysis is based on the following four assumptions: (1) decisions can be quantified; (2) all possible courses of action can be identified and evaluated; (3) the different values of outcomes, viewed from the perspective of the nurse, patient, payer, and administrator, can be examined; and (4) the analysis allows selection of an optimal course of therapy.

To perform the analysis, the researchers must define the boundaries of the clinical in terms of a logical sequence of events over time. All possible courses of action are then determined. These courses of action usually are represented in a decision tree consisting of a starting point, available alternatives, probable events, and outcomes. Next, the goals and objectives of problem resolution are defined. Researchers calculate the probability of occurrence of each path of the decision tree and ensure that an outcome exists for each potential path. Each outcome is assigned a value. These values may be expressed in terms of money, morbidity incidents, quality-of-life measures, or duration of hospital stay. (Figure 9-11 displays a simplified decision tree for breech delivery in obstetrics.) Researchers can then identify an optimal course of action according to which decision maximizes the chances of the most desirable outcomes (Crane, 1988; Keeler, 1994; Sonnenberg, Roberts, Tsevat, Wong, Barry, & Kent, 1994).

Studies analyzing clinical decisions have primarily used questionnaires and interviews. However, determining the clinical decisions of practitioners is not an easy task. Much of

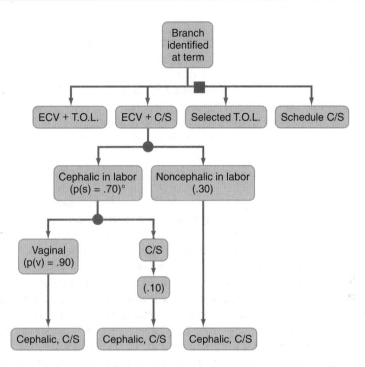

Figure 9-11. Simplified decision tree for breech delivery. Numbers in *parentheses* refer to estimated probability of event. (From Keeler, E. B. [1994]. Decision analysis and cost-effectiveness analysis in women's health care. *Clinical Obstetrics and Gynecology, 37*[1], 208.)

patient care involves the clinician and the patient alone. The underlying theories of care and the processes of care are hidden from view. Thus, it is difficult for clinicians to compare their specific approaches to care. Among physicians, care delivered by other physicians is rarely observed (O'Connor et al., 1993). Studies have found that physicians have difficulty recalling their decisions and providing rationales for them (Chaput de Saintonge & Hattersley, 1985; Kirwan, Chaput de Saintonge, Joyce, Holmes, & Currey, 1986).

Unsworth (2001) describes the following strategies for studying clinical decision making:

> semistructured interviews
> audio-assisted recall (the clinician listens to an audiotape of the clinician-client dialogue and uses this to aid recall of her or his reasoning processes)
> video-assisted recall (the clinician uses video footage to prompt recall of reasoning processes)
> the clinician writing notes as he or she solves a problem
> the think-aloud method (the clinician provides verbal commentary during interaction with the client)
> the clinician presents the reasoning about a clinician-client session afterward from memory
> use of a head-mounted video camera with video-assisted recall.

Chaput de Saintonge and associates (1988) propose a strategy for analyzing clinical decisions using "paper patients." The techniques seem to parallel the decisions made by practitioners in the clinical setting. In their study, 10 common clinical variables used to evaluate the status of patients with rheumatoid arthritis were collected at two points for 30 patients participating in a clinical trial, at the time of entry and 1 year later. Data for 20 of the patients were duplicated throughout the table to check the consistency of responses, making 50 responses in all. The variables were presented to rheumatologists on a single sheet of paper labeled "before" and "after a year." Physicians were asked to indicate the extent of change in each patient's condition using a visual analogue scale (VAS) with the ends labeled "greatest possible deterioration" and "greatest possible improvement." They also were asked whether they considered the change clinically important. Then they were asked to indicate the relative importance of each variable, rating the variables on a scale of 1 to 100.

Regression analyses were performed in which each VAS variable was used as the dependent variable. With increasing VAS values, judgments of clinical importance changed from "not important" to "important." This change occurred over a 5-mm length of the scale or less. (VAS scales traditionally are 100 mm in length.) The researchers designated the midpoint of this transition zone as the "threshold value of clinical importance." Consistency of responses was tested to correlate responses with those of duplicate cases. The researchers then developed a consensus model by weighing each physician's responses on the basis of the correlation. The VAS scores were multiplied by the correlation coefficient. These VAS scores were then used as the dependent variable in another regression analysis. This method is useful in identifying the variables important in the making of clinical decisions and the consistency with which practitioners make their decisions.

Study of the Effectiveness of Interdisciplinary Teams

According to Schmitt, Farrell, and Heinemann (1988), interdisciplinary teams have the following characteristics:

> ...(1) multiple health disciplines are involved in the care of the same patients, (2) the disciplines encompass a diversity of dissimilar knowledge and skills required by the patients, (3) the plan of care reflects an integrated set of goals shared by the providers of care, and (4) the team members share information and coordinate their services through a systematic communication process. (p. 753)

Part of the communication process consists of regularly scheduled face-to-face meetings. The assumption is that collaborative team approaches provide more effective care than that delivered using team approaches or noncollaborative multidisciplinary approaches (parallel care).

Interdisciplinary teams are becoming more common as health care changes. Examples are hospice care teams, home health teams, and psychiatric care teams. Studying the effectiveness of interdisciplinary teams is difficult, however. The characteristics that make team care more effective have not been identified. Studies usually focus on the evaluation of a single team, rather than on conducting comparison studies. The outcomes of team care also are multidimensional, requiring the use of multiple dependent variables.

Evaluation studies examining team care often examine only posttreatment data without baseline data. Comparison of groups will not reveal any evidence that the groups were similar in terms of important variables before the intervention. Involvement of family members with the team has not been examined. Clearly, this is an important focus of research requiring more rigorous designs than have previously been used.

Geographical Analyses

Geographical analyses are used to examine variations in health status, health services, patterns of care, or patterns of use by geographical area and sometimes are referred to as small area analyses. Variations may be associated with sociodemographic, economic, medical, cultural, or behavioral characteristics. Locality-specific factors of a health care system, such as capacity, access, and convenience, may play a role in explaining variations. The social setting, environment, living conditions, and community also may be important factors.

The interactions between the characteristics of a locality and of its inhabitants are complex. The characteristics of the total community may transcend the characteristics of persons within the community and may influence subgroup behavior. High education levels in the community commonly are associated with greater access to information and receptiveness to ideas from outside the community.

Regression analyses commonly are used to develop models using all of the risk factors and the characteristics of the community. Results often are displayed through the use of maps (Kieffer, Alexander, & Mor, 1992). After the analysis, the researcher must determine whether differences in rates are due to chance alone and whether high rates are too high. From a more theoretical perspective, the researcher must then explain the geographical variation uncovered by the analysis (Volinn, Diehr, Ciol, & Loeser, 1994).

Geographical information systems (GISs) can provide an important tool for performing geographic analyses. A GIS uses relational databases to facilitate processing of spatial information. The software tools in a GIS can be used for mapping, data summaries, and analysis of spatial relationships. GISs have the capability of modeling data flows so that the effect of proposed changes in interventions applied to individuals or communities on outcomes can be modeled (Auffrey, 1998).

Economic Studies

Many of the problems studied in health services research address concerns related to the efficient use of scarce resources and, thus, to economics. Health economists are concerned with the costs and benefits of alternative treatments or ways of identifying the most efficient means of care. The economist's definition of efficiency is the least-cost method of achieving a desired end with the maximum benefit to be obtained from available resources. If available resources must be shared with other programs or other types of patients, an economic study can determine whether changing the distribution of resources will increase total benefit or welfare.

To determine the efficiency of a treatment, the economist conducts a cost-effectiveness analysis. This technique uses a single measure of outcomes, and all other factors are expressed in monetary terms as net cost per unit of output (Ludbrook, 1990). Cost-effectiveness analyses compare different ways of accomplishing a clinical goal, such as diagnosing a condition, treating an illness, or providing a service. The alternative approaches are compared in terms of costs and benefits. The purpose is to identify the strategy that provides the most value for the money. Tradeoffs between costs and benefits are unavoidable, however (Oster,

1988). Stone (1998) describes the methodology for performing a cost-effectiveness analysis.

It is time for nurses to take a more active role in conducting cost-effectiveness research. Nurses are well positioned to evaluate health care practices and have the incentive to conduct the studies. Nursing practice is seldom a subject of cost-effectiveness analyses. Nevertheless, such knowledge would enable nurses to refine their practice, substituting interventions that maximize nurses' time to the best advantage, in terms of the patient's health, for interventions that offer less gain (Siegel, 1998).

As Lieu and Newman (1998) point out:

"[C]ost effective" does not necessar[il]y mean "cost-saving" (Doubilet, Weinstein, & McNeil, 1986). Many health interventions, even preventive ones, do not save money (Tengs, Adams, Pliskin, Safran, Siegel, Weinstein, et al., 1995). Rather, a service should be called cost-effective if its benefits are judged worth the costs. Recently, a consensus panel supported by the National Institutes of Health published recommendations that define standards for conducting cost-effectiveness analysis (Gold, Siegel, Russell, & Weinstein, 1996). Cost-effectiveness analysis is only one of several methods that can be used for the economic evaluation of health services (Drummond, Stoddart, and Torrance, 1987). Although these methods are useful, an intervention cannot be cost-effective without being effective" (Lieu & Newman, 1998, p. 1043).

To examine overall benefits, a **cost-benefit analysis** is performed. With this method, the costs and benefits of alternative ways of using resources are assessed in monetary terms, and the use that produces the greatest net benefit is chosen. The costs included in an economic study are defined in exact ways. The actual costs associated with an activity, not prices, must be used. Cost is not the same as price. In most cases, price is greater than cost. **Costs** are a measure of the actual use of resources, rather than the price charged. Charges are a poor reflection of actual costs. Costs typically included in a cost-benefit analysis are costs to the provider, costs to third-party payers (e.g., insurance), out-of-pocket costs, and opportunity costs.

Out-of-pocket costs are those expenses incurred by the patient or family members, or both, that are not reimbursable by the insurance company. Examples are costs of buying supplies, dressings, medications, and special food, transportation expenses, and unreimbursable care expenses.

Opportunity costs are lost opportunities that the patient, family member, or others experience. For example, a family member who must stay at home to care for the patient may lose the opportunity to earn more money. A teenager who needs to drop out of school for a semester to care for a parent may lose the opportunity to advance her education. A husband might have been able to take a better job if the family could have moved to another town, rather than staying in place to enable a member to receive specific medical care.

Opportunity costs often are not included in the consideration of overall costs. This omission results in an underestimation of costs and an overestimation of benefit. For example, caring for an acutely ill patient at home is cost-effective if out-of-pocket costs and opportunity costs are not considered. However, the total costs of providing the care, regardless of who pays or who receives the money, must be included. In performing such a study, it is important to state whose costs are being considered and who is to weigh the benefits against the consequences.

Allred, Arford, Mauldin, and Goodwin (1998) critiqued the seven nursing studies between 1992 and 1996 in which cost-effectiveness analyses were performed. They found these studies to be equivalent in quality to those from other disciplines. They concluded that more emphasis must be placed on cost-effectiveness analyses in nursing research, and they provided guidelines for conducting these studies.

Stone (1998) has described the recommended guidelines for journal reports of cost-effectiveness analyses. Cost-effectiveness studies should be used as aids in decision making, rather than as the end decision. If a cost-effectiveness study is conducted to inform those who make resource allocation decisions, a standard reference case should be presented to allow the decision makers to compare a proposed new health intervention with existing practice.

Ethical Studies

Outcomes studies often result in the development of policies for the allocation of scarce resources. Ethicists take the position that moral principles, such as justice, must be considered as constraints on the use of costs and benefits, to choose treatments that maximize the benefit per unit cost. Value commitments are inherent in choices about research methods and about the selection and interpretation of outcome variables, and these commitments should be acknowledged by researchers.

> The choices researchers make should be documented and the reasons for those choices should be given explicitly in publications and presentations so that readers and other users of the information are enabled and expected to bear more responsibility for interpreting and applying the findings appropriately. (Lynn & Virnig, 1995)

Veatch (1993) proposes that analysis of the implications of rationing decisions in terms of the principles of justice and autonomy will provide more acceptable criteria than outcomes predictors alone. As an example, Veatch performs an ethical analysis of the use of outcome predictors in decisions related to early withdrawal of life support. Ethical studies should play an important role in outcomes programs of research.

Measurement Methods

The selection of appropriate outcome variables is critical to the success of a study (Bernstein & Hilborne, 1993). As in any study, evidence of validity and reliability of the methods of measurement must be evaluated. Outcomes selected for nursing studies should be those most consistent with nursing practice and theory (Harris & Warren, 1995). In some studies, rather than selecting the final outcome of care, which may not occur for months or years, measures of intermediate end points are used. **Intermediate end points** are events or markers that act as precursors to the final outcome. It is important, however, to document the validity of the intermediate end point in predicting the outcome (Freedman & Schatzkin, 1992). In early outcomes studies, researchers selected outcome measures that could be easily obtained, rather than those most desirable for outcomes studies.

Table 9-5 identifies characteristics important to evaluate in selecting methods of measuring outcomes. In evaluating a particular outcome measure, the researcher should consult the literature for previous studies that have used that particular method of measurement, including the publication describing development of the method of measurement. Information related to the measurement can be organized into a table such as Table 9-6, allowing easy comparison of several methods of measuring a particular outcome.

Table 9-5	Characteristics of Outcomes Assessment Instruments	
Characteristic	Considerations in Patient Outcomes Evaluation	References

Applicability	Consider purpose of instruments
	Discriminate between subjects at a point in time
	Predict future outcomes
	Evaluate changes within subjects over time
	Screen for problems
	Provide case-mix adjustment
	Assess quality of care
	Consider whether:
	  Norms are established for clinical population of interest
	  Instrument format is compatible with assessment approach (e.g., observer rated vs. self-administered)
	  Setting in which instrument was developed
		Deyo & Carter, 1992
		Stewart et al., 1989
		Guyatt, Walter, & Norman, 1987
		Feinstein, Josephy, & Wells, 1986
		Deyo, 1984

Practicality (clinical utility)	The instrument: Includes outcomes important to the patient Is short and easy to administer (low respondent burden) Questions are easy to understand and acceptable to patients and interviewers Scores reflect condition severity, condition-specific features, and discriminate those with conditions from those without Is easily scored and scores are readily understandable Level of measurement allows a change score to be determined Provides information that is clinically useful Performance or capacity based Includes patient rating of magnitude of effort and support needed for performance of physical tasks	Leidy, 1991 Nelson, Landgraf, Hays, Wasson, & Kirk, 1990 Stewart et al., 1989 Lohr, 1988 Bombardier & Tugwell, 1987 Feinstein et al., 1986 Kirshner & Guyatt, 1985 Deyo, 1984
Comprehensiveness	Generic measures are designed to summarize a spectrum of concepts applied to different impairments, illnesses, patients, and populations Disease-specific measures are designed to assess specific patients with specific conditions or diagnoses Dimensions of the instrument; a core set of physical, mental, and role function desirable	Nelson et al., 1990 Patrick & Deyo, 1989 Deyo, 1984
Reliability	Can be influenced by day-to-day variations in patients, differences between observers, items in the scale, mode of administration This is the critical determinant of usefulness of an instrument Designed for discriminative purpose	Nelson et al., 1990 Spitzer, 1987 Guyatt et al., 1987 Deyo, 1984

Table 9-5	Characteristics of Outcomes Assessment Instruments—cont'd	
Characteristic	Considerations in Patient Outcomes Evaluation	References
Validity	No consensus of what are scientifically admissible criteria for many indices No "goal standard" exists for establishing criterion validity for many indices	Spitzer, 1987 Deyo, 1984
Responsiveness	Not yet indexed for virtually any evaluative measures Coarse scale rating may not detect changes Aggregated scores may obscure changes in subscales Useful for determining sample size and statistical power Reliable instruments are likely to be responsive but reliability not adequate as sole index of consistent results over time Consider detail in scaling As baseline variability of score changes within stable subjects, may need larger treatment effects to demonstrate efficacy Consider temporal relationship between intervention and outcome	Stewart & Archbold, 1992 Leidy, 1991 Jaeschke, Singer, & Guyatt, 1989 Guyatt et al., 1989 Bombardier & Tugwell, 1987 Guyatt et al., 1987 Deyo & Centor, 1986 Deyo, 1984

From Harris, M. R., & Warren, J. J. (1995). Patient outcomes: Assessment issues for the CNS. *Clinical Nurse Specialist, 9*(2), 82.

Outcomes researchers are moving away from classical measurement theory as a means of evaluating the reliability of measurement methods. They are interested in identifying change in measures over time in a subject, and instruments developed through the use of classical measurement theory are often not sensitive to these changes. The magnitude of change that can be detected also is important to determine. In addition, measures may detect change within a particular range of values but may not be sensitive to changes outside that range. The sensitivity to change of many commonly used outcome measures has not been examined (Deyo & Carter, 1992; Felson, Anderson, & Meenan, 1990). Studies must be conducted specifically to determine the sensitivity of measures before they are used in outcomes studies. As the sensitivity of a measure increases, statistical power increases, allowing smaller sample sizes to detect significant differences.

Creative methods of collecting data on instruments for large outcomes studies must be explored. In a busy office or clinic setting, the typical strategy of having clerks or other staff administer questionnaires or scales to patients is time intensive and costly and may result in lost data. Greist and colleagues (1997) recommend using the computer and the telephone to collect such data. Computers containing the instrument can be placed in locations convenient to patients, so the instrument can be completed with a minimum of staff involvement.

Another option is telephone interviews using the computer. The traditional telephone interview using interviewers to ask questions is costly. The same interactive voice response (IVR) technology used in voice mail, however, can be used in telephone interviewing by computer. IVR allows the patient to respond to yes–no and multiple-choice questions by pressing numbers on the keypad or by saying "yes" or "no" or a number from 0 to 9. Patients can record answers in their own voice.

Table 9-6	Characteristics of the Katz Activities of Daily Living (ADL) Scale: A Proposed Outcome Instrument	

Characteristic	Reference(s)
Applicability	
Purpose is to objectively evaluate results of treatment in chronically ill and aging populations	Katz et al., 1970
Predicts service utilization in elderly population	Winner et al., 1990
Used in case-mix adjustments	Fries, 1990
Scale discriminates well on disability in elderly population, norms easily referenced	Spector, 1990
Ratings judgment based on direct observation and caregiver reports, known differences in observed vs. reported ratings	Spector, 1990 / Burns, 1992
Practicality	
Brief, 6 items with 3 levels of dependency	Katz et al., 1970
Can be used by clinicians and non-clinicians	Spector, 1990
Measures performance (not ability)	Katz et al., 1970
Aggregate score represents increasing level of dependency	Spector, 1990
Comprehensiveness	
Includes bathing, dressing, toileting, transfer, continence, and eating	Katz et al., 1970
Does not explain etiology of level of performance	Kane & Bayer, 1991
Reliability	
Performance may be influenced by motivational, social, and environmental factors	Kane & Bayer, 1991
High internal consistency reported	Spector, 1990
Validity	
Content and construct validity assessments are acceptable	Spector, 1990
Responsiveness	
No published reports that quantify relationship of scale change to minimal clinically important change	

From Harris, M. R., & Warren, J. J. (1995). Patient outcomes: Assessment issues for the CNS. *Clinical Nurse Specialist, 9*(2), 85.

Measuring the frequency and nature of care activities of various staff has been problematic in studies of the process of care. Strategies commonly used are chart review, time and motion studies, work sampling, and retrospective recall. None of these is a satisfactory indicator of the actual care that occurs (Hale, Thomas, Bond, & Todd, 1997). Holmes, Teresi, Lindeman, and Glandon (1997) recommend the use of barcode methodology to measure service inputs. Scanning the barcodes captures what care is provided, for whom, by whom, and at what time. Barcoded service sheets and a portable barcode reader are used with an accompanying database management system.

The Analysis of Measurement Reliability

Estimating the reliability of outcome measures through the use of classical measurement theory may be problematic. The traditional concept of measurement reliability was developed to evaluate quantities that were not expected to change over time for an individual subject. This assessment of reliability is irrelevant or only partially relevant to assessing the suitability or precision of measures selected because of their sensitivity to change within the subject over time. Traditional evaluations of measurement methods assume that any change in group values is a result of interindividual variation. Patient change, however, results in changes within the subject. With classical measurement theory analysis, a measure that did not vary between individual subjects is considered to have zero (or poor) reliability. This measure, however, may be an excellent measure of change over time if individual subjects change on that measure (even if group averages do not change much). Thus, it is inappropriate to assess the reliability of difference scores according to the internal consistency of measures (Collins & Johnston, 1995).

Some outcomes researchers use measures obtained from individual subjects as indicators of characteristics of a group. The data from the measures are aggregated to reflect the group. In this case, the researcher must assess the extent to which the responses represent the group. Although the group mean usually is expected to serve this purpose, it may not adequately represent the group. Verran, Mark, and Lamb (1992) describe techniques for examining the psychometric properties of instruments used to describe group-level phenomena. Items of the instrument should be assessed for content validity to determine how well they measure group-level concepts. Reliability and validity must be assessed at the aggregated level, rather than at the individual level.

Commonly, multiple outcomes measures are used in outcomes studies. Researchers wish to evaluate all relevant effects of care. However, quantity of measures is not necessarily evidence of the quality of the measures. Researchers should select the measures most relevant to the treatment, avoiding measures that are closely correlated. Interpreting the results of studies in which multiple outcomes have been used can be problematic. For example, Felson and colleagues (1990, p. 141) ask "which is the better therapy, the one that shows a change in 6 outcome measures out of 12 tested or the one that shows a change in 4 of the 12 measures? What if the 4 that demonstrate change with one therapy are not the same as the 6 that show a change in another therapy?" If multiple comparisons are made, it is important to make statistical adjustments for them; the risk of a Type I error is greater when multiple comparisons are made.

Some researchers recommend combining various measures into a single summary score (DesHarnais, McMahon, & Wroblewski, 1991; Felson et al., 1990). Such global composite measures have not been widely used, however. The various measures used in such an index may not be equally weighted and may be difficult to combine. Also, the composite index value may not be readily interpretable by clinicians.

The focus of most measures developed for outcomes studies has been the individual patient. However, a number of organizations are now developing measures of the quality of performance of systems of care. In 1990, the Consortium Research on Indicators of System Performance (CRISP) project began to develop indicators of the quality of performance of integrated delivery systems. From the perspective of CRISP, the success of a health system is associated with its ability to decrease the number of episodes of diseases in the population. Therefore, the impact of the delivery system on the community is considered an important measure of performance. CRISP has developed a number of indicators now in use by consortium members, who pay to participate in the studies (Bergman, 1994).

The JCAHO also is applying outcomes data to quality management efforts in hospitals using the IMSystem (Information Management System) (McCormick, 1990; Nadzim, Turpin, Hanold, & White, 1993). The National Committee for Quality Assurance, the organization that accredits managed care plans, has developed a tool (HEDIS—Health plan Employer Data and Information Set) for comparing managed care plans. Comparisons involve more than 60 measures, including patient satisfaction, quality of care, and financial stability (Guadagnoli & McNeil, 1994). Researchers at the Henry Ford Health Systems' Center for Health System Studies in Detroit have evolved 80 performance indicators to evaluate health systems (Anderson, 1991).

Statistical Methods for Outcomes Studies

Although outcomes researchers test for statistical significance of their findings, this determination is not considered sufficient to judge the findings as important. The focus of these researchers' attention is on the *clinical* significance of study findings (see Chapter 12 for more information on clinical significance). In analyzing data, outcomes researchers have moved away from statistical analyses that use the mean to test for group differences. They place greater importance on analyzing change scores and use exploratory methods of examining the data to identify outliers.

The Analysis of Change

With the focus on outcomes studies has come a renewed interest in methods of analyzing change. Gottman and Rushe (1993) reported that the first book addressing change in research, *Problems in Measuring Change*, edited by Harris (1963), is the basis for most current approaches to analyzing change. Since then, a number of new ideas have emerged regarding the analysis of change (e.g., in studies by Collins & Horn, 1991; Rovine & Von Eye, 1991; Von Eye, 1990a, 1990b). Many researchers, however, are unfamiliar with these new ideas and continue to base their reasoning on Harris' 1967 book. Gottman and Rushe (1993) suggest that many beliefs related to the analysis of change are based on little more than the following fallacies:

> *Fallacy 1:* In change, regression toward the mean is an unavoidable law of nature.
> *Fallacy 2:* The difference score between premeasurement and postmeasurement is unreliable.
> *Fallacy 3:* Analysis of covariance (ANCOVA, or related methods such as path analysis) is the way to analyze change.
> *Fallacy 4:* Two points (pretest and posttest) are adequate for the study of change.
> *Fallacy 5:* The correlation between change and initial level is always negative.

Outcomes researchers also are questioning the method of analysis of change. Collins and Johnston (1995) suggest that the recommended analysis method of regressing pretest scores on outcome scores and basing the analysis of change on residual change scores is overly conservative and tends to understate the extent of real change. Serious questions remain about the conceptual meaning of these residual change scores.

For some outcomes, the changes may be nonlinear or may go up and down, rather than always increasing. Thus, it is as important to uncover patterns of change as it is to test for statistically significant differences at various time points. Some changes may occur in relation to stages of recovery or improvement. These changes may occur over weeks, months, or even years. A more complete picture of the process of recovery can be obtained by examining the process in greater detail and over a broader range. With this approach, a recovery curve can be developed, which provides a model of the recovery process and can then be tested (Collins & Johnston, 1995; Ottenbacher, Johnson, & Hojem, 1995).

The Analysis of Improvement

In addition to reporting the mean improvement score for all patients treated, it is important to report what percentage of patients improve. Do all patients improve slightly, or is there a divergence among patients, with some improving greatly and others not improving at all? This divergence may best be illustrated by plotting the data. For example, researchers studying a particular treatment or approach to care may develop a standard or index of various possible degrees of improvement. The index will allow better comparisons of the effectiveness of various treatments. Characteristics of patients who experience various degrees of improvement also are described, and outliers must be carefully examined. This step requires that the study design include baseline measures of patient status, such as demographic characteristics, functional status, and disease severity measures. Analysis of improvement will allow better judgments of the appropriate use of various treatments (Felson, Anderson, & Meenan, 1990).

Variance Analysis

Variance analysis is used to track individual and group variance from a specific critical pathway. The goal is to decrease preventable variance in process, thus helping patients and their families achieve optimal outcomes. Some of the variance is due to the presence of comorbid conditions. Keeping a patient with comorbidity on the desired pathway may require utilization of more resources early in treatment. Thus, it is important to track both variance and comorbidity. Studies examining variations from pathways may facilitate the tailoring of existing critical pathways for a specific comorbid condition.

Variance analysis also can be used to identify at-risk patients who may benefit from the services of a case manager. Variance analysis tracking is expressed through the use of graphics, and the expected pathway is plotted on the graph. The care providers plot deviations (negative variance) on the graph, allowing immediate comparison with the expected pathway. Deviations may be related to the patient, the system, or the provider (Tidwell, 1993).

The Longitudinal Guttman Simplex Model

The Longitudinal Guttman Simplex (LGS) Model is an extension of the Guttman scale that involves points in time, as well as items and persons. For example, an LGS model of mobility may involve the following items:

> *M1:* moving unassisted from bed to chair
> *M2:* moving unassisted from bed to another room
> *M3:* moving unassisted up stairs

Table 9-7 shows hypothetical data collected with this measure on three patients at three points in time, showing a pattern of improving ability over time (Collins & Johnston, 1995).

Table 9-7	Sample Data Using Longitudinal Guttman Scale		
	Functional Items		
	M1	M2	M3
Patient A			
Time 1	Fail	Fail	Fail
Time 2	Pass	Fail	Fail
Time 3	Pass	Pass	Fail
Patient B			
Time 1	Fail	Fail	Fail
Time 2	Pass	Pass	Fail
Time 3	Pass	Pass	Fail
Patient C			
Time 1	Pass	Fail	Fail
Time 2	Pass	Pass	Fail
Time 3	Pass	Pass	Pass

M1, Moving unassisted from bed to chair; M2, moving unassisted from bed to another room; M3, moving unassisted up stairs.

From Collins, L. M., & Johnston, M. V. (1995). Analysis of stage-sequential change in rehabilitation research. *American Journal of Physical Medicine and Rehabilitation, 74*(2), 167.

Latent Transition Analysis

Researchers use latent transition analysis (LTA) when stages or categories of recovery have been defined and transitions between stages can be identified. To use the analysis method, the researchers place each member of the population in a single category or stage for a given point of time. However, stage membership changes over time. The analysis tests stage membership to provide a realistic picture of development. Collins and Johnston (1995) describe an example of latent transition analysis, using a hypothetical model of recovery from functional neglect after stroke, in the following excerpt:

RESEARCH EXAMPLE   **Latent Transition Analysis**

Let's assume that we can define a study subpopulation displaying four latent stages or types of functional neglect: sensory limitations (S), cognitive limitations (C), both (S and C) or patients may recover and adapt to the point that they are functional (F).... Membership in each category is inferred from several clinical symptoms or test items, which supposedly go together but in fact may not for some patients. The items have some error and are imperfect indicators of true (latent) stage membership. Our objective is to estimate in which category a patient probably falls at any point in time and the probability of movement between stages over time, conditional on previous stage membership.... Suppose we use a large number of times periodically to monitor progress, testing the same group of patients at multiple points in time. We record which items the patient passes and which the patient does not. (Collins & Johnston, 1995, p. 47)

After performing LTA by means of a computerized program designed for that purpose, the investigators presented their results in a table (Table 9-A). Data for only two points in time are shown, although the program can handle up to such five points.

TABLE 9-A A Hypothetical Latent Transition Model of Recovery from Neglect Following Stroke

	Latent Status			
	F	**C**	**S**	**S and C**
Total Marginal Proportions				
Time 1 proportions	0.0	0.40	0.30	0.30
Time 2 proportions	0.27	0.25	0.30	0.18
	Time 2 Latent Status			
Time 1 Latent Status	**F***	**C**	**S**	**S and C**
Time 1 to Time 2 Transition				
Proportions with Rows				
Functional (F)	0	0	0	0
Cognitive limitation (C)	0.46	0.54	0.0	0.0
Sensory limitation (S)	0.30	0.0	0.70	0.0
S and C	0.0	0.10	0.30	0.60

From Collins, L. M., & Johnston, M. V. (1995). Analysis of stage-sequential change in rehabilitation research. *American Journal of Physical Medicine and Rehabilitation, 74*(2), 168.

*No patients were functional at Time 1.

The first line of the table contains the estimate of the proportion of patients in each of the four stages at Time 1. In this example, 30% of the sample had both S and C limitations, 30% had S limitations, and 40% had C limitations, and none was functional. At Time 2, the proportion in each functional limitation appears to have declined, except that for S limitations, which is unchanged, and 27% are now in the functional stage. The bottom half of the table is a matrix of transition probabilities that reveals patterns of change. Of patients who started with S, 30% improved; however, the overall percentage at S remained the same because 30% of the patients who started at S and C moved to the S category. Of patients who initially had C problems alone, 46% moved to the functional category.

A third set of quantities estimated by the full LTA model but not shown in the table are the relationships between items and stage memberships. This relationship indicates the probability that when a subject moves from one category to another, each item will also change to reflect the new stage membership. Thus, this relationship is a determination of the effectiveness of the test items or clinical symptoms as indicators of stage membership.

Multilevel Analysis

Multilevel analysis is used in epidemiology to study how environmental factors (aggregate-level characteristics) and individual attributes and behaviors (individual-level characteristics) interact to influence individual-level health behaviors and disease risks. For example, the risk that an adolescent will start smoking is associated with the following variables: (1) attributes of the child (e.g., self-esteem, academic achievement, refusal skills), (2) attributes of the child's family (e.g., parental attitudes toward smoking, smoking behavior of parents), (3) general characteristics of the community (e.g., ease of minors' access to cigarettes, school policies regarding smoking, city smoking ordinances, social norms of students for smoking), and (4) general social factors (e.g., geographical region, economic policies that influence the price of cigarettes). The researchers might ask, "Does smoking status covary with the level of restriction of smoking in public places after we have controlled for the individual-level variables that influence smoking risks?" (Von Korff, Koepsell, Curry, & Diehr, 1992).

Disseminating Outcomes Research Findings

Including plans for the dissemination of findings as a component of a program of research is a new idea within nursing if the process of dissemination is considered to be more than publishing the results in professional journals. The costs associated with dissemination are not included in funding for nursing studies beyond those of publication of the research findings. Strategies for the dissemination of research findings tend to be performed by groups other than the original researchers. The transfer of knowledge from nurse researchers to nurse clinicians has been, for the most part, ineffective.

Nursing, as a discipline, has not yet addressed the various constituencies for nursing research knowledge. A research team conducting a program of outcomes research must identify its constituencies. These should include (1) the clinicians, who will apply the knowledge to practice, (2) the public, members of which may make health care decisions on the basis of the information, (3) health care institutions, which must evaluate care in their facilities on the basis of the information, (4) health policy makers, who or which may set standards on the basis of the information, and (5) researchers, who may use the information in designing new studies. Disseminating information to these various constituencies through presentations at meetings and publications in a wide diversity of journals and magazines, as well as release of the information to the news media, requires careful planning. Mattson and Donovan (1994) suggest that dissemination involves strategies for debunking myths, addressing issues related to feasibility, communicating effectively, and identifying opinion leaders.

KEY CONCEPTS

- Outcomes research was developed to examine the end results of patient care.
- The scientific approaches used in outcomes studies differ in some important ways from those used in traditional research.
- The theory on which outcomes research is based was developed by Donabedian (1987). Quality is the overriding construct of the theory. The three major concepts of the theory are health, subjects of care, and providers of care.
- The goal of outcomes research is the evaluation of outcomes as defined by Donabedian, whose theory requires that identified outcomes be clearly linked with the process that caused the outcome.
- Outcomes research programs are complex and may consist of multiple studies using a variety of designs whose findings must be merged in the process of forming conclusions.
- The researcher must consider the measure's sensitivity to change and the magnitude of change that can be detected.

- Statistical approaches used in outcomes studies include new approaches to examining measurement reliability, strategies to analyze change, and the analysis of improvement.
- Strategies must be developed in nursing to disseminate the findings from outcomes studies to the various constituencies needing the information.

TIPS FOR FURTHER STUDY

- For help determining which studies are outcome studies, complete the Open-Book Quiz in the Evolve Learning Resources and the "Research Strategies for Outcomes Studies" section of your *Study Guide*.
- For help in identifying nursing-sensitive outcomes, work through the Open-Book Quiz and the Bonus Review Questions on http://evolve.elsevier.com/Burns/understanding/.

REFERENCES

Allred, C. A., Arford, P. H., Mauldin, P. D., & Goodwin, L. K. (1998). Cost-effectiveness analysis in the nursing literature, 1992–1996. *The Journal of Nursing Scholarship, 30*(3), 235–242.

American Medical Association (1989). *Journal of the American Medical Association*, 262, 925–930. Copyrighted 1989, American Medical Association.

Anderson, H. J. (1991). Sizing up systems: researchers to test performance measures. *Hospitals, 65*(20), 33–34.

Anderson, R. M., Davidson, P. L., & Ganz, P. A. (1994). Symbiotic relationships of quality of life, health services research, and other research. *Quality of Life Research 3*(5), 367.

Anonymous. (1997). A report on the implementation of a nursing report card for acute care settings executive summary—January 1997. *New Mexico Nurse, 42*(2), 11.

Barton, A. J., Gilbert, L., Erickson, V., Baramee, J., Sowers, D., & Robertson, K. J. (2003). A guide to assist nurse practitioners with standardized nursing language. *Computers, Informatics, Nursing: CIN, 21*(3), 128–135.

Blegen, M. A., Goode, C. J., & Reed, L. (1998). Nurse staffing and patient outcomes, *Nursing Research, 47*(1), 43–50.

Buerhaus, P. I., & Needleman, J. (2000). Pollicy implications of research on nurse staffing and quality of patient care. *Policy, Politics, & Nursing Practice, 1*(1), 5–15.

Bergman, R. (1994). Are my outcomes better than yours? *Hospital Health Network, 68*(15), 113–116.

Bergmark, A., & Oscarsson, L. (1991). Does anybody really know what they are doing? Some comments related to methodology of treatment service research. *British Journal of Addiction, 86*(2), 139–142.

Bernstein, S. J., & Hilborne, L. H. (1993). Clinical indicators: The road to quality care? *Joint Commission Journal on Quality Improvement, 19*(11), 501–509.

Bircumshaw, D., & Chapman, C. M. (1988). A study to compare the practice style of graduate and non-graduate nurses and midwives: The pilot study. *Journal of Advanced Nursing, 13*(5), 605–614.

Campbell-Heider, N., Krainovich-Miller, B., King, K. B., Sedhom, L., & Malinski, V. (1998). Empowering staff nurses to participate in the American Nurses Association's call for quality indicators research. *Journal of the New York State Nurses' Association, 29*(3/4), 21–27.

Chaput de Saintonge, D. M., & Hattersley, L. A. (1985). Antibiotics for otitis media: Can we help doctors agree? *Family Practice, 2*(4), 205–212.

Chaput de Saintonge, D. M., Kirway, J. R., Evans, S. J., & Crane, G. J. (1988). How can we design trials to detect clinically important changes in disease severity? *British Journal of Clinical Pharmacology, 26*(4), 355–362.

Cho, S., Ketefian, S., Barkauskas, V. H., & Smith, D. G. (2003). The effects of nurse staffing on adverse events, morbidity, mortality, and medical costs. *Nursing Research, 52*(2), 71–79.

Clinton, J. J. (1993). Financing medical effectiveness research: Role of the Agency for Health Care Policy and Research. *Annals of the New York Academy of Sciences, 703*, 295–297.

Collins, L. M., & Horn, J. L. (1991). *Best methods for the analysis of change: Recent advances, unanswered questions, future directions*. Washington, DC: American Psychological Association.

Collins, L. M., & Johnston, M. V. (1995). Analysis of stage-sequential change in rehabilitation research. *American Journal of Physical Medicine and Rehabilitation, 74*(2), 163–170.

Crane, V. S. (1988). Economic aspects of clinical decision making: Applications of clinical decision analysis. *American Journal of Hospital Pharmacy, 45*(3), 548–553.

Cummings, G. G., Fraser, K., & Tarlier, D. S. (2003). Implementing advanced nurse practitioner roles in acute care: An evaluation of organizational change. *Journal of Nursing Administration, 33*(3), 139–145.

Davis, K. (1990). Use of data registries to evaluate medical procedures: Coronary Artery Surgery Study and the Balloon Valvuloplasty Registry. *International Journal of Technology Assessment in Health Care, 6*(2), 203–210.

DesHarnais, S., McMahon, L. F., Jr., & Wroblewski, R. (1991). Measuring outcomes of hospital care using multiple risk-adjusted indexes. *HSR: Health Services Research, 26*(4), 425–445.

Deyo, R. A. (1984). Measuring functional outcomes in the therapeutic trials for chronic disease. *Controlled Clinical Trials, 5*(3), 223–240.

Deyo, R. A., & Carter, W. B. (1992). Strategies for improving and expanding the application of health status measures in clinical settings. A research-developer viewpoint. *Medical Care, 30*(5S), MS176–MS186.

Deyo, R. A., Psaty, B. M., Simon, G., Wagner, E. H., & Omenn, G. S. (1997). The messenger under attack—intimidation of researchers by special interest groups. *The New England Journal of Medicine, 336*(16), 1176–1180.

Deyo, R. A., Taylor, V. M., Diehr, P., Conrad, D., Cherkin, D. C., Ciol, M., et al. (1994). Analysis of automated administrative and survey databases to study patterns and outcomes of care. *Spine, 19*(18S), 2083S–2091S.

Donabedian, A. (1976). *Benefits in medical care programs.* Cambridge: Harvard University Press.

Donabedian, A. (1978). *Needed research in quality assessment and monitoring.* Hyattsville, MD: U.S. Department of Health, Education, and Welfare, Public Health Service, National Center for Health Services Research: NCHSR Office of Scientific and Technical Information. [Available from National Technical Information Service, Springfield, VA.]

Donabedian, A. (1980). *Explorations in quality assessment and monitoring.* Ann Arbor, MI: Health Administration Press.

Donabedian, A. (1982). *The criteria and standards of quality.* Ann Arbor, MI: Health Administration Press.

Donabedian, A. (1987). Some basic issues in evaluating the quality of health care. In L. T. Rinke (Ed.), *Outcome measures in home care* (Vol. I, pp. 3–28). New York: National League for Nursing. [Original work published 1976.]

Donohue, R. (2003). Nurse practitioner–client interaction as resource exchange in a women's health clinic: An exploratory study. *Journal of Clinical Nursing, 12*(5), 717–725.

Doran, D. I., Sidani, S., Keatings, M., & Doidge, D. (2002). An empirical test of the Nursing Role Effectiveness Model. *Journal of Advanced Nursing, 38*(1), 29–39.

Doubilet, P., Weinstein, M. C., & McNeil, B. J. (1986). Use and misuse of the term "cost effective" in medicine. *The New England Journal of Medicine, 314*(4), 253–256.

Drummond, M. F., Stoddart, G. L. & Torrance, G. W. (1987). *Method for the economic evaluation of health care programmes.* New York: Oxford University Press.

Evans, R. G., & Stoddart, G. L. (1990). Producing health, consuming health care. *Social Science and Medicine, 31*(12), 1347–1363.

Fardon, D. F., Garfin, S. R., & Saal, J. A. (1997). Intimidation of researchers by special interest groups [Letter; comment]. *The New England Journal of Medicine, 337*(18), 1315–1316.

Feinstein, A. R., Josephy, B. R., & Wells, C. K. (1986). Scientific and clinical problems in indexes of functional disability. *Annals of Internal Medicine 105*(3), 413–420.

Felson, D. T., Anderson, J. J., & Meenan, R. F. (1990). Time for changes in the design, analysis, and reporting of rheumatoid arthritis clinical trials. *Arthritis and Rheumatism, 33*(1), 140–149.

Fowler, F. J., Jr., Cleary, P. D., Magaziner, J., Patrick, D. L., & Benjamin, K. L. (1994). Methodological issues in measuring patient-reported outcomes: The agenda of the Work Group on Outcomes Assessment. *Medical Care, 32*(7 Suppl.), JS65–JS76.

Freedman, L. S., & Schatzkin, A. (1992). Sample size for studying intermediate endpoints within intervention trials or observational studies. *American Journal of Epidemiology, 136*(9), 1148–1159.

Freund, D. A., Dittus, R. S., Fitzgerald, J., & Heck, D. (1990). Assessing and improving outcomes: Total knee replacement. *HSR: Health Services Research, 25*(5), 723–726.

Fullerton, J. T., Hollenbach, K. A., & Wingard, D. L. (1996). Research exchange. Practice styles: A comparison of obstetricians and nurse-midwives. *Journal of Nurse-Midwifery, 41*(3), 243-250.

Gold, M. R., Siegel, J. E., Russell, L. B., & Weinstein, M. C. (Eds.). (1996). *Cost-effectiveness in health and medicine.* New York: Oxford University Press.

Goldberg, H. I., Cummings, M. A., Steinberg, E. P., Ricci, E. M., Shannon, T., Soumerai, S. B., et al. (1994). Deliberations on the dissemination of PORT products: Translating research findings into improved patient outcomes. *Medical Care, 32*(7 Suppl.), JS90–JS110.

Gottman, J. M., & Rushe, R. H. (1993). The analysis of change: Issues, fallacies, and new ideas. *Journal of Consulting and Clinical Psychology, 61*(6), 907–910.

Gray, B. H. (1992). The legislative battle over health services research. *Health Affairs (Project Hope), 11*(4), 38–66.

Greene, R., Bondy, P. K., & Maklan, C. W. (1994). The national medical effectiveness research initiative. The search for what really works in treating common clinical conditions. *Diabetes Care, 17*(Suppl. 1), 45–49.

Greenfield, S., Nelson, E. C., Zubkoff, M., Manning, W., Rogers, W., Kravitz, R. L., et al. (1992). Variations in resource utilization among medical specialties and systems of care: Results from the Medical Outcomes study. *JAMA, 267*(12), 1624–1630.

Greist, J. H., Jefferson, J. W., Wenzel, K. W., Kobak, K. A., Bailey, T. M., Katzelnick, D. J., et al. (1997). The telephone assessment program: Efficient patient monitoring and clinician feedback. *M.D. Computing: Computers in Medical Practice, 14*(5), 382–387.

Guadagnoli, E., & McNeil, B. J. (1994). Outcomes research: Hope for the future or the latest rage? *Inquiry, 31*(1), 14–24.

Guess, H. A., Jacobsen, S. J., Girman, C. J., Oesterling, J. E., Chute, C. G., Panser, L. A., et al. (1995). The role of community-based longitudinal studies in evaluating treatment effects: Example: Benign prostatic hyperplasia. *Medical Care, 33*(4 Suppl.), AS26–AS35.

Guyatt, G., Walter, S., & Norman, G. (1987). Measuring change over time: assessing the usefulness of evaluative investments. *Journal of Chronic Disease. 4*(2) 171–178.

Hale, C. A., Thomas, L. H., Bond, S., & Todd, C. (1997). The nursing record as a research tool to identify nursing interventions. *Journal of Clinical Nursing, 6*(3), 207–214.

Hall, L. M., Doran, D. I., Baker, G. R., Pink, G., Sidani, S., O'Brien, P., et al. (2001). A study of the impact of nursing staff mix models & organizational change strategies on patient, system & caregiver outcomes. Available at: http://www.nursing.utoronto.ca/lmcgillishall/research/nsmos%20summary%20report.pdf

Harris, C. W. (Ed.). (1963). *Problems in measuring change*. Madison: University of Wisconsin Press.

Harris, M. R., & Warren, J. J. (1995). Patient outcomes: Assessment issues for the CNS. *Clinical Nurse Specialist, 9*(2), 82–86.

Head, B. J., Maas, M., and Johnson, M. (2003). Validity and community-health-nursing sensitivity of six outcomes for community health nursing with older clients. *Public Health Nursing, 25*(5), 385–398.

Herrmann, D. (1995). Reporting current, past, and changed health status: What we know about distortion. *Medical Care, 33*(4 Suppl.), AS89–AS94.

Hinshaw, A. S. (1992). Welcome: Patient outcome research conference. In *Patient Outcomes Research: Examining the Effectiveness of Nursing Practice: Proceedings of a Conference Sponsored by the National Center for Nursing Research, September 11–13, 1991* (NIH Publication No. 93–3411). Washington, DC: U.S. Department of Health and Human Services, Public Health Service, National Institutes of Health.

Holmes, D., Teresi, J., Lindeman, D. A., & Glandon, G. L. (1997). Measurement of personal care inputs in chronic care settings. *Journal of Mental Health and Aging, 3*(1), 119–127.

Houser, J. L. (2000). *A model for evaluating the context of nursing care delivery*. Unpublished doctoral dissertation. Greeley: University of Northern Colorado.

Ingersoll, G. L., McIntosh, E., Williams, M. (2000). Nurse-sensitive outcomes of advanced practice. *Journal of Advanced Nursing, 32*(5), 1272–1281.

Irvine, D., Sidani, S., & Hall, L. M. (1998). Linking outcomes to nurses' roles in health care. *Nursing Economics, 16*(2), 58–64, 87.

Irvine, D., Sidani, S., Porter, H., O'Brien-Pallas, L., Simpson, B., Hall, L. M., et al. (2000). Organizational factors influencing nurse practitioners' role implementation in acute care settings. *Canadian Journal of Nursing Leadership, 13*(3), 28–35.

Jennings, B. M., Loan, L. A., DePaul, D., Brosch, L. R., & Hildreth, P. (2001). Lessons learned while collecting ANA indicator data. *Journal of Nursing Administration, 31*(3), 121–129.

Keeler, E. B. (1994). Decision analysis and cost-effectiveness analysis in women's health care. *Clinical Obstetrics and Gynecology, 37*(1), 207–215.

Kelly, K. C., Huber, D. G., Johnson, M., McCloskey, J. C., & Maas, M. (1994). The Medical Outcomes Study: A nursing perspective. *Journal of Professional Nursing, 10*(4), 209–216.

Kieffer, E., Alexander, G. R., & Mor, J. (1992). Area-level predictors of use of prenatal care in diverse populations. *Public Health Reports, 107*(6), 653–658.

Kirwan, J. R., Chaput de Saintonge, D. M., Joyce, C. R., Holmes, J., & Currey, H. L. F. (1986). Inability of rheumatologists to describe their true policies for assessing rheumatoid arthritis. *Annals of the Rheumatic Diseases, 45*(2), 156–161.

Kleinpell-Nowell, R., & Weiner, T. (1999). Measuring advanced practice nursing outcomes. *AACN Clinical Issues, 10*(3), 356–368.

Kozma, C. M., Reeder, C. E., & Schuiz, R. M. (1993). Economic, clinical, and humanistic outcomes: A planning model for pharmacoeromic research. *Clinical Therapeutics, 15*(6), 1125.

Lange, L. L., & Jacox, A. (1993). Using large databases in nursing and health policy research. *Journal of Professional Nursing, 9*(4), 204–211.

Lasker, R. D., Shapiro, D. W., & Tucker, A. M. (1992). Realizing the potential of practice pattern profiling. *Inquiry, 29*(3), 287–297.

Lave, J. R., Pashos, C. L., Anderson, G. F., Brailer, D., Bubloz, T., Conrad, D., et al. (1994). Costing medical care: Using Medicare administrative data. *Medical Care, 32*(7 Suppl), JS77–JS89.

Lee, T. H., & Goldman, L. (1989). Development and analysis of observational data bases. *Journal of the American College of Cardiology, 14*(3, Suppl. A), 44A–47A.

Lewis, B. E. (1995). HMO outcomes research: Lessons from the field. *Journal of Ambulatory Care Management, 18*(1), 47–55.

Lieu, T. A., & Newman, T. B. (1998). Issues in studying the effectiveness of health services for children: Improving the quality of healthcare for children. *HSR: Health Services Research, 33*(4 pt 2), 1041–1058.

Loegering, L., Reiter, R. C., & Gambone, J. C. (1994). Measuring the quality of health care. *Clinical Obstetrics and Gynecology, 37*(1), 122–136.

Ludbrook, A. (1990). Using economic appraisal in health services research. *Health Bulletin, 48*(2), 81–90.

Lynn, J., & Virnig, B. A. (1995). Assessing the significance of treatment effects: Comments from the perspective of ethics. *Medical Care, 33*(4 Suppl) AS292–AS298.

Mark, B. A. (1995). The black box of patient outcomes research. *The Journal of Nursing Scholarship, 27*(1), 42.

Mattson, M. E., & Donovan, D. M. (1994). Clinical applications: The transition from research to practice. *Journal of Studies on Alcohol, 12*(Suppl.), 163–166.

McCloskey, B., Grey, M., Deshefy-Longhi, T., & Grey, L. (2003). APRN practice patterns in primary care. *The Nurse Practitioner, 28*(4), 39–44.

McCormick, B. (1990). Outcomes in action: The JCAHO's clinical indicators. *Hospitals, 64*(19), 34–38.

McDonald, C. J., & Hui, S. L. (1991). The analysis of humongous databases: Problems and promises. *Statistics in Medicine, 10*(4), 511–518.

McNeil, B. J., Pedersen, S. H., & Gatsonis, C. (1992). Current issues in profiling quality of care. *Inquiry, 29*(3), 298–307.

Mitchell, J. B., Bubolz, T., Pail, J. E., Pashos, C. L., Escarce, J. J., Muhlbaier, L. H., et al. (1994). Using Medicare claims for outcomes research. *Medical Care, 32*(7 Suppl.), JS38–JS51.

Mitchell, P. H., Ferketich, S., Jennings, B. M., & American Academy of Nursing Expert Panel on Quality Health Care. (1998). Quality health outcomes model. *The Journal of Nursing Scholarship, 30*(1), 43–46.

Moritz, P. (1991). Innovative nursing practice models and patient outcomes. *Nursing Outlook, 39*(3), 111–114.

Moses, L. E. (1995). Measuring effects without randomized trials? Options, problems, challenges. *Medical Care, 33*(4 Suppl), AS8–AS14.

Nadzim, D. M., Turpin, R., Hanold, L. S., & White, R. E. (1993). Data-driven performance improvement in health care: The Joint Commission's Indicator Measurement System (IMSystem). *The Joint Commission Journal on Quality Improvement, 19*(11), 492–500.

Needleman, J., Buerhaus, P., Mattke, S., Stewart, M., & Zelevinsky, K. (2002a). Nurse staffing and quality of care in hospitals in the United States. *Policy, Politics, & Nursing Practice, 3*(4), 306–308.

Needleman, J., Buerhaus, Pl., Mattke, S., Steward, M., & Zelevinsky, K. (2002b). Nurse-staffing levels and the quality of care in hospitals. *The New England Journal of Medicine, 346*(22), 1715–1722.

O'Connor, G. T., Plume, S. K., & Wennberg, J. E. (1993). Regional organization for outcomes research. *Annals of the New York Academy of Sciences, 703*, 44–51.

One Hundred Sixth Congress of the United States, 1999, S. *580, An Act to Amend title IX of the Public Health Service Act to revise and extend the Agency for Health Care Policy and Research*, pp. 2–3.

Orchard, C. (1994). Comparing healthcare outcomes. *British Medical Journal, 308*(6942), 1493–1496.

Oster, G. (1988). Economic aspects of clinical decision making: Applications in patient care. *American Journal of Hospital Pharmacy, 45*(3), 543–547.

Ottenbacher, K. J., Johnson, M. B., & Hojem, M. (1988). The significance of clinical change and clinical change of significance: Issues and methods. *American Journal of Occupational Therapy, 42*(3), 156–163.

Powe, N. R., Turner, J. A., Maklan, C. W., & Ersek, M. (1994). Alternative methods for formal literature review and meta-analysis in AHCPR Patient Outcomes Research Teams. *Medical Care, 32*(7), JS22–JS37.

Power, E. J., Tunis, S. R., & Wagner, J. L. (1994). Technology assessment and public health. *Annual Review of Public Health, 15*, 561–579.

Rettig, R. (1991). History, development, and importance to nursing of outcomes research. *Journal of Nursing Quality Assurance, 5*(2), 13–17.

Riesenberg, D., & Glass, R. M. (1989). The Medical Outcomes Study. *JAMA, 262*(7), 943.

Rosenfeld, P., McEvoy, M. D., & Glassman, K. (2003). Measuring practice patterns among acute care nurse practitioners. *Journal of Nursing Administration, 33*(3), 159–165.

Rovine, M. J., & Von Eye, A. (1991). *Applied computational statistics in longitudinal research*. San Diego: Academic Press.

Rowell, P. (2001). Lessons learned while collecting ANA indicator data: The American Nurses Association responds. *Journal of Nursing Administration, 31*(3), 130–131.

Sawyer, L. M., Berkowitz, B., Haber, J. E., Larrabee, J. H., Marino, B. L., Martin, K. S., et al. (2002). Expanding American Nurses Association Nursing Quality Indicators

to community-based practices. *Outcomes Management, 6*(2), 53–61.

Schmitt, M. H., Farrell, M. P., & Heinemann, G. D. (1988). Conceptual and methodological problems in studying the effects of interdisciplinary geriatric teams. *The Gerontologist, 28*(6), 753–764.

Sidani, S., & Irvine, D. (1999). A conceptual framework for evaluating the nurse practitioner role in acute care settings. *Journal of Advanced Nursing, 30*(1), 58–66.

Sidani, S., Irvine, D., Porter, H., O'Brien-Pallas, L., Simpson, B., Hall, L. M., et al. (2000). Practice patterns of acute care nurse practitioners. *Canadian Journal of Nursing Leadership, 13*(3), 6–12.

Siegel, J. E. (1998). Cost-effectiveness analysis and nursing research—Is there a fit? *The Journal of Nursing Scholarship, 30*(3), 221–222.

Slade, M., Kuipers, E., & Priebe, S. (2002). Mental health services research methodology, *International Review of Psychiatry, 14*(1), 12–18.

Sledge, C. B. (1993). Why do outcomes research? *Orthopedics, 16*(10), 1093–1096.

Sochalski, J. (2001). Quality of care, nurse staffing, and patient outcomes. *Policy, Politics, & Nursing Practice, 2*(1), 9–18.

Sonnenberg, F. A., Roberts, M. S., Tsevat, J., Wong, J. B., Barry, M., & Kent, D. L. (1994). Toward a peer review process for medical decision analysis models. *Medical Care, 32*(7), JS52–JS64.

Standing, T., Anthony, M. K., & Hertz, J. E. (2001). Nurses' narratives of outcomes after delegation to unlicensed assistive personnel, *Outcomes Management for Nursing Practice, 5*(1), 18–23.

Steinwachs, D. M., Weiner, J. P., & Shapiro, S. (1989). Management information systems and quality. In N. Goldfield & D.B. Nash (Eds.). *Providing quality care: The challenge to clinicians* (pp. 160–180). Philadelphia: ACP.

Stetler, C., & DeZell, A. D. (Contributors) (1989). In M. L. Etheredge (Ed.), *Collaborative care: Nursing case management* (pp. 67–77). Chicago: American Hospital Association.

Stetler, C., Morsi, D., & Burns, M. (2000). Physical and emotional patient safety: A different look at nursing-sensitive outcomes. *Outcomes Management for Nursing Practice, 4*(4), 159–166.

Stewart, A. L., Greenfield, S., Hays, R. D., Wells, K., Rogers, W. H., Berry, S. D., et al. (1989). Functional status and well-being of patients with chronic conditions. Results from the Medical Outcomes Study. *JAMA, 262*(7), 907–913.

Stone, P. W. (1998). Methods for conducting and reporting cost-effectiveness analysis in nursing. *The Journal of Nursing Scholarship, 30*(3), 229–234.

Swaen, G. M., & Meijers, J. M. (1988). Influence of design characteristics on the outcome of retrospective cohort studies. *British Journal of Industrial Medicine, 45*(9), 624–629.

Tanenbaum, S. J. (1994). Knowing and acting in medical practice: The epistemological politics of outcomes research. *Journal of Health Politics, Policy and Law, 19*(1), 27–44.

Temple, R. (1990). Problems in the use of large data sets to assess effectiveness. *International Journal of Technology Assessment in Health Care, 6*(2), 211–219.

Tengs, T. O., Adams, M. E., Pliskin, J. S., Safran, D. G., Siegel, J. E., Weinstein, M. C., et al. (1995). Five hundred life-saving interventions and their cost-effectiveness. *Risk Analysis, 15*(3), 369–390.

Tidwell, S. L. (1993). A graphic tool for tracking variance & comorbidities in cardiac surgery case management. *Progress in Cardiovascular Nursing, 8*(2), 6–19.

Turk, D. C., & Rudy, T. E. (1994). Methods for evaluating treatment outcomes: Ways to overcome potential obstacles. *Spine, 19*(15), 1759–1763.

Unsworth, C. A. (2001). Using a head-mounted video camera to study clinical reasoning. *The American Journal of Occupational Therapy, 55*(5), 582–588.

U.S. Congress, Office of Technology Assessment. (1994). *Identifying health technologies that work: Searching for evidence* (Publication No. OTA-H-608). Washington, DC: U.S. Government Printing Office.

Veatch, R. M. (1993). Justice and outcomes research: The ethical limits. *The Journal of Clinical Ethics, 4*(3), 258–261.

Vermeulen, L. C., Jr., Ratko, T. A., Erstad, B. L., Brecher, M. E., & Matuszewski, K. A. (1995). A paradigm for consensus: The University Hospital Consortium Guidelines for the use of albumin, nonprotein colloid, and crystalloid solutions. *Archives of Internal Medicine, 155*(4), 373–379.

Verran, J. A., Mark, B. A., & Lamb, G. (1992). Psychometric examination of instruments using aggregated data. *Research in Nursing & Health, 15*(3), 237–240.

Vivier, P. M., Bernier, J. A., and Starfield, B. (1994). Current approaches to measuring health outcomes in pediatric research. *Current Opinions in Pediatrics, 6*(5), 531.

Volinn, E., Diehr, P., Ciol, M. A., & Loeser, J. D. (1994). Why does geographic variation in health care practices matter? (and seven questions to ask in evaluating studies on geographic variation). *Spine, 19*(18S), 2092S–2100S.

Von Eye, A. (Ed.). (1990a). *Statistical methods in longitudinal research, Vol. I: Principles and structuring change*. Boston: Academic Press.

Von Eye, A. (Ed.). (1990b). *Statistical methods in longitudinal research, Vol. II: Time series and categorical longitudinal data.* Boston: Academic Press.

Von Korff, M., Koepsell, T., Curry, S., & Diehr, P. (1992). Multi-level analysis in epidemiologic research on health behaviors and outcomes. *American Journal of Epidemiology, 135*(10), 1077–1082.

Wennberg, J. E., Barry, M. J., Fowler, F. J., & Mulley, A. (1993). Outcomes research, PORTs, and health care reform. *Annals of the New York Academy of Sciences, 703*, 52–62.

Werley, H., Devine, E., Zorn, C., Ryan, P., & Westra, B. (1991). The nursing minimum data set: Abstraction tool for standardized, comparable, essential data. *American Journal of Public Health, 81*(4), 421–426.

Werley, H., & Lang, N. (1988). *Identification of the nursing minimum data set*. New York: Springer.

White, K. L. (1993). Health care research: Old wine in new bottles. *The Pharos of Alpha Omega Alpha Honor Medical Society, 56*(3), 12–16.

Wilson, I. B., & Cleary, P. D. (1995). Linking clinical variables with health-related quality of life: A conceptual model of patient outcomes. *Journal of the American Medical Association, 273*(1), 60. Copyright 1995, the American Medical Association.

Wood, L. W. (1990). Medical treatment effectiveness research. *Journal of Occupational Medicine, 32*(12), 1173–1174.

Wray, N. P., Ashton, C. M., Kuykendall, D. H., Petersen, N. J., Souchek, J., & Hollingsworth, J. C. (1995). Selecting disease-outcome pairs for monitoring the quality of hospital care. *Medical Care, 33*(1), 75–89.

Zielstorff, R., Hudgings, C., Grobe, S., & the National Commission on Nursing Implementation Project (NCNIP) Task Force on Nursing Information Systems. (1993). *Next generation nursing information systems: Essential characteristics for professional practice*. Washington, DC: American Nurses Association.

Populations and Samples

Chapter Overview

Learning Outcomes

After completing this chapter, you should be able to:

1. Describe sampling theory, including the concepts of sample, population, subject, target population, sampling criteria, sampling frame, sampling plan, representativeness, sampling error, and systematic bias.

2. Critique the sampling criteria (inclusion and exclusion criteria) used in published studies.

3. Identify the specific type of probability and nonprobability sampling methods used in

published quantitative, qualitative, and outcomes studies.

4. Identify the elements of power analysis in a published quantitative study.

5. Critique the sample size of published quantitative and qualitative studies.

6. Critique the settings used in published quantitative, qualitative, and outcomes studies.

Key Terms

STUDY TOOLS

Be sure to visit http://evolve.elsevier.com/Burns/understanding for additional examples and self-tests. Also, a review of this chapter's concepts and practice exercises can be found in Chapter 10 of the Study Guide for *Understanding Nursing Research: Building an Evidence-Based Practice*, 4th edition.

Students often enter the field of research with preconceived notions about samples and sampling. Many of these notions are acquired through exposure to television advertisements, public opinion polls, market researchers in shopping centers, and newspaper reports of research findings. A television commercial boasts that four of five doctors recommend a particular pain medication; a newscaster announces that John Jones is predicted to win the senate election by a margin of 10%; and a newspaper reports that research has shown that aggressive treatment of hypertension to maintain a blood pressure of 120/80 mm Hg or lower significantly reduces the risk for stroke.

All of these examples include a type of sampling technique. Some of the outcomes from these studies are more valid than others, because of the techniques used to obtain the samples. Thus, when critiquing a study, you must identify the sampling method used and evaluate it for quality. The sample usually is described in the "Methods" section of a published research report. To judge the quality of a sample, you need an understanding of the principles of sampling theory, the types of sampling methods used in research, and the sample size.

This chapter presents the concepts of sampling theory including sampling criteria, sampling frame, and representativeness of a sample. The nonprobability and probability sampling plans or methods and sample size for quantitative and qualitative studies are detailed. The chapter concludes with a discussion of the natural, partially controlled, and highly controlled settings used for conducting research.

Sampling Theory

Sampling involves selecting a group of people, events, behaviors, or other elements with which to conduct a study. A **sampling plan**, or sampling method, defines the selection process, and the **sample** defines the selected group of people (or elements). Samples are expected to represent a population of people. The population might be all people who have diabetes, all patients who have had abdominal surgery, or all persons who receive care from a registered nurse. In most cases, however, it would be impossible for a researcher to study an entire population. Sampling theory was developed to determine the most effective way to acquire a sample that accurately reflects the population under study. Key concepts of sampling theory include elements, populations, sampling or eligibility criteria, representativeness, sampling frames, and sampling plans. This section explains these concepts.

Elements and Populations

An individual unit of a population is called an **element**. An element can be a person, event, experience, behavior, or any other single unit of a study. The element of a study may be the experience of coping with terminal illness or the event of managing health needs following a hurricane disaster. When elements are persons, they are referred to as **subjects**. For example, the subjects may be patients with hypertension who are seen in primary care clinics. The sample is selected to represent the population of hypertensive patients. The **population**, sometimes referred to as the **target population**, is the entire set of persons (or elements) who (or that) meet the sampling criteria (defined in the next section). The sample criteria might be that the subjects are adults 18 years of age, able to read and write English, and a new diagnosis of hypertension in the past 3 months. An **accessible population** is the portion of the target population to which the researcher has reasonable access. The accessible population for this example may be all hypertensive patients seen in primary care clinics within a city, a section of a city, or one clinic.

Researchers obtain a sample from the accessible population, and generalize findings to the target population. **Generalization** extends the findings from the sample under study to the larger population. The extent of the generalization is influenced by the quality of the study and the consistency of the study's findings with the findings from previous research in this area. If a study is of high quality, with findings that are consistent with previous research, then the researchers can be confident in generalizing their findings to the target population. For example, the findings from the study of hypertensive patients in one clinic may be generalized to the target population of all adult patients with hypertension seen in primary care clinics. With this information, a nurse can decide whether it is appropriate to use this evidence in caring for the same type of patients.

Sampling or Eligibility Criteria

Sampling criteria, also referred to as eligibility criteria, include the list of characteristics essential for eligibility or membership in the target population. For example, researchers may choose to study the effect of preoperative teaching on the outcome length of hospital stay after abdominal surgery. In this study the sampling criteria may include (1) age of at least

18 years, (2) ability to speak and read English at the sixth-grade level, (3) absence of history of previous surgeries, and (4) absence of cognitive problems. The sample is selected from the accessible population that meets these sampling criteria. Sampling criteria for a study may consist of inclusion or exclusion sampling criteria, or both. **Inclusion sampling criteria** are the characteristics that the subject or element must possess to be part of the target population. In the example, the inclusion criteria are age older than 18 years and ability to speak and read English at the sixth-grade level. **Exclusion sampling criteria** are those characteristics that can cause a person or element to be excluded from the target population. For example, any subjects with a history of previous surgery or any cognitive problems will be excluded from the preoperative teaching study.

When the study is completed, the findings are generalized from the sample to the target population that meets the sampling criteria. The researcher may narrowly define the sampling criteria to make the sample as **homogeneous** (or similar) as possible or to control for extraneous variables. Conversely, the researcher may broadly define the criteria to ensure that the study sample is **heterogeneous**, with a broad range of values or scores on the variables being studied. If the sampling or eligibility criteria are too narrow and restrictive, the researcher may have difficulty finding subjects who meet the criteria and may not be able to obtain a sufficiently large sample from the accessible population.

In discussing the generalization of findings in a published research report, investigators sometimes attempt to generalize beyond the sampling criteria. The researcher may contend that the sample was limited by the sampling criteria only for convenience in conducting the study but that the findings really apply to a larger population. Using the example preoperative teaching study, the sample may need to be limited to subjects who speak and read English because the preoperative teaching is performed in English and because one of the measurement instruments requires that subjects be able to read English at the sixth-grade level. However, the researcher may believe that the findings can be generalized to non–English-speaking persons. Practicing nurses need to consider carefully the implications of using these findings with non–English-speaking populations. Perhaps such persons, because they come from another culture, do not respond to the teaching in the same way as that observed in the study population.

Generalizing to people unable to read English at the sixth-grade level also may be inappropriate. Poorly educated people, for example, may respond differently than other groups to the preoperative teaching. Subjects unable to read at the sixth-grade level may not be able to read or comprehend written material. They may be reluctant to ask questions when they do not understand something. Many of them may have difficulty organizing their ideas and be unable to express them to another person. They may try to conceal their lack of understanding, making it difficult to clarify misconceptions. Thus, the preoperative teaching program developed for a more educated population may be unlikely to alter the postoperative outcome or length of hospital stay of members of a poorly educated population.

For this study, the population also is limited to patients who have had no previous surgery, because such persons will have the least knowledge of the postoperative experience and how they can best care for themselves. To test differences among groups, the most extreme groups are selected so that the differences are as great as possible, and the statistical procedures are most likely to determine a difference. In this hypothetical study, one group receives standard care, or the small amount of teaching the hospital routinely provides, and the other group receives the treatment. In the treatment group, the researchers can control the subjects' knowledge about how to take care of themselves after surgery by providing the information through a structured preoperative teaching program. The researchers hypothesize that the subjects will use the information to take better care of themselves after surgery, resulting in a shorter hospital stay.

However, the researchers may argue that the findings can be generalized to patients who have had previous surgeries. The effect of the preoperative teaching on patients with past surgical experience may be less than the effect on subjects without past surgical experience, because experienced patients may already know some of the information taught. However, the experienced patients also may be able to use the information to take better care of themselves after surgery and thereby shorten their hospital stay. Therefore, the researchers' claim that the findings can be generalized to patients who have had previous surgery may be justified. However, researchers need to be very cautious not to generalize beyond their sampling criteria, unless a sound rationale for this application can be established on the basis of findings from previous research.

RESEARCH EXAMPLE   Inclusion and Exclusion Sampling Criteria

Simpson and James (2005) studied the effects of immediate versus delayed pushing during second-stage labor on fetal well-being and defined their sampling or eligibility criteria as follows:

Criteria for study inclusion were healthy nulliparous women at term (≥37 weeks' gestation based on last menstrual period and/or early second trimester ultrasound) in the second stage of labor with a singleton fetus in a vertex presentation who were having an elective induction of labor...[and who] had epidural anesthesia providing adequate pain relief...and a reassuring FHR [fetal heart rate] pattern at the time of enrollment. Women with medical or obstetrical complications or a maternal condition that could potentially influence oxygen saturation including history of smoking, asthma, chronic or acute pulmonary or cardiac diseases were excluded. (Simpson & James, 2005, p. 152)

CRITIQUE

Simpson and James (2005) identified specific inclusion and exclusion sampling criteria to precisely designate the subjects in the target population. These sampling criteria probably were narrowly defined by the researchers to promote the selection of a homogeneous sample of healthy pregnant women in their second stage of labor. The researchers also indicated that they limited their sample to nulliparous women because they have a more predictable length of second-stage labor than do multiparous women. The exclusion criteria (medical or obstetrical complications or maternal conditions that may influence oxygen saturation, including history of smoking, asthma, chronic or acute pulmonary diseases, and cardiac diseases) reduced the extraneous variables that might have influenced the oxygen saturation of the fetus. The variable oxygen saturation was measured to indicate fetal well-being. This is a quasi-experimental study that examined the impact of the treatment, delayed pushing, on fetal well-being. Use of increased controls within the study greatly strengthened the likelihood that the study outcome was caused by the treatment and not by extraneous variables.

IMPLICATIONS FOR PRACTICE

The findings from this study suggest that women who delay pushing during their second stage of labor until the urge to push is strong produce a more favorable physiologic fetal well-being, as measured by the fetal oxygen status during labor, than the traditional pushing immediately at 10 centimeters of dilation (Simpson & James, 2005). This study finding can be combined with the findings from previous research to provide evidenced-based care to women during their second stage of labor to improve fetal outcomes.

Representativeness

Representativeness means that the sample, the accessible population, and the target population are alike in as many ways as possible. Representativeness needs to be evaluated in terms of the setting, characteristics of the subjects, and distribution of values on variables measured in the study. Persons seeking care in a particular setting may be different from those who seek care for the same problem in other settings or from those who choose to use self-care to manage their problems. The setting can influence representativeness in a variety of ways. Studies conducted in private hospitals usually exclude the poor. Other settings may exclude older adults or the undereducated. People who do not have access to care are usually excluded from studies. Subjects in research centers and the care they receive are different from patients and the care they receive in community hospitals, public hospitals, veterans' hospitals, or rural hospitals. People living in rural settings may respond differently to a health situation from those who live in urban settings. Obese persons who choose to enter a program to lose weight may differ from those who do not enter such a program. Thus, gathering subjects across a variety of settings provides a more representative sample of the target population than that obtainable by limiting the study to a single setting.

A sample must be representative in terms of characteristics such as age, gender, ethnicity, income, and education, which often influence study variables. These are examples of demographic or attribute variables that might be selected by researchers for examination in their study. Researchers analyze data collected on the demographic variables to produce the sample characteristics—characteristics used to provide a picture of the sample. The sample characteristics in the preoperative teaching study, for example, may be that the mean age of the subjects is 55 years ($SD = 5.6$), a majority of the subjects are female (65%), and they have varied ethnic backgrounds (45% Caucasian, 25% African American, 23% Hispanic, and 7% Asian). The sample characteristics must be reasonably representative of the characteristics of the population. If the study includes groups, the subjects in the groups must have comparable demographic characteristics. Chapter 4 contains a more detailed discussion of demographic variables and sample characteristics.

The sample also needs to be representative relative to the variables being examined in the study. For example, if the study examines attitudes toward acquired immunodeficiency syndrome (AIDS), the sample must be representative of the distribution of attitudes toward AIDS that exist in the specified population. If a study involves blood pressures of patients in a surgical recovery room, the blood pressures of subjects must be representative of those usually noted in a surgical recovery unit.

Measurement values also need to be representative. Measurement values in a study are expected to vary randomly among subjects. **Random variation** is the expected difference in values that occurs when different subjects from the same sample are examined. The difference is random because some values will be higher and others lower than the average (mean) population value. As sample size increases, random variation decreases, improving representativeness.

Systematic variation, or systematic bias—a serious concern in sampling—is a consequence of selecting subjects whose measurement values differ in some specific way from those of the population. This difference usually is expressed as a difference in the average (or mean) values between the sample and the population. Because the subjects have something in common, their values tend to be similar to those of others in the sample but different in some way from those of the population as a whole. These values do not vary randomly around the population mean. Most of the variation from the mean is in the same direction; it is systematic. For example, the sample mean may be higher than the mean of the target population. Increasing the sample size has no effect on systematic variation. For example, if all of the subjects in a study examining some type of knowledge have an intelligence quotient (IQ) above 120, then all of their test scores in the study are likely to be higher than those of the population mean that includes people with a wide variation in IQ scores (but with a mean IQ of 100). The IQs of the subjects will introduce a systematic bias. When a systematic bias occurs in an experimental study, it can lead the researcher to think that the treatment has made a difference, when in actuality the values would have been different even without the treatment.

The probability of systematic variation increases when the sampling process is not random. Even in a random sample, however, systematic variation can occur when a large number of the potential subjects declines participation. As the number of subjects declining participation increases, the possibility of a systematic bias in the study becomes greater. In published studies, researchers may identify a **refusal rate**, which is the percentage of subjects who declined to participate in the study, and the subjects' reasons for not participating. Other studies record an **acceptance rate**, which is the percentage of subjects consenting to participate in a study. The acceptance rate is calculated by dividing the number of subjects consenting to participate in a study by the number of subjects approached and multiplying that answer by 100%. For example, if 80 potential subjects are approached to participate in the hypothetical study about the effects of preoperative teaching and 76 patients accept, then

$$\text{Acceptance rate} = 76 \div 80 = 0.95 \times 100\% = 95\%$$

The refusal rate is calculated by dividing the number refusing to participate in a study by the number of potential subjects approached and then multiplying that answer by 100%. In the hypothetical preoperative teaching study, 76 of 80 potential subjects consented to participate—so 4 refused. Plugging these numbers into the stated formula gives

$$\text{Refusal rate} = 4 \div 80 = 0.05 \times 100\% = 5\%$$

The refusal rate also can be calculated as follows: 100% − acceptance rate = refusal rate, or 100% − 95% = 5%. In this example, the refusal rate is low, only 5%, so the chance for systematic variation is less, and the sample is more representative of the target population.

Systematic variation also may occur in studies with high sample mortality, or attrition. **Sample mortality** is the withdrawal or loss of subjects from a study. Systematic variation is greatest when a large number of subjects withdraw from the study before data collection is completed or when a large number of subjects withdraw from one group but not the other(s) in the study. In studies involving a treatment, subjects in the comparison group who do not receive the treatment may be more likely to withdraw from the study. Sample mortality or attrition must be reported in the published study. For example, in the hypothetical study of preoperative teaching, 31 subjects—12 from the treatment group and 19 from the comparison group—may withdraw, for various reasons. Loss of 31 subjects means a 40.79% sample mortality rate ($31 \div 76 \times 100\%$), with much higher withdrawal rate in the comparison group than in the treatment group. The overall sample mortality rate was considerable (greater than 40%), and the rates differed for the two groups to which the subjects were assigned—both of which increase the potential for systematic variation and result in a sample less representative of the target population.

RESEARCH EXAMPLE   Refusal Rate and Sample Mortality

Simpson and James (2005), in their study of the effects of immediate versus delayed pushing on fetal well-being, indicated that 60 women were eligible for participation in the study. Four of the 60 women declined to participate, resulting in a 6.7% ($4 \div 60 = 0.0667 \times 100\%$) refusal rate, or a 93.3% acceptance rate, for the study. In addition, 56 women consented to participate in the study while in early labor. However, 11 of these subjects required cesarean delivery before reaching the second stage of labor. Thus, the sample mortality rate for the original sample was 19.6% ($11 \div 56 = 0.196 \times 100\%$). Of the 45 subjects who remained in the study, 22 were assigned to the immediate pushing group (comparison group) and 23 to the delayed pushing group (treatment or experimental group). These 45 subjects completed the study, with no withdrawal once they were assigned to groups.

CRITIQUE

In this study (Simpson & James, 2005), the refusal rate was small, only 6.7% (4 women), but the researchers did not specify reasons for refusal to participate in the study. However, 2 of the 4 women who refused to participate later required cesarean delivery and would have not been included in the final sample. The sample mortality rate for this group of women was high at 19.6%, so that only a very small number of subjects were assigned to either the treatment or the comparison group. However, a strength of the study is that all 45 subjects who were assigned to the treatment and the comparison groups finished the study. The small refusal rate and the equal group sizes at the end of the study decreased the potential for systematic variation, but the large sample mortality rate of 19.6% associated with cesarean delivery increased the potential for systematic variation. Thus, the study results obtained from this sample probably are less representative than those for the target population.

IMPLICATIONS FOR PRACTICE

According to the key study findings, delayed pushing is more protective of fetal well-being than is immediate pushing during second-stage labor. However, the small sample size resulting from the refusal rate and sample mortality rate means that additional studies are needed with larger samples, to develop sound evidence for making decisions about pushing during the second stage of labor.

Random Sampling

From a sampling theory perspective, each person or other element in the population should have an opportunity to be selected for the sample. One method of providing this opportunity is referred to as **random sampling**. The purpose of random sampling is to increase the extent to which the sample is representative of the target population. However, random sampling must take place in an accessible population that is representative of the target population. It is rarely possible to obtain a random sample for clinical nursing studies because of informed consent requirements. People who volunteer to participate in a study may differ in important ways from those not willing to participate. (Methods of achieving random samples are described later in the chapter.) The use of the term **control group** is limited to those studies using random sampling methods. If nonrandom methods are used for sample selection, the group not receiving a treatment is referred to as a **comparison group** because there is an increased possibility of preexisting differences between the experimental and comparison groups. In addition, the subjects in the control group receive no intervention, where as the subjects in the comparison group usually receive standard care provided for a condition and the experimental group receives the treatment adding to the preexisting differences between the two groups.

Sampling Frames

For everyone in the accessible population to have an opportunity for selection in the sample, each person in the population must be identified. To accomplish this, a list of every member of the population must be acquired, using the sampling criteria to define eligibility. This list is referred to as the **sampling frame**. Subjects are then selected from the sampling frame using a sampling plan. In some studies the sampling frame cannot be identified, because it is not possible to list all members of the population.

Sampling Plans

A **sampling plan** or method outlines strategies used to obtain a sample for a study. Like a design, a sampling plan is not specific to a study. The plan is designed to increase representativeness and decrease systematic variation or bias. The sampling plan may use probability (random) or nonprobability (nonrandom) sampling methods. When critiquing a study, identify the study sampling plan as either probability or nonprobability, and determine the specific method used to select a sample. The different types of probability and nonprobability sampling methods are introduced next.

Probability Sampling Methods

Probability sampling methods have been developed to increase the representativeness of the sample. In **probability sampling**, every member (element) of the population has a probability higher than zero of being selected for the sample. To achieve this probability, the sample is obtained randomly. All the subsets of the population, which may differ from each other but contribute to the parameters (such as the mean and standard deviation) of the population, have a chance to be represented in the sample. The opportunity for systematic bias is less

Table 10–1	Probability and Nonprobability Sampling Methods	
Sampling Method	**Common Application(s)**
Probability	
Simple random sampling	Quantitative research
Stratified random sampling	Quantitative research
Cluster sampling	Quantitative research
Systematic sampling	Quantitative research
Nonprobability	
Convenience sampling	Quantitative and qualitative research
Quota sampling	Quantitative and rarely qualitative research
Purpose sampling	Qualitative and sometimes quantitative research
Network sampling	Qualitative and sometimes quantitative research
Theoretical sampling	Qualitative research

when subjects are selected randomly, although it is possible for a systematic bias to occur by chance.

Without random sampling strategies, the researcher, who has a vested interest in the study, will tend (consciously or unconsciously) to select subjects whose conditions or behaviors are consistent with the study hypotheses. The researcher may decide that person X is a better subject for the study than person Y. As another possibility, the researcher may exclude a subset of people because he or she does not agree with them, does not like them, or finds them hard to deal with. Potential subjects may be excluded because they are too sick, not sick enough, coping too well, not coping adequately, uncooperative, or noncompliant. By using random sampling, however, researchers leave the selection to chance, thereby increasing the validity of their studies.

Four sampling designs have been developed to achieve probability sampling: simple random sampling, stratified random sampling, cluster sampling, and systematic sampling (Table 10-1). Probability sampling methods are used more often in quantitative research and outcomes research than in qualitative research.

Simple Random Sampling

Simple random sampling is the most basic of the probability sampling plans, and it is achieved by randomly selecting elements from the sampling frame. Random selection can be accomplished in a variety of ways, limited only by the imagination of the researcher. If the sampling frame is small, names can be written on slips of paper, which are then placed in a container, mixed well, and then drawn out one at a time until the desired sample size has been reached. The most common method for randomly selecting subjects for a study is use of a computer program. The sampling frame can be entered into a computer, and then subjects can be randomly selected by the computer until the desired sample size is achieved.

Another method for randomly selecting a study sample is use of a table of random numbers. Table 10-2 displays a section from a random numbers table. To use a table of

Table 10–2		Section from a Random Numbers Table							
06	84	10	22	56	72	25	70	69	43
07	63	10	34	66	39	54	02	33	85
03	19	63	93	72	52	13	30	44	40
77	32	69	58	25	15	55	38	19	62
20	01	94	54	66	88	43	91	34	28

random numbers, the researcher places a pencil or finger on the table with eyes closed. That number is the starting place. Then, by moving the pencil or finger up, down, right, or left, numbers are identified in order until the desired sample size is obtained. Table 10-2 can be used in the following way to select 5 subjects from a population of 100. If the pencil is initially placed on 58 in the table, which is the entry in the fourth column from the left and in the fourth row down, and then moved across the columns to the right, the subject numbers are 58, 25, 15, 55, and 38. Table 10-2 is useful only when the population number is less than 100. Full tables of random numbers are available in other sources (e.g., Burns & Grove, 2005, Appendix A).

RESEARCH EXAMPLE Simple Random Sampling

Manojlovich (2005) used simple random sampling to study how certain environmental factors and personal characteristics could be used to predict professional nursing practice behaviors in hospital settings. She described her sampling method as follows.

The sample consisted of 500 nurses randomly selected from a list of 1,509 names provided by the Michigan Nurses Association (MNA). A list of medical-surgical nurses was specified from the MNA to achieve a more homogeneous sample. Of the 365 individuals who responded, 308 provided usable surveys and demographic information and signed informed consent forms. Ten of the 308 surveys were completed by nurses who did not work in hospitals. These 10 cases were dropped from the sample, because the study purpose was to investigate the effect of environmental and personal influences on hospital nurses only. To achieve further sample homogeneity, managers, supervisors, and nursing faculty were not included in the final sample; thus, an additional 32 cases were dropped. (Manojlovich, 2005, p. 43)

CRITIQUE

The sampling frame was a list of all medical-surgical nurses in the state of Michigan provided by the MNA. The list included 1,509 names, from which 500 nurses were selected for surveying. A total of 365 subjects responded to the survey for a 73% return rate, which is very high for surveys. However, only 308 of the surveys were complete, reducing the response rate to 61.6% (308 ÷ 500 = .616 × 100% = 61.6%). Manojlovich (2005) made the study sample more homogeneous by omitting the 10 nurses who did not work in a hospital and the 32 nurses who were managers or faculty members. A homogeneous sample decreases the influence of extraneous variables and increases the focus on the purpose of the study. The sampling method was random, resulting in a strong sample size of 266 nurses. The researcher used a strong random sampling method, identified a complete sampling frame, obtained a strong response rate to surveys of 61.6%, selected a homogeneous sample, and included 266 subjects in the study. These aspects of the sample indicate only limited potential for systematic variation or bias, which increases the likelihood that the study sample is representative of the accessible and target populations.

IMPLICATIONS FOR PRACTICE

Manojlovich (2005) found that nurses

…may practice more professionally when the environment provides opportunities and power through resources, support, and information. Self-efficacy may contribute to professional practice behaviors, especially in an environment that has the requisite factors that provide empowerment. (p. 41)

On one hand, organizational changes to improve the hospital work environment for nursing practice may be simplified by using structural empowerment as a blueprint for improvement. On the other hand, it may be that the impetus for a satisfactory work environment has to be initiated by staff nurses, rather than by hospital administrators. (p. 46)

Additional research is needed in this area but the importance of structural empowerment is described in this study and provides a basis for making productive changes in hospitals' work environments. Also nurses need to have a more active role in promoting satisfactory work environments.

Stratified Random Sampling

Stratified random sampling is used in situations in which the researcher knows some of the variables in the population that are critical for achieving representativeness. Variables commonly used for stratification include age, gender, ethnicity, socioeconomic status, diagnosis, geographical region, type of institution, type of care, type of registered nurse, nursing area of specialization, and site of care. Stratification ensures that all levels of the identified variables are adequately represented in the sample. With stratification, the researcher can use a smaller sample size to achieve the same degree of representativeness relative to the stratified variable than can be derived for a large sample acquired through simple random sampling. One disadvantage is that a large population must be available from which to select subjects.

If the researcher has used stratification, categories (strata) of the variables selected for stratification must be defined in the published report. For example, using ethnicity for stratification, the researcher may define four strata: Caucasian, African American, Mexican American, and other. The population may be 60% Caucasian, 20% African American, 15% Hispanic, and 5% other. The researcher may select a random sample for each stratum equivalent to the target population proportions of that stratum. Alternatively, equal numbers of subjects may be randomly selected for each stratum. For example, if age is used to stratify a sample of 100 subjects, the researcher may obtain 25 subjects 8 to 34 years of age, 25 subjects 35 to 50 years of age, 25 subjects 51 to 66 years of age, and 25 subjects older than 66 years of age.

RESEARCH EXAMPLE Stratified Random Sampling

Ulrich, Soeken, and Miller (2003) used a stratified random sampling method to obtain their sample of nurse practitioners (NPs) to examine their ethical conflict associated with managed care. The following excerpt from this study described the sampling method used to obtain the final sample of 254 NPs.

> Following Institutional Review Board approval, a stratified random sample of 700 NPs licensed and certified to practice in the state of Maryland listed in the primary care specialties of Family Health, Pediatrics, Obstetrics/Gynecology, and Adult Health was selected from the Maryland State Board of Nursing. The NPs who were no longer practicing, practicing less than 20 hours per week, had no direct or indirect affiliation with managed care, or had a lack of forwarding address or insufficient mailing address were excluded. Responses were obtained from 254 of the 585 (43%) subjects eligible to participate. This response rate is consistent with studies that directly focus on ethical issues in healthcare, with response rates ranging from slightly greater than 30% to over 70%. (Ulrich et al., 2003, p. 170)

CRITIQUE

The study sampling frame listing all NPs practicing in Maryland was obtained from the Board of Nurse Examiners for that state. The sample was stratified by areas of specialty practice, including family, pediatrics, obstetrics/gynecology, and adult. The sample is likely to be representative of the target population because of the large size of the sample ($N = 254$) and the adequate response rate (43%) for this type of survey research.

IMPLICATIONS FOR PRACTICE

The study findings indicate that NPs are experiencing an ethical conflict when practicing in a managed care environment. The NPs are conflicted by their commitment to quality patient care and the goals of managed care. The NPs in the study indicated that sometimes they had to ignore their clinical judgment and follow the insurance guidelines regarding patient care (Ulrich et al., 2003). The goals of managed care do limit the practice of NPs to illness management with limited time for health promotion and illness prevention. So additional research is needed to identify health care delivery models that might improve the work environment of NPs and expand their role in health promotion and illness prevention, which could ultimately decreased health care costs.

Cluster Sampling

In **cluster sampling**, a researcher develops a sampling frame that includes a list of all the states, cities, institutions, or organizations with which elements of the identified population can be linked. A randomized sample of these states, cities, institutions, or organizations can then be used in the study. In some cases, this randomized selection continues through several stages and is then referred to as multistage sampling. For example, the researcher may first randomly select states and then randomly select cities within the sampled states. Next, hospitals within the randomly selected cities may be randomly selected. Within the hospitals, nursing units may be randomly selected. At this level, all of the patients on the nursing unit who fit the criteria for the study may be included, or patients can be randomly selected.

Cluster sampling is used in two types of research situations. In the first such situation, the researcher considers it necessary to obtain a geographically dispersed sample but recognizes that obtaining a simple random sample will require too much travel time and expense. In the second, the researcher cannot identify the individual elements making up the population and therefore cannot develop a sampling frame. For example, a list of all people in the United States who have had open-heart surgery does not exist. Nevertheless, it often is possible to obtain lists of institutions or organizations with which the elements of interest are associated—in this example, perhaps cardiology clinics and/or university medical centers with large, well-funded cardiology departments—and then randomly select institutions from which subjects may be acquired.

RESEARCH EXAMPLE Cluster Sampling

Golding (1996) used multistage probability sampling in her study "Sexual Assault History and Limitations in Physical Functioning in Two General Population Samples." The following excerpt describes her use of a cluster sampling technique to identify adults in mental health catchment areas in Los Angeles and North Carolina.

> Respondents were selected using multistage area probability sampling from household residents 18 years of age and older at each site. The Los Angeles sample was selected to represent adults in two mental health catchment areas in Los Angeles County, one of which was 83% Latino and the other 21% Latino. The Latino residents were largely of Mexican cultural or ethnic origin.... The North Carolina sample was selected to represent adults in two mental health catchment areas in North Carolina, one consisting of Durham County, which is primarily urban, and the other four contiguous rural counties. (Golding, 1996, p. 34)

CRITIQUE

The author used pooled data obtained from two sites of a five-site program initiated by the National Institute of Mental Health (NIMH). Information provided about the sampling method is sparse. The researcher does not provide a rationale for the use of multistage sampling or reasons for choosing the selected sites. Although the author indicates that this is a probability sample, she does not indicate how the sites or subjects were randomly chosen. The original study may have intentionally chosen one area with a large Hispanic population, but no mention is made of a similar effort to include other minority groups. Evidently, an effort also was made to include both urban and rural sites. The available information is insufficient to judge the adequacy of the sampling plan.

IMPLICATIONS FOR PRACTICE

The researchers found that physical symptoms are associated with sexual assault and are related to impairment in physical functioning.

Clinically, it is important to recognize that sexual assault history may contribute to a pattern of multiple symptoms associated with functional limitations. Primary care settings are key locations for

(continues)

IMPLICATIONS FOR PRACTICE *(continued)*

intervention with affected patients, and nurse practitioners are qualified to assess past and recent sexual assault history. (Golding, 1996, p. 42)

This study provides important evidence that supports the need for a comprehensive history to determine patient problems. With a detailed history, individuals who have experienced sexual assaults in their lives might be recognized and provided appropriate interventions. However, this study does have some weaknesses and limited research has been conducted in this area so additional study is needed to generate evidence for the assessment, diagnosis and management of individuals with a history of sexual assault.

Systematic Sampling

Systematic sampling can be conducted when an ordered list of all members of the population is available. The process involves selecting every kth individual on the list, using a starting point selected randomly. If the initial starting point is not random, the sample is not a probability sample. To use this design, the researcher must know the number of elements in the population and the size of the sample desired. The population size is divided by the desired sample size, giving k, the size of the gap between elements selected from the list. For example, if the population size is $N = 1200$ and the desired sample size is $n = 100$, then $k = 12$. Every 12th person on the list would be included in the sample. This value is obtained by using the following formula: k = population size ÷ by the desired sample size = $1200 ÷ 100 = 12$. Some argue that this procedure does not truly give each element of a population an opportunity to be included in the sample; it provides a random but not equal chance for inclusion.

RESEARCH EXAMPLE   Systematic Sampling

Rambur, McIntosh, Val Palumbo, and Reinier (2005) conducted a comparative descriptive study of job satisfaction and career retention in two groups of registered nurses (RNs) whose highest degrees were the associate degree in nursing (ADN) or the bachelor's degree in nursing (BSN). These researchers obtained their sample using systematic sampling technique:

The study population was drawn from the roster of registered nurses by the Vermont Board of Nursing in September 2002 ($n = 7,028$). For this study, advanced practice, inactive, out-of-state, foreign, and deceased nurses were excluded with a resulting population of approximately 6,000. To select a sample of 3,000 nurses for the study sample, the remaining list was ordered by license number and a systematic sample of every second nurse was conducted to identify the proposed sample of 3,000 participants. These 3,000 nurses, therefore, were a systematic sample of active RNs in Vermont in September 2002.... Seven percent of the 3,000 surveys were returned because of inaccurate postal addresses ($n = 220$) or because the nurse was deceased ($n = 2$). Of the remaining 2,778 surveys, the final overall response rate was 56.7% ($n = 1,574$). (Rambur et al., 2005, pp. 188–189)

CRITIQUE

The systematic sampling plan used by Rambur et al. (2005) has more strengths than weaknesses. The researchers made the sample more homogeneous and eliminated potential for bias by excluding advanced-practice, inactive, foreign, and deceased nurses. This resulted in a sampling frame of 6,000 RNs. These researchers desired a sample size of $N = 3,000$ RNs, so they systematically selected every second RN. A potential area for bias is that only 56.7%, or $N = 1574$, subjects returned their surveys and 43.3% did not. Those nurses who did not return their survey may be different in some way from those who did participate, which decreases the sample's representativeness of the target population. The return rate on surveys often is low, however, and the 56.7% is above the average survey return rate of 25-35% (Burns & Grove, 2005). In addition, the representativeness of the sample is strengthened by the large sample size, $N = 1574$, and the use of a probability sampling method.

IMPLICATIONS FOR PRACTICE

Compared with ADN nurses, BSN nurses started their careers earlier, were employed longer, and held more positions. BSN nurses also had significantly higher job satisfaction related to autonomy and growth, job stress and physical demands, and job and organizational security. Thus, this study supports preparation of nurses with BSNs for stronger individual and social return on educational investment. Thus, hospitals need to consider this when hiring nurses that BSN prepared nurses might have a more productive, satisfying, and longer career than ADN nurses.

Nonprobability Sampling Methods Used in Quantitative Research

In nonprobability sampling, not every element of the population has an opportunity for selection in the sample. Although this approach decreases a sample's representativeness of a population, it commonly is used in nursing studies. In an analysis of nursing studies published in six nursing journals from 1977 to 1986, only 9% used probability or random sampling (Moody, Wilson, Smyth, Schwartz, Tittle, & Van Cott, 1988). It appears that this trend continues today, because most of the nursing studies use nonprobability sampling methods. Thus, it is important to be able to discriminate among the various nonprobability sampling plans used in research.

The five nonprobability sampling plans used most frequently in nursing research are convenience sampling, quota sampling, purposive sampling, network sampling, and theoretical sampling. Convenience and quota sampling often are used in quantitative and outcomes studies (see Table 10-1). Purposive, network, and theoretical sampling are used more frequently in qualitative research and are discussed later in this chapter.

Convenience Sampling

Convenience sampling, also called "accidental sampling," is considered a weak approach because it provides little opportunity to control for biases; subjects are included in the study merely because they happen to be in the right place at the right time (Burns & Grove, 2005;

Kerlinger & Lee, 2000). A classroom of students, patients who attend a clinic on a specific day, subjects who attend a support group, patients hospitalized with specific medical diagnoses or nursing problems, and a sample composed of every fifth person who enters the emergency room on a given day are examples of convenience samples. Available subjects are simply entered into the study until the desired sample size is reached. Multiple biases may exist in the sample, some of which may be subtle and unrecognized. However, serious biases are not always present in convenience samples.

Convenience samples are inexpensive, accessible, and usually less time-consuming to obtain than other types of samples. This type of sampling provides a means to conduct studies on topics that cannot be examined with probability sampling. According to Kerlinger and Lee (2000), a convenience sample is not that bad when it is used with reasonable knowledge and care in implementing a study.

The convenience sampling method commonly is used in health care studies. Because the sampling frames are not available for many populations and it is difficult to find adequate subjects for studies, researchers often use a sample of convenience. Most researchers conducting quasi-experimental studies and clinical trials in both medicine and nursing use the convenience sampling method. As a component of these study designs, subjects usually are randomly assigned to groups. This random assignment to groups, which is not a sampling method but a design strategy, does not alter the risk of biases resulting from convenience sampling but does strengthen the equivalence of the study groups. With these potential biases and the narrowly defined sampling criteria used to select subjects in most clinical trials, representativeness of the sample is a concern.

RESEARCH EXAMPLE Convenience Sampling

DeVon, Penckofer, & Zerwic (2005) studied the symptoms of unstable angina (UA) in patients with and without diabetes and used convenience sampling to obtain their sample.

A convenience sample of 50 women and 50 men, hospitalized with UA, were recruited. Subjects were eligible for study if they met the following criteria: (a) an admitting diagnosis of; (b) acute MI [myocardial infarction] ruled out according to standard electrocardiographic parameters and serum cardiac markers; (c) at least 21 years of age; (d) fluent in English; (e) admitted through the emergency department (ED); and (f) pain free for at least 12 hours.... Forty percent of the patients ($n = 40$) in the study were diabetic.... Participants were recruited from an urban and a suburban medical center in the Chicago area. The sites were chosen in order to increase the likelihood of recruiting a heterogeneous sample encompassing a broad array of racial and ethnic groups, and income levels.... Potential participants were identified through computerized census data and were recruited from the intensive care unit, the coronary care unit, post-interventional recovery unit, and cardiac step-down unit. (DeVon et al., 2005, pp. 138–139)

CRITIQUE

Devon et al. (2005) attempted to make the sample as representative of the accessible and target populations as possible by recruiting a large sample of 100 subjects from both urban and suburban medical centers. The sample included equal numbers of male and female subjects (50 female and 50 male) so that the findings could be generalized to both genders. In addition, the researcher recruited a heterogeneous sample encompassing an array of racial and ethnic groups and income levels, which also increases the generalizability of findings to the target population. The sample included 40 subjects with diabetes. The subjects with and without diabetes were compared on the demographic variables of age, race, gender, risk factors, and cardiac and related health history and found to be similar. Convenience sampling can be strengthened, as in this study, but still has a potential for bias that can influence study outcomes and decrease the sample's representativeness of the target population.

IMPLICATIONS FOR PRACTICE

DeVon et al. (2005) found that patients with diabetes were more likely to have a history of high cholesterol, prior history of preexisting heart disease, and prior history of having had an angiogram to diagnose their cardiac condition. Patients with diabetes reported having less nausea, less pain of the squeezing and aching type, and more hyperventilation than the patients without diabetes. On the basis of the evidence from this study, the researchers recommended more research on patients with diabetes to determine their presenting symptoms for UA and myocardial infarction, because morbidity and mortality rates associated with cardiac disease are very high among such patients.

Quota Sampling

Quota sampling uses a convenience sampling technique with an added feature—a strategy to ensure the inclusion of subject types likely to be underrepresented in the convenience sample, such as females, minority groups, and the elderly, poor, rich, and undereducated. The goal of quota sampling is to replicate the proportions of subgroups present in the population. The technique is similar to that used in stratified random sampling. Quota sampling requires that the researcher be able to identify subgroups in the target population that are important for achieving representativeness in the problem being studied. In addition, the researcher must determine what proportion of the target population each identified subgroup represents. Quota sampling offers an improvement over convenience sampling and tends to decrease potential biases.

RESEARCH EXAMPLE Quota Sampling

McCain and colleagues (2003) used quota sampling in their quasi-experimental study of the effects of stress management on the psychoneuroimmunology outcomes in persons with human immunodeficiency virus (HIV) disease. They described their sampling method as follows:

Quota sampling was used to achieve appropriate sample representation by gender, at a ratio of 4 males: 1 female (20%). Gender subgroups were next stratified by prebaseline CD4$^+$ cell counts [indicating the seriousness of HIV disease] to equilibrate study groups by initial CD4$^+$ counts and, indirectly, by stage of illness....

Enrolled in the study were 148 individuals, 29 females (20%) and 119 males.... Study attrition was within the expected range, with 112 participants completing the intervention groups or initial waiting period (76% retention) and 102 individuals completing the 6-month follow-up visit (69% retention). The attrition rate did not differ among study groups. (McCain et al., 2003, pp. 105–106)

(continues)

CRITIQUE

McCain and colleagues (2003) used quota sampling to ensure a gender distribution of 80% males and 20% females for their study sample (to match that in the population of all persons with HIV disease) and also equivalent CD4$^+$ counts and stages of illness among the patients in the two study groups. The stratification by gender and CD4$^+$ count decreased the potential for bias in the sampling method, promoted equality in the study groups, and improved the sample's representativeness of the target population. The researchers also addressed the attrition rate in terms of the total sample and the groups and indicated that this probably did not affect the study findings.

IMPLICATIONS FOR PRACTICE

McCain et al. (2003) found that a stress management intervention did improve the emotional well-being and quality-of-life scores for patients with HIV disease. The researchers recommend the testing of additional interventions that may promote the quality of life and improve the illness trajectory of patients living with HIV disease.

Sample Size in Quantitative Studies

One of the most troublesome questions that arise during the critique of a study is whether the sample size was adequate. If the study was designed to make comparisons and significant differences were found, the sample size, or number of subjects participating in the study, was adequate. Questions about the adequacy of the sample size occur only when no significance is found. Thus, when critiquing a quantitative study in which no significance was found for at least one of the hypotheses or research questions, be sure to evaluate the adequacy of the sample size. Is there really no difference? Or was an actual difference not found because of inadequacies in the research methods, such as a small sample size?

Currently, the adequacy of the sample size is evaluated using a power analysis. Power is the capacity of the study to detect differences or relationships that actually exist in the population. Expressed another way, it is the capacity to correctly reject a null hypothesis. The minimum acceptable level of power for a study is 0.8, or 80% (Cohen, 1988). This power level results in a 20% chance of a Type II error, in which the study fails to detect existing effects (differences or relationships). An increasing number of researchers are performing a power analysis before conducting their study to determine an adequate sample size. The results of this analysis usually are included in the sample section of the published study. Researchers also should perform a power analysis to evaluate the adequacy of their sample size for all nonsignificant findings and include this in the "Discussion" section of their published study.

Polit and Sherman (1990) evaluated the sample size in 62 studies published in 1989 in *Nursing Research* and *Research in Nursing & Health*. They found that most of the studies examined had inadequate sample sizes for making comparisons between groups. The studies needed an average of 218 subjects per group to have a power level of 0.8. Therefore, in most of these studies, the risk of a Type II error—saying something is nonsignificant when it was not—was extremely high.

Other factors that influence the adequacy of sample size (because they affect power) include effect size, type of quantitative study, number of variables, sensitivity of the measurement tools, and data analysis techniques. When critiquing the adequacy of the sample size, consider the influence of all of these factors.

Effect Size

The effect is the presence of the phenomenon examined in a study. **Effect size** is the extent to which the null hypothesis is false. In a study in which two populations are compared, the null hypothesis states that the difference between the two populations is zero. However, if the null hypothesis is false, an identifiable effect is present—a difference between the two groups does exist. If the null hypothesis is false, it is false to some degree; this is the effect size (Cohen, 1988). The statistical test tells you whether there is a difference between groups, or whether variables are significantly related. The effect size tells you the *size* of the difference between the groups or the *strength* of the relationship between two variables.

When the effect size is large (e.g., considerable difference between groups or very strong relationship between two variables), detecting it is easy and requires only a small sample; when the effect size is small (e.g., only a small difference between groups or a weak relationship between two variables), detecting it is more difficult and requires larger samples. It is generally agreed that a small effect size is less than 0.30, a medium effect size is 0.30 to 0.60, and a large effect size is greater than 0.60 (Cohen, 1988). Effect size is smaller with a small sample, so effects are more difficult to detect. Increasing the sample size also increases the effect size, making it more likely that the effect will be detected.

In the nursing studies examined by Polit and Sherman (1990), 52.7% of the effect sizes computed were small. These researchers found that in nursing studies, for small effects, average power was less than 0.30. That is, the probability that acceptance of the null hypothesis was correct was less than 30%, instead of the standard power of 0.8, or 80%, recommended for a study. In most cases, this flaw was due to an insufficient sample size. Even when the effect size was moderate, the average power in the nursing studies examined was only 0.7, or 70%, with a 30% chance for error. The nursing studies reached an acceptable level of power only when the effect size was large, and 11% of these studies were underpowered. Only 15% of the studies had sufficient power for all of their analyses. When critiquing a study, determine whether the study sample size was adequate by noting whether a power analysis was done and what power was achieved.

Types of Quantitative Studies

Descriptive studies (particularly those using survey questionnaires) and correlational studies often require very large samples. In these studies, multiple variables may be examined, and extraneous variables are likely to affect subject response(s) to the variables under study. Researchers often make statistical comparisons on multiple subgroups in a sample, requiring that an adequate sample be available for each subgroup being analyzed. Quasi-experimental and experimental studies use smaller samples more often than descriptive and correlational studies do. As control in the study increases, the sample size can decrease and the sample still will approximate the target population. Instruments in these studies tend to be more refined, with stronger reliability and validity. Designs that use blocking or stratification usually increase the total sample size required. Designs that use matched pairs of subjects have increased power and thus require a smaller sample (Burns & Grove, 2005).

Number of Variables

As the number of variables under study increases, the sample size needed may increase. Including variables such as age, gender, ethnicity, and education in the data analyses can increase the sample size needed to detect differences between groups. Using them only to describe the sample does not cause a problem in terms of power. A number of the studies analyzed by Polit and Sherman (1990) had sufficient sample size for the primary analyses but failed to plan for analyses involving subgroups, such as analyzing the data by age category or ethnic group. The inclusion of multiple dependent variables also increases the sample size needed.

Measurement Sensitivity

Well-developed physiological instruments measure phenomena with accuracy and precision. A thermometer, for example, measures body temperature accurately and precisely. Tools measuring psychosocial variables tend to be less precise. However, a tool that is reliable and valid measures more precisely than a tool that is less well developed. Variance tends to be higher with a less well-developed tool than with one that is well developed. For example, if anxiety is being measured and the actual anxiety score of several subjects is 80, measures ranging from 70 to 90 may be obtained with a less well-developed tool. Much more variation from the true score occurs than when a well-developed tool is used, which will tend to show a score closer to the actual score of 80 for each subject. As variance in instrument scores increases, the sample size needed to obtain significance increases (see Chapter 11 on measurement).

Data Analysis Techniques

Data analysis techniques vary in their capability to detect differences in the data. Statisticians refer to this as the "power of the statistical analysis." An interaction also occurs between the measurement sensitivity and the power of the data analysis technique. The power of the analysis technique increases as precision in measurement increases. Larger samples are needed when the power of the planned statistical analysis is weak.

For some statistical procedures, such as the *t*-test and analysis of variance (ANOVA), equal group sizes will increase power because the effect size is maximized. The more unbalanced the group sizes are, the smaller the effect size is. Therefore in unbalanced groups, the total sample size must be larger (Kraemer & Theimann, 1987). The chi-square test is the weakest of the statistical tests and requires very large sample sizes to achieve acceptable levels of power. As the number of categories increases, the sample size needed increases. Also, if some of the categories contain small numbers of subjects, the total sample size must be increased. The *t*-test, ANOVA, and chi-square statistical analysis techniques will be described in more detail in Chapter 12 Understanding Statistics in Research.

CRITIQUE GUIDELINES Adequacy of the Sample in Quantitative Studies

When critiquing the sample of quantitative studies, address the following questions:

1. Are the sampling inclusion criteria, sampling exclusion criteria, or both clearly identified and appropriate for the study?
2. Is the sample size identified? If groups were included in the study, is the sample size for each group discussed?
3. Is a power analysis reported? Was sample size appropriate as indicated by the power analysis?
4. Are the refusal and sample mortality rates addressed? If the refusal rate or sample mortality rate is high, does the researcher provide reasons?
5. Are the characteristics of the sample detailed? If two or more groups are used in the study, do the groups have comparable characteristics?
6. Is the sampling method probability or nonprobability? Identify the specific sampling method used in the study to obtain the sample. Is the sampling method adequate to achieve a representative sample?
7. Is the sample representative of the accessible and target populations?
8. What was the possibility of Type II error?
9. Are the potential biases in the sample discussed?
10. Does the researcher define the target population to which the findings are generalized?

RESEARCH EXAMPLE Quantitative Study Sample

McFarlane, Groff, O'Brien, and Watson (2005) conducted a study of the behaviors of children exposed to intimate partner violence against their mother following a treatment program for their mother. The abused women were selected using a convenience sampling method, and the children of these women were identified, with one child of each woman being randomly selected for inclusion in the study. The study sample and setting are described in the following excerpts:

> The study was conducted in primary care public health clinics and Women, Infants, and Children (WIC) clinics in a large urban area. The primary care clinics serve between 5,000 and 6,000 female clients, age 18 to 45 years, and each WIC clinic serves almost 4,000 female clients annually [study settings]. An estimated 50% of the women at each clinic are Hispanic, most of whom are first-generation immigrants from Mexico [ethnicity of the sample]....
>
> Sample size needed to detect a small to medium sample effect size of .30, $\alpha = .05$, 80% power, and allowing for a possible attrition rate of 30% was 360 women [power analysis]....
>
> All women between the ages of 18 and 44 who spoke English or Spanish were screened by one of three bilingual research nurses for intimate-partner (i.e., spouse/common-law husband, ex-spouse/ex-common-law husband, boyfriend/girlfriend, or ex-boyfriend/ex-girlfriend) physical or sexual assaults, occurring within the past 12 months [sample inclusion criteria for mothers], until a sample of 360 abused women [sample size] were entered into the study. A list of all children between the ages of 18 months and 18 years was composed for each woman [sample inclusion criteria for children], and one child was chosen at random for the child behavior study [sampling method for children]. Children younger than 18 months were not included in the study because the age limitations of the measurement instrument selected [sample exclusion criteria for children]. (McFarlane et al., 2005, p. 8)

(continues)

CRITIQUE

McFarlane and colleagues (2005) described the important aspects of the sample, such as the sampling criteria, sample size based on power analysis, and setting. The researchers might have clearly identified the sampling method for the women of the study, which appeared to be a sample of convenience. The researchers did provide details on the sample settings, and these clinics provided an ethnically diverse, large sample of 360 women. The size of the sample seems adequate as indicated by the power analysis conducted by the researchers. However, the study refusal and sample mortality rates are needed to determine the adequacy of the sample size. The sampling criteria for the women ensured that they have experienced physical or sexual assaults to be included in the study. The number of children included in the study is not clearly addressed, but the criteria for selecting the children were broad enough to include a variety of children of abused mothers. The research article also included a description of the women and children in the study (sample characteristics) that was not included in this study excerpt.

Sampling in Qualitative Research

Qualitative research is conducted to gain insights and discover meaning about a particular experience, situation, cultural element, or historical event (Burns & Grove, 2005; Patton, 2002). The intent of qualitative research is an in-depth understanding of specially selected sample and less on the generalization of the findings from a randomly selected sample to a target population, as in quantitative research. The sampling in qualitative research focuses more on experiences, events, and incidents than on people (Sandelowski, 1995). The researcher attempts to select subjects who are able to provide extensive information about the experience or event being studied. For example, if the goal of the study is to describe the phenomenon of living with chronic pain, the researcher will select those subjects who are articulate and reflective, have a history of chronic pain, and are willing to share their chronic pain experience (Coyne, 1997).

Three common sampling methods used in qualitative research are purposive sampling, network or snowball sampling, and theoretical sampling (see Table 10-1). These sampling methods enable the researcher to select the specific subjects who will provide the most extensive information about the phenomenon, event, or situation being studied (Clifford, 1997; Munhall, 2001). The sample selection process can have a profound effect on the quality of the research and should be described in enough depth to promote the interpretation of the findings and the replication of the study.

Purposive Sampling

With **purposive sampling**, sometimes referred to as "judgmental" or "selective sampling," the researcher consciously selects certain subjects, elements, events, or incidents to include in the study. Efforts may be made to include typical or atypical subjects or situations. The researcher may select subjects who are of various ages, those who have differences in diagnoses or severity of illness, or those who received an ineffective treatment rather than an effective treatment for their illness. This sampling method has been criticized because it is difficult to evaluate the accuracy of the researcher's judgment. Thus, researchers must indicate the characteristics that they desired in subjects and provide a rationale for selecting these types of subjects to obtain essential data for their study. In qualitative research, this sampling method seems to be the best way to gain insight into a new area of study or to obtain in-depth understanding of a complex experience or event.

RESEARCH EXAMPLE   Purposive Sampling

Kindy, Petersen, and Parkhurst (2005) conducted a phenomenological study to describe nurses' experiences in working in psychiatric units with high risk for assault. The researchers used purposive sampling to obtain 8 of their subjects, and 2 were obtained by network sampling; all of the subjects were registered nurses (RNs).

Following human subjects review by a university internal review board, advertisements soliciting a purposive sample of registered nurses willing to be interviewed about working or having worked in psychiatric or psychiatric/forensic facilities were placed in newspapers of three towns in northern California. Calls of inquiry were received in one location and referred to the researcher living closest to the inquirers. In addition, two participants were referred by other participants [network sampling].... Taped interviews were listened to multiple times to ensure verbatim transcription. Transcriptions were then divided among the researchers who individually analyzed the data. When individual theme analysis was complete, the researchers met. Themes were similar among the researchers, signifying a high degree of interrater reliability and saturation. The researchers collectively used the themes to generate categories and subcategories, providing the structure for an exhaustive description and an essential structure. (Kindy et al., 2005, pp. 170–171)

CRITIQUE

Kindy and colleagues (2005) clearly identified their use of a purposive sampling plan to obtain a sample of RNs who work in psychiatric units with high risk for assaults. However, the researchers needed to indicate that network sampling was used to identify two RN participants, who were identified as potential subjects by the existing study participants. Purposive and network sampling methods enabled the researchers to identify an adequate number of RNs with the unique perilous work experiences in psychiatric facilities. The data analysis indicated interrater reliability, and saturation of data [no new data were obtained with additional subjects] was achieved, resulting in an exhaustive description of the lived experience of working in assaultive psychiatric environments.

IMPLICATIONS FOR PRACTICE

Kindy and colleagues' (2005) analysis of transcripts of the taped interviews

...generated four categories and 13 subcategories subsumed under the primary construct of "perilous work," providing the frame for the exhaustive description and essential structure of participants' lived experiences. Outcomes suggest that serious work-related hazards exist and provide insight into possible remedies and a springboard for follow-up studies. (p. 169)

The researchers recommended additional studies with larger samples to determine if support exists for the evidence generated from this study. So addition research is needed to generate evidence to be used in practice to manage nurses exposed to high risk assault situations in the psychiatric work place.

Network Sampling

Network sampling, sometimes referred to as "snowball sampling," holds promise for locating subjects who would be difficult or impossible to obtain in other ways or who have not been previously identified for study. Network sampling takes advantage of social networks and the fact that friends tend to have characteristics in common. When the researcher has found a few subjects with the necessary criteria, he or she asks their assistance in finding others with similar characteristics (Patton, 2002). The first few subjects often are obtained through a convenience or purposive sampling method, and the sample size is expanded using network sampling, as in the Kindy et al. (2005) study. This sampling method is used in quantitative studies but more commonly is used in qualitative studies.

In qualitative research, network sampling is an effective strategy for identifying subjects who can provide the greatest insight and essential information about an experience or event that is being studied (Munhall, 2001). This strategy also is particularly useful for finding subjects in socially devalued populations, such as persons who are dependent on alcohol, abuse children, commit sexual offenses, are addicted to drugs, or commit criminal acts. These persons seldom are willing to make themselves known. Other groups, such as widows, grieving siblings, or persons successful at lifestyle changes, also may be located using this strategy. Such persons typically are outside the existing health care system and are difficult to find.

RESEARCH EXAMPLE   Network Sampling

Coté-Arsenault and Morrison-Beedy (2001) conducted a phenomenological study entitled "Women's Voices Reflecting Changed Expectations for Pregnancy after Perinatal Loss." They described the sampling plan for their study as follows:

> Following IRB [institutional review board] approval, a snowball sampling approach was used to recruit women who had experienced at least one perinatal loss and a minimum of one subsequent pregnancy. Recruitment was accomplished using various sources: personal contacts, the local perinatal loss support group, and flyers placed within the university community and local community health settings.... The sample consisted of 21 women with diverse pregnancy and loss histories.
>
> The diversity of childbearing experiences was extensive, encompassing one woman who was currently pregnant, a woman who had given birth 14 weeks before, and women whose last birth was more than two decades prior to this study. The women had experienced from 1 to 7 losses which occurred throughout the three trimesters of pregnancy and at birth. All currently had living children. (Coté-Arsenault & Morrison-Beedy, 2001, p. 241)

CRITIQUE

The researchers clearly identified the networks (personal contacts, loss support group, and flyers) that were used to recruit subjects. This sampling plan successfully identified women with diverse childbearing experiences, who provided detailed data on the expectations for pregnancy after perinatal loss. This sample seems to be adequate to describe women's expectations for pregnancy after perinatal loss.

IMPLICATIONS FOR PRACTICE

Coté-Arsenault and Morrison-Beedy (2001) found that

[w]omen's stories portrayed perinatal loss as a life-altering event. Women did not feel emotionally safe in their pregnancies after loss and were afraid that those babies too would die. Despite the differences in their obstetrical and loss histories and time since loss, similarities in their responses to pregnancy far outweighed their differences. These commonalities are contained in six themes: (a) dealing with uncertainty, (b) wondering if the baby is healthy, (c) waiting to lose the baby, (d) holding back their emotions, (e) acknowledging that loss happened and that it can happen again, and (f) changing self.... Care providers should acknowledge women's past losses, address their concerns during a current pregnancy, and recognize the potentially life-long effect perinatal loss may have on these women. (p. 239)

Theoretical Sampling

Grounded theory research frequently uses **theoretical sampling** to develop a selected theory through the research process (Munhall, 2001). The researcher gathers data from any person or group able to provide relevant data for theory generation. The data are considered relevant if they include information that generates, delimits, and saturates the theoretical codes in the study needed for theory generation (Huberman & Miles, 2002). A code is saturated if it is complete and the researcher can see how it fits in the theory. Thus, the researcher continues to seek sources and gather data until the codes are saturated, and the theory evolves from the codes and the data. Diversity in the sample is encouraged, so the theory developed covers a wide range of behavior in varied situations and settings (Patton, 2002).

RESEARCH EXAMPLE Theoretical Sampling

Rew (2003) conducted a grounded theory study to develop a theory of self-care that was grounded in the experiences of homeless youth. The study incorporated theoretical sampling, and the sampling method was described as follows:

Theoretical sampling of homeless youths living temporarily in an urban area was used to insure a wide range of self-care experiences. Potential participants were recruited from youths seeking health and social services from a street outreach program (i.e., a clinic set up in a church basement) in central Texas. Criteria for inclusion were: (a) 16-20 years of age, (b) ability to understand and speak English, and (c) willingness to volunteer for an interview. This age group represented the majority of youths seeking services from this program. Fifteen youths (7 males, 6 females, and 2 transgendered) who were an average of 18.8 years of age volunteered to participate. Saturation (sufficient or adequate data had been collected to meet the goal of the study) was reached at the end of 12 interviews; three additional participants were recruited to verify the findings (Morse, 1998). These participants had been homeless for an average of 4.0 years. In the past year, the majority ($n = 13$) had lived in "squats," which are temporary campsites claimed by youths and other homeless persons. Demographic data and personal characteristics of these participants were summarized and pseudonyms were used to protect the identity of all participants. (Rew, 2003, p. 235)

(continues)

CRITIQUE

Rew (2003) clearly identified the theoretical sampling method used to obtain the 15 subjects and the sampling criteria that indicated the specific subjects required for participation in the study. The subjects were recruited from an urban area to ensure a wide range of self-care experiences. The researchers addressed the number of participants interviewed to reach data saturation and conducted three additional interviews to verify the findings. Adequate data were collected and codes were saturated to ensure the development of a grounded theory.

IMPLICATIONS FOR PRACTICE

Rew (2003) conducted a grounded theory study about the experiences of homeless youth and developed a theory of "Taking Care of Oneself in a High Risk Environment." This descriptive theory of self-care for homeless/street youth included three categories: (1) becoming aware of oneself, (2) staying alive with limited resources, and (3) handling one's own health. The study increased current understanding of the homeless experience for youth and provided a basis for further research to generate support and care for the homeless.

Sample Size in Qualitative Studies

In quantitative research, the sample size must be large enough to identify relationships among variables or to determine differences between groups. The larger the sample size and the effect size, the greater the power to detect relationships and differences in quantitative and outcomes studies. However, qualitative research focuses on the quality of information obtained from the person, situation, or event sampled, rather than on the size of the sample (Huberman & Miles, 2002; Sandelowski, 1995).

The purpose of the study determines the sample size and sampling plan. The depth of information that is obtained and needed to gain insight into a phenomenon, describe a cultural element, develop a theory, or understand a historical event determines the number of people, sites, artifacts, or documents sampled. The sample size can be too small when the data collected lack adequate depth or richness. Thus, an inadequate sample size can reduce the quality and credibility of the research findings. Many qualitative researchers use purposive sampling plans to select the specific subjects, events, or situations that they believe will provide the rich data needed to gain insights and discover new meaning in an area of study (Munhall, 2001).

The number of participants in a qualitative study is adequate when saturation of information is achieved in the study area. Saturation of data occurs when additional sampling provides no new information, only redundancy of previous collected data. Important factors that need to be considered in determining sample size to achieve saturation of data are

(1) scope of the study, (2) nature of the topic, (3) quality of the data, and (4) design of the study (Morse, 2000; Munhall, 2001; Patton, 2002).

Scope of the Study

If the scope of the study is broad, then extensive data will be needed to address the study purpose, and it will take longer to reach saturation. Thus, a study with a broad scope requires more sampling of participants, events, or documents than is needed for a study with a narrow scope (Morse, 2000). A study that has a clear focus and provides focused data collection usually has richer, more credible findings. When critiquing a qualitative study, determine whether the sample size was adequate for the identified scope of the study.

Nature of the Topic

If the topic of study is clear and easily discussed by the subjects, then fewer subjects are needed to obtain the essential data. If the topic is difficult to define and awkward for people to discuss, then an increased number of participants probably will be needed to achieve data saturation (Morse, 2000; Munhall, 2001). For example, a phenomenological study of the experience of an adult living with a history of child sexual abuse is a very sensitive, complex topic to investigate. This type of topic probably will require increased participants and interview time to collect essential data. When critiquing published studies, be sure to consider whether the sample size was adequate based on the complexity and sensitivity of the topic studied.

Quality of the Data

The quality of information obtained from an interview, observation, or document review influences the sample size. When the quality of the data is high, with a rich content, few participants are needed to achieve saturation of data in the area of study. Quality data are best obtained from articulate, well-informed, and communicative participants (Sandelowski, 1995). Such participants are able to share richer data in a clear and concise manner. In addition, participants who have more time to be interviewed usually provide data with greater depth and breadth. Remember to consider these factors in your critique of a qualitative study: the quality of the participants, events, or documents; the richness of the data collected; and the adequacy of the sample based on the findings obtained.

Study Design

Some studies are designed to increase the number of interviews with each participant. When more interviews are conducted with a person, better-quality data are collected. For example, with a study design that includes an interview both before and after an event, more data are produced than with a single-interview design. Designs that involve interviewing families rather than individual people produce more data than can be obtained using designs with single-participant interviews. In critiquing a qualitative study, determine the adequacy of the sample size for the chosen design (Huberman & Miles, 2002).

> ## CRITIQUE GUIDELINES Adequacy of the Sample in Qualitative Studies
>
> When critiquing the sample in qualitative studies, use critical reasoning to address the following questions:
>
> 1. Are the sampling inclusion criteria, sampling exclusion criteria, or both appropriate?
> 2. Is the sampling plan adequate to address the purpose of the study? If purposive sampling was used, does the researcher provide a rationale for the sample selection process? If network sampling was used, does the researcher identify the networks used to obtain the sample and provide a rationale for their selection? If theoretical sampling is used, does the researcher indicate how participants are selected to promote the generation of a theory?
> 3. Is the sample size adequate, based on the scope of the study, nature of the topic, quality of the data, and study design?
> 4. Are the sample refusal rate and the participant mortality rate for the study sample discussed?
> 5. Are the characteristics of the sample adequately described?
> 6. Does the researcher discuss the quality of the study participants? Were the participants articulate, well informed, and willing to share information relevant to the study topic?
> 7. Did the sample produce saturation of data in the area of the study?
> 8. Does the researcher identify the study setting?

RESEARCH EXAMPLE   Qualitative Study Sample

O'Brien (2001) conducted a qualitative study to "examine the experience of providing long-term home care for the child who is technology dependent from the family's viewpoint" (p. 14). Technology dependence was defined as dependence of the child on a medical device to compensate for a loss of vital body function and the need for ongoing nursing care to avert death or further disability. O'Brien (2001) described her sample as follows and the particular aspects of the sample have been identified in brackets):

> A purposive sample [sampling plan or method] of 15 families [sample size], which included a child who was technology dependent was obtained through family response to an introductory letter about the study distributed by health care agencies, social service agencies, and parent support groups [participant selection process]. The child who was technology dependent was 3 to 12 years of age, had been dependent on technology and living at home for at least 1 year, and was medically stable at the time of the study [sample inclusion criteria]. The sample selection continued until there was evidence of thick data description and no new data were being obtained [saturation of data]. A total of 11 mothers and 4 parent couples (mother and father) were interviewed [description of the participants], and all chose to be interviewed in their homes [setting]. One family who had originally indicated interest in the study decided not to participate because of the ongoing issues related to the pending adoption of the child who was technology dependent [refusal rate].
>
> The demographic characteristics of the children who were technology dependent and their families varied considerably [quality of the data]. One exception was race: All of the parents were European-American, and all of the children who were technology dependent were also European-American with the exception of one African-American child [sample characteristics]. (O'Brien, 2001, p. 14)

CRITIQUE

O'Brien (2001) provided extensive detail of her sample and sampling plan, as set forth in the foregoing excerpt. The article also included three additional paragraphs that detailed the characteristics of the sample and the quality of the study participants that were not quoted in this study excerpt. The focus of the purposive sampling plan was addressed, with a limited rationale for selecting this sampling plan. The sample size of 15 seemed adequate, because saturation of data was achieved by interviewing these families. The scope of the study, nature of the topic, quality of the data, and study design were addressed and seemed to support the sample size obtained. The refusal rate was minimal—1 family out of 16 families approached—with no participant mortality. The setting of the study was identified as the home and was described in more detail with the discussion of the participants and sample characteristics. O'Brien provided a detailed discussion of a quality sampling plan that she implemented in this phenomenological study.

IMPLICATIONS FOR PRACTICE

This study provided a detailed description of the problems that parents and children encounter with home care of a technology dependent child. This study will help nurses realize the amount and type of educational, emotional, and social support that is needed in providing care of this type of child. Also additional research is need to develop interventions to improve the home care of technologically dependent children.

Research Settings

The **setting** is the location in which a study is conducted. Three common settings for conducting nursing research are natural, partially controlled, and highly controlled.

Natural Setting

A **natural setting**, or **field setting**, is an uncontrolled, real-life situation or environment. Conducting a study in a natural setting means that the researcher does not manipulate or change the environment for the study. Descriptive and correlational quantitative studies and qualitative studies often are conducted in natural settings.

RESEARCH EXAMPLE **Natural Setting**

Wongvatunyu and Porter (2005) conducted a phenomenological study to describe mothers' experience of helping their young adult children with traumatic brain injury (TBI). This study included 7 subjects who were obtained using a convenience sample. The natural settings for the study were the subjects' home and a meeting room at the university.

Interested volunteers contacted the first author. If the inclusion criteria were met, a preliminary interview was arranged. After informed consent was obtained, the first interview began. The interview guide was used to establish the scope of the discussion. Each mother was asked all the questions, but non-directive techniques were used so that each mother could describe her experiences in her own words.... Interviews took place in the participants' homes at their convenience, or in private meeting rooms of the university. (Wongvatunyu & Porter, 2005, p. 50)

CRITIQUE

The data, which focused on the mothers' descriptions of the young adult children with TBI, were collected in the participants' homes and at the university. No attempts were made during the study to manipulate, change, or control these environments of the participants' homes and the meeting rooms at the university. Thus, the researchers' intent was to study these women in a natural, real-life environment that was accessible and convenient for the participants.

IMPLICATIONS FOR PRACTICE

The five phenomena of the mothers' experiences were: reconnecting my child's brain, considering my child's safety, making our lives as normal as possible, dealing with our biggest problem, and advocating for my child.... The mothers continued rehabilitation efforts with the young adults, even when only minimal services were available to support their efforts. Mothers needed interventions to enhance their knowledge, and they and the young adults with TBI needed expanded community services. (Wongvatunyu & Porter, 2005, p. 48)

The evidence generated from this study provides an understanding of the needs and coping patterns of families with TBI children and how these patients are managed in the home setting. Additional research is needed to verify these needs and coping patterns in families with TBI children and also research needs to focus on interventions to improve the health outcomes for parents and their children.

Partially Controlled Setting

A **partially controlled setting** is an environment that is manipulated or modified in some way by the researcher. An increasing number of nursing studies, usually correlational, quasi-experimental, and experimental studies, are being conducted in partially controlled settings.

RESEARCH EXAMPLE   Partially Controlled Setting

Rivers, Aday, Frankowski, Felknor, White, and Nichols (2003) conducted a predictive correlational study to determine predictors of nurses' acceptance of an intravenous (IV) catheter safety device. These researchers described their setting as follows:

> A 900-bed urban teaching hospital in Texas implemented a new intravenous Protectiv® Plus IV catheter safety needle device in September 1999. Data collection was implemented in December 2000 to ensure that all training had been accomplished and that the device was implemented in all areas. All the nurses on the various 36 nursing units/areas where RNs initiate IV therapy were surveyed by a 34-item, self-administered questionnaire. The units included medical surgical units, intensive care, cardiovascular transplant units, surgical preoperative and post-operative, day surgery, maternal and neonatal units, emergency and urgent care areas, oncology clinic and others.... (Rivers et al., 2003, p. 250)

CRITIQUE

Rivers and colleagues' (2003) study was conducted in a teaching hospital, which provides a partially controlled setting in terms of the units that use IV lines, nurses' training within the hospital and in particular for the IV safety device, and the safety climate or requirements of the workplace. However, the researchers did not control other aspects of the environment, such as the nurses' previous work experience; interactions of the nurses regarding their training and use of the IV safety device on different units; and the data collection process, which was a self-administered questionnaire.

IMPLICATIONS FOR PRACTICE

Rivers and colleagues (2003) confirmed widespread, although not universal, acceptance of the Protectiv® Plus IV catheter safety needle device at a major urban teaching hospital in Texas. The acceptance of this device was based on four main predictors: (1) perception of adequate training, (2) perception of appropriate timing between training and first use of the device, (3) a strong safety climate in the hospital, and (4) a lack of attachment to earlier IV technology. These study results provide direction to other hospitals wanting to implement the Protectiv® Plus IV catheter safety needle device.

Highly Controlled Setting

A **highly controlled setting** is an artificially constructed environment developed for the sole purpose of conducting research. Laboratories, research or experimental centers, and test units in hospitals or other health care agencies are highly controlled settings in which experimental studies often are conducted. This type of setting reduces the influence of extraneous variables, which enables the researcher to examine accurately the effect of one variable on another. Highly controlled settings commonly are used in the conduct of experimental research.

RESEARCH EXAMPLE   Highly Controlled Setting

Rasmussen and Farr (2003) conducted an experimental study of the effects of morphine and time of day on pain and beta-endorphin (BE) level in a sample of dilute brown Agouti (DBA) mice. The study was conducted in a laboratory setting, described as follows:

The mice were housed individually in clear styrene cages in a private, controlled-access room in the laboratory animal facilities of the Comparative Medicine Department. Individual housing was used to reduce social conflict and stress, which have been shown to bring about stress-induced analgesia.... The presence of other mice in the room prevented isolation stress. Food and water were allowed ad libitum. A 12:12 light/dark cycle, with lights on at 0600, and a room temperature of 22 ± 1° C were maintained throughout the study. Experiments timed for the dark phase were performed under dim red lights. (Rasmussen & Farr, 2003, p. 107)

CRITIQUE

The study included the use of a highly controlled laboratory setting in terms of the housing of the mice, the light and temperature of the environment, implementation of the treatments, and the measurements of the dependent variables. Only with animals can this type of setting control be achieved in the conduct of a study. This type of highly controlled setting removes the impact of numerous extraneous variables, so that the effects of the independent variables on the dependent variables can be clearly determined.

IMPLICATIONS FOR PRACTICE

Rasmussen and Farr (2003) found that morphine

...is used frequently to control pain, yet it also alters the endogenous BE response to acute pain. In addition, the magnitude of the increase in pain tolerance provided by morphine is not equal at all times of day. The appropriate timing of morphine administration for the treatment of acute pain should enhance the effect of the endogenous opioid system, which may decrease the need for large doses of morphine at some time points. Specifically, it may be appropriate to decrease morphine dosages during the client's active period or day to achieve this goal. (p. 113)

Because this research was conducted on animals, however, the findings cannot be generalized to humans, and additional research is needed to determine the effects of the independent variables of morphine and time of day on the dependent variables of pain and BE level in humans.

KEY CONCEPTS

- Sampling involves selecting a group of people, events, behaviors, or other elements with which to conduct a study.
- Sampling theory was developed to determine the most effective way of acquiring a sample that accurately reflects the population under study.
- Important concepts in sampling theory include population, population elements, sampling criteria, representativeness, randomization, sampling frame, and sampling plan.
- In quantitative research a sampling plan is developed to increase representativeness, decrease systematic bias, and decrease sampling error.
- The two main types of sampling plans are probability and nonprobability.
- Four sampling designs have been developed to achieve probability sampling: simple random sampling, stratified random sampling, cluster sampling, and systematic sampling.
- The five nonprobability designs discussed in this chapter are convenience sampling, quota sampling, purposive sampling, network sampling, and theoretical sampling.
- Convenience and quota sampling frequently are used in quantitative research.
- Purposive, network, and theoretical sampling are more commonly used in qualitative than in quantitative research.
- Factors that must be considered in making decisions about sample size in quantitative studies include the type of study, number of variables, sensitivity of the measurement tools, data analysis techniques, and expected effect size.
- The number of participants in a qualitative study is adequate when saturation of information is achieved in the study area.
- Important factors that need to be considered in determining sample size to achieve saturation of data are (1) scope of the study, (2) nature of the topic, (3) quality of the data collected, and (4) design of the study.
- Three common settings for conducting nursing research are natural, partially controlled, and highly controlled.

TIPS FOR FURTHER STUDY

- Review the content on determining adequate sample size in quantitative and qualitative studies. Examine the studies in your *Study Guide*. Determine if the sample size is adequate for each of the studies. Provide a rationale for your answer.
  - Determine which sampling method is the strongest to use in conducting a quantitative study.
  - Consider settings commonly used for nursing studies. Do these settings seem appropriate to generate the research evidence for use in practice?
- To practice identifying sampling methods, try the Bonus Review Questions at http://evolve.elsevier.com/Burns/understanding/.

REFERENCES

Burns, N., & Grove, S. K. (2005). *The practice of nursing research: Conduct, critique, and utilization* (5th ed.). Philadelphia: Saunders.

Clifford, C. (1997). *Qualitative research methodology in nursing and healthcare*. New York: Churchill Livingstone.

Cohen, J. (1988). *Statistical power analysis for the behavioral sciences* (2nd ed.). New York: Academic Press.

Coté-Arsenault, D., & Morrison-Beedy, D. (2001). Women's voices reflecting changed expectations for pregnancy after perinatal loss. *The Journal of Nursing Scholarship, 33*(3), 239–244.

Coyne, I. T. (1997). Sampling in qualitative research. Purposeful and theoretical sampling: Merging or clear boundaries. *Journal of Advanced Nursing, 26*(3), 623–630.

DeVon, H. A., Penckofer, S. M., & Zerwic, J. J. (2005). Symptoms of unstable angina in patients with and without diabetes. *Research in Nursing & Health, 28*(2), 136–143.

Golding, J. M. (1996). Sexual assault history and limitations in physical functioning in two general population samples. *Research in Nursing & Health, 19*(1), 33–44.

Huberman, A. M., & Miles, M. B. (2002). *The qualitative researcher's companion*. Thousand Oaks, CA: Sage Publications.

Kerlinger, F. N., & Lee, H. B. (2000). *Foundations of behavioral research*. New York: Harcourt Brace.

Kindy, D., Petersen, S., & Parkhurst, D. (2005). Perilous work: Nurses' experiences in psychiatric units with high risks of assault. *Archives of Psychiatric Nursing, 19*(4), 169–175.

Kraemer, H. C., & Theimann, S. (1987). *How many subjects? Statistical power analysis in research*. Newbury Park, CA: Sage.

Manojlovich, M. (2005). Predictors of professional nursing practice behaviors in hospital settings. *Nursing Research, 54*(1), 41–47.

McCain, N. L., Munjas, B. A., Munro, C. L., Elswick, R. K., Jr., Robins, J. L. W., Ferreira-Gonzalez, A., et al. (2003). Effects of stress management on PNI-based outcomes in persons with HIV disease. *Research in Nursing & Health, 26*(2), 102–117.

McFarlane, J. M., Groff, J. Y., O'Brien, J. A., & Watson, K. (2005). Behaviors of children exposed to intimate partner violence before and 1 year after a treatment program for their mother. *Applied Nursing Research, 18*(1), 7–12.

Moody, L. E., Wilson, M. E., Smyth, K., Schwartz, R., Tittle, M., & Van Cott, M. L. (1988). Analysis of a decade of nursing practice research: 1977–1986. *Nursing Research, 37*(6), 374–379.

Morse, J. M. (1998). Designing funded qualitative research. In N. K. Denzin & Y. S. Lincoln (Eds.), *Strategies of qualitative inquiry* (pp. 56–85). Thousand Oaks, CA: Sage Publications.

Morse, J. M. (2000). Determining sample size. *Qualitative Health Research, 10*(1), 3–5.

Munhall, P. L. (2001). *Nursing research: A qualitative perspective* (3rd ed.). Boston: National League for Nursing Press.

O'Brien, M. E. (2001). Living in a house of cards: Family experiences with long-term childhood technology dependence. *Journal of Pediatric Nursing, 16*(1), 13–22.

Patton, M. Q. (2002). *Qualitative evaluation and research methods* (3rd ed.). Thousand Oaks, CA: Sage.

Polit, D. F., & Sherman, R. E. (1990). Statistical power in nursing research. *Nursing Research, 39*(6), 365–369.

Rambur, B., McIntosh, B., Val Palumbo, M., & Reinier, K. (2005). Education as a determinant of career retention and job satisfaction among registered nurses. *The Journal of Nursing Scholarship, 37*(2), 185–192.

Rasmussen, N. A., & Farr, L. A. (2003). Effects of morphine and time of day on pain and beta-endorphin. *Biological Research for Nursing, 5*(2), 105–116.

Rew, L. (2003). A theory of taking care of oneself grounded in experiences of homeless youth. *Nursing Research, 52*(4), 234–241.

Rivers, D. L., Aday, L. A., Frankowski, R. F., Felknor, S., White, D., & Nichols, B. (2003). Predictors of nurses' acceptance of an intravenous catheter safety device. *Nursing Research, 52*(4), 249–255.

Sandelowski, M. (1995). Focus on qualitative methods: Sample size in qualitative research. *Research in Nursing & Health, 18*(2), 179–183.

Simpson, K. R., & James, D. C. (2005). Effects of immediate versus delayed pushing during second-stage labor on fetal well-being: A randomized clinical trial. *Nursing Research 54*(3), 149–157.

Ulrich, C. M., Soeken, K. L., & Miller, N. (2003). Ethical conflict associated with managed care: Views of nurse practitioners. *Nursing Research, 52*(3), 168–175.

Wongvatunyu, S., & Porter, E. J. (2005). Mothers' experience of helping young adults with traumatic brain injury. *The Journal of Nursing Scholarship, 37*(1), 48–56.

Measurement and Data Collection in Research

Chapter Overview

Learning Outcomes

After completing this chapter, you should be able to:

1. Use measurement theory and the relevant concepts—directness of measurement, measurement error, levels of measurement, reliability, and validity—in critiquing published studies.
2. Identify possible sources of measurement error in published studies.
3. Critique the levels of measurement—nominal, ordinal, interval, and ratio—used in published studies.
4. Determine the types and extent of validity of measurement techniques reported in published studies.
5. Critique the precision and accuracy of physiological measures used in published studies.
6. Examine the measurement approaches—physiological measures, observations, interviews, questionnaires, and scales—used in published studies.
7. Critique the measurement section in a research article.
8. Critique the data collection section in a research article.

Key Terms

STUDY TOOLS

Be sure to visit http://evolve.elsevier.com/Burns/understanding for additional examples and self-tests. Also, a review of this chapter's concepts and practice exercises can be found in Chapter 11 Yes of the Study Guide for *Understanding Nursing Research: Building an Evidence-Based Practice*, 4th edition.

The purpose of measurement is to produce trustworthy data that can be used in statistical analyses. Trustworthy data are essential if a study is to contribute to the evidence base to guide nursing practice. In critiquing a published study, you must judge the trustworthiness of the measurement methods used in the study. To produce trustworthy measures, rules have been established to ensure that values or categories will be assigned consistently from one subject (or event) to another and, eventually, if the measurement strategy is found to be meaningful, from one study to another. The rules of measurement established for research are similar to those used in nursing practice. For example, for pouring a liquid medication, the rule is that the measuring container must be placed at eye level. This ensures accuracy and consistency in the dose of medication. In measuring abdominal girth to detect changes in ascites, the skin on the abdomen is marked to ensure that the measure is always taken the same distance below the umbilicus. With use of this method, any change in measurement can be attributed to a change in ascites, rather than to an inadvertent change in the measurement site. Understanding the logic of measurement is important for critiquing the adequacy of measurement methods in a nursing study. This chapter includes a discussion of some of the concepts of measurement theory, measurement strategies in nursing, and the process of data collection.

Concepts of Measurement Theory

Measurement theory guides the development and use of measurement methods. Measurement theory was developed many years ago by mathematicians, statisticians, and other scholars and includes rules that guide how things are measured. These rules allow everyone to be consistent in how they perform measurements, so that a measure used by one person is the same as that measure used by another person. This section discusses some of the basic concepts and rules of measurement theory, including directness of measurement, measurement error, level of measurement, reliability, and validity.

Directness of Measurement

To measure, the researcher must first identify the object, characteristic, or element to be measured. In some cases, identifying the object to measure and determining how to measure it are quite simple, such as when the researcher measures a person's height or wrist circumference. These are referred to as **direct measures**. Direct measures of concrete things such as height, weight, temperature, elapsed time, space, movement, heart rate, and respiration commonly are used in nursing. Technology is available to measure many bodily functions and biological and chemical characteristics. The focus of measurement in these instances is on the precision of measurement. Nurses Researchers also are experienced in gathering direct measures of variables such as age, gender, ethnic origin, diagnosis, marital status, income, and education.

However, in many cases in nursing research, the thing to be measured is not a concrete object but an abstract idea, a characteristic, or a concept such as stress, caring, coping, anxiety, compliance, or pain. Researchers cannot directly measure the abstract idea, but they can capture some elements of it in their measurements. These measures are referred to as **indirect measures** or **indicators** of the concepts. Rarely, if ever, can a single measurement strategy measure all aspects of an abstract concept. Therefore, multiple indicators are needed, and even then they cannot be expected to measure all elements of an abstract concept. Indicators of coping, for example, may be the frequency or accuracy of problem identification, the speed or effectiveness of problem resolution, level of optimism, and types of self-actualization behaviors.

CRITIQUE GUIDELINES Directness of Measurement

In critiquing a study, be sure to include the following:

1. Determine the variables that were measured.
2. Identify the methods used to measure each variable.
3. Determine whether the type of measurement is direct or indirect.

Measurement Error

The ideal, perfect measure is referred to as the **true measure or score**. However, error is inherent in any measurement strategy. **Measurement error** is the difference between the true measure and what is actually measured. The amount of error in a measure varies. Thus, there may be considerable error in one measurement and very little in the next. Measurement error exists in both direct and indirect measures and can be random or systematic. With direct measures, both the object and the measurement are visible. Direct measures, which generally are expected to be highly accurate, are subject to error. For example, a weight scale may not be accurate, a precisely calibrated thermometer may decrease in precision with use, or a tape measure may not be held at exactly the same tightness with each patient.

With indirect measures, the element being measured cannot be seen directly. For example, you cannot see hope. You may see behavior or hear words that you think represent hope. But hope is a feeling that is not always recognized or clearly expressed by the person experiencing it. The measure of hope usually is a scale that is intended to reflect the amount of hope a person feels. The scale gives numerical values of the extent of hope, based on the person's responses to the scale. Efforts to measure concepts such as hope usually result in measuring only part of the concept. Sometimes measures may identify one aspect of the concept but may include other elements that are not part of the concept. For example, an instrument designed to measure anxiety also may measure aspects of fear.

Two types of error are of concern in measurement: random error and systematic error. The difference between random and systematic error is in the direction of the error. In **random error**, the difference between the measured value and the true value is without pattern or direction (random). In one measurement, the actual value obtained may be lower than the true value, whereas in the next measurement, the actual value obtained may be higher than the true value. A number of situations can occur during the measurement process that can result in random error. For example, the person taking the measurements may not use the same procedure every time; a subject completing a paper-and-pencil scale may accidentally mark the wrong column; or the person entering the data into a computer may punch the wrong key. The purpose of measuring is to estimate the true value, usually by combining a number of values and calculating an average. Thus an average value, such as the mean, is an estimate of the true measurement. As the number of random errors increases, the precision of the estimate decreases.

Measurement error that is not random is referred to as systematic error. In **systematic error**, the variation in measurement values from the calculated average is primarily in the same direction. For example, most of the variation may be higher or lower than the average that was calculated. Systematic error occurs because something else is being measured in addition to the concept. A scale that always shows a weight that is 2 pounds more than the true weight will give measures with systematic error. All of the measured weights will be high, and as a result the mean will be higher than if an accurate scale is used. Some systematic error occurs in almost any measure. Because of the importance of this type of error in a study, researchers spend considerable time and effort refining their measuring instruments to minimize systematic error.

CRITIQUE GUIDELINES Measurement Error

In critiquing a published study, you will not be able to judge the extent of measurement error directly. However, you may find clues to the amount of error in the published report. For example, if the researcher has described the method of measurement in great detail, and provided evidence of accuracy and consistency of measurement, the probability of error typically is reduced. If weight scales are recalibrated periodically during data collection, error tends to be reduced. Measurement will be more precise if the researcher has used a well-developed, reliable, and valid "paper-and-pencil" scale, instead of a newly developed scale.

RESEARCH EXAMPLE   Measurement Error

Accuracy of measurement is important in both research and clinical practice. Craft and Moss (1996) discuss error in the measurement of infant emesis volume.

Liquid amounts are particularly difficult to verify because of the instability of the configuration from event to event. When visualized, the variety in edges, colors, and direction of the liquid in each occurrence makes a template for comparison difficult.

Liquid volumes in the form of emesis are often estimated in nurseries and pediatric units at hospitals. The smaller the patient, the more crucial is accurate fluid output assessment. Infants demand the accurate estimation of fluid loss, and measures to increase accuracy in visual processing are needed. The emesis of infants is particularly difficult to estimate because the infant cannot verbalize the presence of nausea, which would help nurses anticipate vomiting. Therefore nurses are often unable to preweight bibs, spit cloths, or bed linen, or to catch the fluid in a container for objective measurement. (p. 3)

The non-experimental study was conducted using 109 subjects who had a large range of experience in assessing infant emesis volume. Practicing pediatric nurses were invited to participate in the study by displaying posters on pediatric and neonatal areas in a large university hospital. Nursing students from the university also were invited to participate. (p. 4)

Because the purpose of this study was to determine the accuracy of assessing infant emesis volume, a realistic situation was provided, using displays of actual formula volumes on receiving blankets that were all folded to one eighth of their original size. Subjects were asked to write down the correct volume perceived and to state whether they had picked up the blanket to evaluate the weight of the display. (p. 4)

Twenty receiving blankets were used as displays. The amounts of formula to be poured on the blankets were randomly selected by writing amounts on slips of paper.... Subjects were then read the following scenario: "You have just fed Timmy 50 mL of formula before he vomits. You are to determine how much he has vomited." Subjects began at display 1 and walked to display 20, writing down their volume estimations. (p. 4)

Absolute accuracy was defined as subject choosing the exact number of milliliters corresponding to what was measured and poured on the display. The investigators were concerned about the small number of displays that were assessed accurately. This small number necessitated a change from analyzing accuracy to analyzing relative error. Relative error was determined by the range of milliliters chosen on either side of the exact amount.... The findings showed that novice subjects, or students, overestimated an average of 1% of the correct volume, whereas more experienced subjects underestimated an average of 16% of the volume. Subjects who stated they were unsure of what method they used underestimated an average of 60%, and subjects who said they used experience as a method underestimated an average of 50% of the correct volume. (pp. 5–6)

Thus, the amount of error in judging amounts of emesis is high. Such error is problematic both clinically and in nursing studies. Experience alone does not increase accuracy, although teaching a method for estimating volume is related to accuracy in judgments about volume.

CRITIQUE

The purpose of Craft and Moss' (1996) study was to assess the extent of error in measuring emesis volume in infants. Their study indicated that measurement error was high. This finding suggests that using an estimate of the amount of infant emesis in a study is inherently problematic. A search of CINAHL using infant emesis as the search term yielded no further articles after the publication of this paper. Accuracy of measurement is so critical that studies cannot be conducted until a method of accurately measuring infant emesis can be developed. This study demonstrates the importance of critiquing the accuracy of measurements used in a study.

IMPLICATIONS FOR PRACTICE

Accuracy of measurements is equally important in clinical practice. Craft and Moss (1996) point out the need to develop strategies for teaching student nurses how to improve the accuracy of their estimates of infant emesis. Their study found that the estimates of experienced nurses were even less accurate than those of students. They recommend that staff education strategies be developed to improve the accuracy of estimates of all persons employed in the care of hospitalized infants. This study contributes to the body of nursing knowledge primarily by identifying a problem that needs to be addressed through further research.

Levels of Measurement

The traditional levels of measurement were developed by Stevens in 1946. Stevens organized the rules for assigning numbers to objects so that a hierarchy in measurement was established. The levels of measurement, from low to high, are nominal, ordinal, interval, and ratio.

Nominal-Scale Measurement

Nominal-scale measurement is the lowest of the four measurement categories. It is used when data can be organized into categories of a defined property but the categories cannot be compared. For example, you may decide to categorize potential study subjects by diagnosis. However, the category "kidney stone," for example, can't be rated higher than the category "peptic ulcer"; likewise, across categories, "ovarian cyst" is no closer to "kidney stone" than to "peptic ulcer." The categories differ in quality but not quantity. Therefore, it's not possible to say that subject A possesses more of the property being categorized than does subject B. (RULE: The categories must not be orderable.) Categories must be established in such a way that a datum will fit into only one of the categories. (RULE: The categories must be exclusive.) All of the data must fit into the established categories. (RULE: The categories must be exhaustive.) Data such as gender, ethnicity, marital status, and diagnoses are examples of nominal data.

Ordinal-Scale Measurement

With ordinal-scale measurement, data are assigned to categories that can be ranked. To rank data, one category is judged to be (or is ranked) higher or lower, or better or worse, than another category. Rules govern how the data are ranked. As with nominal data, the categories must be exclusive and exhaustive. With ordinal data, the quantity also can be identified. For example, if you are measuring intensity of pain, you may identify different levels of pain. You probably will develop categories that rank these different levels of pain, such as excruciating, severe, moderate, mild, and no pain. However, in using categories of ordinal measurement, you cannot know with certainty that the intervals between the ranked categories are equal. A greater difference may exist between mild and moderate pain, for example, than between excruciating and severe pain. Therefore, ordinal data are considered to have unequal intervals.

Many scales used in nursing research are ordinal levels of measurement. For example, it's possible to rank degrees of coping, levels of mobility, ability to provide self-care, or daily amount of exercise on an ordinal scale. For daily exercise, the scale could be 0 = no exercise, 1 = moderate exercise with no sweating, 2 = exercise to the point of sweating, 3 = strenuous exercise with sweating for at least 30 minutes a day, and 4 = strenuous exercise with sweating for at least 1 hour per day. The measurement is ordinal because it's not possible to claim that equal distances exist between the rankings. A greater difference may exist between the ranks of 1 and 2 than between the ranks of 2 and 3.

Interval-Scale Measurement

Interval-scale measurement uses interval scales, which have equal numerical distances between intervals. These scales follow the rules of mutually exclusive categories, exhaustive categories, and rank ordering and are assumed to represent a continuum of values. Thus, the magnitude of the attribute can be more precisely defined. However, it is not possible to provide the absolute amount of the attribute, because the interval scale lacks a zero point. Temperature is the most commonly used example of an interval scale. The difference between the temperatures of 70° and 80° F is the same as the difference between the temperatures of 30° and 40° F. Changes in temperature can be precisely measured. However, a temperature of 0° does not indicate the absence of temperature.

Ratio-Scale Measurement

Ratio-scale measurement is the highest form of measurement and meets all of the rules of other forms of measurement: mutually exclusive categories, exhaustive categories, ordered ranks, equally spaced intervals, and a continuum of values. In addition, ratio-level measures have absolute zero points. Weight, length, and volume are commonly used as examples of ratio scales. All three have absolute zero points, at which a value of zero indicates the absence of the property being measured; zero weight means the absence of weight. Because of the absolute zero point, such statements as "Object A weighs twice as much as object B" or "Container A holds three times as much as container B" can be justified.

CRITIQUE GUIDELINES   **Level of Measurement**

In critiquing a published study, determine the level of each measurement used in the study. In some studies, the researcher will indicate the level of measurement used. In others, you will need to determine the level of measurement from the description of the measurement method used.

Reliability

Reliability is concerned with the consistency of the measurement technique. For example, if a scale is being used to weigh a subject, the scale should indicate the same weight each time the subject steps on and off the scale. A scale that does not show the same weight every time is unreliable.

Reliability testing is a measure of the amount of random error in the measurement technique. It takes into account such characteristics as dependability, consistency, accuracy, and comparability. Because all measurement techniques contain some random error, reliability exists in degrees and usually is expressed as a correlation coefficient, with a coefficient of 1.00 indicating perfect reliability and a coefficient of 0.00 indicating no reliability. A reliability of 0.80 is considered the lowest acceptable coefficient for a well-developed measurement tool. For a newly developed instrument, a reliability of 0.70 is considered acceptable. Estimates of reliability are specific to the sample being tested. Thus, high reliability values reported for an established instrument do not guarantee that reliability will be satisfactory in another sample or with a different population. Therefore, reliability testing needs to be performed on each instrument used in a study before other statistical analyses are performed. The results of reliability tests must be included in published reports of the study. Cronbach's alpha coefficient is the most commonly used measure of reliability.

Validity

The **validity** of an instrument is a determination of how well the instrument reflects the abstract concept being examined. Validity, like reliability, is not an all-or-nothing phenomenon; it is measured on a continuum. No instrument is completely valid. Thus, one determines the degree of validity of a measure rather than whether validity exists. Validity will vary from one sample to another and from one situation to another; therefore, validity testing evaluates the use of an instrument for a specific group or purpose, rather than the instrument itself. An instrument may be valid in one situation but not in another. For example, Beck's Hopeless Scale was developed to measure the hopelessness of hospitalized suicidal patients. Will the same scale be valid as a measure of the hopelessness of cancer patients? This is determined by pilot testing the scale to test for validity of the instrument in a new population.

In critiquing a study, you need to judge the validity of the measures that were used. However, you cannot consider validity apart from reliability. If a measurement method does not have acceptable reliability, its validity becomes a moot issue. Unfortunately, not all published studies include information on the validity and reliability of measurement instruments used in the study.

CRITIQUE GUIDELINES Reliability and Validity

When critiquing the reliability and validity of an instrument used in a published study, consider the following guidelines:

1. What reliability information is provided from previous studies and for this study?
2. Does the author include reports of the validity of the instrument from previous studies? Unfortunately, in some cases, the researcher will simply state that previous research has found validity of the measurement method to be acceptable. This statement does not provide the information you need to judge validity. In such cases, simply state that you had insufficient information, other than the author's statement that the validity was acceptable, on which to judge validity.

(continues)

CRITIQUE GUIDELINES *(continued)*

3. Did the author perform pilot studies to examine the reliability and validity of the instrument?
4. In the discussion of findings near the end of the report, did the researcher report the use of data from the present study to examine instrument reliability and validity?

RESEARCH EXAMPLE Instrument Reliability and Validity

In a study titled "Changes in Well-Being of Women Cancer Survivors Following a Survivor Weekend Experience," Rutledge and Raymon (2001) report reliability and validity information on an instrument used to measure quality of life in women who have breast cancer.

Quality of Life–Breast Cancer (QOL-BC) (Ferrell et al., 1996) was a newly developed instrument based on the reliable and valid Quality of Life–Cancer Survivors (QOL-CS) Tool (Ferrell, Dow, Leigh, et al., 1995). The 46-item QOL-BC included items dealing with issues of concern to breast cancer survivors. Items represent the four domains of QOL: psychological well-being (22 items), physical well-being (8 items), social well-being (9 items), and spiritual well-being (7 items). Individual items, subscale, and total QOL responses ranged from 0–10. Higher scores indicated better QOL. Documented reliability and validity of the QOL-CS included test-retest reliability over two weeks ($r = 0.89$), internal consistency reliability using Cronbach's alpha coefficient (subscale scores, 0.81–0.93), content validity with a panel of QOL researchers and oncology nurses, and both convergent and divergent validity with known groups (Ferrell, Dow, & Grant, 1995). In the current study, alpha reliabilities for the well-being subscales pre-retreat ($N = 59$) were physical (0.78), psychological (0.93), social (0.87), and spiritual (0.71) and for total QOL it was 0.95. (p. 87)

Conclusions

The Healing Odyssey Retreats enhanced women cancer survivors' total QOL-BC specifically their well-being in four dimensions. (p. 85)

CRITIQUE

The information provided about the tool is sufficient for the reader to critique the reliability and validity of the tool. In total scores, values of 0.80 or higher are considered good. Values of 0.70 to 0.80 are considered acceptable but marginal. Values below 0.70 indicate problems with reliability. In subscale scores, lower values than 0.70 can be acceptable, but the lower the values, the lower the reliability of the subscale. Basically, a value of 0.70 indicates that you can trust the reliability or consistency of the scale score or subscale score 70% of the time—so 30% of the time, you cannot trust the score value. Thus, as the reliability value decreases, the total scores become less trustworthy.

The QOL-BC was first described in the literature in 1996 (Ferrell, Grant, Funk, Garcia, Otis-Green, & Schaffner, 1996) and is based on a broader tool measuring quality of life of cancer survivors. New items were added that are of specific concern to breast cancer survivors. The validity testing addresses values reported for QOL-CS, not QOL-BC, which is the tool used in the study. QOL-BC was tested, but numerical results of the testing were not reported by Rutledge and Raymon (2001). However, references are provided for readers who want to obtain specific results of validity testing. The added items represent 4 domains of Quality of Life and thus adds to the validity of the instrument. Reliability of subscales and of total score in the present study is high. The researchers report item analyses in the discussion of the study findings.

IMPLICATIONS FOR PRACTICE

The information provided is not sufficient to serve as evidence for practice. The tool must first undergo further testing. The study must be replicated, or the results of multiple studies testing the effectiveness of the treatment (Healing Odyssey Retreats) on quality of life of women with breast cancer must be carefully examined, before it can be concluded that the treatment is effective.

Precision and Accuracy of Physiological Measures

Precision and accuracy of physiological and biochemical measures tend not to be reported in published studies. The assumption is made, which is not always correct, that routine physiological measures are precise and accurate. The most common physiological measures used in nursing studies are blood pressure, heart rate, weight, and body temperature. These measures often are obtained from the patient's record, with no consideration of their accuracy. How many times have you heard a nurse ask a patient his or her weight, rather than weighing the patient? Researchers using physiological measures must provide evidence of the accuracy or validity of those measures. The precision or consistency of physiologic measures also need to be addressed when they are used in a study.

CRITIQUE GUIDELINES Precision and Accuracy of Physiological Measures

When critiquing a study, judge the accuracy and precision of any physiological measures used in the study. However, remember that initial attempts to measure a physiological element important to nursing practice are likely to be less accurate than those that have been refined in several studies. Much work is needed to clarify specific elements of physiological assessment in nursing practice; the use of physiological measures in research requires even more rigor than those used in nursing practice (Burns & Grove, 2005).

RESEARCH EXAMPLE Precision and Accuracy of Physiological Measures

Engle and Graney (2000) used the total pulse amplitude in a study of the biobehavioral effects of therapeutic touch (TT). One suggested effect of TT is relaxation. Relaxation occurs because of responses of the autonomic nervous system. How can changes in the autonomic nervous system be measured? These investigators used a very sensitive physiological measure: blood flow of small arteries in the deep dermal layers of the skin in the extremities. This blood flow, affected by the sympathetic autonomic nervous system, is referred to as pulse amplitude. A higher total pulse amplitude is correlated with vasodilation (associated with relaxation), and a lower amplitude is correlated with vasoconstriction (associated with tension).

(continues)

RESEARCH EXAMPLE *(continued)*

The researchers describe the measurement as follows:

Medasonics™ infrared light sensor was lightly taped to the pad of the third finger of the left hand. To prevent arm movement (Goetz, 1940), the participant's arm was stabilized by placing the arm fully extended and palm upward on a 45-degree tilt board using Hartwig and colleagues (1994) protocol. An 8-channel Grass™ polygraph and integrator channel converted signals from the sensor into uniform composite wave forms up to 40 mm in height to represent pulsation. The average of three total pulse amplitude wave form measurements, calculated at the beginning, middle, and end of each time period, was used for data analysis. Test-retest reliability of this measurement protocol for total pulse amplitude for vasoconstriction with ice water has been estimated to be r = .90 for healthy, middle-aged volunteers (Hartwig et al., 1994) (Engle & Graney, 2000, p. 289)

CRITIQUE

The total pulse amplitude was able to demonstrate the occurrence of some physiological change, apparently as a result of TT. However, it is not clear that this measure is reliable or valid. To demonstrate its reliability and validity as a measure of TT, multiple studies using this method of measurement must be conducted to test TT provided by different therapists in a variety of populations. The extent to which the instrument is a valid measure of autonomic responses (used as a proxy for relaxation) is unclear. When compared with the value before TT, the total pulse amplitude changed significantly after TT. The researchers expected that TT would cause vasodilation, but instead they found that vasoconstriction occurred in response to the TT. The researchers speculated that "vasodilation may have occurred in subjects' mesenteric plexus, the area directly under the TT therapist's hands, with a corresponding reflex vasoconstriction in subjects' peripheral circulation" (pp. 291–292). The effect was present in the subjects who received TT, but not in subjects who were in the mimic therapeutic touch group. Other variables examined, such as mean arterial blood pressure, pulse rate, and skin temperature, were not affected by TT.

IMPLICATIONS FOR PRACTICE

Synthesis of multiple studies demonstrating the effectiveness of TT must be available before the use of TT as a nursing intervention can be justified. To determine other methods of measuring the effectiveness of TT and of studies testing the effectiveness of TT as a nursing intervention, search the Cochrane Collection and www.guidelines.gov. Key in therapeutic touch to search these databases.

Measurement Strategies in Nursing

Nursing studies examine a wide variety of phenomena and thus require an extensive array of measurement tools. Many nursing phenomena have not been examined because no one has thought of a way to measure them. This has implications for both clinical practice and research. This section describes some of the most common measurement approaches used in nursing research, including physiological measurement, observational measurement, interviews, focus groups, questionnaires, and scales.

Physiological Measurements

Because of measurement problems, physiological nursing research has lagged behind studies of the psychosocial dimensions of nursing practice. Some of the first physiological nursing studies examined basic care activities, such as mouth care, decubitus ulcer care, the effect of preoperative teaching on postoperative recovery, and infection control related to urinary bladder catheterization, intravenous therapy, and tracheotomy care. Even at this fairly simple level, developing valid methods to measure the variables of interest was difficult and required considerable time and expense. For example, how can changes in a decubitus ulcer be measured? What criteria can be used to determine the effectiveness of a mouth care regimen? Creativity and attention to detail are needed to develop effective physiological measurement strategies.

An increased need for means to measure the outcomes of nursing care also has generated more nursing studies that include physiological measures. The outcome of interest may be the outcome of all nursing care received for a particular care episode or the outcome of a particular nursing intervention. An important focus of **physiological measurement** is finding means to quantify changes, either directly or indirectly, that occur in physiological variables as a result of nursing care. This upsurge of interest in outcome measures has broadened the base of physiological research beyond nurse physiologists to include nurse clinicians. The number of nursing studies including physiological measures has increased dramatically in recent years. The detailed description of physiological measures in a research report need to include the exact procedures followed and specific descriptions of equipment used in measurement, as can be seen from some of the following examples.

A variety of approaches to obtaining physiological measures are possible. Some measurements are relatively easy to make and are an extension of the measurement methods used in nursing practice, such as those used to obtain weight and blood pressure. Other measurements are not difficult to make, but the method requires an imaginative approach. For example, some phenomena are traditionally only observed in clinical practice, but not measured. Some physiological measures are obtained using self-report or paper-and-pencil scales.

Text continues on p. 375.

RESEARCH EXAMPLE **Physiological Measure Using Self Report**

Phaladze, Human, Dlamini, Hulela, Hadebe, et al. (2005) used the Revised Sign and Symptom Checklist for Persons with HIV Disease (Holzemer, Hudson, Kirksey, Hamilton, & Bakken, 2001), which comprises 64 items, to determine the frequency and intensity of human immunodeficiency virus (HIV) disease–related signs and symptoms that the participants were experiencing on a particular day.

The items are rated on an ordinal, three-point Likert-type scale (1 = mild, 2 = moderate, 3 = severe). Calculations included the total number of symptoms (with a range of 0–64) and the mean intensity of symptoms (with a range of 1–3). Validity and reliability of the instrument have been reported previously for a U.S. sample (Holzemer et al., 2001). The instrument was translated into seven languages (Sesotho, Setswana, Siswati, Tswana, Venda, Xhosa, and Zulu) and were [sic] pilot tested before the study. (p. 123)

The question for study was: How do people with HIV/AIDS in sub-Saharan Africa view their quality of life? With a descriptive, cross-sectional design, adults living with HIV/AIDS [acquired immunodeficiency syndrome] in Botswana, Lesotho, South Africa, and Swaziland were the target population. A convenience,

(continues)

RESEARCH EXAMPLE *(continued)*

community-based purposefully selected sample (n = 743) provided data that were collected in 2002 in face-to-face interviews.... Each country-level team—consisting of experts in HIV/AIDS care, nurses working directly in home-based care, and university faculty—reviewed the sign and symptom checklist for its relevance to their communities and confirmed the instrument's content validity. (p. 123)

Participants in this study were people with HIV/AIDS who were not taking antiretroviral medications. Those with higher life satisfaction scores had lower levels of education, had disclosure and financial worries, did not have AIDS diagnoses or comorbidities, had lower symptom intensity, had higher levels of functioning, and had fewer health worries. (p. 125)

These findings indicate the need for greater understanding of the factors associated with the quality of life of people living with HIV/AIDS in sub-Saharan Africa. Further, they illustrate several critical factors that must be addressed to improve their quality of life. Not surprisingly, poverty was directly related to lower quality of life. Poorer functional status was significantly related to lower life satisfaction. If antiretroviral medications improve functional ability, as demonstrated in other areas of the world, many people in sub-Saharan Africa can anticipate a substantial increase in life satisfaction. (p. 126)

IMPLICATIONS FOR PRACTICE

These findings, part of an ongoing program of research on HIV/AIDS at the University of California, San Francisco, contribute to the evidence base for nursing practice and probably will be cited in reviews of evidence-based practice in the Cochrane Reviews and at www.guidelines.gov. The researchers make the following recommendations for practice:

Nurses are in direct contact with people with HIV/AIDS infection and have unique opportunities to influence their quality of life. Nurses can adopt positive attitudes and educate their patients toward "living well" with HIV/AIDS. Nurses can teach and support strategies to reduce functional disability, such as exercise and nutrition. Nurses can provide patient education materials on how to assess, manage, and control HIV-related symptoms. Nurses can provide support for self- and family-care interventions designed to enhance the quality of life for people with HIV/AIDs in sub-Saharan Africa through understanding and supporting the concept of "living well" with HIV/AIDS. (p. 126)

RESEARCH EXAMPLE Physiological Measure Using Observation

Algase, Kupferschmid, Beel-Bates, and Beattie (1997) measured wandering behavior of cognitively impaired elders using observational methods. The following is a description of their observational methods.

Ambulation cycles were measured using time-study techniques. Observers recorded time of onset and cessation for each ambulation episode on the Datamyte 1010 (Allen-Bradley, Minnetonka, MN). The Datamyte 1010 is a portable terminal with programmable clock, solid-state memory, and storage capacity to 64K characters in computer-readable format. Each locomoting phase was also coded for impetus (self- or other-directed starts) and pattern (direct, lapping, pacing, or random).

Data were downloaded directly to a microprocessor for analysis. Cycle period was computed as the time elapsed from the onset of one ambulation episode to the onset of the next. Locomoting phase duration was the time elapsed from the onset of an episode of locomotion to its cessation; nonlocomoting phase was the time elapsed from the cessation of an episode of locomotion to the onset of the next episode. Percent-of-cycle-locomoting was the locomoting phase divided by the cycle period (× 100). All ambulation episodes were observed, but only those coded as self-initiated were analyzed. Of those, lapping, pacing, and random patterns were considered wandering, while the direct pattern was not. (p. 174)

CRITIQUE

Algase and colleagues (1997) used observational measurement methods to provide nursing with an excellent approach to measuring and understanding the wandering behaviors of persons with Alzheimer's disease. Movements are categorized by phases and cycles. The measures are performed in a very detailed and systematic way. The methods provide a valid and reliable means to measure wandering, which has been further developed in more recent studies.

IMPLICATIONS FOR PRACTICE

The measurements used by Algase and colleagues (1997) in this study are not in a form that would be practical for use in clinical studies or in clinical practice. To understand what these researchers have contributed to the nursing body of knowledge related to wandering, you must be aware of the entire program of research that has been published over a period of years. Algase and colleagues have built the body of knowledge needed and synthesized it into an evidence-based practice that includes prescriptive interventions. Evidence-based practice requires the dedication of scholars committed to an ongoing series of studies to build knowledge needed by nursing. Evidence of the scholarship and the body of work can be seen in the references below.

Developing New Physiologic Measures

Nurse clinicians are often the first to identify the need to measure some aspect of nursing care that could be improved if a physical phenomenon could be measured. The effort to develop a new physiologic measure required considerable imagination and creativity, as well as time. The following study describes a physiologic measure developed by physical therapists; however, the process is the same as that used in nursing to develop new physiologic measures.

References

Algase, D. L. (1988). *Cognitive and social discriminants of wandering behavior among cognitively impaired nursing home residents.* Unpublished doctoral dissertation. Case Western Reserve University, Cleveland, Ohio.

Algase, D. L. (1992). Cognitive discriminates of wandering among nursing home residents. *Nursing Research, 41*(2), 78–81.

Algase, D. L. (1992). A century of progress: Today's strategies for responding to wandering behavior. *Journal of Gerontological Nursing, 18*(11), 28–34.

Algase, D. L., Beck, C., Kolanowski, A., Whall, A., Berent, S., Richards, K., & Beattie, E. (1996). Need-driven dementia-compromised behavior: An alternate view of disruptive behavior. *American Journal of Alzheimer's Disease, 11*(6), 10, 12–19.

Algase, D. L., Kupferschmid, B., Beel-Bates, C. A., & Beattie, E. R. A. (1997). Estimates of stability of daily wandering behavior among cognitively impaired long-term care residents. *Nursing Research, 46*(3), 172–178.

(continues)

IMPLICATIONS FOR PRACTICE *(continued)*

Algase, D. L. (1999). Wandering in dementia. *Annual Review of Nursing Research, 17*, 185–217.

Algase, D. L. (1999). Wandering: A dementia compromised behavior. *Journal of Gerontological Nursing, 25*(9), 10–16, 46–51.

Scisney-Matlock, M., Algase, D. L., Boehm, S., Coleman-Burns, P., Oakley, D., Rogers, A. E., Yeo, S., Young, E., & Yu, M. (2000). Clinical methods. Measuring behavior: Electronic devices in nursing studies. *Applied Nursing Research, 13*(2), 97–102.

Algase, D. L., Beattie, E., & Therrien, B. (2001). Impact of cognitive impairment on wandering behavior. *Western Journal of Nursing Research, 23*(3), 283–295.

Algase, D. L., Beattie, E., Bogue, E., & Yao, L. (2001). The Algase Wandering Scale: Initial psychometrics of a new caregiver reporting tool. *American Journal of Alzheimer's Disease and Other Dementias, 16*(3), 141–152.

Beattie, E., & Algase, D. L. (2002). Improving table-sitting of wanderers through substruction: Designing an intervention. *Journal of Gerontological Nursing, 28*(10), 6–11.

Algase, D. L., Beattie, E., Beel-Bates, C. A., & Futrell, M. (2002). Wandering studies: Different purposes, different perspectives...Peatfield, Futrell, and Cox in the April 2002 issue of the Journal (Vol. 27, No. 4, pp. 44–50). *Journal of Gerontological Nursing, 28*(10), 4, 52.

Algase, D. L., Beel-Bates, C. A., & Beattie, E. R. A. (2003). Wandering in long term care. *Annals of Long Term Care, 11*(1), 33–39.

Algase, D. L., Beattie, E. R. A., Leitsch, S. A., & Beel-Bates, C. A. (2003). Biomedical activity devices to index wandering behavior in dementia. *American Journal of Alzheimer's Disease and Other Dementias, 18*(2), 85–92.

Song, J., Algase, D. L., Beattie, E. R. A., Milke, D. L., Duffield, C., & Cowan, B. (2003). Comparison of U. S., Canadian, and Australian participants' performance on the Algase Wandering Scale–Version 2 (AWS-V2). *Research and Theory for Nursing Practice, 17*(3), 241–256).

Algase, D. L., Beattie, E. R. A., Song, J., Millke, D. L., Duffield, C., & Cowan, B. (2004). Validation of the Algase Wandering Scale (version 2) in a cross cultural sample. *Aging & Mental Health, 8*(2), 133–142.

Beattie, E. R. A., Algase, D. L., & Song, J. (2004). Keeping wandering nursing home residents at the table: Improving food intake using a behavioral communication intervention. *Aging & Mental Health, 8*(2), 109–116.

Siders, C., Nelson, A., Brown, L. M., Joseph, I., Algase, D. L., Beattie, E., & Verbosky-Cadena, S. (2004). Evidence for implementing nonpharmacological interventions for wandering. *Rehabilitation Nursing, 29*(6), 195–206.

RESEARCH EXAMPLE   Developing A New Physiological Measure

Tyson & DeSouza (2004). Development of the Brunel Balance Assessment: A new measure of balance disability post stroke.

The restoration of balance skills is a cornerstone of stroke physiotherapy (Ballinger, Ashburn, Low, & Roderick, 1999; Lennon, & Ashburn, 2000). In this study the authors' ultimate aim is to assess the effectiveness of stroke physiotherapy interventions, therefore we needed to identify suitable outcome measures. If a measurement tool is to assess the effects of physiotherapy, in addition to the basic psychometric properties (reliability and validity), it needs to be sensitive to short-term changes due to physiotherapy, relevant to and reflective of physiotherapy practice, suitable for use with all the types of patients and all settings in which physiotherapists work. It also needs to be quick, simple, portable and cheap to be attractive for use in clinical practice (Sackley & Lincoln, 1996) (Tyson & DeSouza, 2004, p. 801-802).

We undertook an extensive review of outcome measures to test balance disability post stroke but none fulfilled these criteria. Ordinal scales were reliable and valid but insensitive to short-term changes (Tyson & DeSouza, 2002a). Functional performance tests (such as the 10-m walk or forward reach tests) were reliable, valid, sensitive and user-friendly but each was only suitable for a narrow range of abilities (Tyson & DeSouza, 2002b). Instrumented measures, such as postural sway equipment, have limited reliability and validity as tests of balance disability and are only suitable for a narrow range of abilities. They are also expensive and unsuitable for use in a community setting (Tyson & DeSouza, 2002c). We therefore needed to develop a new measurement tool which would meet the criteria for use as an outcome measure for stroke physiotherapy interventions (Tyson & DeSouza, 2004, p. 802).

When physiotherapists assess balance in people with stroke they observe the patient's ability to perform a series of increasingly demanding balance tasks. These tasks are progressed by reducing the size of the base of support (from sitting to standing to stepping and single stance tasks) and increasing the complexity of the task (from supported to static and dynamic tasks and changing the base of support) (Tyson & DeSouza, 2002) (Tyson & DeSouza, 2004, p. 802).

A functional performance test was developed to operationalize each level of the hierarchy. . . The idea was that the physiotherapist would identify where on the hierarchy the patient's abilities lay and then use the corresponding functional performance test as a sensitive and specific measure of the patient's abilities. As the patient's abilities changed, they would progress (or regress) to different levels of the hierarchy. Different patients would therefore use different tests but as they were all going through the same series, they would be comparable. To decide where a patient's abilities lay on the hierarchy, there needed to be a basic cut-off point for each test to say whether the patient had passed or failed at that level. These 'pass marks' were based on the measurement error for each test. . . For instance, the minimum score to pass level 8 (dynamic standing balance) is 7 cm. If the patient could reach forwards more than 7 cm beyond arm's length in standing, he or she would pass this level of the ordinal scale. Then the actual score for the forward reach test would be used as a more sensitive measure of changes in performance. The use of the pass marks converted the hierarchy to an ordinal scale (Tyson & DeSouza, 2004, p. 802).

Having chosen items for the prototype scale, the appropriateness of these choices needed to be considered. There are a number of ways that a scale can be constructed. One method is to arrange the items into a hierarchy so the difficulty increases with each item. If the scale forms a true hierarchy, then when a subject fails an item, he or she can be assumed to fail all the following, higher items, or if the subject passes an item, it can be assumed that he or she would pass all the lower items (Wade, 1992). This means that not all the items need to be tested each time the subject is assessed. Testing can stop once the subject has failed an item; alternatively it can start at a level the subject would find reasonably challenging. This reduces the time and effort required for testing for both tester and subject. Another advantage of a hierarchical scale is that it gives information about what a patient can or cannot do, rather than now many activities he or she can do (Eakin, 1989) (Tyson & DeSouza, 2004, p. 803).

If this limited testing of items is used then it is essential that all the items are homogeneous, that is they all test the same basic trait, in this case balance (Barer, & Nouri, 1989. If the items are homogeneous then they should all be moderately correlated to each other and each should correlate to the total score. These two factors form the basis for testing homogeneity or internal consistency (Streiner & Norman, 1997). If, however, one or more items were very highly correlated to another, such item(s) would not add any new information, and would be unnecessary or redundant (Streiner & Norman, 1997). Having redundant items would not only increase the time and effort required for testing but also artificially inflate the internal consistency of the scale, and should be discarded (Streiner & Norman, 1997) (Tyson & DeSouza, 2004, p. 803).

(continues)

RESEARCH EXAMPLE *(continued)*

It takes approximately 10 minutes to complete, uses minimal equipment (a ruler and stand, step-up block and stopwatch), is portable and has been successfully used in the research, hospital and community setting (Tyson & DeSouza, 2004, p. 807). The Brunel Balance Assessment, in its final version is shown below.

The Revised Brunel Balance Assessment

During the scale development level 2 (independent sitting balance) and level 6 (independent standing balance) were found to be redundant. They were therefore removed from the final version which is shown below, leaving a 12-point hierarchical ordinal scale.

Level of balance	Performance test
1) Static sitting balance with upper limb support	Timed for 30 s (Yes/No)
2) Static sitting balance	Arm raise test
3) Dynamic sitting balance	Forward reach test
4) Static standing balance with upper limb support	Time for 30 s (Yes/No)
5) Static standing balance	Arm raise test
6) Dynamic standing balance	Forward reach test
7) Static double stance (stride standing)	Timed for 30 s (Yes/No)
8) Supported single stance	Timed 5-m walk with an aid
9) Dynamic double stance (stride stand)	Weight-shift test
10) Changing the BoS (between double and single stance)	Timed 5-m walk without aid
11) Maintaining static single stance	Tap test
12) Advanced change of the BoS	Step-up test

(Tyson & DeSouza, 2004, p. 810)

References

Ballinger, C., Ashburn, A., Low, J., & Roderick, P. (1999). Unpacking the black box of therapy—A pilot study to describe occupational therapy and physiotherapy interventions for people with stroke. *Clinical Rehabilitation, 13*(4), 301-309.

Barer, D., & Nouri, F. (1989). Measurement of activities of daily living. *Clinical Rehabilitation, 3*(X), 179-187.

Eakin, P. (1989). Assessment of activities of daily living: A critical review. *British Journal of Occupational Therapy, 52*(1), 179-187.

Lennon, S., & Ashburn, A. (2000). The Bobath Concept in stroke rehabilitation: A focus group study of experienced physiotherapists' perspective. *Disability & Rehabilitation, 22*(15), 665-674.

Sackley, C., & Lincoln, N. (1996). Physiotherapy treatment for stroke patients: A survey of current practice. *Physiotherapy Theory & Practice, 12*( ), 87-96.

Streiner, D., & Norman, G. (1997). *Health measurement scales: A practical guide to their development and use*, second edition. Oxford: Oxford Medical Publications.

Tyson, S., & DeSouza, L. (2002a). The assessment of balance and walking post stroke: Part 1 ordinal scales. *Physical Therapy Review. 7*, 87-91.

Tyson, S., & DeSouza, L. (2002b). The assessment of balance and walking: Part 2 functional performance tests. *Physical Therapy Review, 7*, 231-241.

Tyson, S., & DeSouza, L. (2002c). The assessment of balance post stroke: Part 3 instrumented measurement tools. *Physical Therapy Review, 7*, 231-241.

Tyson, S., & DeSouza, L. (2003). A clinical model for the assessment of posture and balance post stroke. *Disability & Rehabilitation, 25*, 120-126.

Wade, D. T. (1992). *Measurement in neurological rehabilitation*. Oxford: Oxford University Press.

CRITIQUE

Tyson and DeSouza, 2004 (2004) provide a clear description of the reason the new measure was developed and the process of development. In a section not quoted above, the careful testing of validity and reliability were tested. Although the focus of much instrument testing is accuracy and precision, when validity and reliability can reasonable be tested, it is used to verify the performance of the measure.

IMPLICATIONS FOR PRACTICE

The implications for practice in this study are focused on physical therapists. However, there might be some instances in which the measurement method might be used as an element of nursing practice. However, the greatest implication for nurses is the description of the development process and the imagination used in it's development. Nurse clinicians at the Baccalaureate level, perhaps working in partnership with master's or doctoral level nurses, can contribute to the development of new measures needed for nursing practice.

Observational Measurements

Although observational measurement is most commonly used in qualitative research, it is used to some extent in all types of studies. Unstructured observations involve spontaneously observing and recording what is seen. Although unstructured observations give the observer freedom, they carry the risk that objectivity will be lost; furthermore, the observer may not remember all of the details of the observed event. In structured observational measurement, the researcher carefully defines what is to be observed and how the observations are to be made, recorded, and coded. In most cases a category system is developed for organizing and sorting the behaviors or events being observed. Checklists often are used to indicate whether a behavior occurred. Rating scales allow the observer to rate the behavior or event. This provides more information for analysis than dichotomous data, which indicate only whether or not the behavior occurred.

Observation tends to be more subjective than other types of measurement and thus often is considered less credible. However, in many cases this approach is the only way to obtain important data for nursing's body of knowledge. As with any means of measurement, consistency is very important; thus, reporting interrater reliability is essential.

CRITIQUE GUIDELINES **Observational Measurements**

When critiquing observational measures, consider the following questions.

1. Is the object of observation clearly identified and defined?
2. Is interrater reliability described?
3. Are the techniques for recording observations described?

RESEARCH EXAMPLE Observational Measurement

Holditch-Davis, Miles, Burchinal, O'Donnell, McKinney, and Lim (2001) used observational methods to record mother-infant interactions in a study of parental caregiving and developmental outcomes of infants of mothers with HIV. The observations were made during home visits when the infants were 12, 18, and 24 months of age. Data were collected during periods when the infant was awake and not due for a feeding.

During the 1-hour observation, the occurrences of 17 maternal and 12 infant behaviors during each 10-second period were recorded onto paper, using a one-zero sampling method. The end of each 10-second period was signaled audibly to the observer through an earphone from a small electronic timer (Holditch-Davis & Thoman, 1988; Miller & Holditch-Davis, 1992; Tesh & Holditch-Davis, 1997). Five mother variables were used in this study: negative (directing negative affect toward the child), positive (directing positive affect toward the child), play with child, talk, and interaction (talking to, touching, gesturing toward, or playing with child). To adjust for variations in the lengths of observations, these variables were measured as percentages of the total observation. The percentages were calculated by dividing the number of 10-second periods during which a behavior occurred by the number of 10-second periods in the observation.

Four observers conducted the observations. Before beginning observations, each observer achieved interrater reliability of at least 85% exact agreement on occurrences by coding live observations on volunteer children or study participants along with an investigator who was experienced in behavioral observation. It took 3 to 6 months of practice before initial reliability was achieved. Ongoing interrater reliability for the observation was assessed approximately every other observation throughout the study by having two observers score an observation together. Cohen's kappas were 0.75 for negative, 0.90 for positive, 0.85 for play, 0.85 for talk, and 0.82 for interaction. (p. 7)

The authors found that mental development and adaptive behavior decreased as the child grew older. Infants who changed their primary caregiver had lower motor and adaptive behavior. More positive attention and more negative control were associated with higher mental, motor, and adaptive behavior.

CRITIQUE

Holditch-Davis and colleagues (2001) clearly identified and defined the observations to be recorded. The frequency of observations was timed electronically at 10-second intervals for 1 hour. The techniques for recording observations are carefully described. Observers were trained for a 3- to 6-month period before initiating the study and then were trained repeatedly during the data collection period. Interrater reliability was high, indicating that the observational training was very successful. The observer recorded observations every 10 seconds onto paper, using the codes written on the paper, and indicating a 1 if the coded behavior was occurring and 0 if it was not. This allowed the observer to record multiple behaviors during the 10 seconds.

IMPLICATIONS FOR PRACTICE

Nurses who provide care for mothers with HIV disease and their infants are in a position to support and guide the mothers in parent-child interactions to promote optimal child development. Suggestions can be given for giving positive attention to the infant and for using negative control measures. Changing the primary caregiver is not always possible to avoid if the mother becomes physically unable to provide care for the infant or dies.

Interviews

An **interview** involves verbal communication between the researcher and the subject during which information is provided to the researcher. Although this measurement strategy most commonly is used in qualitative and descriptive studies, it also can be used in other types of studies. A variety of approaches can be used to conduct an interview, ranging from a totally unstructured interview, in which the content is completely controlled by the subject, to a structured interview, in which the content is similar to that of a questionnaire, with the possible responses to questions carefully designed by the researcher.

Unstructured interviews may be initiated by asking a broad question, such as "Describe for me your experience with…." After the interview has begun, the role of the interviewer is to encourage the subject to continue talking, using techniques such as nodding the head or making sounds that indicate interest. In some cases, the subject may be encouraged to elaborate further on a particular dimension of the topic of discussion.

During **structured interviews**, the researcher uses strategies to control the content of the interview. Questions the interviewer asks are designed by the researcher before the initiation of data collection, and the order of the questions is specified. In some cases the interviewer can elaborate on the meaning of the question or modify the way in which the question is asked so that the subject can understand it better. In more structured interviews, the interviewer is required to ask the question precisely as it has been designed.

Because nurses frequently use interviewing techniques in nursing assessment, the dynamics of interviewing are familiar; however, using the technique for measurement in research requires greater sophistication. Interviewing is a flexible technique that allows the researcher to explore meaning in greater depth than is possible with other techniques. Interpersonal skills can be used to facilitate cooperation and elicit more information. Because the response rate for interviews is higher than for questionnaires, interviewing often allows a more representative sample to be obtained. Interviewing allows collection of data from subjects who are unable or unlikely to complete questionnaires, such as those who are very ill or whose ability to read, write, and express themselves is marginal.

Interviews are a form of self-report, and it must be assumed that the information provided is accurate. Because of time and costs, sample size usually is limited. Subject bias is always a threat to the validity of the findings, as is inconsistency in data collection from one subject to another.

CRITIQUE GUIDELINES   Interviews

When critiquing interview methods of measurement in studies, consider the following questions.

1. Do the interview questions address concerns expressed in the research problem?
2. Are the interview questions relevant for the research purpose and objectives, questions, or hypotheses?
3. Does the design of the questions tend to bias subjects' responses?
4. Does the sequence of questions tend to bias subjects' responses?

RESEARCH EXAMPLE Interviews

Schumacher, Koresawa, West, Dodd, Paul, Tripathy, et al. (2002) conducted interviews to determine the usefulness of a daily pain management diary for outpatients with cancer-related pain. The study was funded by a grant from the National Cancer Institute.

The diary was used as a component of a randomized clinical trial of the PRO-SELF© Pain Control Program. At the completion of the last home visit, patients and family caregivers in both the treatment and control group were asked if they had found the pain management diary useful. Responses to this query provided the data for analysis of the interview. Two end-of-study questions were asked: (1) "Tell me about the help-fulness or unhelpfulness of the pain diary" and (2) "Do you have any suggestions about modifying the diary?" Responses were tape-recorded and transcribed verbatim.... Content analysis was used for data analysis. Two members of the research team coded all data independently and then met to compare results and resolve differences through consensus. Responses were sorted into clearly positive, clearly negative, or other categories. When patients and family caregivers elaborated on their positive or negative responses, researchers did line-by-line coding and categorization of their narratives to better understand how patients and family caregivers found the diary useful or not useful. Categories and subcategories were allowed to emerge from the data rather than from an investigator-generated, a priori coding scheme.... Differences in responses between groups were evaluated using t-tests or chi square analyses. Differences were considered significant at the $p < 0.05$ level. (Schumacher et al., 2002, p. 1307)

One hundred fifteen (74%) patients clearly said that they found the diary useful, and 16 (10%) gave clearly negative responses. Nine others (6%) found no current benefit from the diary, although they could see how it might be useful in the future. Most of the patients in this group were experiencing low levels of pain intensity, which suggests that patients with higher levels of pain may be more motivated to use a pain management diary. Fifteen (10%) of the patients gave no response or an ambiguous response to the question about the diary's usefulness (e.g., "Well, yes and no").... No significant difference was found between the proportion of patients in the PRO-SELF and the control groups who found the diary useful. (p. 1307)

Four major categories emerged from the content analysis of patients' and family caregivers' comments about how they found the pain management diary useful: (a) it heightened awareness of the pain experience, (b) it provided a guide to self-care behaviors, (c) it facilitated communication, and (d) it enhanced their sense of control.... Very few patients and caregivers found the diary to be burdensome. (p. 1308)

CRITIQUE

The interview questions addressed concerns expressed in the research problem. The interview questions were relevant for the research purpose, which was to describe the usefulness of the daily pain management diaries to patients and caregivers. The questions asked were relevant to the purpose and were designed to avoid biasing subject responses. The responses suggest that such diaries may be helpful to patients with chronic pain who are being cared for at home.

IMPLICATIONS FOR PRACTICE

The diary was used in the PRO-SELF Pain Control Program as an integral part of patients' self-care activities, rather than for research purposes. Thus, it was a component of the intervention. Its purpose was to improve cancer pain management. Family caregivers also found the pain diary useful. "Patients seemed to have discovered on their own, as opposed to being taught, that organizing and recording medications is useful" (Schumacher et al., 2002, p. 1311). "However, the results indicate that patients may need more explicit education and coaching on how to use a diary to its fullest potential" (p. 1312).

Focus Groups

The use of focus groups is a relatively recent strategy in nursing studies, beginning in the late 1980s. However, they have been in use in other fields for a long time. The technique serves several purposes in nursing research. **Focus groups** are used to study qualitative issues, analyze policy, assess consumer satisfaction, evaluate quality of care, examine the effectiveness of public health programs, make professional decisions, develop instruments, explore patient care problems, develop effective interventions and education programs, study various patient populations, and gather data for participatory research projects. A study using focus groups usually includes between 1 and 50 groups.

Focus groups are designed to obtain the participants' perceptions of a narrow subject in a setting that is permissive and nonthreatening. One of the assumptions underlying the use of focus groups is that the group dynamics can encourage people to express and clarify their views in ways that are less likely to occur in a one-to-one interview. The group may give a sense of "safety in numbers" to persons who are wary of researchers or are anxious. Many different forms of communication are used in focus groups, including teasing, arguing, joking, and telling anecdotes. Nonverbal approaches, such as gesturing, facial expressions, and other body language, are used as well. Everyday forms of communication may tell as much, if not more, about what people know or experience.

Recruiting the appropriate participants for each of the focus groups is critical. Recruitment is the most common source of failure in research using focus groups. Each focus group must include 6 to 10 participants. Fewer participants tend to result in inadequate discussion. In most cases, participants should be unknown to each other. However, in targeting professional groups such as clinical nurses or nurse educators, this usually is not possible. The researcher may use purposive sampling, in which persons known to have the desired expertise are sought. In other cases, participants may be sought through the media, posters, or advertisements.

Segmentation is the process of sorting participants into focus groups with common characteristics. Selecting participants who are similar to each other, in lifestyle or experiences, views, and characteristics, facilitates more open discussion. Validity is increased by conducting multiple focus groups with participants of differing characteristics in separate groups. Such characteristics may include age, gender, social class, ethnicity, culture, lifestyle, and health status. Groups with a unifying characteristic may be naturally occurring, as in the case of several people who work together.

Selecting effective moderators is as critical as selecting appropriate participants. The moderator must be successful at encouraging participants to talk about the topic. In some cases, adding an assistant moderator may be helpful. A successful moderator encourages participants to interact with one another, formulate ideas, and draw out cognitive structures not previously articulated. Moderators must remain neutral and nonjudgmental. If the topic is sensitive, the moderator works to put the participants at ease. In such instances, choosing a moderator who shares certain characteristics with the group's participants is recommended.

The setting for the focus group should be relaxed, with space for each participant to sit comfortably in a circle and maintain eye contact with all other participants. The group should meet in a room with good acoustics, so that a high-quality tape recording of the session can be made. Sessions usually last 1 to 2 hours, although some may extend to an entire afternoon or continue to a series of meetings.

Data collected from focus groups are analyzed the same way as for data collected from qualitative studies. However, data from focus groups are complex, so analysis is required at several levels: across responses given by the same person, among people in the same group, and among different groups. It is important to attend to the degree of consensus and interest in the topics generated in the discussion. Analysis of deviance and of minority opinions also is important. Paying attention to the context within which statements were made is critical to the analysis (Morgan, 1995).

CRITIQUE GUIDELINES Focus Groups

When critiquing a focus group study, consider the following questions:

1. What was the aim of the focus group?
2. Was the group size appropriate for the focus group method?
3. Was the group sufficiently homogeneous for its members to speak candidly?
4. Was the moderator successful in keeping the discussion focused?
5. Was the aim of the focus group achieved?
6. Did the conclusions appear to be a valid representation of the discussion?
7. Were minority positions identified and explored?

RESEARCH EXAMPLE Focus Groups

Jones and Broome (2001) conducted focus groups with African American adolescents to obtain recommendations for strategies that could enhance recruitment and retention in intervention studies. They describe their process as follows:

Fifteen African American adolescents, ages 13 to 17 years, participated in this study. Adolescents attended one of three focus groups, which varied by size, gender, and type of chronic condition. The three focus groups consisted of adolescents who were well (n = 7), had sickle cell disease (SCD, n = 5), or diabetes (n = 3). The well group (WG) of adolescents without any known health problem or illness served as a comparison group. The groups consisted of adolescents diagnosed with SCD, and adolescents in the diabetes group (DG) all had Type I insulin-dependent diabetes. The teens with SCD were recruited because the large intervention study to be implemented later was developed for teens with a chronic pain condition. The teens with diabetes were targeted to compare their responses with those teens that were well and those with SCD to determine whether their concerns were disease focused or could be generalized to adolescents with a chronic health condition.

A structured focus group interview guide was developed that included 15 questions that elicited adolescents ideas about strategies, perceptions, and concerns related to recruitment and retention of adolescents into research. The interview guide was an important factor in controlling variability across the three focus group discussions. Questions elicited adolescents' perceptions and recommendations about potential symptom management interventions (self-management of a disease, art, relaxation, and imagery), class structure and content, teacher characteristics, and specific incentives/disincentives. Probe questions were included to gain more specific and detailed information (e.g., to clarify a statement such as "someone who can speak our language").

Each focus group discussion was audiotaped and transcribed. Audiotapes were erased by the investigator after they have been listened to, transcribed, and the accuracy of transcribed content validated. Confidentiality of transcribed data was addressed by using adolescents' first names only. After each focus group session the investigator also recorded field notes that documented her thoughts, impressions, and events capturing the context and the processes of the group. (pp. 90–91)

After analyzing the data, the researchers summarized their findings.

Important factors to consider in "getting adolescents there" included straightforward communication about how they or others would benefit from the research, what would be expected of them, incentives, and accessing them where they were. Suggestions for keeping teens interested in a research study included honest, open communication between the investigators, the teen and their parents, incentives, and allowing for exercise of choice and active involvement in the research intervention. Employing honest and respectful communication strategies with the teens, showing respect for their contributions and a willingness to listen were viewed as critical to keeping them coming back The adolescents also thought investigators need to recognize the potential for family problems (e.g., lack of transportation or the need for a teen to babysit) that might interfere with their attendance. (pp. 92–93)

CRITIQUE

The aim of the focus groups was to obtain recommendations from the adolescents on strategies to enhance recruitment and retention in intervention studies. The group sizes seemed small for the focus group method. However, the groups were sufficiently homogeneous to facilitate candid remarks. The moderator followed a focused group interview guide with 15 questions that seemed successful in keeping the discussion focused. The aim of the focus groups was achieved. The conclusions appear to validly represent the discussion. Minority positions were not identified, perhaps because of the small group sizes.

IMPLICATIONS FOR PRACTICE

The implications are primarily for recruiting African American adolescents into clinical trials. However, some findings are relevant to the needs of African American adolescents who have illness requiring care within the health care system. African American adolescents wanted opportunities to have relationships with each other during their care, whether it be treatments or hospitalization. They were concerned about fewer social activities and less intimate relationships because of their chronic illnesses. They wanted to get to know other adolescents with the same chronic conditions as theirs. They wanted to learn about their illnesses in safe, friendly, nurturing environments, rather than in the structured teaching environments provided for adults. They want to be able to talk about some things other than their disease. They wanted honesty, choice, and "realness" from the health care providers. These desires seem generalizable to most adolescents receiving care within the health care system and could provide direction for all caregivers of adolescents.

Questionnaires

A **questionnaire** is a printed self-report form designed to elicit information through written or verbal responses of the subject. Questionnaires are sometimes referred to as surveys, and a study using a questionnaire may be referred to as survey research. The information obtained from questionnaires is similar to that obtained by an interview, but the questions tend to have less depth. The subject is not permitted to elaborate on responses or ask for clarification of questions, and the data collector cannot use probing strategies. However, questions are presented in a consistent manner to each subject, and opportunity for bias is less than in an interview. Questionnaires often are used in descriptive studies to gather a broad spectrum of information from subjects, such as facts about the subject; facts about persons, events, or situations known by the subject; or beliefs, attitudes, opinions, knowledge, or intentions of the subject. Like interviews, questionnaires can have various structures. Some questionnaires ask open-ended questions, which require written responses from the subject. Other questionnaires ask closed-ended questions, which have only answers selected by the researcher. A modification is the use of computers to gather questionnaire data.

Stotts, Henderson, and Burns (1988) used a questionnaire to examine smoking patterns of nurses in the state of Texas. Items from that questionnaire are shown in Figure 11-1.

Although questionnaires can be distributed to very large samples, either directly or through the mail, the response rate for questionnaires generally is lower than that for other forms of self-report, particularly if the questionnaires are mailed. If the response rate is lower than 50%, the representativeness of the sample is seriously in question. The response rate for mailed questionnaires usually is small (25% to 30%), so the researcher frequently is unable to obtain a representative sample, even with random sampling methods. Respondents commonly fail to mark responses to all of the questions, especially on long questionnaires. The incomplete nature of the data can threaten the validity of the instrument.

CRITIQUE GUIDELINES Questionnaires

When critiquing a published study that used a questionnaire, evaluate the adequacy of the questionnaire to measure the concepts important to the study (content-related validity evidence). In most studies, only a brief description of the questionnaire is provided. Usually, the questionnaire itself will not be available for you to examine in the published report.

1. Compare the description of the contents of the questionnaire with the conceptual definitions the questions are intended to reflect.
2. Search for information on content-related validity. If the CVI (Content Validity Index) was used, the value obtained should be reported.

With most questionnaires, researchers analyze data at the level of individual items, rather than adding the items together and analyzing the total scores. Responses to items usually are measured at the nominal or ordinal level.

1. Do you currently smoke cigarettes?
   a. No
   b. Yes

2. How old were you when you started smoking?
   a. Under 15 years   e. 18 years   h. 21 years
   b. 15 years   f. 19 years   i. 22 years
   c. 16 years   g. 20 years   j. Over 22 years
   d. 17 years

3. Before entering your basic (GENERIC) nursing education program, on average, about how many cigarettes a day did you smoke?
   a. Did not smoke at all   d. 15 to 24 cigarettes per day
   b. Did not smoke every day   e. 25 to 39 cigarettes per day
   c. Less than 15 cigarettes per day   f. 40 or more cigarettes per day

4. During your basic (GENERIC) nursing education program, on average, about how many cigarettes a day did you smoke?
   a. Did not smoke at all   d. 15 to 24 cigarettes per day
   b. Did not smoke every day   e. 25 to 39 cigarettes per day
   c. Less than 15 cigarettes per day   f. 40 or more cigarettes per day

5. How many organized programs have you attended to help you quit smoking?
   a. None   d. Three   g. Six
   b. One   e. Four   h. Seven
   c. Two   f. Five   i. More than seven

6. What is the longest single period you have stopped smoking?
   a. Have never stopped   e. More than 1 month but less than 1 year
   b. Less than a day   f. More than 1 year but less than 3 years
   c. Less than a week   g. 3 years or more
   d. Less than a month

7. Aside from what you think you actually could do, which would you most like to do?
   a. Quit smoking   d. Not sure at this time
   b. Cut down   e. Smoke as much as now
   c. Cut down just a little

Figure 11-1. Examples of items from a smoking questionnaire.

RESEARCH EXAMPLE   Questionnaires

Willaing and Ladelund (2005) used a questionnaire in their study titled "Nurse Counseling of Patients with an Overconsumption of Alcohol." They describe the questionnaire as follows:

The questionnaire included age, sex, type of ward, type of job, self-rated qualifications for counseling patients and relatives about alcohol, self-rated knowledge of the deleterious effects of alcohol, self-reported clinical practice in relation to patients with an overconsumption of alcohol, attitudes toward caring for and counseling of patients with an overconsumption of alcohol, self-reported priorities for different types of lifestyle counseling in the ward (alcohol, smoking, diet, and physical activity), and their need for education. A Likert-type scale with four response categories was used to assess whether nurses regarded caring for and counseling patients with an overconsumption of alcohol as an exciting and worthwhile challenge.

(continues)

RESEARCH EXAMPLE *(continued)*

FINDINGS

The response rate was 77% (n = 565 of the 734 nurses employed in the hospital).

Important findings in this study were that self-rated qualifications, ward, and attitudes toward care were significantly related to the self-reported clinical care of patients with an overconsumption of alcohol. Psychiatric nurses were consistently most active and knowledgeable, medical nurses were less active, and surgical nurses were least active. (p. 33).

This study indicated that nurses' self-efficacy was an important determinant for actions regarding overconsumption of alcohol. (p. 34).

IMPLICATIONS FOR PRACTICE

Awareness of overconsumption of alcohol is a prerequisite for changing negative attitudes toward dealing with the problem. Hospital nurses need to be convinced that an active role does not interfere negatively with the nurse-patient relationship. Alcohol screening and brief interventions could be integrated in the more general context of preventive health services (Babor & Higgins-Biddle, 2000). (Willaing & Ladelund, 2005, p. 34)

Scales

The **scale**, a form of self-report, is a more precise means of measuring phenomena than the questionnaire. Most scales measure psychosocial variables. However, scaling techniques can be used to obtain self-reports on physiological variables such as pain, nausea, or functional capacity. The various items on most scales are summed to obtain a single score. These are referred to as *summated scales*. Fewer random and systematic errors occur when the total score of a scale is used. The various items in a scale increase the dimensions of the concept that are reflected in the instrument. The types of scales described next include rating scales, Likert scales, semantic differential scales, and visual analogue scales.

Rating Scales

Rating scales are the crudest form of measure using scaling techniques. A rating scale lists an ordered series of categories of a variable and is assumed to be based on an underlying continuum. A numerical value is assigned to each category. The subtlety of the distinctions among categories varies with the scale. Rating scales commonly are used by the general public. In conversations, one can hear statements such as "On a scale of one to ten, I would rank that…." This type of scale often is used in observational measurement to guide data collection. Burns (1974) used the rating scale in Figure 11-2 to examine differences in communication among nurses and both cancer patients and other medical-surgical patients.

CRITIQUE GUIDELINES Rating Scales

When critiquing a rating scale, ask the following questions.

1. Is the instrument clearly described?
2. Are the techniques that were used to administer and score the scale provided?
3. Is information about validity and reliability of the scale described from previous studies?
4. Is information about validity and reliability of the scale described for the present sample?
5. If the scale was developed for the study, was the instrument development process described?

RESEARCH EXAMPLE Rating Scales

Lenz and Perkins (2000) used a rating scale to measure functional health in their study titled "Coronary Artery Bypass Graft Surgery Patients and Their Family Member Caregivers: Outcomes of a Family-Focused Staged Psychoeducational Intervention." Their description of the rating scale is as follows:

The patient's functional health status was measured using the COOP charts (Nelson, Wasson, & Kirk, 1987), a standardized, 10-item pictorial self-report instrument. For each aspect of functioning, the subject rates himself/herself on a 5-point scale in which higher values reflect poorer functional status. The measure has physical (fitness, daily activities, and pain items) and emotional (feelings, social activities, and quality-of-life items) subscales, as well as a total score that ranges from 10 to 50. The instrument developers reported test-retest reliability alpha values ranging from .73 to .98. Both convergent and divergent validity have been satisfactory in multiple populations; however the COOP charts have sacrificed both sensitivity and specificity in the interest of brevity and ease of administration (Nelson, Landgraf, Hays, Wasson, & Kirk, 1990; Wasson et al., 1992). The internal consistency of the scale ranged from .63 to .81 in the study sample of patients. (p. 145)

FINDINGS

Differences in the number of self-reported complications/symptoms were not in the predicted direction. Improvement occurred in clinical, functional, and emotional outcomes; however, several symptoms, such as fatigue and pain, persisted. Family caregivers reported more depressive symptoms than patients preoperatively and at later stages of recovery. (p. 142)

CRITIQUE

The instrument, an established scale with good validity and reliability, was clearly described. Techniques used to administer and score the scale were provided. Validity and reliability information was reported from previous studies but not for the current study. Techniques for administering and scoring the scale were provided.

IMPLICATIONS FOR PRACTICE

Information obtained from this study will contribute to evidence-based practice, but results from this study need to be synthesized with other studies before being applied to practice situations.

1. Nurses come into my room
   a. Rarely
   b. Sometimes
   c. Whenever I call them
   d. Frequently just to speak or check on me

2. I would *like* nurses to come into my room
   a. Rarely
   b. Sometimes
   c. Whenever I call them
   d. Frequently just to speak or check on me

3. When a nurse enters my room, he/she usually
   a. Talks very little
   b. Tries to talk about things I do not wish to discuss
   c. Talks only about casual things
   d. Is willing to listen or discuss what concerns me

4. When a nurse enters my room, I would *prefer* that he/she
   a. Talk very little
   b. Talk only when necessary
   c. Talk only about casual things
   d. Be willing to listen or discuss what concerns me

5. When a nurse talks with me, he/she usually seems
   a. Not interested
   b. In a hurry
   c. Polite but distant
   d. Caring for me as a person

6. When a nurse talks with me, I would *prefer* that he/she be
   a. Not interested
   b. In a hurry
   c. Polite but distant
   d. Caring for me as a person

7. When a nurse talks with me, he/she usually
   a. Stands in the doorway
   b. Stands at the foot of the bed
   c. Stands at the side of the bed
   d. Sits beside the bed

8. When a nurse talks with me, I would *prefer* that he/she
   a. Stand in the doorway
   b. Stand at the foot of the bed
   c. Stand at the side of the bed
   d. Sit beside the bed

9. When a nurse talks with me, he/she is
   a. Strictly business
   b. Casual
   c. Friendly but does not talk about feelings
   d. Open to talking about things I worry or think about

10. When a nurse talks with me, I would *prefer* that he/she keep the conversation
    a. Strictly business
    b. Casual
    c. Friendly but not talk about feelings
    d. Open to talk about things I worry or think about

Figure 11-2. A rating scale used to measure the nature of nurse-patient communications.

11. Nurses talk with me about things important to me
    a. Rarely
    b. Sometimes
    c. Frequently
    d. As often as I need to talk

12. I would *like* for the nurse to talk with me about things important to me
    a. Rarely
    b. Sometimes
    c. Frequently
    d. As often as I need to talk

13. The nurse looks me in the eye when he/she talks with me
    a. Rarely
    b. Sometimes
    c. Frequently
    d. Very frequently

14. I would *prefer* that the nurse look me in the eye when he/she talks with me
    a. Rarely
    b. Sometimes
    c. Frequently
    d. Very frequently

15. When a nurse talks to me, he/she touches me
    a. Rarely
    b. Sometimes
    c. Frequently
    d. Very frequently

16. When a nurse talks to me, I would *prefer* that he/she touches me
    a. Rarely
    b. Sometimes
    c. Frequently
    d. Very frequently

17. My feelings about nurses talking to me are which of the following?
    a. They should do their work well and otherwise leave me alone.
    b. They may talk if they need to; it does not bother me.
    c. I enjoy talking with the nurses.
    d. When the nurse lets me talk with him/her about things important to me, I feel that he/she cares for me as a person.

On question 18, please mark as many answers as you wish.

18. I would like to feel free to talk with the nurse about my
    a. Illness
    b. Future
    c. Financial problems
    d. Feelings about myself
    e. Feelings about my family
    f. Life up to this time

Figure 11-2, cont'd

The Likert Scale

The **Likert scale**, which was designed to measure the opinion or attitude of a subject, contains a number of declarative statements with a scale after each statement. The Likert scale is the most commonly used scaling technique. The original version of the scale consisted of five categories. However, the number of categories may range from four to seven. Values are placed on each response, with a value of 1 on the most negative response and a value of 5 on the most positive response (Nunnally & Bernstein, 1994). Response choices on a Likert scale most commonly address agreement, evaluation, or frequency. Agreement responses may include options such as strongly agree, agree, uncertain, disagree, and strongly disagree. Evaluation responses ask the respondent for a categorical rating along a good-to-bad continuum, such as positive to negative or excellent to terrible. Categorical options may include such responses as rarely, seldom, sometimes, occasionally, and usually. The values from each item are summed to provide a total score. Figure 11-3 illustrates the form used for this type of scale.

RESEARCH EXAMPLE The Likert Scale

Badger, McNiece, and Gagan (2000) used a Likert-type scale to measure depression in their study of the incidence of depression, need for services, and use of services in vulnerable populations. The following is a description of their instrument.

Depression was measured using the 20-item Center for Epidemiological Studies–Depression Scale (CES-D) (Radloff, 1977). The CES-D has been used in both general and clinical populations to measure the frequency and severity of depression symptomatology. Participants were asked to rate each depressive symptom experienced in the past week on a 4-point Likert-type scale, ranging from 0 (rarely or none of the time) to 3 (most or all of the time). Scores are then summed and range from 0 to 60, with higher scores reflecting greater depressive symptoms. Although scores >16 are typically used to indicate significant depressive symptoms, in this study the more conservative criterion of >27 was used. The more conservative score is recommended when the participants have multiple chronic illnesses or disabling conditions (Schulberg et al., 1985). Adequate reliability and validity with other community samples have been established (Davidson, Feldman, & Crawford, 1994: Schulberg et al., 1985). Cronbach's alpha in this study was .92. (p. 29)

FINDINGS

Significant differences were found between the 2 groups for predisposing characteristics, enabling characteristics, need for care, service use, and satisfaction with services. (p. 173)

CRITIQUE

The researchers used a previously developed scale with established validity and reliability. The instrument is clearly described, with methods used to complete and score the scale provided. The researchers state that the scale has established reliability and validity but do not provide sufficient information to judge the validity and reliability. A Cronbach's alpha value of 0.92 is reported for the present study, which indicates that the study has good reliability for the present sample; however, no validity information was provided.

IMPLICATIONS FOR PRACTICE

The study results are descriptive and do not provide information to guide practice. However, this information is important to include in syntheses of studies for purposes of describing population characteristics.

	Strongly Disagree	Disagree	Uncertain	Agree	Strongly Agree
People with cancer almost always die					
Chemotherapy is very effective in treating cancer					
We are close to finding a cure for cancer					
I would work next to a person with cancer					
Nurses take good care of patients with cancer					

Figure 11-3. Example of items that could be included in a Likert scale.

Semantic Differential Scales

The **semantic differential scale** measures attitudes and beliefs. A semantic differential scale consists of two opposite adjectives with a 7-point scale between them. The subject is asked to select one point on the scale that best describes his or her view of the concept being examined. Values of 1 to 7 are assigned to each space, with 1 being the most negative response and 7 being the most positive. The placement of negative responses to the left or right of the scale needs to be randomly varied to avoid global responses (in which the subject places checks in the same column of each scale item). Values that are reversed are transposed before the values are added. The values for the scales are summed to obtain one score for each subject. Burns (1981, 1983) developed a semantic differential scale that uses descriptive phrases to measure beliefs about cancer. Figure 11-4 includes descriptive phrases from this 23-item scale.

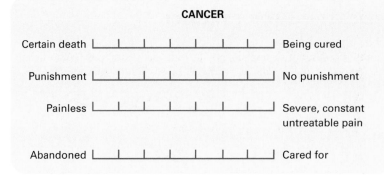

Figure 11-4. Example of items from the Burns Cancer Beliefs Scale.

CRITIQUE GUIDELINES Semantic Differential Scales

When critiquing a semantic differential, ask the following questions.

1. Is the instrument clearly described?
2. Are the techniques to administer and score the scale provided?
3. Is information about validity and reliability of the scale described from previous studies?
4. Is information about validity and reliability of the scale described for the present sample?
5. If the scale was developed for the study, is the instrument development process described?

Visual Analogue Scales

The **visual analogue scale** is a line that is 100 mm long, with right angle "stops" at either end. The line may be oriented horizontally or vertically. Bipolar anchors are placed beyond either end of the line. These end anchors must include the entire range of sensations possible for the phenomenon being measured (e.g., all and none, best and worst, no pain and most severe pain).

The subject is asked to place a mark through the line to indicate the intensity of the stimulus. A ruler is then used to measure the distance between the left end of the line (on a horizontal scale) and the subject's mark. This measure is the value of the stimulus. The visual analogue scale has been used to measure pain, mood, anxiety, alertness, craving for cigarettes, quality of sleep, attitudes toward environmental conditions, functional abilities, and severity of clinical symptoms (Wewers & Lowe, 1990). An example of a visual analogue scale is shown in Figure 11-5.

Strategies commonly used to evaluate the reliability of scales are not useful for visual analogue scales. Because these scales are used to measure phenomena that are erratic over time, test-retest reliability is inappropriate; and because each scale contains a single item, other methods of determining reliability cannot be used.

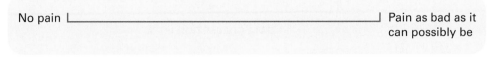

Figure 11-5. Example of a visual analogue scale.

CRITIQUE GUIDELINES **Visual Analogue Scales**

When critiquing a visual analogue scale, consider the following questions:

1. Is the instrument clearly described?
2. Are the techniques needed to administer and score the scale provided?
3. Is information about validity of the scale described from previous studies?
4. Is information about validity of the scale described for the present sample?
5. If the scale was developed for the study, is the instrument development process described?

Process of Data Collection

Data collection is the process of acquiring the subjects and collecting the data for the study. The actual steps of collecting the data are specific to each study and depend on the research design and measurement techniques. During the data collection period, the researcher focuses on obtaining subjects, training data collectors, collecting data in a consistent way, maintaining research controls, protecting the integrity (or validity) of the study, and solving problems that threaten to disrupt the study.

Good research reporting dictates that the researcher describe the data collection process in the published study. The strategies used to approach potential subjects who meet the sampling criteria are made clear. The number and characteristics of subjects who decline to participate in the study are specified. The approach used to perform measurements, and the time and setting at which measurements are taken, also are described. The result is a step-by-step description of exactly how, where, and in what sequence the data were collected.

In many studies, data collection forms are used to gather data. These forms may be used to record data from the patient record, or to ask the subject for such information as demographic data. The form itself is not a measurement tool. In many cases, each item on these forms is a separate measurement. Thus, the researcher needs to report the source of information and describe the method and level of measurement of each item on the form. Figure 11-6 shows an example of a data collection form.

DATA COLLECTION FORM

Subject identification number _____ Date _____

A. Age _____ B. Gender: ☐ Male ☐ Female

C. Weight _____ pounds D. Height _____ inches

E. Surgical diagnosis _____

F. Surgery date _____ Time _____

G. Narcotics order after surgery _____

_____

H. Narcotic administration:

Date	Time	Type of narcotic	Dose
1.			
2.			
3.			
4.			
5.			

I. Patient instructed on Pain Scale: Date _____ Time _____
   Comments:

J. Type of treatment: ☐ TENS ☐ Placebo-TENS ☐ No treatment control

K. Treatment implemented: Date _____ Time _____
   Comments:

L. Dressing change: Date _____ Time _____
   Hours since surgery _____

M. Score on Visual Analogue Pain Scale _____
   Date _____ Time _____

Data collector's name _____
   Comments:

Figure 11-6. Hypothetical data collection form for Hargreaves and Lander's (1989) study, "Use of Transcutaneous Nerve Stimulation Electric for Postoperative Pain."

Data Collection Tasks

During either quantitative or qualitative research, the investigator performs five tasks during the data collection process. These tasks are interrelated and run concurrently, rather than in sequence. These tasks are

- Selecting subjects
- Collecting data in a consistent way
- Maintaining research controls as indicated in the study design
- Protecting the integrity (or validity) of the study
- Solving problems that threaten to disrupt the study

Recruiting Subjects

Subjects may be recruited only at the initiation of data collection or throughout the data collection period. The design of the study determines the method of selecting subjects. Recruiting the number of subjects originally planned is critical because data analysis and interpretation of findings depend on having an adequate sample size. Factors related to subject recruitment and selection should be continually examined to determine possible biases in the sample obtained.

Recruiting subjects for research is becoming more difficult for a variety of reasons, including the following: (1) an increasing number of nurses are conducting research, (2) clinical agencies are placing constraints on the time staff nurses can be released from patient care for research activities, (3) patients are being protected from participating in too many investigations, and (4) access to patients is being limited so that agency personnel can use these patients for their own research (Cronenwett, 1986). Thus, nurse researchers will need to be creative and persistent in recruiting adequate numbers of subjects.

In recruiting subjects, researchers have found that direct contact with potential subjects is the most effective method, telephone contact is less effective, and mail contact is least effective. Direct contact in small groups usually is more effective for subject recruitment than contact in large groups (Crosby, Ventura, Finnick, Lohr, & Feldman, 1991). The researcher must determine the most effective recruitment approach as indicated by the purpose of the study, the type and number of subjects required, and the design of the study.

Maintaining Consistency

The key to accurate data collection in any study is consistency. Consistency involves maintaining the data collection pattern for each collection event as it was developed in the research plan. A good plan will facilitate consistency and maintain the validity of the study. However, developing a consistent plan is easier than implementing it. Deviations, even if they are minor, should be noted and evaluated for their impact on the interpretation of the findings. When data collectors are used in a study, they should be trained to note deviations during the data collection process.

Maintaining Controls

Research controls should be built into the plan, to minimize the influence of intervening forces on study findings. Maintenance of these controls is essential; many controls are not natural in a field setting, and maintaining them is not easy. In some cases the controls slip without the researcher's realizing it. In addition to maintaining the controls identified in the plan, the researcher needs to continually look for previously unidentified, extraneous variables that might have an impact on the data being collected. This type of variable often is specific to a study and tends to become apparent during the data collection period. The extraneous variables identified during data collection must be considered during data analysis and interpretation. These variables also must be noted in the research report, so that future researchers can be aware of and attempt to control them.

Protecting Study Integrity

Maintaining consistency and controls during subject selection and data collection protects the integrity or validity of the study. In addition, the integrity of the study must be considered in a broad context. To accomplish this, the researcher needs to view the process of data collection as a whole, instead of examining single elements of data collection. Changes in one small component of data collection can modify other elements, thereby altering the entire process in ways that threaten the validity of the outcomes.

RESEARCH EXAMPLE Data Collection

Harrison, Wells, Fisher, and Prince (1996) conducted a study to evaluate evidence of the effectiveness of practice guidelines for the prediction and prevention of pressure ulcers. They used a Demographic and Clinical Profile Form to capture information about age and gender of the subjects, length of hospital stay, reason for admission, diagnosis of medical problem, use of pressure relief devices, and type of nursing unit in which the subject was treated. The Prevalence Grid was used to identify 20 sites to assess skin integrity. If ulcers were present, a staging classification system was used to categorize ulcers from Stage I to Stage IV. The Braden Scale (Bergstrom, Braden, Laguzza, & Holman, 1987) was used to assess the risk of pressure ulcers. The authors described their data collection procedure as follows:

A survey team of 23 registered nurses conducted a head-to-toe skin assessment and administered the Braden Scale to consenting subjects. The surveyors were prepared through an education workshop that included an orientation to the study purpose and procedures, the use of data collection instruments, and a theoretical and practical hands-on component to stage ulcers and conduct risk assessment. The training films developed by Bergstrom and Braden were included in the workshop format. Reliability was assessed on a range of known cases where team members went to clinical areas, staged ulcers, and then had these assessments checked by a clinical expert (enterostomal therapist).

On prevalence day [days of the week selected to assess skin integrity of all subjects], the surveyors were divided into four data collection teams plus a validation team. Each had a team leader who was not directly involved in data collection to attend to administrative tasks, such as tracking admissions and discharges, and deploying surveyors. The team members were assigned to clinically familiar areas (e.g., critical care nurses to critical care areas) but not to their home units where they would know the patients. The enterostomal therapist was on call at all times if the surveyors required a second opinion on an assessment of ulcer stage.

The validation team, [composed] of two registered nurse surveyors, reassessed a randomly selected subsample of 10% of the prevalence population to assess reliability. Correlation of the survey team and validation team on total Braden scores was calculated using Pearson's product-moment correlation. Correlation of the survey team and validation team assessments was r = 0.87. The degree of association indicates a strong relationship between assessments.

The surveyors conducted a full skin examination and administered the Braden Scale for risk assessment on prevalence day. The risk assessment was completed using the chart, plan of care, clinical assessment, and consultation with the patient's assigned nurse to complete the data collection. The Braden Scale was administered in this manner because it closely emulates the way in which clinical staff would use such a scale if implemented institution-wide.

To determine the Braden Scale's accuracy in the setting, the same data (full skin assessment and administration of the Braden Scale) was collected in a 20-week follow-up on a Monday-Wednesday-Friday schedule by a subsample of the surveyors. They had no information of the subjects' prior risk scores, and with the number of surveyors, computer calculation of total scores, and the large number of patients in the study, the likelihood of bias by remembering an assessment was minimal.

To evaluate the Braden Scale and the risk cut-off scores, the sensitivity (i.e., percentage of all subjects who developed a pressure ulcer and were so predicted by the scale), specificity (i.e., percentage of all subjects who did not develop pressure ulcers and were so predicted by the scale), positive predictive value (i.e., percentage of subjects who were predicted to be at risk and did develop a pressure ulcer), and the negative predictive value (i.e., percentage of subjects who were predicted to be at low risk and did not develop a pressure ulcer) were calculated. The calculations are well described by Bergstrom, Demuth, and Braden (1987). (pp. 12–13)

CRITIQUE

As can be seen in the report, Harrison and colleagues (1996) took careful steps to maintain the rigor of their data collection plan. Data collectors were carefully trained. Data collection forms were developed for the study. They built in multiple cross-checks and avoided biases by not assessing patients they had personally cared for. The reliability of the skin assessments were validated by a second assessment team that cross-checked measures of 10% of the sample. The way subjects were obtained was described but is not included in the excerpt. The researchers identify measures taken to avoid possible threats to validity.

IMPLICATIONS FOR PRACTICE

The study was designed to evaluate practice guidelines current at the time of the study. It provides a good example of how to validate current guidelines in a clinical study. In some cases, guidelines that are based on excellent study results are problematic to apply in clinical settings.

Solving Problems

Problems can be perceived either as a source of frustration or as a challenge. The fact that the problem occurred is not as important as the success of problem resolution. Therefore, the final and perhaps most important task of the data collection period may be problem resolution. Little has been written in the scientific literature about the problems encountered by nurse researchers. The research reports often read as though everything went smoothly. The implication is that good researchers have no problems, which is not true. Research journals generally do not provide sufficient space to allow description of the problems encountered, and the absence of such information may give a false impression to the inexperienced researcher. A more realistic picture can be obtained through personal discussions with researchers about the data collection process.

Serendipity

Serendipity is the accidental discovery of something useful or valuable. During the data collection phase of studies, researchers often become aware of elements or relationships that they had not previously identified. In some published studies, therefore, the researcher has gathered data, made observations, or recorded events that were not originally planned. These new-found aspects may or may not be closely related to the planned study. Because the researcher is focused on close observation, other elements in the situation can come into clearer focus and take on new meaning. Serendipitous findings are important for the development of new insights in nursing, and they can lead to new areas of research that generate knowledge.

KEY CONCEPTS

- The purpose of measurement is to produce trustworthy evidence that can be used in evaluating the outcomes of research.
- The rules of measurement ensure that the assignment of values or categories is performed consistently from one subject (or event) to another and, eventually, if the measurement strategy is found to be meaningful, from one study to another.
- The levels of measurement from low to high are nominal, ordinal, interval, and ratio.
- Reliability in measurement is concerned with the consistency of the measurement technique.
- The validity of an instrument is a determination of the extent to which the instrument reflects the abstract concept being examined.
- Common measurement approaches used in nursing research include physiological measures, observation, interviews, questionnaires, and scales.
- The researcher performs five tasks during the process of data collection: (1) obtaining subjects, (2) collecting data in a consistent way, (3) maintaining research controls, (4) protecting the integrity (or validity) of the study, and (5) solving problems that threaten to disrupt the study.
- It is important to critique the description of the data collection process for threats to validity.
- During data collection, the researcher may make an accidental discovery of valuable information unrelated to the planned study; this is called serendipity.

TIPS FOR FURTHER STUDY

- Are you having difficulty differentiating the levels of measurement? Complete the "Matching Questions" in the Open-Book Quiz on http://evolve.com/Burns/understanding.
- Determine the level of measurement of various things you are required to measure in the clinical setting.
- Look for things in your clinical setting that would improve clinical practice if they could be measured.
- Ask the nurse manager in your clinical setting about data that is being collected on the unit. Inquire about the data collection process.

REFERENCES

Algase, D. L., Kupferschmid, B., Beel-Bates, C. A., & Beattie, E. R. (1997). Estimates of stability of daily wandering behavior among cognitively impaired long-term care residents. *Nursing Research, 46*(3), 172–178.

Babor, T. F., & Higgins-Biddle, J. C. (2000). Alcohol screening and brief intervention: Dissemination strategies for medical practice and public health. *Addiction, 95*(5), 677–686.

Badger, T. A., McNiece, C., & Gagan, M. J. (2000). Depression, service need, and use in vulnerable populations. *Archives of Psychiatric Nursing, 14*(4), 173–182.

Bergstrom, N., Braden, B. H., Laguzza, A., & Holman, V. (1987). The Braden Scale for predicting pressure sore risk. *Nursing Research, 36*(4), 205–210.

Bergstrom, N., Demuth, P. J., & Braden, B. J. (1987). A clinical trial of the Braden Scale for predicting pressure sore risk. *Nursing Clinics of North America, 22*(2), 417–428.

Burns, N. (1974). *Nurse-patient communication with the advanced cancer patient.* Unpublished master's thesis. Texas Woman's University, Dallas.

Burns, N. (1981). *Evaluation of a supportive-expressive group for families of cancer patients.* Unpublished doctoral dissertation. Texas Woman's University, Denton, TX.

Burns, N. (1983). Development of the Burns Cancer Beliefs Scale. *Proceedings of the American Cancer Society Third West Coast Cancer Nursing Research Conference* (pp. 308–329).

Burns, N., & Grove, S. K. (2005). *The practice of nursing research: Conduct, critique, and utilization* (5th ed.). Philadelphia: Saunders.

Craft, M. J., & Moss, J. (1996). Accuracy of infant emesis volume assessment. *Applied Nursing Research, 9*(1), 2–8.

Cronenwett, L. (1986). Research reflections: Access to research subjects. *Journal of Nursing Administration, 16*(2), 8–9.

Crosby, F., Ventura, M. R., Finnick, M., Lohr, G., & Feldman, M. J. (1991). Enhancing subject recruitment for nursing research. *Clinical Nurse Specialist, 5*(1), 25–30.

Davidson, H., Feldman, P. H., & Crawford, S. (1994). Measuring depressive symptoms in the frail elderly. *Journal of Gerontology, 49*(4), 159.

Engle, V. F., & Graney, M. J. (2000). Biobehavioral effects of therapeutic touch. *The Journal of Nursing Scholarship, 32*(3), 287–293.

Ferrell, B. R., Dow, K. H., & Grant, M. (1995). Measurement of quality of life in cancer survivors. *Quality of Life Research, 4*(6), 523–531.

Ferrell, B. R., Dow, K. H., Leigh, S., Ly, J., & Gulasekaram, P. (1995). Quality of life in long-term cancer survivors. *Oncology Nursing Forum, 22*(6), 915–922.

Ferrell, B. R., Grant, M., Funk, B., Garcia, N., Otis-Green, S., & Schaffner, M. L. (1996). Quality of life in breast cancer. *Cancer Practice, 4*(6), 331–340.

Goetz, R. H. (1940). Plethysmography of the skin in the investigation of peripheral vascular diseases. *British Journal of Surgery, 27,* 506–520.

Hargreaves, A., & Lander, J. (1989). Use of transcutaneous electrical nerve stimulation for postoperative pain. *Nursing Research, 38*(3), 159–161.

Harrison, M. B., Wells, G., Fisher, A., & Prince, M. (1996). Practice guidelines for the prediction and prevention of pressure ulcers: Evaluating the evidence. *Applied Nursing Research, 9*(1), 9–17.

Hartwig, M. S., Cardoso, S. S., Hathaway, D. K., & Gaber, A. O. (1994). Reliability and validity of cardiovascular and vasomotor autonomic function tests. *Diabetes Care, 17*(12), 1433–1440.

Holditch-Davis, D., Miles, M. S., Burchinal, M., O'Donnell, K., McKinney, R., & Lim, W. (2001). Parental caregiving and developmental outcomes of infants of mothers with HIV. *Nursing Research, 50*(1), 5–14.

Holditch-Davis, D., & Thoman, E. (1988). The early social environment of premature and full term infants. *Early Human Development, 17*(2), 221–232.

Holzemer, W. L., Hudson, A., Kirksey, K. M., Hamilton, M. J., & Bakken, S. (2001). The revised sign and symptom check-list for HIV (SSC-HIVrev). *Journal of the Association of Nurses in AIDS Care, 12*(5), 60–70.

Jones, F. C., & Broome, M. E. (2001). Focus groups with African American adolescents: Enhancing recruitment and retention in intervention studies. *Journal of Pediatric Nursing, 16*(2), 88–96.

Lenz, E. R., & Perkins, S. (2000). Coronary artery bypass graft surgery patients and their family member caregivers: Outcomes of a family-focused staged psychoeducational intervention. *Applied Nursing Research, 13*(3), 142–150.

Miller, D. B., & Holditch-Davis, D. (1992). Interactions of parents and nurses with high-risk preterm infants. *Research in Nursing & Health, 15*(3), 187–197.

Morgan, D. L. (1995). Why things (sometimes) go wrong in focus groups. *Qualitative Health Research, 5*(4), 516–523.

Nelson, E. C., Landgraf, J. M., Hays, R. D., Wasson, J. H., & Kirk, J. W. (1990). The functional status of patients: How can it be measured in physicians' offices? *Medical Care, 28*(12), 1111–1126.

Nelson, E. C., Wasson, J. H., & Kirk, J. W. (1987). Assessment of function in routine clinical practice: Description of the COOP chart method and preliminary findings. *Journal of Chronic Diseases, 49*(Suppl. 1), 55S–63S.

Nunnally, J. C., & Bernstein, I. H. (1994). *Psychometric theory* (3rd ed.). New York: McGraw-Hill.

Phaladze, N. A., Human, S., Dlamini, S. B., Hulela, E. B., Hadebe, I. M., Sukati, N. A., Makoae, L. N., Seboni, N. M., Moleko, M., & Holzemer, W. L. (2005). Quality of life and the concept of "Living Well" with HIV/AIDS in Sub-Saharan Africa. *The Journal of Nursing Scholarship, 37*(2), 120–126.

Radloff, L. S. (1977). The CES-D scale: A self report depression scale for research in the general population. *Applied Psychological Measures, 1,* 385–394.

Rutledge, D. N., & Raymon, N. J. (2001). Changes in well-being of women cancer survivors following a survivor weekend experience. *Oncology Nursing Forum, 28*(1), 85–91.

Schulberg, H. C., Saul, M., McClelland, M., Ganguli, M., Christy, W., & Frank, R. (1985). Assessing depression in primary medical and psychiatric practices. *Archives of General Psychiatry, 42*(12), 1164–1170.

Schumacher, K. L., Koresawa, S., West, C., Dodd, M., Paul, S. M., Tripathy, D., et al. (2002). The usefulness of a daily pain management diary for outpatients with cancer-related pain. *Oncology Nursing Forum, 29*(9), 1304–1313.

Schumacher, K. L., Koresawa, S., West, C., Dodd, M., Paul, S. M., Tripathy, D., Koo, P., & Miaskowski, C. (2005). Qualitative research contribution to a randomized clinical trial. *Research in Nursing & Health, 28*(3), 268–280.

Stevens, S. S. (1946). On the theory of scales of measurement. *Science, 103*(2684), 677–680.

Stotts, C., Henderson, A., & Burns, N. (1988). *Health exemplar? Nurses, nursing students and smoking behavior.* XIII World Conference on Health Education, Houston, August 28–September 2.

Tesh, E. M., & Holditch-Davis, D. (1997). HOME Inventory and NCATS: Relation to mother and child behaviors during naturalistic observations. *Research in Nursing & Health, 20*(4), 295–307.

Tyson, S. F., & DeSouza, L. H. (2004). Development of the Brunel Balance Assessment: A new measure of balance disability post stroke. *Clinical Rehabilitation, 18*(7), 801–810.

Wasson, J., Keller, A., Rubenstein, L., Hays, R., Nelson, E., Johnson, D., & The Dartmouth Primary COOP Project. (1992). Benefits and obstacles of health status assessment in ambulatory settings. *Medical Care, 30*(5 Suppl.), 42–S49.

Wewers, M. E., & Lowe, N. K. (1990). A critical review of visual analogue scales in the measurement of clinical phenomena. *Research in Nursing & Health, 13*(4), 227–236.

Willaing, I., & Ladelund, S. (2005). Nurse counseling of patients with an overconsumption of alcohol. *The Journal of Nursing Scholarship, 37*(1), 30–35.

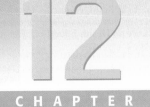

Understanding Statistics in Research

Learning Outcomes

After completing this chapter, you should be able to:

1. Identify the purposes of statistical analysis.
2. Describe the process of data analysis:
  (a) preparing the data for analysis;
  (b) describing the sample; (c) testing the reliability of the measurement methods;
  (d) conducting exploratory analysis of the data;
  (e) conducting confirmatory analyses guided by objectives, questions, or hypotheses; and
  (f) conducting posthoc analyses.
3. Differentiate probability theory from decision theory.

4. Describe the process of inferring from a sample to a population.
5. Discuss the distribution of the normal curve.
6. Compare and contrast Type I and Type II errors.
7. Differentiate a one-tailed test of significance from a two-tailed test of significance.
8. Compare the clinical and the statistical significance of findings.

9. Differentiate the ungrouped frequency distribution from the grouped frequency distribution.

10. Describe the three measures of central tendency: mean, median, and mode.

11. Discuss the purpose of measures of dispersion.

12. Discuss the purposes and interpretation of results of chi-square analysis, *t*-test, analysis of variance, Pearson correlation, and regression analysis.

13. Critique the use of chi-square analysis, *t*-test, analysis of variance, Pearson correlation, and regression analysis in published studies.

14. Describe the five types of results obtained from quasi-experimental and experimental studies that are interpreted within a decision

theory framework: (a) significant and predicted results, (b) nonsignificant results, (c) significant and unpredicted results, (d) mixed results, and (e) unexpected results.

15. Differentiate among the results, findings, and conclusions in a study.

16. Critique findings for statistical significance and practical clinical significance in a study.

17. Identify the following elements of a research report: findings, conclusions, significance of findings, generalization of findings, implications, and suggestions for further study.

18. Given a study, critique the results, findings, conclusions, generalizations, implications, and suggestions for further study.

Key Terms

Analysis of covariance, p. 432

Analysis of variance, p. 430

Between-group variance, p. 430

Bivariate correlation, p. 423

Chi-square test of independence, p. 420

Clinical significance, p. 438

Coefficient of multiple determination, p. 427

Conclusions, p. 437

Confirmatory analysis, p. 405

Correlation matrix, p. 425

Decision theory, p. 406

Degrees of freedom, p. 412

Dependent groups, p. 433

Descriptive statistics, p. 413

Effect size, p. 412

Empirical generalizations, p. 439

Explained variance, p. 424

Exploratory analysis, p. 404

Factor, p. 426

Factor analysis, p. 426

Findings, p. 436

Frequency distribution, p. 413

Generalization, p. 408

Grouped frequency distributions, p. 413

Implications, p. 437

Independent groups, p. 432

Inference, p. 408

Level of statistical significance, p. 407

Line of best fit, p. 427

Mean, p. 417

Measures of dispersion, p. 417

Measures of central tendency, p. 415

Median, p. 415

Mixed results, p. 435

Mode, p. 415

Multiple regression, p. 426

Negative relationship, p. 423

Nonsignificant results, p. 435

Normal curve, p. 408

One-tailed test of significance, p. 409

Outliers, p. 404

Pearson product-moment correlation, p. 423

Percentage distribution, p. 414

Positive relationship, p. 423

Posthoc analyses, p. 405

Power, p. 412

Power analysis, p. 412

Probability theory, p. 406

Range, p. 417

Regression analysis, p. 426

Scatterplot, p. 418

Significant and unpredicted results, p. 435

Significant results, p. 433

Standard deviation, p. 418

Standardized scores, p. 418

Symmetrical, p. 423

Total variance, p. 430

t-test, p. 428

Two-tailed test of significance, p. 409

Type I error, p. 410

Type II error, p. 411

Unexpected results, p. 435

Unexplained variance, p. 424

Ungrouped frequency distribution, p. 443

Variance, p. 417

Within-group variance, p. 430

X axis, p. 418

Y axis, p. 418

Z-score, p.418

STUDY TOOLS

Be sure to visit http://evolve.elsevier.com/Burns/understanding for additional examples and self-tests. Also, a review of this chapter's concepts and practice exercises can be found in Chapter 12 of the Study Guide for *Understanding Nursing Research: Building an Evidence-Based Practice*, 4th edition.

The expectation that the practice of nursing be evidence-based has made it more important that clinical nurses acquire skills in reading and evaluating the results of statistical tests. Nurses probably have more anxiety about statistical results and data analysis than they do about any other aspect of the research process. We hope that this chapter will dispel some of that anxiety and facilitate your critique of studies. The statistical information in this chapter is provided from the perspective of reading, understanding, and critiquing published quantitative studies, rather than from that of selecting statistical procedures or performing statistical analyses. To critique a quantitative study, you need to be able to (1) identify the statistical procedures used; (2) judge whether these procedures were appropriate for the hypotheses, questions, or objectives of the study, and for the level of measurement of the variables; (3) comprehend the discussion of data analysis results in the study; (4) judge whether the author interpretation of the results is appropriate; and (5) evaluate the clinical significance of the findings.

The chapter begins with a discussion of some of the more pragmatic aspects of quantitative data analysis procedures: the purposes of statistical analysis and the process of performing data analysis. The reasoning behind statistics is explained, and some of the more common statistical procedures used to describe variables, examine relationships, and predict and test causal hypotheses are introduced. The chapter concludes with strategies for judging statistical suitability and evaluating the interpretation of statistical outcomes.

Process of Data Analysis

Statistical procedures are used to examine the numerical data gathered in a study. In critiquing a study, it may be helpful to understand the process the researcher uses to perform data analyses. The quantitative data analysis process consists of several stages: (1) preparing the data for analysis; (2) describing the sample; (3) testing the reliability of measurement methods; (4) conducting exploratory analysis of the data; (5) conducting confirmatory analysis guided by the hypotheses, questions, or objectives; and (6) conducting posthoc analysis. Although not all of these stages are equally reflected in the final published report of the study, they all contribute to the insights that can be gained from analysis of the data.

Preparing the Data for Analysis

Except in very small studies, researchers almost always use computers for data analyses. The first step of the process is entering the data into the computer. The researcher uses a systematic plan for data entry designed to reduce errors during the entry phase. After entry, the data are cleaned. This process is time intensive and tedious but essential for ensuring accuracy of the data. If the data file is small enough, every datum on the printout is cross-checked with the original datum for accuracy. Otherwise, data points are randomly checked for accuracy. All identified errors are corrected. Missing data points are identified. If the information can be obtained, the missing data are entered into the data file. If enough data are missing for certain variables, the researcher may have to determine whether the data are sufficient to perform analyses using those variables. In some cases, subjects must be excluded from an analysis because data considered essential to that analysis are missing.

CRITIQUE GUIDELINES Preparing the Data for Analysis

When critiquing a study look for clues to the accuracy of the data.
Search for information about the amount of missing data.

Describing the Sample

Next, the researcher obtains as complete a picture of the sample as possible. First, frequencies of descriptive variables related to the sample are obtained. Estimates of central tendency (such as the mean) and dispersion (such as the standard deviation) of variables relevant to the sample are calculated. Variables relevant to the sample might include age, education level, health status, gender, and ethnicity. If the study includes more than one group (e.g., treatment group and comparison group), the researcher might compare the various groups in relation to these variables. For example, it might be important to know whether the age distribution of the various groups was similar. If the groups being compared are not equivalent in ways important to the study, the groups cannot justifiably be compared through statistical procedures. Thus the researcher must decide whether to continue the analysis process.

CRITIQUE GUIDELINES Describing the Sample

When critiquing a study, judge the representativeness of the sample.
    If the sample is divided into groups that are compared in the statistical analyses, determine the equivalence of the groups.
    Determine the variables used to describe the sample.
    Identify the statistical procedures used to describe the sample.

Testing the Reliability of Measurement

After describing the sample, the researcher examines the reliability of the measurement methods used in the study. Reliability of observational or physiological measures may have been determined during the data collection phase, but will be noted again at this point. If paper-and-pencil scales were used to collect data, the Cronbach statistical procedure will be performed on the scale items to determine the alpha coefficient value. If the Cronbach alpha coefficient is unacceptably low (below 0.70), the researcher must decide whether to analyze the data collected with the instrument. A value of 0.70 is considered marginally acceptable. A Cronbach alpha coefficient value of 0.80 to 0.89 indicates that the measurement is sufficiently reliable to use in a study. The *t*-test or Pearson's Correlation statistics may be used to determine test-retest reliability.

CRITIQUE GUIDELINES **Testing the Reliability of Measurement**

When critiquing a study, search for information on the reliability of measures used to gather data for the analyses.
Identify the statistical procedures used to determine the reliability of measures.

Conducting Exploratory Analyses

The next step, **exploratory analysis**, is used to examine all of the data descriptively. This step is discussed in more detail later in the section "Using Statistics to Describe." The researcher must become as familiar as possible with the nature of the data obtained on variables that will be used to test hypotheses, research questions, or objectives. Data on each variable are examined using measures of central tendency and dispersion to determine the nature of variation in the data and to identify **outliers**, which are subjects or data points with extreme values (values that lie far from other plotted points on a graph) that seem unlike the rest of the sample. The most valuable insights from a study often come from careful examination of outliers (Tukey, 1977). In many studies, relationships among variables and differences between groups are explored using statistical procedures that also are used in confirmatory studies. However, when these procedures are used for exploratory purposes, the results are not generalized to a larger population. The results are used to give a better understanding of the data.

CRITIQUE GUIDELINES **Exploratory Analyses**

In critiquing a study, examine the values obtained for the study variables. Ask yourself the following questions:

1. Do they appear to be representative of values you would expect to find in the population under study?
2. Is the full range of values for each variable represented in the data?
3. What is the nature of outliers in the sample?
4. Is it likely that data from outliers affected the results of the analyses?
5. Are analyses used for exploratory or confirmatory purposes?

Conducting Confirmatory Analyses

Researchers use **confirmatory analysis** to confirm expectations regarding data that are expressed as hypotheses, questions, or objectives. When performing confirmatory analyses, investigators generalize findings from the sample to appropriate populations. Statistical procedures designed for the purpose of making inferences (inferential statistical procedures) are used. To justify generalization of the results of confirmatory analyses, a rigorous research methodology is needed, including a strong research design, reliable and valid measurement methods, and a large sample size.

> **CRITIQUE GUIDELINES** Confirmatory Analyses
>
> When critiquing a study, identify the confirmatory analyses performed. Is the research methodology sufficiently rigorous to warrant using confirmatory analyses?

Conducting Posthoc Analyses

Some statistical analyses, such as chi-square analysis and analysis of variance (ANOVA), are used to test for differences among groups in studies including more than two groups. These statistical procedures indicate significant differences among groups but do not specify which groups are different. For example, a study may examine the proportion of the sample in four occupational groups of workers who are smokers to determine differences in smoking behavior among the groups. Chi-square analysis or ANOVA may show significant differences among the groups, but the researcher will not be able to determine which groups were different. In such studies, when significant differences are found, **posthoc analyses** are performed after the initial statistical analysis to identify which groups are significantly different.

> **CRITIQUE GUIDELINES** Posthoc Analyses
>
> When critiquing a study, identify the specific posthoc analyses that were done. These should be indicated in the research report.
> Determine which groups were statistically different.
> Determine which groups were not statistically different.

Reasoning behind Statistics

One reason that nurses tend to avoid statistics is that many were taught only the mathematical procedures of calculating statistical equations, with little or no explanation of the logic behind those procedures or the meaning of the results. Computation is a mechanical process usually performed by a computer, and information about the calculation procedure is not necessary to begin understanding statistical results. Here we present an approach to data analysis that will enhance your understanding of the statistical analysis process. You can then use this understanding to critique data analysis techniques in the "Results" section of research reports.

This section presents a brief explanation of some concepts that commonly are used in statistical theory. The concepts include probability theory, decision theory, hypothesis testing, level of significance, inference, generalization, the normal curve, tailedness, Type I and Type II errors, power, and degrees of freedom. More extensive discussion of these topics can be found in other sources; we recommend our own recent textbook (Burns & Grove, 2005).

Probability Theory

Probability theory, which is deductive, is used to explain the extent of a relationship, the probability that an event will occur in a given situation, or the probability that an event can be accurately predicted. The researcher might want to know the probability that a particular outcome will result from a nursing action. For example, the researcher may want to know how likely it is that urinary catheterization during hospitalization will lead to a bladder infection after discharge from the hospital. The researcher also may want to know the probability that subjects in the experimental group are members of the same larger population from which the control group subjects were taken. Probability is expressed as a lowercase letter p, with values expressed as percentages or as a decimal value ranging from 0 to 1. For example, if the probability is 0.23, then it is expressed as $p = 0.23$. This means that there is a 23% probability that a particular outcome (such as a bladder infection) will occur. Probability values also can be stated as less than a specific value, such as 0.05, expressed as $p < 0.05$. (The symbol < means "less than.") A research study may find that the probability that the experimental group subjects were members of the same larger population as the control group subjects was less than or equal to 5% ($p \leq 0.05$). In other words, it is NOT very likely that the control group and the experimental group are from the same population. Put another way, you might say that there is a 5% chance that the two groups are from the same population and a 95% chance that they are not from the same population. Probability values often are stated with the results of statistical analyses. In critiquing studies, it is useful to recognize these symbols and understand what they mean.

Decision Theory, Hypothesis Testing, and Level of Significance

Decision theory, which is inductive, assumes that all of the groups in a study (e.g., experimental and control groups) used to test a particular hypothesis are components of the same population relative to the variables under study. This expectation (or assumption) traditionally is expressed as a null hypothesis, which states that there is no difference between (or among) the groups in a study, in terms of the variables included in the hypothesis. It is up to the researcher to provide evidence for a genuine difference between the groups. For example, the researcher may hypothesize that the frequency of urinary tract infections that occurred after discharge from the hospital in patients who were catheterized during hospitalization is no different from the frequency of such infections in those who were not catheterized. To test the assumption of no difference, a cutoff point is selected before data collection. The cutoff point, referred to as alpha (α), or the **level of statistical significance**, is the probability level at which the results of statistical analysis are judged to indicate a statistically significant difference between the groups. The level of significance selected for most nursing studies is 0.05. This means that if the level of significance found in the statistical analysis is 0.05 or less, the experimental and the control groups are considered to be significantly different (members of different populations). In some studies, the more rigorous level of significance of 0.01 may be chosen. This may be written as $\alpha = 0.01$, particularly in tables and figures.

Decision theory requires that the cutoff point selected for a study be absolute. *Absolute* means that even if the value obtained is only a fraction above the cutoff point, the samples are considered to be from the same population, and *no* meaning can be attributed to the differences. Thus, it is inappropriate when using decision theory to state that the findings approached significance at the 0.051 level if the alpha level was set at 0.05. Using decision theory rules, this finding indicates that the groups tested are not significantly different, and the null hypothesis is not rejected. On the other hand, once the level of significance has been set at 0.05 by the researcher, if the analysis reveals a significant difference of 0.001, this result is not considered more significant than the 0.05 originally proposed (Slakter, Wu, & Suzaki-Slakter, 1991). The level of significance is dichotomous, which means that the difference is either significant or not significant; there are no "degrees" of significance. However, some people, not realizing that their reasoning has shifted from decision theory to probability theory, indicate in their research report that the 0.001 result makes the findings more significant than if they had obtained only a 0.05 level of significance. The researcher may even state that the findings are highly significant, which is unacceptable from the perspective of decision theory.

From the perspective of probability theory, there is considerable difference in the risk of occurrence of a Type II error (defined and discussed later) when the probability is between 0.05 and 0.001. If $p = 0.001$, the probability that the two groups are components of the same population is 1 in 1000; if $p = 0.05$, the probability that the groups belong to the same population is 5 in 100. In other words, if $p = 0.05$, then in 5 times out of 100, groups with statistical values such as those found in these statistical analyses actually are members of the same population, and the conclusion that the groups are different is erroneous.

In computer analysis the probability value obtained from each data analysis (e.g., $p = 0.03$ or $p = 0.07$) frequently is provided on the printout and often is reported by the researcher in the published study, along with the level of significance set before data analysis was done. In summary, the probability (p) value reveals the risk of a Type II error. The alpha (α) value reveals whether the probability value for a particular analysis met the cutoff point for deciding whether there is a significant difference between or among groups.

CRITIQUE GUIDELINES Level of Significance

When critiquing a study, be sure to include the following:

1. Identify the level of significance and determine whether the findings show statistically significant differences.
2. Judge the risk of a Type II error.

Inference and Generalization

An **inference** is a conclusion or judgment based on evidence. Statistical inferences are made cautiously and with great care. The decision theory rules used to interpret the results of statistical procedures increase the probability that inferences are accurate. A **generalization** is the application of information that has been acquired from a specific instance to a general situation. Generalizing requires making an inference; both require the use of inductive reasoning. Inductively, an inference is made from a specific case and extended to a general truth, from a part to the whole, from the concrete to the abstract, and from the known to the unknown. In research, an inference is made from the study findings obtained from a specific sample and applied to a more general population, using the results from statistical analyses. Thus, a researcher may conclude in a research report that a significant difference was found in the number of urinary tract infections found between two samples, one in which the subjects had been catheterized during hospitalization and another in which the subjects had not. The researcher also may conclude that this difference can be expected in all patients who have been cared for in hospitals. The findings are generalized from the sample in the study to all previously hospitalized patients. Statisticians and researchers can never prove something using inference; they can never be certain that their inferences and generalizations are correct. For example, the researcher generalization of the incidence of urinary tract infection may not have been carefully thought out; the findings may have been generalized over too broad a population. It is possible that in the more general population, there is no difference in the incidence of urinary tract infection that is based on whether the patient was catheterized.

CRITIQUE GUIDELINES   Inference and Generalization

When critiquing a study, judge whether generalizations made by the researcher are justified on the basis of the study results.

Normal Curve

The theoretical **normal curve** is an expression of statistical theory (Figure 12-1). A normal curve is a theoretical frequency distribution of all possible values in a population; however, no real distribution exactly fits the normal curve. The idea of the normal curve was developed by an 18-year-old mathematician, Johann Gauss, in 1795. He found that data from variables (e.g., the mean of each sample) measured repeatedly in many samples from the same population can be combined into one large sample. From this large sample, a more accurate representation can be developed of the pattern of the curve in that population than is possible with only one sample. Surprisingly, in most cases the curve is similar, regardless of the specific variables examined or the population studied.

Levels of significance and probability are based on the logic of the normal curve. The normal curve presented in Figure 12-1 shows the distribution of values for a single population. Note that 95.5% of the values are within 2 standard deviations of the mean, ranging

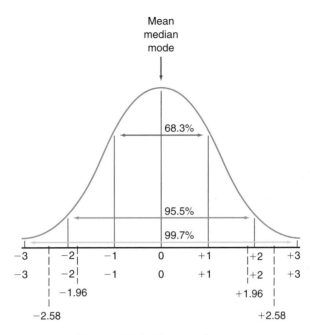

Mean
median
mode

68.3%

95.5%

99.7%

−3   −2   −1   0   +1   +2   +3

−3   −2   −1   0   +1   +2   +3

−1.96   +1.96

−2.58   +2.58

Figure 12-1. The normal curve.

from −2 to +2 standard deviations. (Standard deviations are defined and discussed later in the chapter under "Using Statistics to Describe.") Thus, there is approximately a 95% probability that a given measured value (e.g., the mean of a group) would fall within 2 standard deviations of the mean of the population, and there is a 5% probability that the value would fall in the tails of the normal curve (the extreme ends of the normal curve, below −2 standard deviations [2.5%] or above +2 standard deviations [2.5%]). If the groups being compared were from the same population (not significantly different), you would expect the value (e.g., the mean) of each group to fall within the 95% range of values on the normal curve. If the groups were from (significantly) different populations, you would expect one of the group values to be outside the 95% range of values. A statistical analysis performed to determine differences between or among groups, using a level of significance set at 0.05, would test that expectation. If the statistical test demonstrates a significant difference (the value of one group does not fall within the 95% range of values), the groups are considered to belong to different populations. However, in 5% of the statistical tests, the value of one of the groups can be expected to fall outside the 95% range of values but still belong to the same population (a Type I error).

Tailedness

Nondirectional hypotheses usually assume that an extreme score (obtained because the group with the extreme score did not belong to the same population) can occur in either tail of the normal curve (Figure 12-2). The analysis of a nondirectional hypothesis is called a **two-tailed test of significance**. In a **one-tailed test of significance**, the hypothesis is directional, and

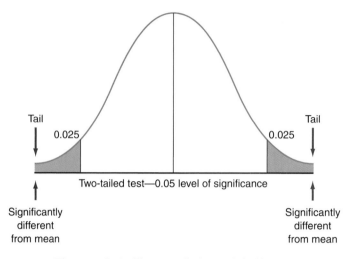

Figure 12-2. The two-tailed test of significance.

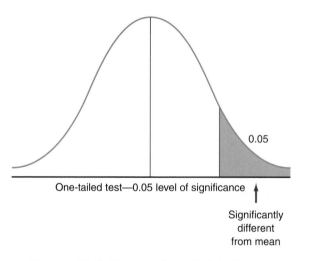

Figure 12-3. The one-tailed test of significance.

extreme statistical values that occur on a single tail of the curve are of interest (see Chapter 4 for discussion of directional and nondirectional hypotheses). The hypothesis states that the extreme score is higher or lower than that for 95% of the population, indicating that the sample with the extreme score is not a member of the same population. In this case, 5% of statistical values that are considered significant will be in one tail, rather than two. Extreme statistical values occurring in the other tail of the curve are not considered significantly different. In Figure 12-3, which shows a one-tailed figure, the portion of the curve in which statistical values will be considered significant is the right tail. Developing a one-tailed hypothesis requires that the researcher have sufficient knowledge of the variables to predict whether the difference will be in the tail above the mean or in the tail below the mean. One-

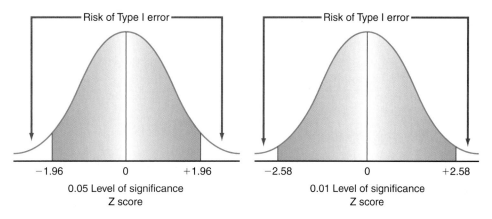

Figure 12-4. Risk of Type I error.

tailed statistical tests are uniformly more powerful than two-tailed tests, decreasing the possibility of a Type II error.

CRITIQUE GUIDELINES Tailedness

When critiquing a study, determine whether there are one-tailed or two-tailed hypotheses. If the researcher states a one-tailed hypothesis, judge whether there is sufficient knowledge on which to base a one-tailed statistical test.

Type I and Type II Errors

According to decision theory, two types of error can occur when a researcher is deciding what the result of a statistical test means: Type I and Type II. A **Type I error** occurs when the null hypothesis is rejected when it is true (e.g., when the results indicate that there is a significant difference, when, in reality, there is not). The risk of a Type I error is indicated by the level of significance. There is a greater risk of a Type I error with a 0.05 level of significance than with a 0.01 level of significance. As the level of significance becomes more extreme, the risk of a Type I error decreases, as illustrated in Figure 12-4.

A **Type II error** occurs when the null hypothesis is regarded as true but it is in fact false. For example, a statistical analyses may indicate no significant differences between groups, but in reality the groups are different. There is a greater risk of a Type II error when the level of significance is 0.01 than when it is 0.05. However, Type II errors often are caused by flaws in the research methods. In nursing research, many studies are conducted with small samples and with instruments that do not precisely measure the variables under study. In many nursing situations, multiple variables interact to cause differences within populations. However, when only a few of the interacting variables are examined, small differences may be overlooked, which can lead to the false conclusion that there are no differences between the samples. Thus, the risk of a Type II error is high in many nursing studies.

CRITIQUE GUIDELINES Type I and Type II Errors

When critiquing a study, evaluate the risk of a Type I or Type II error.
What elements of the study have resulted in the risk?

Power: Controlling the Risk of a Type II Error

Power is the probability that a statistical test will detect a significant difference that exists. The risk of a Type II error can be determined using power analysis. Cohen (1988) has identified four parameters of a **power analysis:** the level of significance, sample size, power, and effect size. If three of the four are known, the fourth can be calculated using power analysis formulas. The minimum acceptable power level is 0.80. The researcher determines the sample size and the level of significance. **Effect size** is "the degree to which the phenomenon is present in the population, or the degree to which the null hypothesis is false" (Cohen, 1988, pp. 9–10). For example, if changes in anxiety level are measured in a group of patients before surgery, with the first measurement taken when the patients are still at home, and the second taken just before surgery, effect size will be large if a great change in anxiety occurs in the group between the two time periods. If the effect of a preoperative teaching program on the level of anxiety is measured, the effect size will be the difference in the posttest level of anxiety in the experimental group compared with that in the control group. If only a small change in the level of anxiety is expected, the effect size will be small. In most nursing studies, only small effect sizes can be expected. In such a study, a sample of 200 or more is needed to detect a significant difference. This small effect size occurs because nursing studies tend to use samples that are small, study designs in which threats to the validity of the design are not tightly controlled, and measurement methods that measure only large changes. The power level is required to be reported in studies that fail to reject the null hypothesis (or have nonsignificant findings). If the power level is below 0.80, you need to question the validity of nonsignificant findings.

CRITIQUE GUIDELINES Power Level

When critiquing a study, look for reports of the effect size and the power level.
Judge the adequacy of the sample size.
Judge the adequacy of the design.
Judge the adequacy of measurements used in the study.

Degrees of Freedom

The concept of **degrees of freedom** (*df*) is important for calculating statistical procedures and interpreting the results using statistical tables. However, this concept is difficult to explain because of the complex mathematics involved. Degrees of freedom involve the freedom of a score value to vary given the other existing scores' values and the established sum of these scores. Degrees of freedom often are reported with statistical results.

Using Statistics to Describe

In any study in which the data are numerical, data analysis begins with descriptive statistics (also called "summary statistics"). For some descriptive studies, researchers limit data analyses to descriptive statistics. For other studies, researchers use descriptive statistics primarily to describe the characteristics of the sample from which the data were collected and to describe values obtained from the measurement of variables. Descriptive statistics presented in this book include frequency distributions, measures of central tendency, measures of dispersion, and standardized scores.

Frequency Distributions

Frequency distribution usually is the first method used to organize the data for examination. There are two types of frequency distributions: ungrouped and grouped.

Ungrouped Frequency Distributions

Most studies have some categorical data that are presented in the form of an ungrouped frequency distribution, in which a table is developed to display all numerical values obtained for a particular variable. This approach generally is used on discrete rather than continuous data. Examples of data commonly organized in this manner are gender, ethnicity, marital status, diagnostic category of study subjects, and values obtained from the measurement of variables. In Table 12-1, LoBiondo-Wood, Williams, Wood, and Shaw (1997) present the ungrouped frequency of subject characteristics in their study of the impact of liver transplantation on quality of life.

Grouped Frequency Distributions

Grouped frequency distributions are used when continuous variables, such as age, are being examined. Many measures taken during data collection, including body temperature, vital lung capacity, weight, scale scores, and time, are measured using a continuous scale. Any method of grouping results in loss of information. For example, if age is grouped, a breakdown into two groups, under 65 years of age and over 65 years of age, provides less information about the data than groupings of 10-year age spans. As with levels of measurement, rules have been established to guide classification systems. There should be at least 6 but not more than 20 groups. The classes established must be exhaustive; each datum must fit into one of the identified classes. The classes must be exclusive; each datum must fit into only one. A common mistake occurs when the ranges contain overlaps that would allow a datum to fit into more than one class. For example, a researcher may classify age ranges as 20 to 30, 30 to 40, 40 to 50, and so on. By this definition, subjects aged 30, 40, and so on can be classified into more than one class. The range of each class must be equivalent; with age, for example, if 10 years is the range, each class must include 10 years of ages. This rule is violated in some cases to allow the first and last categories to be open-ended and worded to include all scores above or below a specified point. In Table 12-1, income is a grouped frequency.

Table 12-1	Subject Characteristics		
Characteristic	Variable	*n*	Percentage
Gender	Male	19	46.3
	Female	22	53.7
Marital status	Single	4	9.8
	Married	32	78.0
	Divorced	4	9.8
	Widowed	1	2.4
Education	High school	18	43.9
	Attended/completed college	12	29.3
	Attended/completed graduate school	10	24.4
Income—family	Below $20,000	14	34.4
	$20,001–30,000	6	14.6
	$30,001–40,000	7	17.1
	$40,001–50,000	5	12.2
	$50,001–60,000	3	7.3
	Above $60,000	3	7.3
Diagnosis	Cirrhosis	24	58.5
	Primary biliary cirrhosis	8	19.5
	Primary sclerosing cholangitis	7	17.1
	Secondary biliary cirrhosis	1	2.4
	Malignancy	1	2.4
Occupation	Unemployed	20	48.8
	Laborer	6	14.6
	Semiskilled	2	4.9
	Skilled	1	2.4
	Clerical	2	4.9
	Semiprofessional	2	4.9
	Minor/lesser professional	6	14.6
	Professional	3	7.3

From LoBiondo-Wood, G., Williams, L., Wood, R. P., & Shaw, B. W. (1997). Impact of liver transplantation on quality of life: A longitudinal perspective. *Applied Nursing Research, 10*(1), 29, with permission.

Percentage Distributions

A **percentage distribution** indicates the percentage of subjects in a sample whose scores fall into a specific group and the number of scores in that group. Percentage distributions are particularly useful for comparing the present data with findings from other studies that have different sample sizes. The percentage distribution is provided for each variable in Table 12-1. A cumulative distribution is a type of percentage distribution in which the percentages and frequencies of scores are summed, as one moves from the top of the table to the bottom. Thus, the bottom category would have a cumulative frequency equivalent to the sample size and a cumulative percentage of 100 (Table 12-2). Frequency distributions also are displayed using tables or graphs (e.g., pie charts, bar charts, histograms, frequency polygons). Graphic

Table 12-2	Example of a Cumulative Frequency Table			
Score	Frequency	Percent	Cumulative Frequency (*f*)	Cumulative Percent
1	4	8	4	8
3	6	12	10	20
4	8	16	18	36
5	14	28	32	64
7	8	16	40	80
8	6	12	46	92
9	4	8	$n = 50$	100

displays of the grouped frequency distribution of data from Table 12-2 are presented in Figure 12-5.

Measures of Central Tendency

A **measure of central tendency** frequently is referred to as an "average," which is a lay term not commonly used in statistics because it is vague. The measures of central tendency are the most concise statement of the nature of the data; the three that are commonly used in statistical analyses are the mode, median, and mean. For a data set that has a normal distribution, these values are equal (see Figure 12-1); however, they usually are different for data obtained from real samples.

Mode

The **mode** is the numerical value or score that occurs with greatest frequency; it does not necessarily indicate the center of the data set. The mode can be determined by examination of an ungrouped frequency distribution of the data. In Table 12-2, the mode is the score of 5, which occurred 14 times in the data set. The mode can be used to describe the typical subject or to identify the most frequently occurring value on a scale item. The mode is the appropriate measure of central tendency for nominal data. A data set can have more than one mode. If two modes exist, the data set is referred to as "bimodal," as illustrated in Figure 12-6. A data set with more than two modes is said to be multimodal.

Median

The **median** is the score at the exact center of the ungrouped frequency distribution—the 50th percentile. The median is obtained by rank ordering the scores. If the number of scores is uneven, exactly 50% of the scores are above the median and 50% are below it. If the number of scores is even, the median is the average of the two middle scores; thus, the median may not be one of the scores in the data set. Unlike the mean, the median is not affected by extreme scores in the data (outliers). The median is the most appropriate measure of central tendency for ordinal data. The median for the data in Table 12-2 is 5.

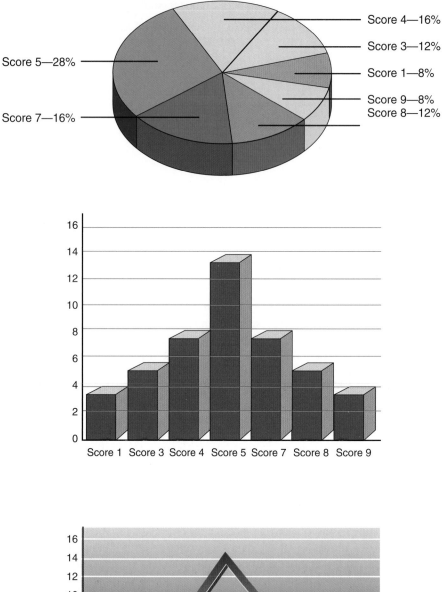

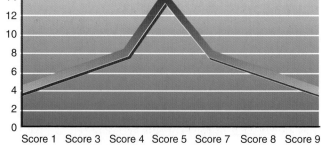

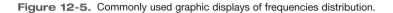

Figure 12-5. Commonly used graphic displays of frequencies distribution.

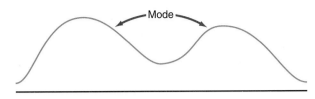

Figure 12-6. Bimodal distribution.

Mean

The most commonly used measure of central tendency is the mean. The **mean** is the sum of the scores divided by the number of scores being summed. Thus, like the median, the mean may not be a member of the data set. The mean is the appropriate measure of central tendency for interval and ratio-level data. The mean for the data in Table 12-2 is 5.28.

Measures of Dispersion

Measures of dispersion, or variability, are measures of individual differences of the members of the sample. They give some indication of how scores in a sample are dispersed around the mean. These measures provide information about the data that is not available from measures of central tendency. They indicate how different the scores are, or the extent to which individual scores deviate from one another. If the individual scores are similar, measures of variability are small, and the sample is relatively homogeneous, or similar, in terms of those scores. A heterogeneous sample has a wide variation in scores. The measures of dispersion most commonly used are range, variance, and standard deviation. Standardized scores may be used to express measures of dispersion. Scatterplots frequently are used to illustrate the dispersion in the data.

Range

The simplest measure of dispersion is the **range**, which is obtained by subtracting the lowest score from the highest score. The range for the scores in Table 12-2 is calculated as follows: $9 - 1 = 8$. The range is a difference score, which uses only the two extreme scores for the comparison. It is a very crude measure and is sensitive to outliers.

Variance

The **variance** is calculated with a mathematical equation. The numerical value obtained from the calculation depends on the measurement scale used; the calculated variance value has no absolute value and can be compared only with data obtained using similar measures. Generally, however, the larger the variance value, the greater the dispersion of scores. The variance for the data in Table 12-2 is 4.94.

Standard Deviation

The **standard deviation** is the square root of the variance. Just as the mean is the average value, the standard deviation is the average difference (deviation) value. The standard deviation provides a measure of the average deviation of a value from the mean in that particular sample. It indicates the degree of error that would result if the mean alone were used to interpret the data. In the normal curve, 68% of the values will be within 1 standard deviation above or below the mean, 95% will be within 2 standard deviations above or below the mean, and 99% will be within 3 standard deviations above or below the mean (see Figure 12-1).

The standard deviation for the data in Table 12-2 is 2.22. The mean is 5.28, so the value of a subject 1 standard deviation below the mean would be 5.28 – 2.22, or 3.06. The value of a subject 1 standard deviation above the mean would be 5.28 + 2.22, or 7.50. So approximately 68% of the sample (and perhaps the population from which it was derived) can be expected to have values in the range of 3.06 to 7.50. Extending this calculation further, the value of a subject 2 standard deviations above the mean would be 5.28 + 2.22 + 2.22 = 9.72. Using this strategy, the entire distribution of values can be estimated. The value of a single individual can be compared with the value calculated for the total sample (e.g., mean, median, or mode). Standard deviation is an important measure, both for understanding dispersion within a distribution and for interpreting the relationship of a particular value to the distribution.

Standardized Scores

Because of differences in the characteristics of various distributions, comparing a value in one distribution with a value in another is difficult. For example, perhaps you want to compare test scores from two classroom examinations. The highest possible score in one test is 100 and in the other, 70; the scores will be difficult to compare. To facilitate this comparison, a mechanism was developed to transform raw scores into **standardized scores**. Numbers that make sense only within the framework of measurements used within a specific study are transformed into numbers (standardized scores) that have a more general meaning. Transformation into standardized scores allows an easy conceptual grasp of the meaning of the score. A common standardized score is called a **Z-score**. It expresses deviations from the mean (difference scores) in terms of standard deviation units (see Figure 12-1). A score that falls above the mean will have a positive Z-score, whereas a score that falls below the mean will have a negative Z-score. The mean expressed as a Z-score is zero. The standard deviation is equal to the Z-score. Thus, a Z-score of 2 indicates that the score from which it was obtained is 2 standard deviations above the mean. A Z-score of –0.5 indicates that the score is 0.5 standard deviation below the mean.

Scatterplots

A **scatterplot** has two scales: horizontal and vertical. Each scale is referred to as an axis. The vertical scale is called the **Y axis**; the horizontal scale is the **X axis**. A scatterplot can be used to illustrate the dispersion of values on a variable. In this case, the X axis represents the possible values of the variable. The Y axis represents the number of times each value of the variable occurred in the sample. Scatterplots also can be used to illustrate the relationship between values on one variable and values on another. Then each axis will represent one variable. For example, if a graph is developed to illustrate the relationship between the number of days a patient has been hospitalized and the stage of the patient's decubitus ulcer, the horizontal axis represents days and the vertical axis, decubitus ulcer stage. For each unit or subject, there is a value for X and a value for Y. The point at which the values of X and Y for a single subject intersect is plotted on the graph (Figure 12-7). When the values for each subject in the sample have been plotted, the degree of relationship between the variables is revealed (Figure 12-8).

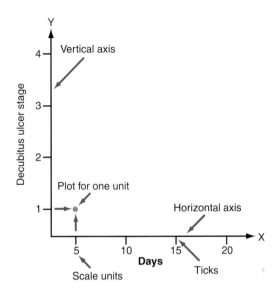

Figure 12-7. Structure of a plot.

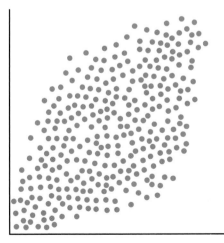

Figure 12-8. Example of a scatterplot.

Table 12-3	Comparison of Findings for Enema Composition Study			
	Amount Instilled (g)	Net Output[a] (g)	PEG[b] (g/L)	Recovery[c]
Tap water group (n = 12)	M: 939 SD: 70 Range: 723 to 980[d]	M: −175.3 SD: 185.6 Range: −556 to +147	M: 1.7 SD: 0.45	68%
Soapsuds group (n = 13)	M: 918 SD: 202 Range: 400 to 976[e]	M: +10.5 SD: 106.1 Range: −205 to +173	M: 1.4 SD: 0.35	72%
Statistical significance (α = 0.05)	No significant difference (α = 0.05)	t = −3.039 df = 17 p = 0.007	No significant difference (α = 0.05)	No significant difference

[a]Weight of enema returns minus weight of enema instilled.

[b]Concentration of a PEG marker in the enema returns.

[c]Percentage of original polyethylene glycol marker added to the enema that was recovered in the enema returns.

[d]One man retained less than 900 g total tap water; he retained 723 g.

[e]Four people retained less than 900 g of soapsuds enema. Two women received 400 g and 718 g, and two men received 448 g and 794 g of solution.

df, degrees of freedom; M, mean; p, probability; PEG, polyethylene glycol 3350; SD, standard deviation; t, t-test.

From Schmelzer, M., Case, P., Chappell, S. M., & Wright, K. B. (2000). Colonic cleansing, fluid absorption, and discomfort following tap water and soapsuds enemas. *Applied Nursing Research, 13*(2), 88.

Understanding Descriptive Statistical Results

In a published study, investigators often report descriptive statistics in the text of the "Results" section, usually as part of the description of the sample. It also is important to report the values obtained on study variables, as well as the measures of central tendency and dispersion of each variable. In some studies, descriptive statistics may be summarized in a table. Schmelzer, Case, Chappell, and Wright (2000) used a table to report descriptive statistics in a study that compared the effectiveness of two enema solutions. Table 12-3 presents the results of descriptive analysis of these data.

Additionally, descriptive statistics can be used to describe differences between either groups or variables. Examining differences between variables also reflects their relatedness. From a descriptive perspective of descriptive analyses, the purpose is not to test for causality but rather to describe their differentness. One statistical procedure used for this purpose is the chi-square test.

Chi-Square Test of Independence

The **chi-square test of independence** determines whether two variables are independent or related; the test can be used with nominal or ordinal data. The procedure examines the frequencies of observed values and compares them with the frequencies that would be expected if the data categories were independent of each other. The procedure is not very powerful; thus, the risk of a Type II error is high, and large samples are needed to reduce this risk. Therefore, most studies using this procedure place little importance on results in which no differences are found. Researchers frequently perform multiple chi-square tests in a sample. However, results generally are presented only when a chi-square analysis shows a significant difference.

Interpreting Results

The result of the mathematical calculation is a chi-square statistic, which is compared with the chi-square values in a statistical table. If the value of the statistic is equal to or greater than the value identified in the chi-square statistical table (see the textbook by Burns & Grove, 2005, p. 707, for a statistical table), the researcher can conclude that there are significant differences between the two variables. The exact location of specific differences among categories of variables cannot be determined from this analysis. Posthoc analyses can be used to identify the categories where the differences lie. In some published studies, the researchers discuss the results as if they knew where the differences were without having performed posthoc analyses. As a reader, you should view these reports with skepticism.

RESEARCH EXAMPLE **Chi-Square Results in Text**

In a published study, chi-square test results may be reported in the text of the results section. In a study examining depression, service needs, and service use in vulnerable populations, Badger, McNiece, and Gagan (2000) compared enabling characteristics that assist or inhibit persons seeking health care. For the analysis, subjects were assigned to one of two groups: depressed people and nondepressed people. A 0.05 level of significance was set for the study. The authors report their findings as follows:

There were significant differences between the 2 groups for work status (χ^2 [4] = 18.10, p = 0.001). More depressed participants (70%) were disabled compared to nondepressed participants (43%). There were also fewer retirees among depressed participants. (p. 178)

Often the first reaction to a sentence about "significant differences" by those unfamiliar with reading statistical results is panic. (The next reaction may be to skip to the next sentence—maybe that one will make more sense!) However, a sentence that looks "dense" with statistics, such as in the foregoing excerpt, provides a great deal of information in a small amount of space. Rather than trying to take in the entire sentence in one glance, examine the component parts first. In the component "(χ^2 [4] = 18.10, p = 0.001)," the author is using chi-square (χ^2) analysis to compare the depressed and nondepressed groups. The author provides the degrees of freedom (df = 4), so that the reader can validate the accuracy of the results using a statistical chi-square table (Burns & Grove, 2005, p. 707). The numerical value after the first equal sign, 18.10, is the chi-square value obtained from calculating the chi-square equation (probably using a computer). This value has no inherent meaning other than to determine significance on a statistical table. As noted earlier, the symbol p is the abbreviation for probability. The groups were significantly different because p = 0.001, which is below the cutoff point of 0.05. The phrase also indicates that the probability is 0.1% (i.e., 0.001), or 1 in 1000, that these groups come from the same population. Thus, the two groups are significantly different since there is only 1 chance in 1000 the study results are an error.

RESEARCH EXAMPLE   Chi-Square Results in Table

Chi-square results sometimes are provided within a table. Fitch, Gray, Franssen, and Johnson (2000) used a table and text to report chi-square test results from their study. Their table (Table 12-A) displays the results of chi-square analyses examining differences in the adequacy of help received for a variety of problems in two groups of men, all of whom had prostate cancer. One group was composed of men who had not experienced a recurrence of cancer, and the other group was composed of men who had. The following excerpt discusses the results presented in the table.

Table 12-A provides the percentage of men in each group who indicated that they had received adequate help for the most frequently identified problems they experienced. For the entire sample of men who had experienced a particular problem since their diagnosis, approximately two-thirds indicated that they had received adequate help for their problems with side effects (56%) and pain (60%). Approximately one-third (37%) reported that they received adequate help for problems with incontinence, whereas one-fourth or less received adequate help related to fear of dying (25%), anger (22%), and sexual function (19%). A higher percentage of men with recurrent disease reported receiving adequate help with pain (72% versus 28%, $\chi^2 = 5.9$, $df = 1$, $p < 0.001$). (p. 1258)

Table 12-A Problems Identified Since Diagnosis

Problem Cited	No Recurrent Disease (*n* = 845)	Recurrent Disease (*n* = 120)	Whole Group (*n* = 965)
Sexual function	49%	56%	50%
Side effects*	32%	60%	35%
Incontinence	25%	29%	25%
Anger†	12%	26%	14%
Fear of dying	13%	18%	14%
Pain‡	12%	30%	14%
Getting around	8%	20%	9%
Diet	5%	13%	6%
Self blame/guilt	5%	9%	6%
Feeling isolated	5%	12%	6%
Change in family relationships	4%	12%	4%
Household responsibilities	4%	9%	5%
Get to out-of-town appointments	4%	7%	5%
Change in friend relationship	4%	9%	5%
Bathing	4%	8%	5%
Social relations	4%	15%	5%
Feeling stigmatized	3%	5%	4%
Financial	3%	8%	4%
Get to in-town appointments	3%	7%	3%
Feeling discriminated against	2%	3%	2%
Dressing	2%	10%	3%
Loss of employment	2%	9%	3%

*$p < 0.001$; †$p < 0.01$; ‡$p < 0.05$.

Using Statistics to Examine Relationships

Investigators use correlational analyses to identify relationships between or among variables. The purpose of the analysis may be to describe relationships between variables, clarify the relationships among theoretical concepts, or assist in identifying possible causal relationships, which can then be tested by causal analyses. All of the data for the analysis need to be from a single population from which values were available on all variables to be examined in a correlational analysis. Data measured at the interval level provide the best information on the nature of the relationship. However, analysis procedures are available for most levels of measurement. Data for a correlational analysis also need to span the full range of possible values on each variable used in the analysis. For example, if values for a particular variable can range from a low of 1 to a high of 9, each of the values from 1 to 9 will probably be found in subjects in the data set. If all or most of the values are in the middle of that scoring range (4, 5, and 6) and few or none have extreme values, a full understanding of the relationship cannot be obtained from the analysis. Thus, large samples with diverse scores are desirable for correlational analyses.

Pearson Product-Moment Correlation

Pearson product-moment correlation is a parametric test used to determine relationships among variables. **Bivariate correlation** measures the extent of relationship between two variables. Data are collected from a single sample, and measures of the two variables to be examined must be available for each subject in the data set. Less commonly, data are obtained from two related subjects, such as breast cancer incidence in mothers and daughters. Correlational analysis provides two pieces of information about the data: the nature of a relationship (positive or negative) between the two variables and the magnitude (or strength) of the relationship. Scatterplots sometimes are presented to illustrate the relationship graphically. The outcomes of correlational analyses are symmetrical, rather than asymmetrical. **Symmetrical** means that the analysis gives no indication of the direction of the relationship. It's not possible to establish from the analysis that variable A leads to or causes variable B, or that B causes A.

Interpreting Results

The outcome of the Pearson product-moment correlation analysis is a correlation coefficient (r) with a value between -1 and $+1$. This r value indicates the degree of relationship between the two variables. A value of 0 indicates no relationship. A value of -1 indicates a perfect negative (inverse) correlation. In a **negative relationship**, a high score on one variable is correlated with a low score on the other variable. A value of $+1$ indicates a perfect positive relationship. In a **positive relationship**, a high score on one variable is correlated with a high score on the other variable. A positive correlation also exists when a low score on one variable is correlated with a low score on the other variable. The variables vary or change in the same direction, either increasing or decreasing together. As the negative or positive values of

r approach 0, the strength of the relationship decreases. Traditionally, an r value of 0.1 to 0.29 is considered to indicate a weak relationship; a value between 0.3 and 0.5, a moderate relationship; and if the r value is above 0.5, it is considered to indicate a strong relationship (Burns & Grove, 2005). However, this interpretation of the r value depends to a great extent on the variables being examined and the situation in which they were measured. Therefore, interpretation requires some judgment on the part of the researcher.

When Pearson's correlation coefficient is squared (r^2), the resulting number is the percentage of variance explained by the relationship. Even when two variables are related, values of the two variables will not be a perfect match. For example, if two variables show a strong positive relationship, a high score on one variable can be expected to be associated with a high score on the other variable. However, a subject who has the highest score on one value will not necessarily have the highest score on the other variable. Thus, r^2 indicates the variance that is known by correlating two variables. There will be some variation in the relationship between values for the two variables for individual subjects. Some of the variation in values is explained by the relationship between the two variables. This is called **explained variance**. The amount of explained variation is indicated by r^2 and is expressed as a percentage. The author may state, for example, that the relationship of the two variables, as expressed by r^2, explained 43% of the variance of scores in the two variables. However, part of the variation is the result of things other than the relationship. This is called **unexplained variance**. In the example provided, 57% of the variation in scores is due to something other than the relationship studied—perhaps variables not examined in the study. A strong correlation has less unexplained variance than a weak correlation.

There has been a tendency to disregard weak correlations in nursing research. This approach can result in overlooking a relationship that may in fact have some meaning within nursing knowledge if the relationship is examined in the context of other variables. Three common reasons for this situation, which is similar to that of a Type II error, have been recognized. First, many nursing measurements are not powerful enough to detect fine discriminations. Some instruments may not detect extreme scores, and a relationship may be stronger than is indicated by the crude measures available. Second, correlational studies must have a wide range of scores for relationships to be detected. If the study scores are homogeneous or the sample is small, relationships that exist in the population may not show up as clearly in the sample. Third, in many cases, bivariate analysis does not provide a clear picture of the dynamics in the situation. A number of variables can be linked through weak correlations, but together they provide increased insight into situations of interest. Statistical procedures (such as regression analysis, discussed later) are available for examining the relationships among multiple variables simultaneously.

Testing the Significance of a Correlation Coefficient

Before inferring that the sample correlation coefficient applies to the population from which the sample was taken, statistical analysis must be performed to determine whether the coefficient is significantly different from zero (no correlation). With a small sample, a very high correlation coefficient can be nonsignificant. With a very large sample, the correlation coefficient can be statistically significant when the degree of association is too small to be clinically significant. Therefore, in judging the significance of the coefficient, both the size of the coefficient and its statistical significance need to be considered.

RESEARCH EXAMPLE Correlation Results in Text

Lyon and Munro (2001) reported the results of correlations in a study of disease severity and symptoms of depression in black Americans infected with human immunodeficiency virus (HIV). In the study, five measures were correlated: HIV RNA viral load (measures the number of human immunodeficiency viral particles in plasma), CD4+ T-lymphocyte count (crucial control cells in the acquired immune response), CDC (Centers for Disease Control and Prevention) stage of disease (1993 Revised Classification System for HIV Infection), number of years the subject had been seropositive for HIV, and the CES-D (Center for Epidemiologic Studies–Depression Scale) score. The results were reported as follows:

Of the HIV disease severity measures, viral load was the only laboratory or clinical indicator that was correlated with depressive symptoms at a statistically significant level. CD4+ T-lymphocyte counts were not associated with depressive symptom[s] nor was CDC HIV stage. There was no trend in the data consistent with a higher frequency of depressive symptoms according to time of known HIV-seropositivity or at certain potential crisis points such as initial diagnosis or at late-stage immune compromise. Depressive symptoms were prominent at all levels of HIV disease. (Lyon & Munro, 2001, p. 7)

Tables sometimes are used to report the results of correlations, particularly when several variables have been correlated.

RESEARCH EXAMPLE Correlation Results in Table

Lyon and Munro (2001) presented their findings in a table (Table 12-B). Correlational results for a number of variables presented in table form are referred to as a correlation matrix. The numbers from the variables listed on the left side of the table indicate the same variables as the numbers across the top of the table. For example, the variable "CDC stage" is number 3, both on the left side and at the top. The blank spaces in the table are typical of a correlational matrix. A blank space is present just to the right of variable 1, viral load, and below the number 1. This space indicates the relationship between variable 1 and variable 1, which will always be a perfect relationship of +1. By tradition, this space is left blank rather than showing the perfect relationship value of +1. The spaces that show the relationship of each of the other variables to itself also are blank. The table contains other blanks as well. For example, variable 3, "CDC stage" (on the left), has a blank in the first column, which should show the value between variables 1 and 3. The value that should be shown here can be found on the first line of variable 1 (viral load) under 3. This value is 0.217. For each one of the variables, there are two places on the matrix in which the same value could be given. These unseen values are referred to as mirror images and are left blank to keep the table as simple as possible. You can determine the percentage of variance explained by each relationship by squaring the values shown in Table 12-B. For example, viral load explained 4.95% of the variance in the relationship with CD4+ count.

Table 12-B Intercorrelations Among HIV Disease Measures and Depressive Symptoms

	1	2	3	4	5
1. Viral load		−0.225	0.217	0.262*	0.252*
2. CD4[†]			−0.589[†]	−0.078	0.075
3. CDC stage				0.060	−0.09
4. Years HIV[†]					0.054
5. CES-D score					

*Correlation is significant at the 0.05 level (two-tailed test).

[†]Correlation is significant at the 0.01 level (two-tailed test).

Lyon, D. E., & Munro, C. (2001). Disease severity and symptoms of depression in Black Americans infected with HIV. *Applied Nursing Research*, *14*(1), p. 7.

Factor Analysis

Factor analysis examines interrelationships among large numbers of variables and disentangles those relationships to identify clusters of variables that are most closely linked. Intellectually, you might do this by identifying categories and sorting the variables according to your judgment of the most appropriate category. Factor analysis sorts the variables into categories according to how closely related they are to the other variables. Closely related variables are grouped together into a **factor**. Several factors may be identified within a data set. Once the factors have been identified mathematically, the researcher must interpret the results by explaining why the analysis grouped the variables in a specific way. Statistical results will indicate the amount of variance in the data set that can be explained by a particular factor, and the amount of variance in the factor that can be explained by a particular variable.

Factor analysis aids in the identification of theoretical constructs; it also is used to confirm the accuracy of a theoretically developed construct. For example, a theorist may state that the concept (or construct) of "hope" consists of the following elements: (1) anticipation of the future, (2) belief that things will work out for the best, and (3) optimism. Ways can then be developed to measure these three elements, and a factor analysis can be conducted on the data to determine whether subject responses clustered into these three groupings.

Factor analysis frequently is used in the process of developing measurement instruments, particularly those related to psychological variables, such as attitudes, beliefs, values, and opinions. The instrument operationalizes a theoretical construct. Factor analysis also can be used to sort out meaning from large numbers of questions on survey instruments.

Using Statistics to Predict

The ability to predict future events is becoming increasingly important in today's world. People are interested in predicting who will win the football game, what the weather will be like next week, or what stocks are likely to rise in the near future. In nursing practice, as in the rest of society, the capacity to predict is crucial. For example, nurse researchers would like to be able to predict the length of a hospital stay for patients with illnesses of different severity, as well as the response of patients with a variety of characteristics to nursing interventions. Nurses also need to know what factors play an important role in a patient response to rehabilitation. Predictive analyses are based on probability theory, rather than decision theory. Prediction is one approach to examining causal relationships between or among variables.

Regression Analysis

Regression analysis is used to predict the value of one variable when the value of one or more other variables is known. The variable to be predicted in a regression analysis is referred to as the dependent variable. The dependent variable usually is measured at the interval level. The goal of the analysis is to explain as much of the variance in the dependent variable as possible. In regression analysis, variables used to predict values of the dependent variable are referred to as independent variables. If there is more than one independent variable, the analysis is referred to as **multiple regression**. In regression analysis, the symbol for the dependent variable is Y, and the symbol for the independent variable(s) is X. Scatterplots and a bivariate correlation matrix often are developed before regression analysis is per-

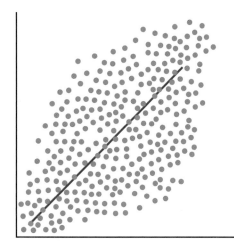

Figure 12-9. Overlay of scatterplot and best-fit line.

formed, to examine the relationships that exist in the variables. The purpose of the regression analysis is to develop a **line of best fit** that will best reflect the values on the scatterplot. The line of best fit is often illustrated as an overlay on the scatterplot (Figure 12-9). Many types of regression analyses have been developed to analyze various types of data. One type, logistic regression, was developed to predict values of a dependent variable measured at the ordinal level. Logistic regression is being used with increasing frequency in nursing studies.

Interpreting Results

The outcome of a regression analysis is the regression coefficient, R. When R is squared (R^2), it indicates the amount of variance in the data that is explained by the equation. When more than one independent variable is being used to predict values of the dependent variable, R^2 is sometimes referred to as the **coefficient of multiple determination**. The test statistic used to determine the significance of a regression coefficient may be t or F. Small sample sizes decrease the possibility of obtaining statistical significance. Values for R^2, t, and F are reported with the results of a regression analysis. The calculated coefficient values may also be expressed as an equation. Many studies using regression analysis are complex, including multiple independent variables and involving more than one regression procedure. Understanding the discussion of complex results requires reading each sentence carefully for comprehension before proceeding to the next sentence.

RESEARCH EXAMPLE Regression Analysis

Craft and Moss (1996) used regression analysis in their study of how accurately the volume of infant emesis could be assessed. In their study, carefully measured amounts of baby formula were poured on receiving blankets. Nurses and nursing students were asked to estimate the volume poured on each of 20 receiving blankets. Each nurse examined the blankets in the same order so that the researchers could determine if accuracy changed as the number of blankets examined by each nurse increased. Error was

(continues)

RESEARCH EXAMPLE *(continued)*

calculated as the difference between the volume actually poured on the blanket and the volume estimated by the nurse. The authors report the results of the regression analysis as follows:

> Analysis with stepwise multiple regression using relative error per subject as the dependent measure showed that subject practice status (student versus practicing nurse), the nature of subject clinical experience, and number of displays assessed for weight accounted for a significant proportion of variance (Table 12-C). Nurses from large newborn nurseries underestimated 23% to 30%, whereas nurses from units with sick toddlers had a lower percentage of underestimation ($M = -0.13$). These data show that the nature of experience, rather than the length of experience, could be important. Only a small portion of the variance ($R^2 = .19$) in mean relative error per subject was accounted for by the variables studied, indicating the need for further study of other variables that must also influence the accuracy of visual assessment in emesis volume determination. (p. 6)

Table 12-C Stepwise Multiple Regression of Independent Variables on Mean Relative Error

Variable	R	R^2	R^2 Increase	F	p
Subject practice (student versus practicing nurse)	0.26	0.07	0.07	7.55	0.007
Nature of clinical practice	0.36	0.13	0.06	7.53	0.001
Number of displays assessed for weight	0.36	0.19	0.06	7.21	0.001

From Craft, M. J., & Moss, J. (1996). Accuracy of infant emesis volume assessment. *Applied Nursing Research, 9*(1), 6, with permission.

Using Statistics to Examine Causality

Causality is a way of knowing that one thing causes another. Because they can be used to understand the effects of interventions, statistical procedures that examine causality are critical to the development of nursing science. These statistics examine causality by testing for significant differences between or among groups.

t-Tests

One of the most common analyses used to test for significant differences between two samples is the *t*-test. A variety of *t*-tests have been developed for various types of samples. Frequently, researchers misuse the *t*-test by using multiple *t*-tests to examine differences in various aspects of data collected in a study. This misapplication will result in an escalation of significance that increases the risk of a Type I error. The Bonferroni procedure, which controls for the escalation of significance, may be used when multiple *t*-tests must be performed on different aspects of the same data.

Interpreting Results

The result of the mathematical calculation is a *t* statistic. This statistic is compared with the *t* values in a statistical table (Burns & Grove, 2005, p. 702). The table is used to identify the critical value of *t*. If the computed statistic is greater than or equal to the critical value, the groups are significantly different.

RESEARCH EXAMPLE   *t*-Tests

Stover, Skelly, Holditch-Davis, and Dunn (2001) used a *t*-test to compare subjects who reported symptoms with subjects who did not report symptoms. The SF-20, a measure of symptoms and other health perceptions, was used. They reported the results of the *t*-test in the text as follows.

The mean of each of the 6 subscales of the SF-20 [a measure of health perceptions] were compared [between] subjects reporting symptoms and those that did not using student *t* tests. Mental health is the first column across the top of Table IV. The *t* values, degrees of freedom, and *p* values are shown in the last three rows of the table (bottom three lines of the left column). On average, African American women with Type 2 diabetes and symptoms of upper and lower neuropathy and/or peripheral vascular disease rated their perceptions of general health, physical role, social functioning, and bodily pain as poorer, compared with subjects without these symptoms. (p. 65)

Because they provided a table (Table 12-D) with the statistical results, these were not provided in the text. If the results of comparing mental health, for example, had been presented in text form, the investigators might have stated: "There was no significant difference in mental health (because $t = 1.3$, $df = 71.6$, $p = 0.18$) between subjects who did not report symptoms in the past 2 weeks and subjects who did."

The phrase "$t = 1.3$, $df = 71.6$, $p = 0.18$" tells you that the value of t was 1.3, the df value was 71.6, and the results were not significant, because $p = 0.18$ is above the 0.05 cutoff. The t value, 1.3, has no meaning other than to determine the level of significance on a statistical table. In Table 12-D, the authors provide the mean (M) and standard deviation (SD) for each variable, the t value, and the p value. The mean is not clearly labeled. However, examine the values for Mental Health. The mean for the subjects with no symptoms in past 2 weeks is 60.1. The Standard Deviation just below is (6.5). Providing this information allows another researcher to check the accuracy of the analyses reported in the study, to perform a power analysis, or to use the data in a meta-analysis. Because the authors used more than one t-test to examine data in the same sample, there is an increased risk of a Type I error. Researchers will have less risk of a Type I error if they analyze their data using the Bonferroni procedure for multiple t-tests.

Table 12-D SF-20 and Symptoms of Upper or Lower Neuropathy or Peripheral Vascular Disease in the Past 2 Weeks

		Subscale of the SF-20					
	n	Mental Health	General Health	Physical Function	Role Function	Social Function	Bodily Pain
Subjects with no symptoms in past 2 weeks	29 (SD)	60.1 (6.5)	45.5 (27.2)	78.7 (23.5)	74.1 (41.3)	83.5 (28.8)	62.8 (29.1)
Subjects with symptoms in past 2 weeks	46 (SD)	57.7 (9.0)	29.8 (21.6)	50.0 (34.6)	41.3 (47.5)	63.0 (35.0)	49.1 (26.9)
t values		1.3	2.6	4.3	3.1	2.6	2.1
Degrees of freedom		71.6	49.8	72.5	65.6	67.8	56.1
p values		18.0	<0.01	<0.01	<0.01	<0.01	<0.05

From Stover, J. C., Skelly, A. H., Holditch-Davis, D., & Dunn, P. F. (2001). Perceptions of health and their relationship to symptoms in African American women with type 2 diabetes. *Applied Nursing Research, 14*(2), 76.

Analysis of Variance

Analysis of variance (ANOVA) tests for differences between means. ANOVA is more flexible than other analyses, because it can be used to examine data from two or more groups. There are many types of ANOVA, some developed for analysis of data from complex experimental designs, such as those using blocking or repeated measures. Rather than focusing just on differences between means, ANOVA tests for differences in variance. One source of variance is the variance within each group, because individual scores in the group will vary from the group mean. This variance is referred to as the **within-group variance**. Another source of variation is variation of the group means around the grand mean, which is referred to as the **between-group variance**. The assumption is that if all of the samples are drawn from the same population, these two sources of variance will exhibit little difference. When these two types of variance are combined, they are referred to as the **total variance**. The test for ANOVA is always one-tailed.

Interpreting Results

The results of an ANOVA are reported as an *F* statistic. The *F* distribution table is used to determine the level of significance of the *F* statistic. (*F* statistical tables are provided in the textbook by Burns and Grove, 2005, pp. 703–706.) If the *F* statistic is equal to or greater than the appropriate table value, there is a significant difference between the groups. If only two groups are being examined, the location of a significant difference is clear. However, if more than two groups are under study, it is not possible to determine from the ANOVA where the significant differences lie. The researcher cannot assume that all of the groups examined are significantly different. Therefore, posthoc analyses are conducted to determine the location of the differences among groups. The frequently used posthoc tests are Bonferroni procedure, Newman-Keuls' test, Tukey's Honestly Significantly Different (HSD) test, Scheffé's test, and Dunnett's test (Burns & Grove, 2005).

RESEARCH EXAMPLE ANOVA

In their study of perceptions of health and their relationship to symptoms in African American women with type 2 diabetes, Stover and colleagues (2001) also reported the results of an ANOVA to determine the effects of the number of complications reported by the subjects. The researchers report their findings as follows:

To determine the effects of the number of complications, we placed subjects into three groups according to the number of complications listed in their medical records (specifically, nephropathy, retinopathy, neuropathy, peripheral vascular disease [PVD], and amputation) and then compared these groups using one-way analysis of variance (ANOVAs) for each subscale. (p. 75)

The three groups were (1) no complications, (2) one complication, and (3) more than one complication. The subscales of the SF-20 used were mental health, general health, physical function, role function, social function, and bodily pain.

A significant difference was found in the mean perceived bodily pain scores of subjects with varied number of complications using one-way ANOVA ($F[2,72] = 4.2$; $p = 0.02$). (p. 75)

F is the statistic reported in ANOVA; [2,72] specifies the degrees of freedom. The value 4.2 is the statistical *F* value obtained from the analysis; $p = 0.02$ is the probability that the groups are different.

We then calculated the Tukey's Honest Square Difference (sic) posthoc analysis, which showed that individuals with two or more of the provider-defined complications experienced more pain than individual[s] with only 1 complication. (p. 77)

RESEARCH EXAMPLE   ANOVA Results in Table

Froman and Owen (1997) used a table (Table 12-E) to report the results of an ANOVA in their study on the validity of the AIDS Attitude Scale. They proposed that pediatric nurses would have more positive attitudes (higher empathy, lower avoidance) than nurses caring for adults. They administered the instrument to 28 pediatric nurses and 36 nurses caring for adults. Half of each group worked in an intensive care unit (ICU), and the other half worked in a floor setting. Table 12-E is an ANOVA summary table summarizing their findings. The three sources of variance analyzed in ANOVA (between groups, within groups, and total) are given, as are the degrees of freedom for each source of variance. The sum of squares (SS) and mean square (MS) values, which are used in the process of performing an ANOVA, are provided. With these values, others could recalculate the F value to verify its accuracy. The p value is indicated by an asterisk beside the F value if the value is significant at the 0.05 level. Two ANOVAs were performed, one with "avoidance" as the dependent variable and one with "empathy" as the dependent variable. The authors discuss their results as follows.

The results of the ANOVAs conducted...reveal a more complex relationship than had been expected, showing a joint effect of intensity of care and patient age on attitude. With further consideration, this finding is understandable in the context of construct validity. Nurses caring for children, regardless of their own risk of exposure, maintain similarly therapeutic and accepting attitudes. These attitudes are adequately sturdy and young patients are sufficiently attractive to counteract influences on attitude that might result from increased risks associated with ICU care. Nurses caring for noncritically ill adults (those experiencing illnesses requiring hospitalization but not fully debilitated) hold similar attitudes. Nurses in the non-ICU setting are likely to interact with their adult AIDS patients and know them as individuals. It is only the combination of adult patients and ICU setting, with its assumed advanced illness condition, that is associated with notably negative attitudes. In discussing these findings with practicing nurses they were not surprised at such results. Their interpretation, put simply, was that adult AIDS patients in ICU settings are repellent as a result of many diseases associated with AIDS (e.g., Kaposi sarcoma, pneumocystic pneumonia). They are usually uncommunicative either because of apparatus (i.e., ventilator) or disease processes. Given these characteristics, the adult ICU AIDS patients lose opportunity to elicit the accepting attitudes that pediatric patients or alert adult patients experience. (Froman & Owen, 1997, p. 167)

Table 12-E ANOVA Summaries for Avoidance and Empathy

Dependent Variable	Source	SS	df	MS	F
Avoidance	Patient age	0.01	1	0.01	0.02
	Intensity	1.07	1	1.07	2.19
	Age × intensity	2.02	1	2.02	4.14*
	Error	29.25	60	0.49	
Empathy	Patient age	0.59	1	0.59	1.63
	Intensity	0.79	1	0.79	2.19
	Age × intensity	1.96	1	1.96	5.43*
	Error	21.66	60	0.36	

*$p < 0.05$.

Analysis of Covariance

Analysis of covariance (ANCOVA) allows the researcher to examine the effect of a treatment apart from the effect of one or more potentially confounding variables (see Chapter 4 for a discussion of confounding variables). Potentially confounding variables that commonly are of concern include pretest scores, age, education, social class, and anxiety level. These variables would be confounding if they were not measured and if their effects on study variables were not statistically removed by performing regression analysis before performing ANOVA. This strategy removes the effect of differences among groups that is due to a confounding variable. Once this effect is removed, the effect of the treatment can be examined more precisely. This technique sometimes is used as a method of statistical control when it is not possible to design the study so that potentially confounding variables are controlled. However, control through careful planning of the design is more effective than statistical control.

ANCOVA may be used in pretest-posttest designs in which differences occur in groups on the pretest. For example, people who achieve low scores on a pretest tend to have lower scores on the posttest than those whose pretest scores were higher, even if the treatment had a significant effect on posttest scores. Conversely, if a person achieves a high pretest score, it is doubtful that the posttest will indicate a strong change as a result of the treatment. ANCOVA maximizes the capacity to detect differences in such cases.

Judging Statistical Suitability

Multiple factors are involved in determining the suitability of a statistical procedure for a particular study. These include the study's (1) purpose; (2) hypotheses, questions, or objectives; (3) design; and (4) level of measurement. Determining the suitability of various statistical procedures for a particular study is not straightforward. Regrettably, there is not usually one "right" statistical procedure for a particular study.

CRITIQUE GUIDELINES   Statistical Suitability

When critiquing suitability, you not only must be familiar with the statistical procedure used in the study but also must be able to compare that procedure with others that could have been used, perhaps to greater advantage. You must judge whether the procedure was performed appropriately and the results interpreted correctly.

Evaluating statistical procedures requires that you make a number of judgments about the nature of the data and what the researcher wanted to know. You need to determine (1) whether the data for analysis were treated as nominal, ordinal, or interval; (2) how many groups were in the study; and (3) whether the groups were dependent or independent. In **independent groups**, the selection of one subject is totally unrelated to the selection of other subjects. For example, if subjects are randomly assigned to treatment and control groups, the groups are independent. In **dependent groups**, subjects or observations selected for data collection are related in some way to the selection of other subjects or observations. For example, if subjects serve as their own control by using the pretest as a control, the observations (and therefore the groups) are dependent. Also, if matched pairs of subjects are used for control and treatment groups, the observations are dependent. For example, in a study of twins, one twin may be placed in the control group and the other in the treatment group. Because they are twins, they are matched on several variables.

One approach to judging the appropriateness of an analysis technique for a critique is to use an algorithm, which directs you by gradually narrowing the number of appropriate statistical procedures as you make judgments about the nature of the study and the data. An algorithm that has been helpful in judging the appropriateness of statistical procedures is presented in Figure 12-10. This algorithm identifies four factors related to the appropriateness of a statistical procedure: the research question, level of measurement, design, and type of sample. To use the algorithm in Figure 12-10, you would (1) determine whether the research question focuses on differences (I) or associations (relationships) (II), (2) determine the level of measurement (A, B, or C), (3) select the design listed that most closely fits the study you are critiquing (1, 2, or 3), and (4) determine whether the study samples are independent (a), dependent (b), or mixed (c). The lines on the algorithm are followed through each selection to identify the appropriate statistical procedure.

Interpreting Statistical Outcomes

To be useful, the evidence from data analysis must be carefully examined, organized, and given meaning. Evaluating the entire research process, organizing the meaning of the results, and forecasting the usefulness of the findings, all of which are involved in interpretation, require high-level intellectual processes. In this segment of a study, the researcher translates the results of analysis into findings and then interprets them by attaching meaning to the findings.

Within the process of interpretation are several intellectual activities that can be isolated and explored, including examining evidence, forming conclusions, considering implications, exploring the significance of the findings, generalizing the findings, and suggesting further studies. This information usually is included in the final section of published studies, which often is entitled "Discussion."

Types of Results

Interpretation of results from quasi-experimental and experimental studies traditionally is based on decision theory, with five possible results: (1) significant results that agree with those predicted by the researcher, (2) nonsignificant results, (3) significant results that are opposite those predicted by the researcher, (4) mixed results, and (5) unexpected results. In critiquing a study, you need to identify which types of results were presented in the study.

Significant and Predicted Results

Significant results agree with those predicted by the researcher and support the logical links developed by the researcher between the framework, questions, variables, and measurement

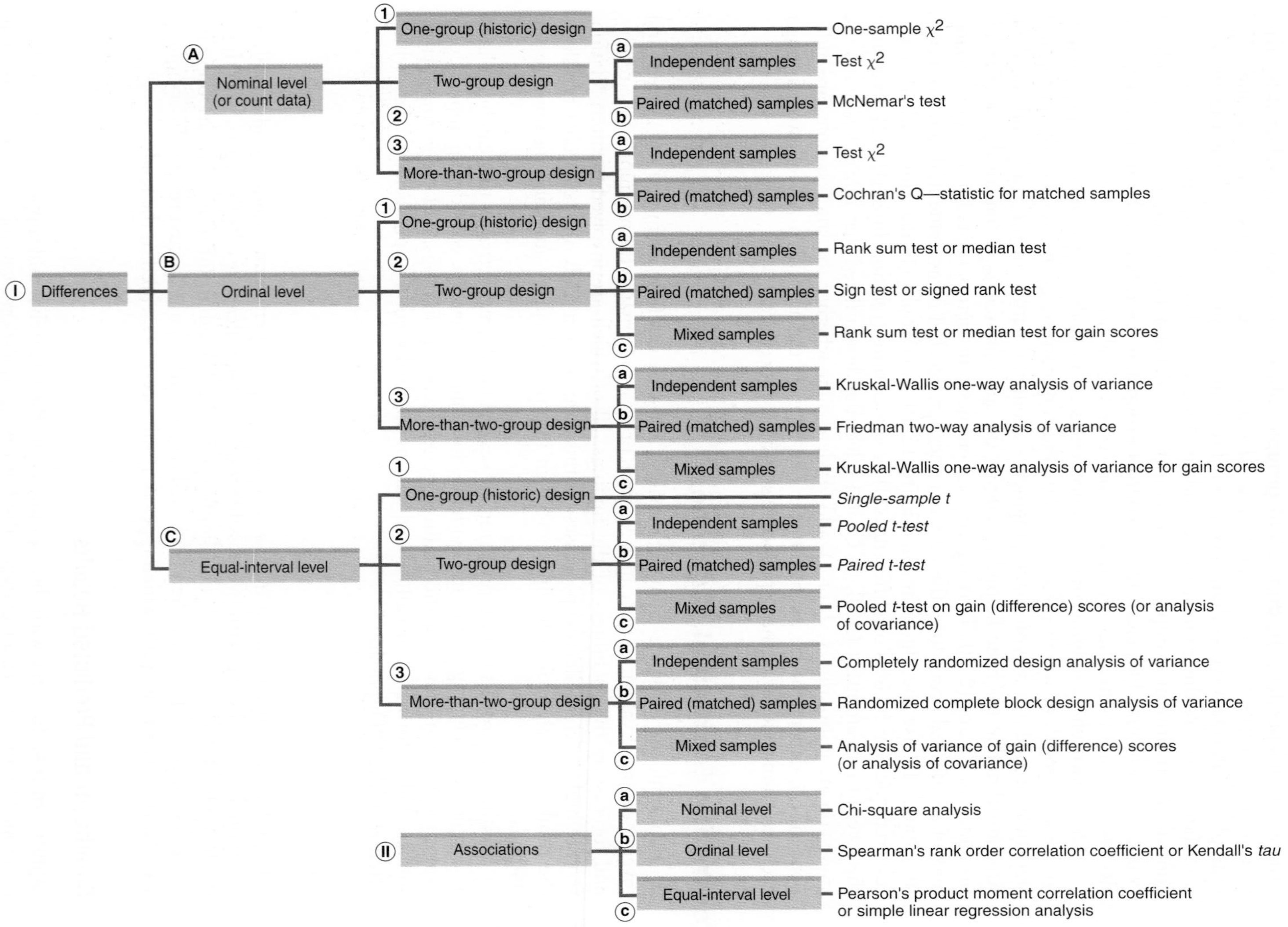

Figure 12-10. Algorithm for choosing a statistical test. (From Knapp, R. B. [1985]. *Basic statistics for nurses*. Albany, NY: Delmar. Reproduced with permission.)

tools. In examining the results, however, you need to consider the possibility of alternative explanations for the positive findings. What other elements could possibly have led to the significant results?

Nonsignificant Results

Nonsignificant (or inconclusive) **results**, often referred to as "negative" results, may be a true reflection of reality. In that case, the reasoning of the researcher or the theory used by the researcher to develop the hypothesis is in error. If it is, the negative findings are an important addition to the body of knowledge. But the results also may stem from a Type II error due to inappropriate methodology, a biased sample, a small sample, problems with internal validity, inadequate measurement, weak statistical measures, or faulty analysis. In such instances, the reported results could introduce faulty information into the body of knowledge (Angell, 1989). Negative results do not mean that no relationships exist among the variables. Negative results indicate only that the study failed to find any. Nonsignificant results provide no evidence of either the truth or the falsity of the hypothesis.

Significant and Unpredicted Results

Significant and unpredicted results are the opposite of those predicted by the researcher and indicate that flaws are present in the logic of both the researcher and the theory being tested. If the results are valid, however, they constitute an important addition to the body of knowledge. For example, a researcher may propose that social support and ego strength are positively correlated. If the relevant study shows instead that high social support is correlated with low ego strength, the result is opposite that predicted.

Mixed Results

Mixed results probably are the most common outcome of studies. In this case, one variable may uphold predicted characteristics whereas another does not; or two dependent measures of the same variable may show opposite results. These differences may be due to methodology problems, such as differing reliability or sensitivity of two methods of measuring variables. The mixed results also may indicate that existing theory should be modified.

Unexpected Results

Unexpected results usually are relationships found between variables that were not hypothesized and not predicted from the framework being used. Most researchers examine as many elements of data as possible, in addition to those directed by the questions. These findings can be useful in the modification of existing theory and in the development of both new theories and later studies. In addition, serendipitous results are important evidence for developing the implications of the study. However, serendipitous results must be interpreted carefully, because the study was not designed to examine these results.

Findings

Results in a study are translated and interpreted; then they become **findings**, which are a consequence of evaluating evidence. Although much of the process of developing findings from results occurs in the mind of the researcher, evidence of the author's thought processes can be found in published research reports.

CRITIQUE GUIDELINES   Findings

When critiquing a study, identify the findings and evaluate the linkages between statistical results and the findings expressed by the researcher.

RESEARCH EXAMPLE   Findings

In their study "Perceptions of Health and Their Relationship to Symptoms in African American Women with Type 2 Diabetes," Stover and colleagues (2001) present the following results and findings.

Results

The most common symptoms that the subjects experienced in the preceding two weeks were headache, abdominal pain, dizziness, fatigue, and knee pain. There were no subjects who were asymptomatic. The range of symptoms per subject was from 1 to 12 with a mean of 4 symptoms. (p. 75)

The mean general health score for all subjects was 35.9% (SD of 24.9%), based on a scale of 0 to 100. The mean physical functioning score was 61.1% (SD 33.7%), role functioning was 54% (SD 47.8%) and social functioning was 70.9% (SD 34.1%). The mean mental health score was 70.9% (SD 22.8%) and the mean pain score was 54.4% (SD of 28.4%). Perception of health scores were found to be generally lower than those previously reported in chronically ill and non-chronically ill subjects. (p. 76)

On average, African American women with Type 2 diabetes and symptoms of upper and lower neuropathy and/or peripheral vascular disease rated their perceptions of general health, physical role, social functioning, and bodily pain as poorer, compared with subjects without these symptoms. African American women with symptoms of visual change rated their mental health, general health, role functioning, and bodily pain perceptions poorer than the ratings of subjects without these symptoms. Visual change (retinopathy) was the only variable we analyzed that had a statistically significant relationship to mental health perception. (p. 77)

A significant difference was found in the mean perceived bodily pain scores of subjects with varied number of complications We also found a significantly lower physical functioning score in subjects with peripheral vascular disease (PVD) when compared with subjects without PVD. There were no other significant differences in the mean scores of the SF-20 by complication type. We found a significant relationship between age at diagnosis and mean scores on both the general health and social functioning subscales. (p. 77)

Findings

The major finding of this study is that African American women with Type 2 diabetes have poorer perceptions of their health status when compared with other women with chronic illnesses. These women also have a poorer perception of health when compared with other individuals with diabetes as noted in previous studies (Glasgow et al, 1997; Stewart et al, 1989). This finding may reflect the symptoms they were experiencing. (p. 78)

As can be seen in this example, the findings are related to findings from previous research and theoretical literature.

Conclusions

Conclusions are a synthesis of the findings. In forming conclusions, the researcher uses logical reasoning, creates a meaningful whole from pieces of information obtained through data analysis and findings from previous studies, remains receptive to subtle clues in the data, and considers alternative explanations of the data. One of the risks in developing conclusions is going beyond the data, or forming conclusions that are not warranted by the data. This occurs more frequently in published studies than one would like to believe.

CRITIQUE GUIDELINES Conclusions

When critiquing a study, identify the conclusions and judge whether they are warranted by the data.

Stover and colleagues (2001) concluded the following from their findings: "Data show that African American women with Type 2 diabetes have a wide variety of symptoms and poor perceptions of their general health and physical functioning" (p. 72).

Considering Implications

Implications are the meanings of conclusions from scientific research for the body of nursing knowledge, theory, and practice. Implications are based on but are more specific than conclusions, and they provide specific suggestions for implementing the findings. For example, a researcher may suggest how nursing practice should be modified. If a study indicates that a specific solution is effective in decreasing stomatitis, the implications will state how the care of patients with stomatitis needs to be modified.

CRITIQUE GUIDELINES Implications

When critiquing a study, identify the implications indicated by the researcher. In addition, you may be able to identify implications not considered by the author.

RESEARCH EXAMPLE Implications

A study by Stover and colleagues (2001) suggested the following implications:

Although quality of life is often an elusive concept to define and/or describe, there is some evidence that symptom distress and quality of life are linked (Germino, 1987). Our findings indicate that individuals with diabetes experience frequent symptoms that influence how they appraise the quality of their lives. Patients

(continues)

RESEARCH EXAMPLE *(continued)*

live with symptoms (e.g., toe pain, foot numbness) and understand symptoms more readily than the more abstract concepts of glycosylated hemoglobin and target blood sugar ranges. Health care providers need to address symptoms with as much attention and concern as is paid to "object data," such as blood glucose levels and cardiograms. As health care providers, we need to re-evaluate the content of the information we provide when educating patients. Improved self-care practices can be presented as a strategy for symptom relief. More emphasis needs to be placed on helping patients differentiate among their current or past pattern of symptoms and increasing their repertoire of strategies to assess their problems and identify patterns of change in serious symptoms. Effective symptom-focused diabetes care has the potential to improve the quality of life for persons with diabetes. (p. 79)

Exploring the Significance of Findings

The significance of a study is associated with its importance to the nursing body of knowledge. Significance is not a dichotomous characteristic because studies contribute in varying degrees to the body of knowledge. Significance may be associated with the amount of variance explained, the degree of control in the study design to eliminate unexplained variance, or the ability to detect statistically significant differences. To the extent possible at the time the study is reported, the researcher is expected to clarify the significance.

A few studies, referred to as "landmark studies," become important reference points in the discipline (Johnson, 1972; Van Aernam & Lindeman, 1971; Passos & Brand, 1966; Williams, 1972). The true importance of a particular study may not become apparent for years after publication. Certain characteristics, however, are associated with the significance of studies: Significant studies make an important difference in people's lives; it is possible to generalize the findings far beyond the study sample so that the findings have the potential of affecting large numbers of people. The implications of significant studies go beyond concrete facts to abstractions and lead to the generation of theory or revisions of existing theory. A very significant study has implications for one or more disciplines in addition to nursing. The study is accepted by others in the discipline and frequently is referenced in the literature. Over a period of time, the significance of a study is measured by the number of other studies it generates.

Clinical Significance

The findings of a study can have statistical significance but not clinical significance. **Clinical significance** is related to the practical importance of the findings. There is no common agreement in nursing about how to evaluate the clinical significance of a finding. The effect size, however, can be used to determine clinical significance. For example, one group of patients may have a body temperature 0.1° F higher than that of another group. Data analysis may indicate that the two groups are statistically significantly different, but the findings have no clinical significance. The difference is not sufficiently important to warrant changing patient care. In many studies, however, it is difficult to judge how much change would constitute clinical significance. In studies testing the effectiveness of a treatment, clinical significance may be demonstrated by the proportion of subjects who showed improvement or the extent to which subjects returned to normal functioning. But how much improvement do subjects need to demonstrate for the findings to be considered clinically significant? Questions also arise regarding who should judge clinical significance: the patients and their families, the clinician, the researcher, or society at large? At this point in the development of nursing knowledge, clinical significance is ultimately a value judgment (LeFort, 1993).

CRITIQUE GUIDELINES Significance

When critiquing a study, be sure to address the element of significance:

1. Judge the significance of the study.
2. Indicate factors that make it significant.
3. Evaluate its clinical significance.

Generalizing the Findings

Generalization extends the implications of the findings from the sample studied to a larger population. For example, if the study was conducted on diabetic patients, it may be possible to generalize the findings to persons with other illnesses or to healthy people. In their 2001 study, Stover and colleagues cautioned that "[b]ecause this was an exploratory study and we did not perform a correction for multiple tests, it is possible that an isolated finding might be due to chance and need to be confirmed" (p. 79). In such a study it would be unwise to suggest generalization of the findings without further confirmatory studies.

How far can generalizations be made? From a very narrow perspective, it's not feasible to generalize from the sample on which the study was conducted; any other sample is likely to be different in some way. Researchers with a conservative view consider generalization particularly risky if the sample was not randomly selected. According to Kerlinger and Lee (1999), unless special precautions are taken and efforts made, the research results frequently are not representative and therefore are not generalizable. Most nurse researchers are not this conservative in making generalizations.

Empirical generalizations are based on accumulated evidence from many studies and are important for the verification of theoretical statements or the development of new theory. Empirical generalizations constitute the base of a science and contribute to scientific conceptualization. Nursing has few empirical generalizations at this time.

CRITIQUE GUIDELINES Generalizing the Findings

When critiquing a study, be sure to consider generalization of the findings:

1. Determine the populations to which the researcher has generalized.
2. Judge the appropriateness of the generalization.

You may be able to identify other populations to which the findings should be generalized.

Suggesting Further Studies

In every study, the researcher gains knowledge and experience that can be used to design a better study next time. Therefore, the researcher often will make suggestions for future studies that emerge logically from the present study. Recommendations for further study may include replications or repeating the design with a different or larger sample. Recommendations also may include the formation of hypotheses to further test the framework in use.

CRITIQUE GUIDELINES Suggesting Further Studies

When critiquing a study, identify the researcher's recommendations for future research. You may be able to make additional recommendations.

RESEARCH EXAMPLE Suggesting Further Studies

Stover and colleagues (2001) made the following recommendations for future research:

In subsequent investigations, it will be important to obtain information on descriptors of the symptom experience to provide a better basis for interventions. In this initial attempt to look at symptoms and their relationship to perceptions of health and functioning in African American women with Type 2 diabetes, we did not attempt to address the severity, frequency, or duration of their symptoms. We also did not investigate the amount of distress caused by these symptoms (the physical or mental anguish or suffering that results from the experience of a symptom occurrence) (Rhodes & Watson, 1987) or the measures participants used to control and/or alleviate their symptoms. Diabetes is a chronic disorder that necessitates life-long commitment to an often complex self-care regimen. Associated with diabetes is the potential for long-term complications that often significantly affect an individual['s] quality of life. (p. 79)

KEY CONCEPTS

- In critiquing a quantitative study, you will need to (1) identify the statistical procedures used; (2) judge whether these statistical procedures were appropriate for the hypotheses, questions, or objectives of the study and to the data available for analysis; (3) comprehend the discussion of data analysis results; (4) judge whether the author interpretation of the results is appropriate; and (5) evaluate the clinical significance of the findings.
- Quantitative data analysis has several stages: (1) preparing the data for analysis; (2) describing the sample; (3) testing the reliability of measurement methods; (4) conducting exploratory analysis of the data; (5) conducting confirmatory analyses guided by the hypotheses, questions, or objectives; and (6) conducting posthoc analyses.
- You must understand the concepts of statistical theory to critique research effectively.
- Probability theory, which is deductive, is used to explain a relationship, the probability of an event occurring in a given situation, or the probability of accurately predicting an event.
- Decision theory, which is inductive, assumes that all of the groups in a study (such as experimental and control groups) used to test a particular hypothesis are components of the same population in relation to the variables under study.
- A Type I error occurs when the null hypothesis is rejected when it is true; the risk of a Type I error is indicated by the level of significance.
- A Type II error occurs when the null hypothesis is accepted when it is false. Type II errors often are a consequence of flaws in the research methods. The risk of a Type II error can be determined using power analysis.
- Summary statistics include frequency distributions, measures of central tendency, and measures of dispersion.
- In the "Discussion" section of the research report, the researcher examines evidence, forms conclusions, considers implications, explores the significance of the findings, generalizes the findings, and suggests further studies.
- In critiquing a study, you will need to evaluate the appropriateness of the researcher discussion.

TIPS FOR FURTHER STUDY

- Are you having difficulty differentiating the various statistical procedures? Try questions on your Companion CD-ROM and in the Bonus Review at http://evolve.elsevier.com/Burns/unerstanding.
- If you have problems understanding written reports of statistical analyses, see Chapter 12 of your *Study Guide*.
- For help in distinguishing Type 1 and Type 2 errors, review the content on p. 410 and complete the Open-Book Quiz at http://evolve.elsevier.com/Burns/understanding
- Select a quantitative study from the literature and critique the results section. What data analysis techniques were used? Were the test results significant or nonsignificant?

REFERENCES

Angell, M. (1989). Negative studies. *The New England Journal of Medicine, 321*(7), 464–466.

Badger, T. A., McNiece, C., & Gagan, M. J. (2000). Depression, service need, and use in vulnerable populations. *Archives of Psychiatric Nursing, 14*(4), 173–182.

Burns, N., & Grove, S. K. (2005). *The practice of nursing research: Conduct, critique, and utilization* (5th ed.). Philadelphia: Saunders.

Cohen, J. (1988). *Statistical power analysis for the behavioral sciences* (2nd ed.). New York: Academic Press.

Craft, M. J., & Moss, J. (1996). Accuracy of infant emesis volume assessment. *Applied Nursing Research, 9*(1), 2–8.

Fitch, M. I., Gray, R., Franssen, E., & Johnson, B. (2000). Men's perspectives on the impact of prostate cancer: Implications for oncology nurses. *Oncology Nursing Forum, 27*(8), 1255–1263.

Froman, R. D., & Owen, S. V. (1997). Further validation of the AIDS Attitude Scale. *Research in Nursing & Health, 20*(2), 161–167.

Germino, B. B. (1987). Symptom distress and quality of life. *Seminars in Oncology Nursing, 3*(4), 299–302.

Glasgow, R., Dryfoos, J., Ruggiero, L., Chobanin, L., & Eakin, E. (1997). Quality of life and associated characteristics in a large national sample of adults with diabetes. *Diabetes Care, 20*(4), 562–567.

Johnson, J. E. (1972). Effects of structuring patients' expectations on their reactions to threatening events. *Nursing Research, 21*(6), 499–504.

Kerlinger, F. N., & Lee, H. B. (1999). *Foundations of behavioral research*. New York: Harcourt Brace.

Knapp, R. G. (1985). *Basic statistics for nurses*. Albany, NY: Delmar.

LeFort, S. M. (1993). The statistical versus clinical significance debate. *Image—The Journal of Nursing Scholarship, 25*(1), 57–62.

LoBiondo-Wood, G., Williams, L., Wood, R. P., & Shaw, B. W. (1997). Impact of liver transplantation on quality of life: A longitudinal perspective. *Applied Nursing Research, 10*(1), 27–32.

Lyon, D. E., & Munro, C. (2001). Disease severity and symptoms of depression in Black Americans infected with HIV. *Applied Nursing Research, 14*(1), 3–10.

Passos, J. Y., & Brand, L. M. (1966). Effects of agents used for oral hygiene. *Nursing Research, 15*(3), 196–202.

Rhodes, V. A., & Watson, P. M. (Eds.). (1987). Symptom distress. *Seminars in Oncology Nursing, 3*(4), 299–302.

Schmelzer, M., Case, P., Chappell, S. M., & Wright, K. B. (2000). Colonic cleansing, fluid absorption, and discomfort following tap water and soapsuds enemas. *Applied Nursing Research, 13*(2), 83–91.

Slakter, M. H., Wu, Y. B., & Suzaki-Slakter, N. S. (1991). *, **, and ***: statistical nonsense at the 0.00000 level. *Nursing Research, 40*(4), 248–249.

Stewart, A. L., Greenfield, S., Hayes, R. D., Wells, K., Rogers, W. H., Berry, S. D., McGlynn, E. A., & Ware, J. E. (1989). Functional status and well-being of patients with chronic conditions. *Journal of the American Medical Association, 262*(7), 907–913.

Stover, J. C., Skelly, A. H., Holditch-Davis, D., & Dunn, P. F. (2001). Perceptions of health and their relationship to symptoms in African American women with type 2 diabetes. *Applied Nursing Research, 14*(2), 72–80.

Tukey, J. W. (1977). *Exploratory data analysis*. Reading, MA: Addison-Wesley.

Van Aernam, B, & Lindeman, C. A. (1971). Nursing intervention with the presurgical patient: The effects of structured and unstructured preoperative teaching. *Nursing Research, 20*(4), 319–332.

Williams, A. (1972). A study of factors contributing to skin breakdown. *Nursing Research, 21*(3), 238–243.

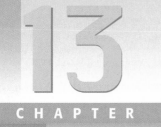

Critiquing Research for Nursing Practice

Learning Outcomes

After completing this chapter, you should be able to:

1. Describe the intellectual research critique process.
2. Apply the basic critique guidelines to research reports.
3. Describe the roles of nurses in critiquing studies to determine the research evidence that is ready for use in practice.
4. Describe the four phases of quantitative research critique: comprehension, comparison, analysis, and evaluation.
5. Conduct a critique of a quantitative research report.
6. Discuss the standards used in critiquing qualitative studies: descriptive vividness, methodological congruence, analytical and interpretative preciseness, philosophical or theoretical connectedness, and heuristic relevance.
7. Conduct a critique of a qualitative research report.

Key Terms

The nursing profession continually strives for evidence-based practice, which includes critiquing studies, synthesizing the findings, and applying the scientific evidence in practice (Brown, 1999; Melnyk & Fineout-Overholt, 2005; Hamer & Collinson, 1999). Thus, critiquing research is an essential step toward basing your practice on empirical evidence. The word **critique** often is linked to *criticize*; a term that frequently is viewed as negative. In the arts and sciences, however, *critique* takes on another meaning: it is associated with critical thinking and appraisal—tasks requiring carefully developed intellectual skills. This type of critique sometimes is referred to as an intellectual critique. An intellectual critique is directed at the element that is created, rather than at the creator. For example, it's possible to conduct an intellectual critique of a work of art, an essay, or a study.

The idea of the intellectual critique was introduced early in this book and has been woven throughout the chapters. As each step of the research process was introduced, guidelines were provided to direct the critique of that step in a research report. This chapter summarizes and builds on previous critique content and provides direction for conducting critiques of both quantitative and qualitative studies. The elements of intellectual critique of research used by nurses are described to assist you in determining the quality of empirical evidence generated by studies. In addition, the steps used to critique quantitative research (comprehension, comparison, analysis, and evaluation) are reviewed in detail. An example critique of a published quantitative study is provided. The chapter concludes with an introduction to the critique process for qualitative research and an example critique of a qualitative study.

Examining the Elements of an Intellectual Research Critique

An **intellectual research critique** is a careful, complete examination of a study to judge its strengths, weaknesses, logical links, meaning, and significance. A high-quality study focuses on a significant problem, demonstrates sound methodology, produces credible findings, and provides a basis for additional studies conducted by other researchers. Ultimately, the findings from several studies can be critiqued and synthesized to provide empirical evidence for use in practice (Stevens, 2005).

CRITIQUE GUIDELINES Intellectual Critique

When conducting an intellectual critique of a study, address questions such as the following:

1. Was the research problem significant? Will the study problem and purpose generate or refine knowledge for nursing practice?
2. What are the major strengths of the study?
3. What are the major weaknesses of the study?
4. Did the researchers use sound methodology?
5. Do the findings from the study accurately reflect reality? Are the findings credible?
6. Are the findings consistent with those from previous studies?
7. Can the study be replicated by other researchers?
8. What are the implications of the findings for nursing practice?

Answering these questions requires careful examination of the problem, purpose, literature review, framework, methods, results, and findings of the study.

An intellectual critique involves the application of some basic guidelines to assist you in answering the preceding questions. These guidelines, presented in Table 13-1, stress the importance of critiquing the entire study and clearly, concisely, and objectively, identifying the study's strengths and weaknesses. All studies have weaknesses or flaws; if every flawed study were discarded, no scientific evidence would be available for use in practice. In fact, science itself is flawed. Science does not completely or perfectly describe, explain, predict, or control reality. However, improved understanding and increased ability to predict and control phenomena depend on recognizing the flaws in studies and in science. Additional studies can then be planned to minimize the weaknesses of earlier studies.

All studies have both strengths and weaknesses. Recognizing these strengths is critical for generating scientific knowledge and using findings in practice. If critiques identify only weaknesses, readers may discount the value of studies and refuse to invest time in examining research. The continued work of the researcher depends on the recognition of the study's strengths and weaknesses. If no study is good enough, why invest time conducting research? Adding together the strong points from multiple studies slowly builds a solid base of evidence for practice.

Two nursing research journals, *Scholarly Inquiry for Nursing Practice: An International Journal* and *Western Journal of Nursing Research*, include commentaries (partial critiques) after some of the published research reports. In these journals, authors receive critiques of their work and have an opportunity to respond to the critiques. Published critiques usually increase the reader's understanding of the study and ability to critique other studies. Another more informal critique of a published study might appear in a letter to the editor. Readers have the opportunity to comment on the strengths and weaknesses of published studies by writing to the editors of journals.

Table 13-1   Steps in Conducting a Research Critique

1. *Read and critique the entire study.* A research critique involves examining the quality of all steps of the research process.
2. *Examine the organization and presentation of the research report.* A well-prepared report is complete, concise, clearly presented, and logically organized. It does not include excessive jargon that is difficult for students and practicing nurses to read. The references need to be complete and presented in a consistent format.
3. *Examine the significance of the problem studied for nursing practice.* The focus of nursing studies needs to be on significant practice problems if a sound knowledge base is to be developed for the profession.
4. *Identify the strengths and weaknesses of a study.* All studies have strengths and weaknesses, so attention must be given to all aspects of the study.
5. *Be objective and realistic in identifying the study's strengths and weaknesses.* Be balanced in your critique of a study. Try not to be overly critical in identifying a study's weaknesses or overly flattering in identifying the strengths.
6. *Provide specific examples of the strengths and weaknesses of a study.* Examples provide evidence for your critique of the strengths and weaknesses of a study.
7. *Provide a rationale for your critique.* Include justifications for your critique, and document your ideas with sources from the current literature. This strengthens the quality of your critique and documents the use of critical thinking skills.
8. *Suggest modifications for future studies.* Modifications in future studies will increase the strengths and decrease the weaknesses identified in the present study.
9. *Discuss the feasibility of replication of the study.* Is the study presented in enough detail to be replicated?
10. *Discuss the usefulness of the findings for practice.* The findings from the study need to be linked to the findings of previous studies. All of these findings need to be examined for use in clinical practice.

Roles of Nurses in Conducting Intellectual Research Critiques

Scientists in every field, including nursing, critique research to broaden their understanding, determine evidence for use in practice, and provide a background for conducting further study. All nurses, including students, practicing nurses, educators, administrators, and researchers, need a background in critiquing studies. Basic knowledge of the research process and the critique process often is provided early in professional nursing education at the baccalaureate level. More advanced critique skills are taught at the master's and doctorate levels, with critique skills increasing as knowledge of the research process increases.

As a student, you are encouraged to critique published studies on relevant clinical topics, to increase your understanding of the research process, promote your interest in reading research articles, and improve your ability to determine how the accumulated empirical evidence can be used in practice. Critiques of studies by practicing nurses are essential for expanding understanding and making changes in practice. Nurses in practice need to constantly update their nursing interventions in response to current research knowledge. In addition, accrediting agencies for health care facilities require that policy and procedure manuals used to direct nursing care be based on research.

Educators critique studies to update their knowledge of research findings. This knowledge provides a basis for developing and refining content taught in classroom and clinical settings. Instructors and textbooks often identify the nursing interventions that were tested through research. Many educators who conduct studies critique research as a basis for planning and implementing their own studies. Researchers often focus on one problem area and update their knowledge base by critiquing new studies in this area. The outcome of the critique influences the selection of research problems, identification of frameworks, development of methodologies, and interpretation of findings in future studies.

Understanding the Quantitative Research Critique Process

Critiquing research involves the use of a variety of critical thinking skills in the application of knowledge of the research process (Burns & Grove, 2005; Miller & Babcock, 1996). The research critique process includes four critical thinking phases: comprehension, comparison, analysis, and evaluation. These phases initially occur in sequence and presume accomplishment of the preceding steps. However, after you gain experience in the critique process, you will be able to perform several of these phases simultaneously. Conducting a critique is a complex mental process that is stimulated by raising questions. Thus relevant questions are provided for each phase of the critique process. The comprehension phase is covered separately because students who are new to critiquing research need to start with this phase. The comparison and analysis phases are presented together because they often occur simultaneously in the mind of the person conducting the critique. Evaluation is covered separately because it requires increased expertise and builds on the knowledge generated from the comprehension, comparison, and analyses phases of the critique process. Each of these critique phases involves examination of the steps of the quantitative research process and identification of the strengths and weaknesses of these steps.

Phase 1: Comprehension

The **comprehension phase** is the first step in the research critique process. This critique phase involves understanding the terms and concepts in the report and identifying the elements or steps of the research process, such as the problem, purpose, framework, and design. It is also necessary to grasp the nature, significance, and meaning of these steps in a research report.

Guidelines for Comprehension of a Research Report

The first steps are reviewing the abstract, reading the entire study, and examining the references. Next, the presentation of the study is evaluated using the following questions: Was the writing style clear and concise? Were the major sections of the research report, such as the literature review, framework, methods, results, and discussion, clearly identified? Were relevant terms clearly defined? (Burns & Grove, 2005). You are encouraged to underline terms you do not understand and look them up in the glossary at the back of this book. Next, it may help to read the article a second time and highlight or underline each step of the research process.

CRITIQUE GUIDELINES   Comprehension

To write a beginning research critique that demonstrates comprehension of the study, concisely identify each step of the research process, and briefly respond to the following questions. Do not answer the questions with a yes or no; rather, provide a rationale or include examples or content from the study to address the questions.

1. What is the study problem?
2. What is the study purpose?
3. Is the literature review presented?
   a. Are relevant previous studies identified and described?
   b. Are relevant theories and models identified and described?
   c. Are the references current? Examine the number of sources in the last five and ten years in the reference list.
   d. Are the studies critiqued by the author?
   e. Is a summary of the current knowledge provided? This summary needs to include what is known and not known about the research problem.
4. Is a study framework identified?
   a. Is the framework explicitly expressed or must it be extracted from the literature review?
   b. Is a particular theory or model identified as a framework for the study?
   c. Does the framework describe and define the concepts of interest?
   d. Does the framework present the relationships among the concepts?
   e. Is a map or model of the framework provided for clarity?

    f. If a map or model is not presented, develop one that represents the study's framework and describe it.

    g. Link the concepts in the framework with the variables in the study.

    h. Is the framework related to nursing's body of knowledge?

5. Are research objectives, questions, or hypotheses used to direct the conduct of the study? Identify these.

6. Are the major variables or concepts identified and defined (conceptually and operationally)? Identify and define the appropriate variables included in the study:

    a. Independent variables

    b. Dependent variables

    c. Research variables or concepts

7. What attribute or demographic variables are examined in the study?

8. Is the research design clearly addressed?

    a. Identify the specific design of the study.

    b. Does the study include a treatment or intervention? If so, is the treatment clearly described and consistently implemented?

    c. If the study has more than one group, how were the subjects assigned to groups?

    d. Are the extraneous variables identified and controlled?

    e. Were pilot study findings used to design the major study? Briefly discuss the pilot study and the findings. Indicate the changes made in the major study based on the pilot.

9. Are the following elements of the sample described?

    a. Identify the inclusion and exclusion sample criteria

    b. Indicate the method used to obtain the sample. Did the researchers identify the sampling frame for the study?

    c. Identify the sample size. Indicate if a power analysis was conducted to determine sample size.

    d. What number and percentage of the potential subjects refused to participate?

    e. Identify the characteristics of the sample.

    f. Identify the sample mortality (number and percentage) or attrition from the study.

    g. Discuss the institutional review board approval obtained from University and/or agency where the study was conducted.

    h. Identify the informed consent obtained from the subjects.

    i. Discuss the setting and whether it was appropriate for the conduct of the study.

10. Are the measurement strategies described?

    a. Identify the author of each measurement strategy.

    b. Identify the type of each measurement strategy (i.e., Likert scale, visual analogue scale, physiological measurement, questionnaire, observation, or interview).

    c. Identify the level of measurement (nominal, ordinal, interval, or ratio) achieved with each instrument.

    d. Discuss how each study instrument was developed.

    e. Report the reliability and validity of each instrument or scale from previous studies and the current study.

    f. Discuss the precision and accuracy of the physiological measurement methods used in a study.

(continues)

CRITIQUE GUIDELINES *(continued)*

You can use the table below to present the essential information on the measurement methods used in a study.

Name of the Instrument	Author	Measurement Strategy	Level of Measurement	Development of Instrument	Reliability or Precision	Validity or Accuracy
Beck Depression Inventory	Beck	Likert Scale	Treated as interval/ratio data	Not addressed in study	Cronbach alpha previous studies 0.82 to 0.89 and for correct study, 0.86	Convergent and divergent validity from previous studies achieved but no details provided in this study

11. How were study procedures implemented and data collected during the study?
12. What statistical analyses are included in the research report?
    a. Identify the analysis techniques used to describe the sample.
    b. Was the level of significance or alpha identified? If so, indicate the level (0.05, 0.01, or 0.001).
    c. Complete the following table with the analysis techniques conducted in the study: (1) identify the focus (description, relationships, or differences) of each analysis technique; (2) list the statistical procedures; (3) list the statistics; (4) identify specific results; and (5) provide a specific probability value (*p*), as shown.

Purpose of Analysis	Statistical Procedure	Statistic	Results	Probability (*p*)
Description of subjects' pulse rate	Mean standard deviation	$\overline{X}$ SD	72.43 5.67	
Difference between males and females on blood pressure	*t*-test	*t*	3.75	*p* = .04
Difference between treatment and comparison groups on weight loss	Analysis of variance	*F*	5.79	*p* = .009
Relationship of pain perception and anxiety for adolescents	Pearson correlation	*r*	0.56	*p* = .03

13. What is the researcher's interpretation of the findings?
    a. Are the results related to the study framework? If so, do the findings support the study framework?
    b. Which findings are consistent with those expected?
    c. Which findings are unexpected?
    d. Are the findings consistent with previous research findings?
14. Are the limitations of the study identified by the researcher?
15. What conclusions did the researcher identify based on this study and previous research?

16. How does the researcher generalize the findings?
17. What implications do the findings have for nursing practice?
18. What suggestions are made for further studies?
19. What are the missing elements of the study?
20. Is the description of the study sufficiently clear to allow replication?

Phases 2 and 3: Comparison and Analysis

Critique phases 2 and 3 (comparison and analysis) are frequently done simultaneously when critiquing a study. The **comparison phase** requires knowledge of what each step of the research process should be like, and then the ideal is compared to the real. During the comparison phase, you must examine the extent to which the researcher followed the rules for an ideal study. Examine the steps of the study, such as the problem, purpose, framework, methodology, and results, based on the content presented in Chapters 4 to 8, and 10 to 12 of this book. Did the researcher rigorously develop and implement the study? What are the strengths of the study? What are the weaknesses of the study?

The **analysis phase** involves a critique of the logical links connecting one study element with another. For example, the presentation of the problem must provide a background and direction for the statement of the purpose. In addition, the overall logical development of the study must be examined. The variables identified in the study purpose should be consistent with the variables identified in the research objectives, questions, or hypotheses. These variables must be conceptually defined in light of the study framework. The conceptual definitions provide the basis for the development of the operational definitions. The study design needs to be appropriate for the investigation of the purpose of the study and for the specific objectives, questions, or hypotheses. The instruments used in the study need to adequately measure the variables. The sample selected should be representative of the population identified in the problem and purpose. Analysis techniques provide results that address the purpose and the specific objectives, questions, or hypotheses. To determine the current knowledge of the study problem, the findings from a study must be linked to the framework and the findings from previous research. These findings are synthesized in the conclusions so that they can be generalized to individuals other than the study subjects. Depending on the quality of the findings, the researcher indicates the use of the findings in nursing practice. All steps of the research process provide a basis for the identification of future research projects. The steps of the research process need to be precisely developed and strongly linked to each other to conduct a quality study.

Guidelines for Comparison and Analysis of a Research Report

To conduct the comparison and analysis steps, review the chapters in this text, as well as other references describing the steps of the research process (Burns & Grove, 2005; Mateo & Kirchhoff, 1999; Munro, 2005; Polit & Beck, 2006; Robinson, 2001). Then compare the steps in the study you are critiquing with the criteria established for each step in this textbook or other sources (phase 2, comparison). Next analyze the logical links among the steps of the study (phase 3, analysis). The guidelines in this section should assist you in implementing the phases of comparison and analysis for each step of the research process. Questions relevant to analysis are identified; all other questions direct the comparison of the steps of the study with the ideal. Use these questions to determine how rigorously the steps of the research process were implemented in published studies. Indicate which steps are strengths and which steps are weaknesses. When labeling a step as a strength or weakness, provide examples from the study and state a rationale, along with documentation to support your conclusions. In addition, identify the strengths in the logical way the steps of the study are linked together or any breaks or weaknesses in the links of a study's steps.

CRITIQUE GUIDELINES Comparison and Analysis

The written critique should be a narrative summary of the strengths and weaknesses that you note in the study. Use the following guidelines to examine the significance of the problem, fit of the framework, rigor of the methodology, and quality and relevance of the findings in published studies.

1. Research problem and purpose
   a. Is the problem sufficiently narrow in scope without being trivial?
   b. Is the problem significant and relevant to nursing?
   c. Does the purpose narrow and clarify the focus or aim of the study and identify the research variables, population, and setting?
   d. Was this study feasible to conduct in terms of money commitment; the researchers' expertise; availability of subjects, facility, and equipment; and ethical considerations?
2. Literature review
   a. Is the literature review organized to demonstrate the progressive development of ideas through previous research? (Analysis)
   b. Is a theoretical knowledge base developed for the problem and purpose? (Analysis)
   c. Does the literature review provide a rationale and direction for the study? (Analysis)
   d. Does the summary of the current empirical and theoretical knowledge provide a basis for the study? (Stone, 2002)
3. Study framework
   a. Is the framework presented with clarity?
   b. Is the framework linked to the research purpose? (Analysis)
   c. Would another framework fit more logically with the study? (Analysis)
   d. Is the framework related to nursing's body of knowledge? (Analysis)
   e. If a proposition from a theory is to be tested, is the proposition clearly identified and linked to the study hypotheses? (Analysis)
4. Research objectives, questions, or hypotheses
   a. Are the objectives, questions, or hypotheses clearly and concisely expressed?
   b. Are the objectives, questions, or hypotheses logically linked to the research purpose? (Analysis)
   c. Are the research objectives, questions, or hypotheses linked to concepts and relationships (propositions) from the framework? (Analysis)

5. Variables
    a. Do the variables reflect the concepts identified in the framework? (Analysis)
    b. Are the variables clearly defined (conceptually and operationally) based on previous research and/or theories?
    c. Is the conceptual definition of a variable consistent with the operational definition? (Analysis)
6. Design
    a. Was the best design selected to direct this study?
    b. Does the design provide a means to examine all of the objectives, questions, or hypotheses and the study purpose? (Analysis)
    c. What are the threats to design validity? Were these threats identified by the researcher?
    d. Have the threats to design validity (statistical conclusion validity, internal validity, construct validity, and external validity) been minimized?
    e. Is the design logically linked to the sampling method and statistical analyses? (Analysis)
    f. If a treatment is implemented, is it clearly defined conceptually and operationally? Is the treatment appropriate for examining the study purpose and hypotheses? (Analysis) (Brown, 2002; Santacroce, Maccarelli, & Grey, 2004)
7. Sample, population, and setting
    a. Is the target population to which the findings will be generalized defined?
    b. Is the sampling method adequate to produce a sample that is representative of the study population?
    c. What are the potential biases in the sampling method?
    d. Is the sample size sufficient to avoid a Type II error? Was the sample size determined by a power analysis?
    e. If more than one group is used, do the groups appear equivalent?
    f. Are the rights of human subjects protected? Are the HIPAA privacy regulations followed in conducting the study? (Olsen, 2003)
    g. Is the setting used in the study typical of clinical settings?
8. Measurements
    a. Do the instruments adequately measure the study variables? (Analysis)
    b. Are the instruments sufficiently sensitive to detect differences between subjects?
    c. Is the reliability of the instruments adequate for use in the study?
    d. Is the validity of the instruments adequate for use in the study?
    e. Do the instruments need further research to evaluate validity and reliability? (Roberts, & Stone, 2003)
    f. Respond to the following questions that are relevant to the measurement approaches used in the study.
    g. Scales and questionnaires
        (1) Are the instruments clearly described?
        (2) Are techniques to administer, complete, and score the instruments provided?
        (3) Is the reliability of the instruments described?
        (4) Is the validity of the instruments described?
        (5) Did the researcher examine the reliability and the validity of the instruments for the present sample?

(continues)

CRITIQUE GUIDELINES *(continued)*

   (6) If the instrument was developed for the study, is the instrument development process described?

h. Observation
   (1) Is what is to be observed clearly identified and defined?
   (2) Are interrater and intrarater reliability described?
   (3) Are the techniques for recording observations described?

i. Interviews
   (1) Do the interview questions address concerns expressed in the research problem? (Analysis)
   (2) Are the interview questions relevant for the research purpose and objectives, questions, or hypotheses? (Analysis)
   (3) Does the design of the questions tend to bias subjects' responses?
   (4) Does the sequence of questions tend to bias subjects' responses?

j. Physiological measures
   (1) Are the physiological measures or instruments clearly described? If appropriate, are the brand names (e.g., Space Labs, Hewlett-Packard) of the instruments identified?
   (2) Are the accuracy, precision, selectivity, sensitivity, and error of the physiological instruments discussed?
   (3) Are the methods for recording data from the physiological measures clearly described?

9. Data collection
   a. Is the data collection process clearly described?
   b. Is the training of data collectors clearly described and adequate?
   c. Is the data collection process conducted in a consistent manner?
   d. Are the data collection methods ethical?
   e. Do the data collected address the research objectives, questions, or hypotheses? (Analysis)

10. Data analyses
   a. Are data analysis procedures clearly described?
   b. Do data analyses address each objective, question, or hypothesis?
   c. Are data analysis procedures appropriate to the type of data collected? (Duffy, 1988)
   d. Are the results presented in an understandable way?
   e. Are tables and figures used to synthesize and emphasize certain findings? (Burns & Grove, 2005)
   f. Are the analyses interpreted appropriately?
   g. If the results were nonsignificant, was the sample size sufficient to detect significant differences? Was a power analysis conducted to examine nonsignificant findings?

11. Interpretation of findings
   a. Are findings discussed in relation to each objective, question, or hypothesis? (Analysis)
   b. Are significant and nonsignificant findings explained?
   c. Were the statistically significant findings also examined for clinical significance?
   d. Does the interpretation of findings appear biased? Are the biases in the study identified?

e. Are there uncontrolled extraneous variables that may have influenced the findings?
f. Do the conclusions fit the results from the analyses? (Analysis)
g. Are the conclusions based on statistically and clinically significant results? (Analysis)
h. Did the researchers identify important study limitations?
i. Are there inconsistencies in the report?

Phase 4: Evaluation

During the **evaluation phase** of a research critique, the meaning and significance of the study findings are examined. The evaluation becomes a summary of the study's quality that builds on conclusions reached during the first three phases (comprehension, comparison, and analysis) of the critique. This level of critique may or may not be conducted by a nursing student in a baccalaureate degree program. The level of critiquing attained during a student's educational program depends on when the research course is taken, during the junior or senior year of the curriculum, and how many credit hours are devoted to research. The guidelines for the evaluation phase are provided for those students who want to perform a more comprehensive critique of the literature to summarize findings for use in practice.

Guidelines for Evaluation of a Research Report

The evaluation phase involves reexamining the findings, conclusions, limitations, implications for nursing, and suggestions for further study, which usually are presented in the "Discussion" section of a research report. All nurses should be able to determine the value of research findings in the development of nursing knowledge and for use in practice.

The evaluation phase involves developing a summary of the study's quality. This summary is a narrative that usually is the last one or two paragraphs of a critique.

CRITIQUE GUIDELINES   Evaluation

Using the following questions as a guide, summarize the quality of the study, the accuracy of the findings, and the usefulness of the findings for nursing practice.

1. How much confidence can be placed in the study findings? Are the findings an accurate reflection of reality?
2. Are the findings related to the framework?
3. Are the findings linked to those of previous studies?
4. What do the findings add to the current body of knowledge?
5. To what populations can the findings be generalized?
6. What research questions emerge from the findings? Are these questions identified by the researcher?
7. What is the overall quality of this study when the strengths and weaknesses are summarized? Could any of the weaknesses have been corrected?
8. Do the findings have potential for use in nursing practice?

A Practice Critique

To serve as a subject for a practice critique, the following Research Example presents a published quantitative study in its entirety: "Oxygen Uptake and Cardiovascular Response in Patients and Normal Adults during In-Bed and Out-of-Bed Toileting," by Winslow, Lane, and Gaffney (1984). This was a seminal study in the development of knowledge about cardiovascular response during activities of daily living, such as toileting and bathing.

An initial critique may focus on comprehension and involve identification of the steps of the research process in the study. The comprehension critique may be written in outline format, with headings identifying the steps of the research process. A more in-depth critique includes not only the comprehension step but also the comparison, analysis, and evaluation phases. The sample critique provided at the end of the article includes all four phases—the comprehension, comparison, analysis, and evaluation—and is presented in a narrative format. Read the article and identify the steps of the research process; then try to list the strengths and weaknesses of the study, including the logical links among the study steps. Use the questions in this chapter to develop a critique of this study, and then compare your critique with the one provided here. Doing your own initial critique and then reading the sample critique can help you expand your critiquing skills.

RESEARCH EXAMPLE **A Quantitative Study**

Oxygen Uptake and Cardiovascular Response in Patients and Normal Adults during In-Bed and Out-of-Bed Toileting

Elizabeth Hahn Winslow, PhD, RN, Lynda Denton Lane, BSN, RN, and F. Andrew Gaffney, MD

Patients dislike using the bedpan and urinal while in bed and often insist that it would be easier and better for them to get out of bed to toilet. Little data are available about the physiologic costs of toileting. Therefore, we measured oxygen uptake (VO_2), peak heart rate (HR_{peak}), peak rate-pressure product (RPP_{peak}), rating of perceived exertion, and preference in 42 women who used the bedpan and bedside commode for urination and in 53 men who used the urinal while in bed and standing. The subjects included 26 healthy volunteers, 16 cardiac outpatients, 27 medical inpatients, and 26 acute post-myocardial infarction patients (two to 28 days postinfarction). No physiologically important differences were found between in-bed and out-of-bed toileting. Both in-bed and out-of-bed toileting produced small increases in energy cost and myocardial work over resting levels, with a mean $VO_2 < 1.6$ times resting VO_2, a mean $HR_{peak} < 100$ beats/min, and a mean $RPP_{peak} < 11,200$. The subjects clearly preferred getting out of bed to toilet. Out-of-bed toileting produces minimal energy expenditure and cardiac stress and can help reduce bed rest-induced orthostatic intolerance. In-bed toileting should be reserved for patients with specific contraindications to postural change.

Over 30 years ago Benton and co-workers[1] reported that using the bedpan required 50% greater energy cost above resting level than did using the bedside commode. Since then, many clinicians have recommended that the myocardial infarction (MI) patient use the bedside commode after hospital admission.[2-6] However, time-honored traditions change slowly, especially when only a single study of the topic is available. Many physicians still wait several days before permitting their acute MI patients to use the bedside commode or stand beside the bed to urinate. Patients often complain about this and insist that it would be easier and better for them to get out of bed to toilet.

To determine which toileting method is more appropriate for the acutely ill medical patient, one should consider both the total energy cost and also the approximate myocardial work of in-bed and out-of-bed toileting methods when performed by patients. Therefore, we measured oxygen uptake (VO_2), peak heart rate (HR_{peak}), peak rate-pressure product (RPP_{peak}) (systolic blood pressure × heart rate), rating of perceived exertion (RPE), and preference in 95 hospitalized and nonhospitalized adults during in-bed (bedpan and urinal) and out-of-bed (bedside commode and standing urinal) toileting. Data on which to base toilet method recommendations for the hospitalized patient are provided.

Materials and Methods

SUBJECTS

The 42 women and 53 men (range 18–79 years) who volunteered for the study consisted of 26 healthy adults, 16 coronary artery disease patients who were participating in a supervised outpatient exercise program, 27 stable medical inpatients with a variety of cardiac and noncardiac disorders, and 26 stable acute MI inpatients who had their MI from 2 to 28 days earlier (8.81 ± 5 days [mean $\pm$ SD]) (Table I). Eight patients had their MI five days or less before the study began. Acute MI was established by history, clinical, electrocardiographic (ECG), and enzyme findings and by myocardial scintigraphy. Nineteen (73%) of the patients had transmural infarctions; seven (27%) had subendocardial infarctions. All medical and cardiac inpatients were ambulatory prior to hospitalization, and none had neural or musculoskeletal problems that would preclude standing unassisted. Six (37%) of the cardiac outpatients, seven (26%) of the medical inpatients, and five (19%) of the acute MI patients were receiving propranolol at the time of the study. The research protocol was approved by the Institutional Review Board, and informed written consent was obtained from all subjects prior to the study.

Table I Subject Characteristics

Subject Group	Sex	N	Age (yr ± SD)	Weight (kg ± SD)	Height (cm ± SD)
Healthy volunteers	Female	11	38 ± 13	65 ± 8	168 ± 4
	Male	15	29 ± 7	77 ± 8	177 ± 4
Cardiac outpatients	Female	6	62 ± 4	58 ± 10	157 ± 6
	Male	10	58 ± 5	76 ± 8	173 ± 3
Medical inpatients	Female	14	57 ± 15	72 ± 16	161 ± 9
	Male	13	51 ± 10	84 ± 17	175 ± 7
Acute MI inpatients	Female	11	63 ± 11	76 ± 18	164 ± 6
	Male	15	61 ± 12	84 ± 17	172 ± 9

METHODS

Oxygen uptake during rest and toileting was determined by open-circuit, indirect calorimetry. The subject had a nose clip and mouthpiece in place. During the timed period, expired air was collected via a one-way respiratory valve (Daniels) and 64-inch plastic tubing into a 30 L (rest) or 150 L (toileting) bag (Douglas). A standard adjustable helmet held the mouthpiece and valve in a comfortable, secure position; the Douglas bag was tied to a rolling intravenous pole. Expired air volume was measured by a Collins Chain Compensated Gasometer (Tissot), and air composition was analyzed by mass spectrometer (Perkin-Elmer Medical Gas Analyzer 1100). The mass spectrometer was calibrated electronically and checked against gases of known concentration. Standard equations were used to derive VO_2.

Gas collection was begun immediately before toileting when the subject was supine and was stopped when the subject had resumed the supine position. A continuous ECG (lead II) was recorded during toileting. Peak HR was the most rapid HR observed during any 15-second period. Blood pressure was measured by

(continues)

RESEARCH EXAMPLE *(continued)*

cuff sphygmomanometer immediately before and after toileting and after each position change. In the eight coronary care unit (CCU) patients, blood pressure was taken before and after toileting only. After each toileting method, the subject selected a number from the Borg scale of perceived exertion.[7] After both toileting methods, the subject completed a questionnaire wherein he ranked each method for comfort, pleasantness, and ease.

PROTOCOL

Oxygen uptake, HR, and RPP were determined during a 3-minute supine rest period and during in-bed and out-of-bed toileting. A 10-minute rest period separated the randomly ordered toileting methods. Women used the bedpan and bedside commode for urinating; men used the urinal while lying in bed and while standing beside the bed. The subject simulated voiding if unable to void during the second toileting trial.

The toileting protocol simulated usual clinical conditions; therefore, toileting duration varied. The investigator assisted the women in lifting their hips for bedpan placement and removal, and placed the bedside commode in a standardized position beside the head of the bed. Subjects used their own techniques to get out of and back into bed and were not lifted by the investigator. The investigator left the room while the subject urinated and returned when given a signal from the subject. Subjects took as much time as they needed for urination.

STATISTICAL ANALYSIS

Oxygen uptake, HR, and RPP results were analyzed for each sex and group by repeated measures analysis of variance (ANOVA). Ratings of perceived exertion and preferences were analyzed by the Friedman two-way ANOVA by ranks. Spearman correlation coefficients were calculated for selected variables including VO_2, age, and toileting duration.

Results

Oxygen uptake, HR, and RPP results during rest and toileting are shown in Table II and Figures I, II, and III. During rest, VO_2 ranged from 2.15 to 4.52 ml/kg/min, HR from 44 to 104 beats/min, and RPP from 5,000 to 14,100. During toileting, VO_2 ranged from 2.77 to 5.84 ml/kg/min, HR_{peak} from 56 to 132 beats/min, and RPP_{peak} from 5,400 to 14,400.

During in-bed toileting, 14 subjects (15%) had a HR_{peak} of 100 beats/min or greater; during out-of-bed toileting, 19 subjects (21%) had a HR_{peak} of 100 beats/min or greater at some time during toileting. Only four subjects had a HR_{peak} over 108 beats/min. The subjects with the highest resting HRs had the highest HRs during toileting. The highest HRs observed during each study condition were 104, 120, and 132 beats/min during rest, bedpan use, and bedside commode use, respectively, in one elderly woman with atrial fibrillation and an uncontrolled ventricular response. None of the subjects experienced chest pain, shortness of breath, lightheadedness, palpitations, or other signs or symptoms of cardiovascular distress during toileting.

Statistically significant differences in VO_2, HR, and RPP between in-bed and out-of-bed toileting were found within some groups of subjects ($p < 0.05$). These differences represent mean differences of less than 1 ml/kg/min, 8 beats/min, and 1,300 units in VO_2, HR_{peak}, and RPP_{peak}, respectively.

Analysis for differences among the four subject groups did not show any statistically significant differences in resting VO_2. However, during toileting, hospitalized patients generally had a significantly lower VO_2 value than did nonhospitalized subjects ($p < 0.05$). Heart rate and RPP responses during rest and toileting did not differ significantly among the four groups of female subjects; however, significant differences in cardiovascular response were found among some male groups. The hospitalized men generally had a significantly higher HR and RPP during rest and toileting than did nonhospitalized men ($p < 0.05$).

Table II Mean Oxygen Uptake ($\dot{V}O_2$), Heart Rate (HR), and Rate-Pressure Product (RPP) during Rest and Mean $\dot{V}O_2$, Peak HR, and RPP_{peak} during In-Bed and Out-of-Bed Toileting

Subject	Activity	Women (W)			Men (M)		
		$\dot{V}O_2$ (ml/kg/min ± SD)	HR (beats/min ± SD)	RPP (SBP × hr/100 ± SD)	$\dot{V}O_2$ (ml/kg/min ± SD)	HR (beats/min ± SD)	RPP (SBP × hr/100 ± SD)
Healthy volunteers (W = 11, M = 15)	Rest In-bed Out-of-bed	3.43 ± 0.42 4.84 ± 0.71 4.66 ± 0.63 (N = 11)	66 ± 10 84 ± 10 85 ± 9 (N = 10)	79 ± 15 92 ± 14 91 ± 15 (N = 11)	3.67 ± 0.41 4.78 ± 0.46 4.66 ± 0.52 (N = 15)	60 ± 7 87 ± 10 84 ± 8 (N = 12)	72 ± 12 79 ± 12 91 ± 14* (N = 15)
Cardiac outpatients (W = 6, M = 10)	Rest In-bed Out-of-bed	3.20 ± 0.35 4.43 ± 0.57 4.36 ± 0.61 (N = 5)	65 ± 12 81 ± 16 81 ± 17 (N = 6)	89 ± 25 104 ± 30 103 ± 24 (N = 6)	3.56 ± 0.36 4.72 ± 0.59 4.77 ± 0.47 (N = 9)	59 ± 8 77 ± 11 77 ± 12 (N = 10)	75 ± 17 86 ± 20 84 ± 15 (N = 10)
Medical inpatients (W = 14, M = 13)	Rest In-bed Out-of-bed	3.14 ± 0.43 3.91 ± 0.61 4.25 ± 0.79* (N = 11)	74 ± 14 85 ± 15 88 ± 16 (N = 14)	97 ± 17 111 ± 17 105 ± 19 (N = 14)	3.32 ± 0.37 3.92 ± 0.53 4.24 ± 0.42* (N = 12)	73 ± 8 89 ± 8 96 ± 9* (N = 13)	90 ± 13 99 ± 18 108 ± 21 (N = 13)
Acute MI inpatients[†] (W = 11, M = 15)	Rest In-bed Out-of-bed	2.90 ± 0.65 3.52 ± 0.59 3.84 ± 0.55 (N = 7)	77 ± 9 89 ± 9 94 ± 9 (N = 11)	101 ± 26 110 ± 22 109 ± 26 (N = 9)	3.22 ± 0.38 3.78 ± 0.56 4.21 ± 0.42* (N = 11)	72 ± 7 84 ± 12 91 ± 9* (N = 15)	89 ± 13 94 ± 15 102 ± 15 (N = 15)

*In-bed versus out-of-bed toileting ($p < 0.05$).

[†]Data from the eight coronary care unit patients (4 W and 4 M) are not included in $\dot{V}O_2$ results because a modified $\dot{V}O_2$ collection protocol was used (see text).

Mean duration for bedpan use (5.8 ± 1.5 min) did not differ significantly from that of bedside commode use (6.2 ± 1.4 min); however, duration for in-bed urinal use (3.6 ± 1.0 min) was significantly shorter than that of out-of-bed urinal use (5.2 ± 0.9 min) ($p < 0.05$). Analysis for group differences did not show a significant difference in duration among the four male groups; the healthy women, however, had a significantly shorter duration than did the other three groups of women ($p < 0.05$).

The rating of perceived exertion (RPE) results showed that in-bed toileting was perceived to require significantly more exertion than out-of-bed toileting ($p < 0.05$). However, most subjects considered both in-bed and out-of-bed toileting light exertion. The mode RPE scores were 9 (very light) for bedpan, bedside commode, and out-of-bed urinal and 11 (fairly light) for in-bed urinal. The median RPE scores were 11 for bedpan, 10 for bedside commode, 11 for in-bed urinal, and 9 for out-of-bed urinal. Both men and women reported significantly higher comfort, pleasantness, and ease of ranking ($p < 0.0005$) for out-of-bed toileting compared with in-bed toileting.

(continues)

RESEARCH EXAMPLE *(continued)*

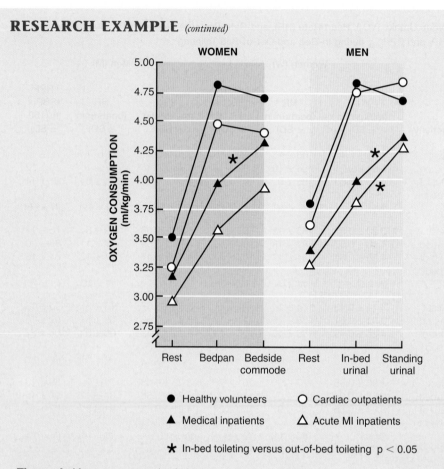

Figure I. Mean oxygen uptake during rest, in-bed toileting, and out-of-bed toileting in four groups of subjects. *MI,* myocardial infarction.

DISCUSSION

Both in-bed and out-of-bed toileting methods produced small increases in energy cost over resting levels. When the energy cost results are expressed as multiples of the subject's resting VO_2 (METs), the energy costs of using the bedpan and bedside commode were 1.3 and 1.4 METs, respectively; and the energy costs of using the urinal while in bed and while standing were 1.2 and 1.3 METs, respectively. These results are comparable with those of Benton and co-workers,[1] who measured VO_2 in 15 cardiac subjects and 13 noncardiac subjects during simulated defecation in the bedpan and bedside commode and found that bedpan use required 1.6 METs and bedside commode use required 1.4 METs. The higher energy cost for bedpan use in the Benton study (1.6 METs) compared with that found in our study (1.3 METs) may be explained by differences in research protocol—the Benton subjects got on and off the bedpan unassisted, whereas our subjects received assistance.

The measured VO_2 values in Benton's study and ours are slightly lower than the actual VO_2 for toileting, because Benton measured VO_2 during toileting as well as during a recovery period following toileting, and we measured VO_2 during the entire toileting process, which included pauses for blood pressure measure-

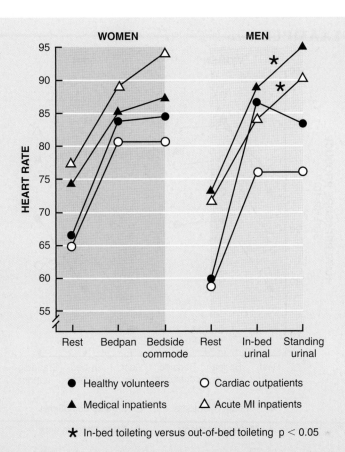

Figure II. Mean heart rate during rest and mean peak heart rate during in-bed and out-of bed toileting in four groups of subjects. *MI,* myocardial infarction.

ment. When the blood pressure pauses were eliminated for the eight coronary care unit patients, the VO_2 values for in-bed and out-of-bed toileting were 4.3 and 4.6 mL/kg/min, respectively, for the women and 4.5 and 4.7 mL/kg/min, respectively, for the men. These results convert to 1.4 METs for bedpan use, 1.5 METs for bedside commode use, 1.3 METs for using the urinal while in bed, and 1.4 METs for using the urinal while standing. Therefore, toileting produces low energy costs, and the differences in energy cost between in-bed and out-of-bed toileting, though statistically significant in some groups of subjects, appear clinically and physiologically unimportant.

The findings of Benton and co-workers[1] have been misunderstood and misquoted in several publications. Gordon[8] erroneously stated that bedside commode use required 3.6 kcal/min (approximately 3 METs) and bedpan use required 4.6 kcal/min (approximately 4 METs). Zohman and Tobias,[9] Acker,[10] the editors of *Exercise Equivalents*,[11] and others quote Gordon's numbers and thus perpetuate Gordon's misinterpretation of the Benton data. In *Exercise Equivalents*,[11] the energy cost of using a bedside commode (3 METs) is shown to be equal to that of scrubbing a floor, and the energy cost of using a bedpan (4 METs) is shown to be equal to that of beating a carpet. Close examination of the Benton data, however, shows that use of the bedpan and bedside commode require only about 1.5 times resting energy cost and not the threefold to fourfold increase subsequently reported.

(continues)

RESEARCH EXAMPLE *(continued)*

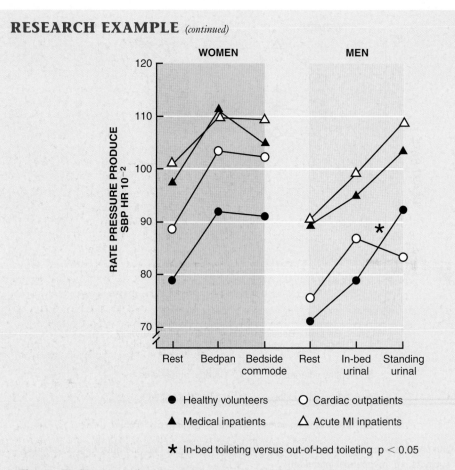

Figure III. Mean rate-pressure product during rest and mean peak rate-pressure product during in-bed and out-of-bed toileting. *HR,* heart rate; *MI,* myocardial infarction; *SBP,* systolic blood pressure.

Our hospitalized patients generally had significantly lower VO_2 values during toileting than did the nonhospitalized subjects. Hospitalized patients also have been reported to have a significantly lower energy cost during bathing than did healthy volunteers.[12,13] Resting VO_2, adjusted for body weight, did not differ significantly among our four groups of subjects. Spearman rank correlation coefficients (r_s) were calculated to determine the relationship of toilet method VO_2 (ml/kg/min) to age and toileting duration. In nonhospitalized women, VO_2 during bedpan use correlated with toileting duration ($r_s = -0.60$, $p = 0.01$). In hospitalized men, age correlated with VO_2 during in-bed urinal use ($r_s = -0.60$, $p = 0.002$), and during standing urinal use ($r_s = -0.41$, $p = 0.05$). No other significant correlations were found. The meaning of the few significant correlations is unclear because of the lack of consistent trends. Conservation of effort may explain the hospitalized patients' lower energy expenditure, because in our study and in the bathing studies[12,13] the hospitalized patients appeared to move more slowly and deliberately than did the nonhospitalized subjects. However, none of the studies used matched groups; thus, other variables may also explain the VO_2 differences.

In addition to quantitating overall energy costs, we measured HR_{peak} and RPP_{peak} during toileting to estimate myocardial work.[14] The statistically significant differences in HR_{peak} and RPP_{peak} between in-bed and out-of-bed toileting in some groups of subjects represent increases of only 8% in HR and 15% in RPP. These differences are quite small and probably not of physiologic importance. The higher values in the hospitalized men can be explained by differences in conditioning, orthostatic tolerance, and the presence of arterial hypertension.

Benton and co-workers[1] recorded blood pressure, HR, and an ECG before, during, and after each toileting method but did not report the data because of their extreme variability. Singman and co-workers[15] recorded continuous ECGs during defecation in 51 CCU patients, including 23 with acute MI. Both bedpan ($N = 15$) and bedside commode ($N = 48$) were used. The ECGs were analyzed for ectopy and for changes in ST segments or of 10 beats/min or greater in HR. Only two patients had ECG changes other than an increased HR; the authors do not describe these changes. The finding that more patients increased HRs by 10 beats/min or more during bedside commode use than during bedpan use is an expected response to the upright posture. The virtual absence of ECG abnormalities supports our findings that the cardiovascular differences in bedpan and bedside commode use are physiologically insignificant.

Acute MI patients treated with strict bed rest for nine to 24 days have pronounced orthostatic intolerance during upright tilt or sitting posture; in contrast, orthostatic tolerance is not impaired in acute MI patients treated for seven to 18 days with modified bed rest—the patients performed active leg exercises, sat on the edge of the bed, and used the commode from the day of admission.[16] Signs of orthostatic intolerance develop after as little as six hours of bed rest[17] and progress as bed rest continues.[18] Orthostatic intolerance needs to be prevented in acute MI patients, because the postural changes in HR and blood pressure are potential causes of cerebral infarction and extension of MI.

Studies by Convertino and associates[19,20] show that orthostatic stress is the most important factor limiting exercise tolerance after bed rest and that exposure to gravitational stress for 3.5 hours daily may obviate much of the deterioration in cardiovascular performance resulting from bed rest. Getting the patient up for eating and toileting should provide the gravitational stress necessary to minimize bed rest-induced orthostatic intolerance.

The results of our study show that both in-bed and out-of-bed toileting methods produce minimal energy cost and cardiovascular stress for healthy volunteers, cardiac outpatients, stable medical inpatients, and stable inpatients who had an acute MI from 2 to 28 days earlier. Clinically or physiologically important differences were not found between staying in bed and getting out of bed to toilet. The subjects clearly preferred getting out of bed to toilet. Findings from other studies show that getting out of bed for short periods minimizes bed rest-induced orthostatic intolerance[16,20] and that the upright posture may even decrease myocardial oxygen demands.[21,22] In-bed toileting should be reserved for those patients with specific contraindications to postural changes. Thus, for medical patients without specific contraindications, we recommend out-of-bed toileting.

The authors thank Cathleen L. Michaels, MSN, PN, Ann McCash, BSN, RN, Jo Cole, MSN, RN, Robert Rude, MD, C. Gunnar Blomqvist, MD, and the nurses of the tenth floor, coronary care unit, and MILIS study at Parkland Memorial Hospital for assistance in the study; Kent Dana, MA, and Nancy Wilson, MS, at the University of Texas Health Science Center for statistical advice; and Carolyn Donahue for preparing the manuscript.

REFERENCES

1. Benton JG, Brown H, Rusk HA: Energy expanded by patients on the bedpan and bedside commode. *JAMA* 1950; 144:1443-1447.
2. Gazes PC, Gaddy JE: Bedside management of acute myocardial infarction. *Am Heart J* 1979; 97:782-796.
3. Levine SA, Lown B: Armchair treatment of acute coronary thrombosis. *JAMA* 1952; 148:1365-1369.

(continues)

RESEARCH EXAMPLE *(continued)*

4. Newman LB, Wasserman, RR, Borden G: Productive living for those with heart disease: The role of physical medicine and rehabilitation. *Arch Phys Med Rehabil* 1956; 37:137-149.
5. Niccoli A, Brammell HL: A program for rehabilitation in coronary heart disease. *Nursing Clin North Am* 1976; 11:237-250.
6. Wenger NK: Rehabilitation of the patient with myocardial infarction: Responsibility of the primary care physician. *Primary Care* 1981; 8:491-507.
7. Borg G: Perceived exertion: A note on history and methods. *Med Sci Sports* 1973; 5:90-93.
8. Gordon EE: Energy costs of activities in health and disease. *Arch Intern Med* 1958; 101:702-713.
9. Zohman LR, Tobias JS: *Cardiac rehabilitation*. New York, Grune and Stratton, 1970.
10. Acker J: Early ambulation of post-myocardial infarction patients: Early activity after myocardial infarction, in Naughton JP, Hellerstein HK (eds): *Exercise testing and exercise training in coronary heart disease*. New York, Academic Press, 1973.
11. *Exercise Equivalents*. Denver Colorado Heart Association.
12. Gordon EE: Energy costs of various physical activities in relation to pulmonary tuberculosis. *Arch Phys Med* 1952; 33:201-209.
13. Winslow EH, Gaffrey L: Oxygen consumption and cardiovascular responses in normal adults and acute myocardial infarction patients during basin bath, tub bath, and shower. *Nurs Res* (submitted for publication).
14. Kilamura K, Jorgensen CR, Gobel FL, Taylor HL, Wang Y: Hemodynamic correlates of myocardial oxygen consumption during upright exercise. *J Appl Physiol* 1972; 32:516-522.
15. Singman H, Kinsella E, Goldberg E: Electrocardiographic changes in coronary care unit patients during defecation. *Vasc Surg* 1975; 9:54-57.
16. Fareeduddin K, Abelmann WH: Impaired orthostatic tolerance after bed rest in patients with myocardial infarction. *N Engl J Med* 1969; 280:345-350.
17. McCally M, Piemme TE, Murray RH: Tilt table responses of human subjects following application of lower body negative pressure. *Aerospace Med* 1966; 37:1247-1249.
18. Chobanian AV, Lille RD, Tercyak A, Blevins P: The metabolic and hemodynamic effects of prolonged bed rest in normal subjects. *Circulation* 1974; 49:551-559.
19. Convertino VA, Hung J, Goldwater D, DeBusk RF: Cardiovascular responses to exercise in middle-aged men after 10 days of bed rest. *Circulation* 1982;65:134-140.
20. Convertino VA, Sandler H, Webb P, Annis JF: Induced venous pooling and cardiorespiratory responses to exercise after bed rest. *J Appl Physiol* 1982; 52:1342-1348.
21. Lecerof H: Influence of body position on exercise tolerance, heart rate, blood pressure, and respiration rate in coronary insufficiency. *Br Heart J* 1971; 33:78-83.
22. Langou RA, Wolfson S, Olson EG, Cohen LS: Effects of orthostatic postural changes on myocardial oxygen demands. *Am J Cardiol* 1977; 39:418-421.

SAMPLE CRITIQUE   A Quantitative Study

COMPREHENSION PHASE

1. *Problem:* "Patients dislike using the bedpan and urinal while in bed and often insist that it would be easier and better for them to get out of bed to toilet. Little data are available about the physiologic costs of toileting" (Winslow et al., 1984, p. 456*).

*Page numbers in this critique refer to the version of the article reprinted in this book.

2. *Purpose:* The researchers "measured oxygen uptake (VO_2), peak heart rate (HR_{peak}), peak rate-pressure product (RPP_{peak}) (systolic blood pressure × heart rate), rating of perceived exertion (RPE), and preference in 95 hospitalized and nonhospitalized adults during in-bed (bedpan and urinal) and out-of-bed (bedside commode and standing urinal) toileting." (pp. 456–457)

3. *Literature review:* A minimal review of literature is presented at the beginning of the article. However, many studies are cited in the "Discussion" section, where the findings from this study are compared and contrasted with the findings from previous studies (see the research article, pp. 460–463). (Often in clinical specialty journals, such as the *Journal of Cardiac Rehabilitation* and *Heart & Lung: Journal of Acute and Critical Care*, studies are cited in the "Discussion" section so that findings can be synthesized to indicate the current knowledge in a problem area. Therefore, when critiquing the review of literature for a study, examine both the beginning of the article and the "Discussion" section.)

The researchers cited several studies, but few focused on the effects of in-bed and out-of-bed toileting (Benton, Brown, & Rusk, 1950; Singman, Kinsella, & Goldberg, 1975). Because limited research has been done in this area, additional study is needed. The references range from 1950 to 1982; most were published in the 1970s. These sources are considered current because the study being critiqued was published in 1984. The findings from studies are synthesized to indicate briefly what is known and not known about the study problem.

4. *Framework:* The framework is not identified by the researchers and must be extracted from the literature review. The key concepts of toileting, acutely ill adults, healthy adults, rehabilitating adults, and energy cost were identified but not defined in the article. The researchers indicate that Levine's Conservation Model, specifically the energy conservation principle and the overload and progression principle of exercise physiology, provided the framework for this study (Winslow, January 2000, personal communication). On the basis of the review of literature and following personal communication with the primary researcher, we developed the map shown in Figure 13-1 to identify the relationships among the concepts relevant to this study.

This map indicates that adults' health status (healthy, acutely ill, or rehabilitating) affects their energy conservation. This is a negative relationship, because the healthier people are, the less likely they are to

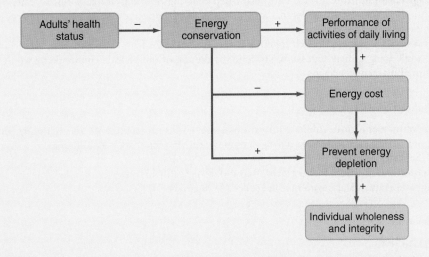

Figure 13-1. Proposed framework for the Winslow, Lane, and Gaffney study based on Levine's Conservation Model.

(continues)

SAMPLE CRITIQUE *(continued)*

conserve energy. When health declines with acute illnesses, adults are more likely to conserve their energy. The energy conservation affects adults' performance of their activities of daily living, such as toileting and bathing. Adults will conserve energy so they can perform their activities of daily living (positive relationship). The activities of daily living result in energy cost (positive relationship). However, a relationship also exists between energy conservation and energy cost. The more adults conserve energy, the less their energy costs for the activities they perform (negative relationship). Energy conservation involves the appropriate use of energy to prevent energy depletion and promote wholeness and integrity of the organism (Schaefer & Pond, 1991). Thus, acutely ill adults with less energy conserve their energy more than do healthy adults. The more they conserve their energy, the smaller their energy costs during activities of daily living such as toileting. When people are ill, they need to use the most appropriate and preferred toileting method to prevent excessive energy costs.

The adults in this study were male and female healthy volunteers, cardiac outpatients, medical inpatients, and acute myocardial infarction (MI) inpatients. The toileting methods examined were the in-bed methods of bedpan and urinal and the out-of-bed methods of bedside commode and standing urinal. The energy costs for different types of patients during toileting were examined by measuring the variables of VO_2, HR_{peak}, RPP_{peak}, and perceived exertion. Individual preference was determined by the preferred toileting method variable.

5. The researchers did not include *objectives*, *questions*, or *hypotheses*. The study purpose was used to direct the conduct of this study.
6. *Variables:* The researchers identified and operationally defined the variables but did not provide conceptual definitions. A possible conceptual definition and the operational definition follow for each variable.

INDEPENDENT VARIABLES

Toileting Methods

Conceptual definition. In-bed and out-of-bed toileting methods are activities of daily living performed by both ill and healthy adults that are influenced by the affected person's level of energy conservation and require greater energy cost than a resting level.

Operational definition. In-bed toileting is the use of the bedpan by women and the urinal by men to urinate while lying in bed. Out-of-bed toileting is the use of the bedside commode by women and the standing urinal by men to urinate.

ADULTS' HEALTH STATUS

Conceptual definition. Adults with various levels of health (acutely ill, rehabilitating, or healthy) conserve their energy appropriately during activities of daily living, such as toileting, to prevent energy depletion (Schaefer & Pond, 1991).

Operational definition. Subjects with four different health statuses were studied: healthy volunteers, cardiac outpatients, medical inpatients, and acute MI inpatients.

DEPENDENT VARIABLES

Oxygen Uptake (VO_2)

Conceptual definition. The amount of oxygen used by the body during an activity of daily living that indicates energy cost or expenditure.

Operational definition. Oxygen uptake was determined by

open-circuit, indirect calorimetry…. Expired air volume was measured by a Collins chain compensated gasometer (Tissot), and air composition was analyzed by mass spectrometer (Perkin-Elmer Medical Gas Analyzer 1100)…. Standard equations were used to derive VO_2. (Winslow et al., 1984, p. 457)

Peak Heart Rate (HR$_{peak}$)

Conceptual definition. The highest HR an adult reaches during an activity of daily living that indicates energy cost or expenditure.
Operational definition. "Peak HR was the most rapid HR observed during any 15-second period" (Winslow et al., 1984, p. 457).

Peak Rate-Pressure Product (RPP$_{peak}$)

Conceptual definition. The myocardial energy cost for an adult during an activity of daily living that indicates energy cost or expenditure.
Operational definition. A product of systolic blood pressure times HR. The highest RPP observed during toileting was defined as the RPP$_{peak}$.

Perceived Exertion

Conceptual definition. An individual's perception of the energy cost during an activity of daily living.
Operational definition. The subjects selected "a number from the Borg Scale of Perceived Exertion" to indicate their perceived level of exertion during toileting" (Winslow et al., 1984, p. 458).

Preferred Toileting Method

Conceptual definition. The toileting method a person likes best that influences how the individual will perform this activity of daily living.
Operational definition. "After both toileting methods, the subject completed a questionnaire wherein he ranked each method for comfort, pleasantness, and ease" (Winslow et al., 1984, p. 458).

7. *Attribute variables:* The attribute variables were gender, age, weight, height, medical diagnosis, date and type of MI, and current medications.
8. *Research design:* The research design is not identified but appears to be a quasi-experimental repeated-measures design, in which each subject was exposed to both treatments (in-bed and out-of-bed toileting). The subjects were randomly assigned to an initial toileting method. The gas collections for VO_2 and HR were measured immediately before, during, and after each toileting method. Blood pressure for RPP was measured before and after each method of toileting (pretest and posttest). The Borg Scale of Perceived Exertion and the questionnaire for toileting preference were completed after each toileting method (posttest only).
   a. *Study procedures:* The following protocol was used to direct the study.
      Protocol: "Oxygen uptake, HR, and RPP were determined during a 3-minute supine rest period and during in-bed and out-of-bed toileting. A 10-minute rest period separated the randomly ordered toileting methods. Women used the bedpan and bedside commode for urinating; men used the urinal while lying in bed and while standing beside the bed. The subjects simulated voiding if unable to void during the second toileting trial." (Winslow et al., 1984, p. 458)
      The toileting protocol simulated usual clinical conditions; therefore, toileting duration varied. The investigator assisted the women in lifting their hips for bedpan placement and removal, and

(continues)

SAMPLE CRITIQUE *(continued)*

placed the bedside commode in a standardized position beside the head of the bed. Subjects used their own techniques to get out of and back into bed and were not lifted by the investigator. The investigator left the room while the subject urinated and returned when given a signal from the subject. Subjects took as much time as they needed for urination. (Winslow et al., 1984, p. 458)

b. *Extraneous variables* are not specifically identified, but the researchers structured the sample criteria, treatment protocols, and data collection process to eliminate extraneous variables. For example, the medical diagnoses of patients were clearly documented, and all patients were ambulatory and had no neural or musculoskeletal problems that might interfere with the toileting treatments. The treatments were randomly implemented, and the protocols for the treatments and measurements were highly structured and consistently implemented.

c. No *pilot study* was identified.

9. Description of the sample

a. *Sample criteria:* The subjects were adult male and female volunteers who were either healthy individuals, coronary artery disease patients who were participating in a supervised outpatient exercise program, stable medical inpatients with a variety of cardiac and noncardiac disorders, or stable acute MI inpatients whose MI had occurred at least 2 days earlier.

"Acute MI was established by history, clinical, electrocardiographic (ECG), and enzyme findings and by myocardial scintigraphy.... All medical and cardiac inpatients were ambulatory prior to hospitalization [inclusion sample criteria], and none had neural or musculoskeletal problems that would preclude standing unassisted" [exclusion sample criteria]. (Winslow et al., 1984, p. 457)

b. *Sampling method:* Nonprobability sample of convenience.

c. *Sample size:* There were 95 hospitalized and nonhospitalized adult subjects. The authors did not indicate that power analysis was used to determine sample size.

d. *Refusal rate:* The authors did not mention the refusal rate when approaching potential subjects.

e. *Characteristics of the sample:*

"The 42 women and 53 men (range 18–79 years) who volunteered for the study consisted of 26 healthy adults, 16 coronary artery disease patients.... 27 stable medical inpatients with a variety of cardiac and noncardiac disorders, and 26 stable acute MI inpatients who had their MI from 2 to 28 days earlier (8.81 ± 5 days [mean ± SD]) Eight patients had their MI five days or less before the study began.... Nineteen (73%) of the patients had transmural infarctions; seven (27%) had subendocardial infarctions.... Six (37%) of the cardiac outpatients, seven (26%) of the medical inpatients, and five (19%) of the acute MI patients were receiving propranolol at the time of the study." (Winslow et al., 1984, p. 457)

Some of the sample characteristics also are presented in a table (see Table I, p. 457).

f. *Sample mortality:* No sample mortality was mentioned; data analyses included all 95 subjects.

g. *Institutional review board and type of consent:* "The research protocol was approved by the Institutional Review Board, and informed written consent was obtained from all subjects prior to the study." (Winslow et al., 1984, p. 457)

10. *Measurement strategies:* The researchers measured five variables—three (VO_2, HR_{peak}, and RPP_{peak}) with physiologic instruments, one (perceived exertion) with a self-report scale, and one (toileting preference) with a questionnaire.

a. "VO_2 was determined by open-circuit, indirect calorimetry. The subject had a nose clip and mouth piece in place. During the timed period, expired air was collected via a one-way respiratory valve

(Daniels) and 64-inch plastic tubing into a 30 L (rest) or 150 L (toileting) bag (Douglas).... Expired air volume was measured by a Collins Chain Compensated Gasometer (Tissot), and air composition was analyzed by mass spectrometer (Perkin-Elmer Medical Gas Analyzer 1100).... Standard equations were used to derive VO_2." (Winslow et al., 1984, p. 457)

The measurement strategy produced ratio-level data. To demonstrate the precision and accuracy of the equipment, the "mass spectrometer was calibrated electronically and checked against gases of known concentration." (Winslow et al., 1984, p. 457)

b. HR_{peak} was identified using a continuous electrocardiogram (ECG) (lead II) that was recorded during toileting. "Peak HR was the most rapid HR observed during any 15-second period" (Winslow et al., 1984, p. 457). This measurement strategy produced ratio-level data. The brand name of the electrocardiographic equipment and the precision, sensitivity, accuracy, and error of the equipment were not addressed.

c. RPP_{peak} was determined by multiplying systolic blood pressure times heart rate and selecting the highest RPP. "Blood pressure was measured by cuff sphygmomanometer immediately before and after toileting and after each position change" (Winslow et al., 1984, pp. 457–458). This measurement strategy produced ratio-level data. The precision, sensitivity, selectivity, accuracy, and error of the blood pressure cuff and sphygmomanometer were not addressed. The manufacturer of this equipment was not identified.

d. *Perceived exertion* was measured using the Borg Scale of Perceived Exertion. The level of data is unclear but probably was ordinal, because nonparametric tests for ordinal data (Friedman two-way analysis of variance [ANOVA] by ranks and Spearman correlation coefficients) were used for analysis. The validity and reliability of the Borg Scale are not discussed, but a reference article is cited.

e. *Preferred toileting method* was measured with a questionnaire that examined the comfort, pleasantness, and ease of each method. The level of data probably was ordinal, because nonparametric tests were used for analysis. The development of this questionnaire was not discussed, and no validity or reliability information was provided.

11. *Data collection procedures:* The data collection process was detailed in the "Methods" and "Protocol" sections of the article (pp. 457–458). Most of this content was presented in the "Measurement" and "Design" sections of this critique.

12. *Statistical analyses:* The analyses were descriptive and inferential. VO_2, HR, and RPP data were analyzed with descriptive statistics, including mean, range, and standard deviation. These results are presented in a table (see Table II, p. 459). Graphs also are presented, allowing the reader to visualize the differences among the four groups (healthy volunteers, medical inpatients, cardiac outpatients, and acute MI inpatients) in VO_2 (see Figure I, p. 460), HR (see Figure II, p. 461), and RPP (see Figure III, p. 462) during rest, in-bed toileting, and out-of-bed toileting.

The inferential statistical analyses were conducted primarily to examine differences between in-bed and out-of-bed toileting methods for four groups of subjects:

"Oxygen uptake, HR, and RPP results were analyzed for each sex and group by repeated measures analysis of variance. Ratings of perceived exertion and preferences were analyzed by the Friedman two-way ANOVA by ranks. Spearman correlation coefficients were calculated for selected variables including VO_2, age, and toileting duration." (Winslow et al., 1984, p. 458)

The repeated-measures ANOVA results indicated that no physiologically important differences were found between in-bed and out-of-bed toileting. Both in-bed and out-of-bed toileting produced small increases in energy cost and myocardial work over resting levels, with a mean VO_2 < 1.6 times resting VO_2, a mean HR_{peak} 100 beats/min, and a mean RPP_{peak} < 11,200. (Winslow et al., 1984, p. 456)

(continues)

SAMPLE CRITIQUE *(continued)*

13. *Interpretation of findings:* The findings from "the study show that both in-bed and out-of-bed toileting methods produce minimal energy cost and cardiovascular stress for healthy volunteers, cardiac outpatients, stable medical inpatients, and stable inpatients who had an acute MI from two to 28 days earlier. Clinically or physiologically important differences were not found between staying in bed and getting out of bed to toilet. The subjects clearly preferred getting out of bed to toilet." (Winslow et al., 1984, p. 463)

    These findings were expected and were consistent with the findings from Benton et al. (1950) and Singman et al. (1975). An unexpected finding was that hospitalized patients had significantly lower VO_2 values than those of nonhospitalized patients. The researchers hypothesized that hospitalized patients with depleted energy reduce their energy expenditure during toileting. No serendipitous findings were identified. Because the study has no clearly designated framework, the findings were not linked to a framework.

14. *Limitations of the study:* Limitations are not identified.

15. *Generalization of findings:* "In-bed toileting should be reserved for patients with specific contraindications to postural change.... For medical patients without specific contraindications, we recommend out-of-bed toileting." (Winslow et al., 1984, p. 463)

16. *Implications for nursing:* Nurses are encouraged to get stable medical inpatients and stable inpatients who have had an acute MI out of bed to toilet. This toileting method has minimal energy cost, is preferred by patients, and minimizes bed rest–induced orthostatic intolerance.

17. *Suggestions for further research:* The researchers provide no specific directions for further research.

18. *Missing elements of the study:* The study lacks a clearly expressed framework; reliability and validity information for one of the scales; precision, accuracy, and sensitivity information for some of the physiologic instruments; limitations; and recommendations for further research.

19. *Replication:* The study is sufficiently clear to replicate. Anyone planning replication should contact the researchers for clarification of parts of the data collection process and the research protocol and for more information regarding some of the measurement methods.

COMPARISON AND ANALYSIS PHASES

This section discusses the strengths and weaknesses of the steps of the research process and the logical links among these steps. The title, abstract, problem, purpose, literature review, framework, methodology, results, and discussion elements of the article are critiqued.

Title and abstract: The title, although a little long, clearly indicates the focus of the study. The abstract includes the study problem, purpose, sample size, sample characteristics, significant results, relevant findings, and implications of the findings for nursing practice. This relevant information is presented in a way that captures the attention of the reader.

Problem and purpose: The problem is clearly identified in the abstract and in the first paragraph of the article. Determining the energy costs of different methods of toileting will provide direction in caring for hospitalized patients. Because toileting is the responsibility of nurses, this is a significant problem and requires investigation.

The purpose is expressed clearly in the abstract and in the second paragraph of the article. The purpose identifies the independent and dependent variables, the population, and the setting. The study was feasible to conduct because of (1) the clinical and research expertise of the investigators; (2) the financial support received for the study (see p. 463); (3) the availability of subjects, facilities, and equipment discussed in the " Methods" section; (4) the cooperation of others (acknowledged at the end of the article); and (5) the ethical considerations given the subjects (informed consent) (Burns & Grove, 2005).

Literature review: The literature review is brief because of the limited number of studies conducted in this area. Additional related research and theoretical sources might have been cited to indicate the current knowledge of the problem. However, journals often limit the length of an article, and researchers must cut information from the literature review and other sections of their research reports to meet publication requirements. A final summary of what is known and not known about the problem studied would have added clarity to the literature review.

Framework: The study lacks a clearly identified framework. The concepts relevant to the study are identified but not defined, and the relationships among the concepts should have been clarified and documented. The variables are clearly defined operationally but are neither conceptually defined nor linked to the concepts identified. The study findings, if linked to Levine's Conservation Model, could have added support to this model and to the understanding of energy conservation in healthy and ill adults (Schaefer & Pond, 1991).

Methods: The "Methods" section is a major strength of the study. The sample size was large (95 subjects) and included a variety of subjects (healthy volunteers, cardiac outpatients, medical inpatients, and acute MI inpatients). The heterogeneity of the subjects increases the generalizability of the findings (Burns & Grove, 2005). A limitation is that the study groups were of unequal size. The cardiac outpatient group had only 16 subjects, but the other three groups were fairly equal, with 26 to 27 subjects per group. The sampling method, sampling criteria, and sample characteristics are clearly presented. The study was ethical, because it was approved for conduct by an institutional review board and informed written consent was obtained from the subjects.

The measurement methods seem appropriate for measuring energy cost, myocardial workload, perceived exertion, and preferred toileting method. The measurement of VO_2 is presented in detail, and the precision and accuracy of the equipment are described. The equipment (electrocardiograph, blood pressure cuff, and sphygmomanometer) for measuring HR and RPP are described, but the accuracy and precision of the equipment are not addressed (DeKeyser & Pugh, 1990). Discussion of the Borg Scale of Perceived Exertion and the questionnaire used to measure toileting preference is limited; discussing the reliability and validity of these instruments would have strengthened the study.

The design is not identified, and the threats to design validity are not discussed. However, the study protocol clearly describes the implementation of the independent variables and the measurement of the dependent variables. The toileting protocol simulated usual clinical conditions, which increases the ability to generalize the findings to patients in clinical practice. The researchers did not indicate who collected the data. If more than one person collected data, the reliability or consistency of the data collection process must be addressed (Burns & Grove, 2005).

Results: The statistical techniques used to analyze data from the measurement of the five dependent variables are clearly identified. The analysis techniques (descriptive and inferential) were appropriate for the level of measurement of the variables (Burns & Grove, 2005; Munro, 2005). The purpose of the study is clearly addressed in the "Results" section. The results are presented in narrative form, tables, and graphs to facilitate understanding.

Discussion: The expected and unexpected findings are explained, and the statistical and clinical significance of the findings is addressed (Burns & Grove, 2005). The findings are consistent with previous research, and this is documented. The generalization of the findings and their implications for nursing are clearly presented. The researchers could have strengthened the report by identifying the study limitations and providing suggestions for further research.

EVALUATION PHASE

This study examines a significant nursing problem and provides important findings that can be used in nursing practice. The findings are consistent with those of previous research (Benton et al., 1950; Singman et al., 1975) and seem to describe accurately the energy costs of toileting for hospitalized and nonhospitalized

(continues)

SAMPLE CRITIQUE *(continued)*

patients. Out-of-bed toileting is recommended for medical patients without specific contraindications. These findings can be generalized to stable medical inpatients and stable inpatients who have had an acute MI.

The following questions might generate further research: What additional dependent variables may be measured to determine the energy costs during toileting? How can these dependent variables be measured? What are the best toileting methods for other types of acutely and chronically ill patients? What are the energy costs for toileting in the bathroom? What are the energy costs for in-bed and out-of-bed toileting during defecation versus urination? Further research in these areas will strengthen the evidence base related to toileting and enable nurses to provide evidence-based practice when assisting patients with toileting.

The strengths of this study greatly outweigh the weaknesses. The weaknesses regarding the framework, design, measurement methods, and suggestions for further research could easily be corrected in future studies. The findings support previous research and provide strong evidence to direct practice.

Introduction to the Critique Process for Qualitative Research

Qualitative studies are appearing more frequently in nursing journals and are providing relevant information for nursing practice. Therefore, nurses in every phase and field of practice need experience in critiquing both qualitative and quantitative studies. However, critiquing a qualitative study involves a different approach and guidelines to identify study strengths and weaknesses.

When critiquing a qualitative study, you must examine differences between the qualitative approaches. For example, in grounded theory the goal is to develop a theory based on participant perspectives, although this goal is inconsistent with other qualitative approaches. In ethnography, the researcher often lives with or spends months interacting with participants to develop a careful understanding of their beliefs and practices. Such a time commitment is not consistent with other qualitative approaches. In Husserlian phenomenology, the researcher "brackets off" or distances himself or herself from any personal knowledge of, beliefs about, or understandings regarding the phenomenon. By contrast, in Heideggerian phenomenology, it is assumed that a researcher cannot bracket off previously acquired knowledge, beliefs, or understandings. Rather, that background understanding is how the researcher—or any observer—develops a richer view of the phenomenon under examination (Benner, 1994). Irrespective of these differences among qualitative methods, common criteria by which qualitative studies can be evaluated have been identified.

A scholarly critique of qualitative studies includes a balanced evaluation of a study's strengths and weaknesses. As discussed next, five standards have been proposed to evaluate qualitative studies: (1) descriptive vividness, (2) methodological congruence, (3) analytical and interpretative preciseness, (4) philosophical or theoretical connectedness, and (5) heuristic relevance (Burns, 1989; Burns & Grove, 2005; Cesario, Morin, & Santa-Donato, 2002).

Standard 1: Descriptive Vividness

To achieve **descriptive vividness**, the study purpose, significance, and interpretations must be articulated in such detail and richness that the reader has the sense of personally experiencing the event and clearly understanding the significance of the findings. For example, Glaser and Strauss (1965, p. 9) believe that the social world studied should be described and interpreted "so vividly that the reader can almost literally see and hear its people."

Threats to descriptive vividness include

- Failure to include essential descriptive information
- Lack of clarity in description
- Inadequate interpretative/analytic skill. Interpretative and narrative skill is vital because good qualitative research seeks to identify what is "most essential, characteristic, and defining" about a given phenomenon (van Manen, 1990, p. 5). The results need to illuminate more than what was provided in participant quotes and more than what was previously understood or reported in the literature.

CRITIQUE GUIDELINES Descriptive Vividness

When critiquing a qualitative study for descriptive vividness, consider the following questions:

1. Was the significance of the study adequately described?
2. Was the purpose of the study clearly described?
3. Were the interpretations presented in a descriptive way that illuminated more than the quotes did?

Standard 2: Methodological Congruence

Evaluation of **methodological congruence** requires knowledge of the methodological approach the researchers used and whether that approach was consistent with the philosophical basis of the study (see Chapter 3). Qualitative researchers need to identify the philosophy and methodological approach they used and cite references for these choices (Munhall, 2001). Methodological excellence has four dimensions: adequate documentation of the participants, careful attention to the procedural approach, adherence to ethical standards, and auditability (Beck, 1993; Burns, 1989; Burns & Grove, 2005; Miles & Huberman, 1994).

Adequate Documentation of the Participants

Adequate documentation of the participants requires a detailed description of the study participants, rationale for why and how the participants were selected, and a description of the context and location where the study was conducted.

Threats to adequate documentation of the participants include

- Failure to describe the participants in detail
- Failure to provide a rationale for selecting the participants
- Failure to describe the context or location of the study so that others can determine if the findings are applicable to their setting

CRITIQUE GUIDELINES   Adequate Documentation of the Participants

When critiquing a qualitative study for adequate documentation of the participants, consider the following questions:

1. Were the study participants described in detail?
2. Was the selection of participants reasonable? Was a rationale provided for participant selection (Miles & Huberman, 1994)?
3. Was the context and location of the study described with sufficient detail to determine if the findings are applicable to other settings?

Careful Attention to the Procedural Approach

Another dimension of methodological congruence is how careful the researcher is in applying selected procedures for the study. To the extent possible, the researcher must clearly state the steps that were taken to ensure that data were accurately recorded and that the data obtained are representative of the data as a whole (Knafl & Howard, 1984). When critiquing a qualitative study, examine the description of assumptions, the data collection process, and role of the researcher for threats to the procedural approach.

Threats to the procedural approach include

- Failure to articulate the assumptions associated with the research
- Failure to establish trust with the participants, open dialogue, and a conversational approach to data collection (Benner, 1994; van Manen, 1990)
- Failure to ask appropriate questions that address the participant's beliefs, experiences, values, or perceptions (Kirk & Miller, 1986)
- Failure to adequately describe the data collection process
- Failure to spend adequate time gathering data or to conduct multiple interviews
- Failure to describe the data collection procedures used by multiple data collectors
- Failure to use appropriate process for selecting and gaining access to participants
- Failure to detail the role of the researcher during the interview process
- Failure to describe the qualitative expertise of the researcher(s)

CRITIQUE GUIDELINES   Careful Attention to Procedural Approach

When critiquing a qualitative study for attention to procedural approach, consider the following questions:

1. Did the researchers identify the philosophical or theoretical base of the study?
2. Were the assumptions underlying the study articulated? Were the assumptions and data collection procedures congruent?
3. Was adequate trust established with the participants? Was there an open dialogue with a conversational approach to data collection?

4. Were research questions articulated? Did the researcher ask questions that explore partici-pant's experiences, beliefs, values, or perceptions?
5. Was the data collection process adequately described?
6. Did the researcher spend sufficient time with participants gathering data? Did the researcher conduct multiple interviews?
7. Was the approach of multiple data collectors similar?
8. Was the method of selecting and gaining access to the study participants reasonable?
9. Was the role of the researcher during the interview process described? Were the researcher(s) qualitative credentials and expertise described?

Adherence to Ethical Standards

Ethical standards require recognition and discussion by the researcher of the ethical implica-tions related to the study. Informed consent is obtained from participants and documented. The report must indicate that the researcher took action to ensure that the rights of the participants were protected during the study. As you critique the study, examine the data-gathering process, and identify potential threats to ethical standards.

Threats to ethical standards include

- Failure to inform the participants of their rights
- Failure to obtain informed consent from the participants
- Failure to protect participant rights

CRITIQUE GUIDELINES Adherence to Ethical Standards

When critiquing a qualitative study for adherence to ethical standards, consider the following questions:

1. Were participants informed of their rights?
2. Was informed consent obtained?
3. Were participant rights protected?

Auditability

A fourth dimension of methodological congruence is the rigorous development of a decision trail (Miles & Huberman, 1994). Guba and Lincoln (1982) refer to this dimension as auditability. The research report needs to be sufficiently detailed to allow a second researcher with a similar background and philosophical approach, using the original data and the decision trail, to arrive at conclusions similar to those of the original researcher.

Threats to auditability include

- Failure of the researcher to record the nature of the decisions made, the data on which they were based, and the decision trail and rules for arriving at conclusions. Other researchers with a similar background and philosophical background are not able to arrive at similar conclusions after applying the decision rules to the data (Beck, 1993; Burns, 1989; Cesario et al., 2002; Hawker, Payne, Kerr, Hardey, & Powell, 2002).

- Failure to include enough participant quotes to support the findings. The interpretative statements developed do not correspond with the findings (Miles & Huberman, 1994).
- Failure to provide quotes that are sufficiently rich or detailed to allow judgments to be made. This flaw also has been described as not achieving saturation or redundancy in the data (van Manen, 1990).
- Failure to provide specific examples of the phenomenon being investigated.

CRITIQUE GUIDELINES   Auditability

When critiquing a qualitative study for auditability, consider the following questions:

1. Was the decision trail used in arriving at conclusions described in adequate detail? Can the findings be linked with the data?
2. Were enough participant quotes included to support the findings?
3. Were the data sufficiently rich to support the conclusions? Were the findings validated by data? Did the participants describe specific examples of the phenomenon being investigated?

Standard 3: Analytical and Interpretative Preciseness

The analytical process in qualitative research involves a series of interpretations and transformations during which concrete data are transformed across several levels of abstraction. The outcome of the analysis imparts meaning to the phenomenon under study. The analytical and interpretative process frequently is poorly described in research reports. **Analytical and interpretative preciseness** requires that the researcher involve others in the interpretative process and present a meaningful picture of the phenomenon under study (Huberman & Miles, 2002; Hawker et al., 2002).

Threats to analytical and interpretative preciseness include

- Failure to present the findings in a way that yields a meaningful picture of the phenomenon under study
- Failure to return the findings to participants or experts in the area or to readers who determine if the results are consistent with common meanings and understandings (Benner, 1994; Madison, 1988; Sandelowski, 1986)
- Failure to involve two or more researchers in data analysis or to describe how disagreements about data analysis were handled (Benner, 1994)

CRITIQUE GUIDELINES   Analytical and Interpretative Preciseness

When critiquing a qualitative study for analytical and interpretative preciseness, consider the following questions:

1. Do the categories, themes, or findings present a whole picture? Did the findings yield a meaningful picture of the phenomenon under study?
2. Were the findings returned to participants or experts in the area?
3. Did two or more researchers participate in data analysis? How were disagreements about data analysis handled?

Standard 4: Philosophical or Theoretical Connectedness

Philosophical or **theoretical connectedness** requires that the findings developed from the study be clearly expressed, logically consistent, and compatible with the knowledge base of nursing. Moreover, the study assumptions, methodological procedures, and interpretative/analytic approach must be consistent with the philosophical or theoretical basis of the study. Citations need to be provided documenting the philosophical or theoretical approach that was used (Cesario et al., 2002; Hawker et al., 2002; Munhall, 2001).

Threats to philosophical or theoretical connectedness include

- Failure to link data to nursing practice
- Failure to identify a philosophical or theoretical basis for the study
- Failure to cite references for the philosophical or theoretical approach used
- Failure to link the philosophical or theoretical basis of the study with the study assumptions, data collection procedures, and analytical and interpretative approach

CRITIQUE GUIDELINES   Philosophical or Theoretical Connectedness

When critiquing a qualitative study for philosophical or theoretical connectedness, consider the following questions:

1. Was a clear connection made between the data and nursing practice?
2. Did the researcher identify the philosophical or theoretical basis for the study? Were citations provided for the philosophical or theoretical approach used?
3. Was the philosophical or theoretical basis of the study consistent with the study assumptions, data collection process, and analysis and interpretative methods used? Were citations provided for the philosophical or theoretical approach used?

Standard 5: Heuristic Relevance

To be of value, the results of a study must have **heuristic relevance** for the reader. This value is reflected in the reader's ability to recognize the phenomenon described in the study, its applicability to nursing practice, and its influence on future research. The dimensions of heuristic relevance include intuitive recognition, relationship to the existing body of knowledge, and applicability.

Intuitive Recognition

Intuitive recognition indicates that the findings will have immediate meaning for readers within their personal knowledge base. Readers immediately recognize the phenomenon, its connection to their personal experience, and its relationship to nursing practice (Denzin & Lincoln, 2002).

Threats to intuitive recognition include

- Failure to present the findings in a way in which the reader can recognize them as being consistent with common meanings and experiences

CRITIQUE GUIDELINES   Intuitive Recognition

When critiquing a qualitative study for intuitive recognition, consider the following questions:

1. Can the reader recognize the phenomenon described in the study?
2. Are the findings consistent with common meanings or experiences?

Relationship to the Existing Body of Knowledge

The existing body of knowledge must be reviewed by the researcher and compared with the study findings. Similarities between the current knowledge base and the study findings add strength to the findings; the researcher also needs to explore reasons for differences. When critiquing a study, you evaluate the degree to which the author(s) compared and contrasted the study findings with the results of other researchers' work.

Threats to the relationship to the existing body of knowledge include

- Failure to examine the existing body of knowledge
- Failure to compare and contrast the study findings with those of other studies
- Failure to describe the lacunae or omissions in current understandings that would account for unique findings (Benner, 1994)

> ### CRITIQUE GUIDELINES   Relationship to the Existing Body of Knowledge
>
> When critiquing a qualitative study for relationship to the existing body of knowledge, consider the following questions:
>
> 1. Did the researcher adequately examine the existing body of knowledge?
> 2. Did the researcher compare and contrast the findings with those of other studies?
> 3. Did the researcher describe the lacunae or omissions in current understandings that would account for unique findings?

Applicability to Nursing Practice, Research, or Education

Nurses need to be able to integrate the research findings into their knowledge base and apply them in nursing practice. In addition, the findings must contribute to nursing practice, education, or research. Researchers also need to outline suggestions for future research in the "Discussion" section of the research report. When critiquing a qualitative study, examine the "Discussion" section for threats to applicability (Burns, 1989; Cesario et al., 2002; Hawker et al., 2002).

Threats to applicability to nursing practice, research, or education include

- Failure to link study findings to nursing practice, research, or education
- Failure to emphasize how the findings extended what was previously reported in the literature
- Failure to identify implications of the study for related cases (Benner, 1994)
- Failure to summarize suggestions for future research

> ### CRITIQUE GUIDELINES   Applicability to Nursing Practice, Research, or Education
>
> When critiquing a qualitative study for applicability to nursing practice, research, or education, consider the following questions:
>
> 1. Are the findings relevant to nursing practice, research, or education?
> 2. Did the reader learn more than had been previously reported in the literature?
> 3. Do the findings have implications for related cases?
> 4. Are suggestions for further study identified?

A Practice Critique

As a basis for a practice critique, the following Research Example presents a published qualitative study (Gordon-Larsen; Griffiths; Bentley; Ward, Kelsey; Shields, et al., 2004), in its entirety. The sample critique provided at the end of the Research Example includes the five standards: descriptive vividness, methodological congruence, analytical and interpretative preciseness, philosophical or theoretical connectedness, and heuristic relevance.

Read the article and critique it using the standards, and then compare your critique with the one provided. Doing your own initial critique and then reading the sample critique can help you expand your critiquing skills.

RESEARCH EXAMPLE   A Qualitative Study

Barriers to Physical Activity: Qualitative Data on Caregiver–Daughter Perceptions and Practices

Penny Gordon-Larsen PhD, Paula Griffiths PhD, Margaret E. Bentley PhD, Dianne S. Ward EdD, Kristine Kelsey PhD, Kenitra Shields BA and Alice Ammerman DrPH

Background

There is little research on household and physical environment barriers to physical activity, particularly in minority populations at high risk for obesity and inactivity. Few studies include data on caregiver and daughter dyads. Formative data were used to develop intervention strategies and pathways for the *Girls Rule!* obesity prevention intervention, in under-studied high-risk pre-adolescents.

Methods

Participants included 12 African-American girls (mean age 7.8 years) and their 11 primary female caregivers (mean age 41.8 years)—eight mother–daughter dyads and three grandmother–granddaughter dyads—for a total of 51 interviews across 23 participants interviewed from April to October 2000. A qualitative approach was used for 51 semistructured in-depth interviews with 11 dyads (female caregiver and girl), consisting of up to three interviews per respondent (mean = 2.4 interviews per respondent). Interviews were transcribed, coded, and systematically analyzed between January 2002 and January 2003 to identify recurrent patterns and themes related to physical activity.

Results

Findings indicate clear preference of the girls for sedentary, rather than active, behaviors. Caregivers were unaware of the amount of TV viewed and found positive benefits of TV viewing, including safe supervision of their daughters. Barriers to physical activity include perceived lack of affordable and accessible recreation facilities and low caregiver motivation. Potential intervention strategies identified by respondents include walking for exercise and transportation and several low-cost, favored physical activities, such as hopscotch, jumping rope, and dance.

Conclusions

These findings point toward several physical activity and obesity intervention strategies that can guide obesity prevention efforts.

Introduction

Childhood obesity has increased dramatically in the United States,[1-4] particularly among African-American females[1,3,5] who have higher inactivity relative to non-Hispanic whites.[6] It is suggested that activity is more important than diet in obesity etiology in this population.[7] Approximately 36.7% of African-American girls aged 6 to 11 years are at risk for or overweight, compared to the population average of 27.8%.[8] Overweight tracks from childhood through adolescence and into adulthood[9]; physical activity declines with age and pubertal development among girls,[10,11] especially African-American girls.[12] Health consequences of childhood overweight include psychosocial and cardiovascular risks.[13]

Overweight parents create obesigenic household environments.[14-16] Diet and lifestyle patterns are initiated during early childhood,[17] and family support and encouragement are strongly and consistently associated with childhood physical activity.[18-20] Intervention research shows positive fitness changes associated with home- and community-based physical activity programs,[21] with recent focus on family-based interventions.[22] However, interventions have not been adequately successful in bringing about health behavior change because of a failure to identify appropriate mediating variables.[23]

Qualitative data are extremely valuable for providing insight into health determinants.[24-27] Collection of qualitative data in **both** caregivers and their children provides a rich description of the context within which diet and activity choices are made.[26,28] Despite these strengths, there is minimal empirical research on patterns of activity among caregiver–daughter dyads. The aim of this qualitative research is to explore perceptions of sedentary behaviors, barriers to and facilitators of physical activity, and directions for intervention factors in this high-risk population.

Methods

STUDY DESIGN

Girls Rule! is a church-based pilot program including formative research (April to October 2000) to inform an obesity prevention program (July 2001 to November 2002) for African-American girls, aged 6 to 9 years, and their primary female caregivers.[29,30] Key elements from the formative data collection were used to design age-appropriate and culturally appropriate intervention strategies to be implemented among African-American caregiver–daughter dyads.

SAMPLE

Participants were recruited in a North Carolina church representative of the subsequent Girls Rule! intervention churches (medium income, suburban neighborhood). Church pastors and liaisons disseminated screening questionnaires in their churches. Study personnel followed with phone calls to further explain the project and to schedule the consent appointment and first interview. Eligible respondents included households with a female caregiver and a female child aged 6 to 9 years; all eligible and willing dyads were included. The formative research sample included multiple face-to-face semistructured, in-depth interviews with 12 African-American girls (mean age 7.8 years) and their 11 primary female caregivers (mean age 41.8 years), for a total of 51 interviews across 23 participants and 11 caregiver–daughter dyads (eight mother–daughter, and three grandmother–daughter pairs). Data collection followed informed consent procedures established by the University of North Carolina's School of Public Health Institutional Review Board.

INSTRUMENTS

Pilot data indicated approximately 180 minutes of interview time, divided into three 60-minute parts, given caregiver schedules and the girls' attention span. The three semistructured interviews included (1) diet and correlates; (2) activity and correlates (including activity and TV recall); and (3) potential intervention activities and strategies. The present study focused on physical activity, neighborhood characteristics, and caregiver–daughter shared activities, largely from the second and third interviews, although all three interviews were searched. Up to three interviews per respondent were conducted (mean of 2.4 interviews per respondent); however, not all dyads completed all three interviews due to completion of all data collection within two interviews or missing data. Four interviewers, working in two pairs (consistent across dyads), used an interview guide to conduct concurrent interviews with caregivers and daughters in separate rooms. Detailed field notes were taken during interviews.

(continues)

RESEARCH EXAMPLE *(continued)*

DATA ANALYSIS

Data were analyzed between January 2002 and January 2003. All interviews were recorded and transcribed, and then entered as text and coded using QRS NUD*IST (NVIVO Software for Qualitative Research, London, 1998). Text data were carefully read and systematically analyzed by investigators to identify recurrent activity-related patterns and themes originating from the research team's original research questions and hypotheses.[31,32] Individual researchers read all interviews and the team evaluated main codes and text samples to support the codes.

Coded text was extracted from all interviews and comparisons made across data using a matrix-based analysis approach,[32] which allows systematic analysis of the data and avoids selectivity. The matrices allow both responses and lack of responses regarding a particular code to be examined across cases.[26] Analysis protocol included checks for consistency between codes and coding of interviews, including double coding (by two coders) half of the interviews to ensure agreement and consistency. Cases of disagreement were discussed to generate consensus on coding.

A total of six major categories related to physical activity were identified: (1) shared activity (two subcategories); (2) barriers to activity (eight subcategories); (3) knowledge of the health-promoting effects of activity (four subcategories); (4) need for change in activity (three subcategories); (5) facilitators to activity (six subcategories); and (6) control of behaviors related to activity by caregivers (three subcategories).

Results

Three important themes (Table III) identified through the six major thematic categories included: (1) sedentary behaviors, (2) barriers to physical activity, and (3) potential intervention strategies. Selective, representative quotations are presented below.

Table III Themes and Subthemes Derived from "Girls Rule!" Caregiver–Daughter Dyad Formative Research

Sedentary Behaviors
Caregivers control quality rather than quantity of TV that their daughters watch.
Caregivers generally are unaware of the amount of TV their daughters watch.
Girls prefer sedentary, rather than physically active, behaviors, with clear preference for TV viewing.
TV is perceived to fill an important role as safe and affordable child supervision.

Barriers to Physical Activity
Perceived environmental barriers, such as lack of affordable and accessible recreational resources, were believed to reduce opportunities for physical activity.
Caregivers are poor role models for a physically active lifestyle, and acknowledge their own low motivation to be physically active.

Directions for Intervention
Girls identified low-cost, low-equipment physical activities as enjoyable, such as hopscotch, jump rope, dancing, swimming, and bicycling.
Walking for exercise and transportation emerged as a potential caregiver-daughter–shared physical activity.

SEDENTARY BEHAVIORS

Findings indicate that caregivers were more concerned with the **types** of TV programs, as opposed to quantity of TV, watched by their daughters. For example, when asked about the amount of time spent watching TV, a caregiver stated, "It's fine as long as she watches kids' shows." Another caregiver stated, "They are limited in what they can watch, but we don't limit how much they can watch." Viewing rules also included completion of homework, without regard for quantity. A daughter noted, "I have to do my homework before I watch TV. If I don't do my homework, I don't watch TV." Caregivers reported that TV filled an important role as a "baby-sitter," indicating no advantages for turning the TV off. For example, a caregiver stated, "So it's [TV] pretty much to pacify them [the children] while I'm getting something done."

Caregivers reported that the girls watched a substantial amount of TV. For example, "I would say an hour or 2 hours at the most [after school] … 1.5 hours [after dinner]," and on the weekend, "If it's raining outside, all day," were reported by two different caregivers. In general, caregivers did not find the quantity of TV that their daughters viewed to be an issue; several caregivers made statements such as, "I don't think she needs to reduce it," "I think it's the right amount," and "I don't think they watch it an excessive amount of time." The girls were under the impression that there were no limits on TV quantity, and statements such as, "I can just stay up and watch TV," and "I don't think so. I don't know [whether there are rules around TV use]." There was also a clear disjunction between the caregivers' perceived control of TV and reported TV viewing. For example, one caregiver stated that her daughter watched 2 to 3 hours TV total on the weekend, while her daughter stated that she watched TV from "8:00 AM … until I fall asleep." One caregiver expressed dismay when she actually counted the number of hours of TV that her daughter watched, stating "3 hours a day, yes, that would be like 8 shows. Wow. I don't think she watches that much."

The majority of girls indicated that they did not like to play outdoors and preferred to watch TV, making statements such as "[my favorite thing is to] lay down and watch TV," and choosing to "[p]lay games, play on the computer…" rather than outdoor activities. Caregivers also stated that although they try to encourage their girls to play outside, they "can't get them to go outside." The girls reported using TV to meet specific needs, such as falling asleep or as a pick-me-up when feeling sad (e.g., "I have to look at the TV when I go to bed because it's the only way to get me to go to sleep"). If not watching TV, there was indication of substitution of other sedentary behaviors. As one caregiver reported, "Oh yeah, she'd find something else to do. If I said 'no TV,' they would run to that computer."

BARRIERS TO PHYSICAL ACTIVITY

Perceived lack of recreation-related neighborhood and household facilities and equipment was an issue. One caregiver stated, "I have tried to get [my daughter] in several activities at the park recreation department. They don't get enough kids so she can't get involved because enough kids don't sign up." Another stated, "[I would like to see] a lot more organization and a lot more availability for minorities. There is nothing around here at all. And what there is to do, half the time we can't afford it." Caregivers reported that their neighborhoods were considerably nonconducive to an active lifestyle. Common statements included: "(The traffic) is very bad … to be honest that's why I don't walk a lot," "I don't feel safe … people fly up and down the hill and act like the children are not there," and "We have also posted on our street 'no 18-wheeler trucks,' but they continue to come up the street." Several caregivers reported lack of sidewalks and streetlights in their neighborhoods, dogs that were not properly restrained, and drinking and vagrancy. Other issues included the lack of same-age children in the neighborhood and unwillingness of parents to allow their children to play outside unsupervised.

The lack of role modeling of an active lifestyle was identified as a key theme. A large number of caregivers reported that despite knowledge of positive health benefits, they did not have the motivation to be physically active. One caregiver stated, "I'm the one who is lazy and I can't make her run outside and make her do exercise while I sit there and watch TV. So I can't blame her if she wants to come inside and watch TV because she learns from example." Another caregiver stated, "I can hear my body telling me to get outside…. I can literally hear it telling me what I need to do and I'm not listening. I enjoy being myself and sitting still." Several caregivers reported that they did not participate in active games or use recreational facilities with their daughters, stating, for example, that while at parks or playgrounds, they just "observe."

(continues)

RESEARCH EXAMPLE *(continued)*

DIRECTIONS FOR INTERVENTION

The girls identified a number of physical activities that they particularly liked and were potentially good candidate intervention activities. Favorite activities included hopscotch, jumping rope, dancing, swimming, and bicycling. Other activities mentioned included soccer, basketball, skating, or riding a scooter.

In addition to the activities that the girls identified that they liked doing on their own or with their peers, the caregivers and girls were also asked to identify activities that they could enjoy participating in together. Interestingly, this question identified far more sedentary activities (e.g., watching TV and eating) than physical activities. The top choice of shared activities, among caregivers of all ages, was walking for exercise and transportation. The caregivers made statements such as the following: "If we are going to the game that day, we will just walk on down to Kenan stadium." "We might walk to the store once or twice a week together." "I think [that] … walking and taking some time for yourself physically and mentally are important." In other cases, walking was seen as a physical activity purely for exercise purposes. One caregiver said, "I think that's very important, family group kind of things where you get exercise." Another caregiver stated, "I only see myself walking [for exercise]."

Despite this interest in walking, walking was not an activity that was regularly included in their schedules because of time, motivation, or pedestrian safety. One caregiver reported, "[Walking] is not a routine." Another caregiver reported, "Now we used to try and walk at least two nights a week…. That didn't last…but a month." While a daughter stated, "Yeah, I love going on walks. But as a matter of fact, you get too hot and sweaty."

Discussion

The findings suggest that there are many household and environmental factors predisposing these girls to inactivity. The girls reported frequent participation in, and enjoyment of, sedentary behaviors, largely watching TV. There were substantial perceived environmental barriers to activity (e.g., lack of facilities, lack of sidewalks, traffic safety) and caregiver and daughter motivational barriers, including preference for sedentary behaviors. However, findings point toward important potential intervention strategies, particularly within the caregiver–daughter relationship, likely to be acceptable in this and similar settings.

Frequency of TV viewing is high among U.S. children,[6,33,34] particularly African-American youth.[6,35] While not without controversy, TV viewing has been shown to be associated with overweight.[33,36,37] That the children in this study already selectively seek out and prefer sedentary pastimes, such as TV viewing, speaks to the critical need for educational and intervention strategies with children (and parents) at a very young age. The caregivers perceive disadvantages to reducing TV time for their daughters; thus, intervention strategies must also involve safe and inexpensive child care and/or supervision.

Inactive children are likely to remain inactive throughout childhood, adolescence, and young adulthood,[38-40] and are at high risk for obesity. Prepubertal girls have lower physical activity levels than do boys,[41,42] with declines in activity starting at around age 9 to 10 years[42] and continuing throughout adolescence and young adulthood.[11,43-46] Minority adolescents, particularly girls, have especially low levels of moderate-to-vigorous physical activity.[6,11,12] Early intervention is critical.

Although the sample is small, this study uses detailed qualitative information from caregivers and daughters that is exceedingly rare. Limitations included no direct measures of physical activity and anthropometrics. However, the aim of the research was to examine the underlying factors related to obesity prevention, sedentary behaviors, barriers to physical activity, and directions for interventions, objectives for which qualitative data are most suited. In addition, accurate behavior data from recall surveys are notoriously difficult to obtain from preadolescent children.[47]

Findings from this qualitative assessment provide significant insight for the development of the Girls Rule! intervention and can help inform similar obesity prevention efforts in this very high-risk and understudied population. Clearly caregivers play a crucial role, both in terms of their own behavior modeling and control or influence over the household environment. Perceived parental enjoyment of physical activity is particularly important in encouraging girls to be active.[20] It is apparent that many caregivers are not aware of the amount of time that their daughters spend watching TV, and actually find TV to fill a beneficial role as safe and inexpensive "baby-sitting." The disadvantages to TV viewing reduction and preferences for sedentary behaviors must be addressed in intervention efforts, as these are strong barriers to reducing inactivity.

There is a perceived lack of affordable and culturally appropriate neighborhood recreational programs and facilities to provide the necessary opportunity and impetus for physical activity for these African-American girls. Indeed, there is great recent attention to such environmental correlates,[48-52] and empirical research shows a positive link between recreation facilities and activity patterns.[53,54] There is also a clear need to address individual barriers, such as motivation for activity and preference for inactivity. Many of the girls stated a preference for sedentary activities, but also described active play and games (such as jumping rope and dance) that they enjoy, particularly when part of a broader social experience.

Responding to these insights, the Girls Rule! intervention included activities of preference and initiation to new activities. Sessions with the caregiver and daughter were held concurrently, providing supervision and activity opportunities for the daughters. Educational efforts for caregivers included positive role modeling, strategies to reduce TV, and fitness sessions. Girls and caregivers were encouraged to go on walks together as a way to motivate each other and enjoy family time together—choosing walking trails, shopping malls, and other avenues where poor sidewalks and traffic issues were not barriers.

Conclusions

Findings highlight considerable individual and environmental barriers to activity among African-American female pre-adolescents. Potential intervention strategies include raising caregiver motivation for physical activity, increasing awareness of the importance of activity, countering perceptions of the positive role of TV, and increasing affordable and accessible physical activity options at the environment (e.g., sidewalks, traffic safety) and individual levels (e.g., low-cost activities, such as jumping rope, hopscotch, and walking).

What This Study Adds

Qualitative data are important to the development of health behavior interventions.

This paper presents qualitative data on household and environment barriers to physical activity in African-American, female caregiver–daughter pairs, providing a rich description of the context within which physical activity choices are made.

We have no competitive interests. Our involvement follows: PGL and PG drafted the manuscript; PGL, PG, MEB, DSW, and AA participated in study design; KK and KCS were involved in data collection; PGL, PG, and MEB were involved with data analysis and interpretation; and all read and approved the final version of the manuscript.

Funding for this study was provided by the National Heart, Lung and Blood Institute (grant R01 HL65131-02); U.S. Department of Health and Human Services, Office of Minority Health (grants 01T051701, 02T030502); and U.S. Department of Health and Human Services, Office of Women's Health (grant 01T40010901D).

We are grateful to staff members at the North Carolina churches as well as the caregivers and their daughters. In addition, we would like to thank Mikisha Brown, Amy Corneli, Mira Katz, and the Girls Rule! team for their contributions to the development of the physical activity codes. We thank the anonymous reviewers for their helpful comments.

References

1. Centers for Disease Control and Prevention, Update: prevalence of overweight among children, adolescents, and adults—United States, 1988–1994, *MMWR* **46** (1997), pp. 199–202.

(continues)

RESEARCH EXAMPLE *(continued)*

2. R.S. Strauss and H.A. Pollack, Epidemic increase in childhood overweight, 1986–1998, *JAMA* **286** (2001), pp. 2845–2848.

3. R.P. Troiano, K.M. Flegal, R.J. Kuczmarski, S.M. Campbell and C.L. Johnson, Overweight prevalence and trends for children and adolescents. The National Health and Nutrition Examination surveys, 1963 to 1991, *Arch Pediatr Adolesc Med* **149** (1995), pp. 1085–1091.

4. R.P. Troiano and K.M. Flegal, Overweight children and adolescents: description, epidemiology and demographics, *Pediatrics* **101** (1998), pp. 497–504.

5. C.L. Ogden, R.P. Troiano, R.R. Briefel, R.J. Kuczmarski, K.M. Flegal and C.L. Johnson, Prevalence of overweight among preschool children in the United States, 1971 through 1994, *Pediatrics* **99** (1997), p. E1.

6. P. Gordon-Larsen, R.G. McMurray and B.M. Popkin, Adolescent physical activity and inactivity vary by ethnicity: the National Longitudinal Study of Adolescent Health, *J Pediatr* **135** (1999), pp. 301–306.

7. P. Gordon-Larsen, Obesity-related knowledge, attitudes, and behaviors in obese and non-obese urban Philadelphia adolescents, *Obes Res* **9** (2001), pp. 112–118.

8. C.L. Ogden, K.M. Flegal, M.D. Carroll and C.L. Johnson, Prevalence and trends in overweight among US children and adolescents, 1999–2000, *JAMA* **288** (2002), pp. 1728–1732.

9. M.K. Serdula, D. Ivery, R.J. Coates, D.S. Freedman, D.F. Williamson and T. Byers, Do obese children become obese adults: a review of the literature, *Prev Med* **22** (1993), pp. 167–177.

10. M.I. Goran, B.A. Gower, T.R. Nagy and R.K. Johnson, Developmental changes in energy expenditure and physical activity in children: evidence for a decline in physical activity in girls before puberty, *Pediatrics* **101** (1998), pp. 887–891.

11. L.G. Bandini, A. Must, J.L. Spadano and W.H. Dietz, Relation of body composition, parental overweight, pubertal state and race-ethnicity to energy expenditure among premenarcheal girls, *Am J Clin Nutr* **76** (2002), pp. 1040–1047.

12. S.Y. Kimm, N.W. Glynn and A.M Kriska *et al.*, Decline in physical activity in black girls and white girls during adolescence, *N Engl J Med* **347** (2002), pp. 709–715.

13. W.H. Dietz, Health consequences of obesity in youth: childhood predictors of adult disease, *Pediatrics* **101** (1998), pp. 518–525.

14. J. Wardle, C. Guthrie, S. Sanderson, L.L. Birch and R. Plomin, Food and activity preferences in children of lean and obese parents, *Int J Obes Relat Metab Disord* **25** (2001), pp. 147–157.

15. K.K. Davison and L.L. Birch, Obesigenic families: parents' physical activity and dietary intake patterns predict girls' risk of overweight, *Int J Obes Relat Metab Disord* **26** (2002), pp. 1186–1193.

16. L.A. Francis, Y. Lee and L.L. Birch, Parental weight status and girls' television viewing, snacking, and body mass indexes, *Obes Res* **11** (2003), pp. 143–151.

17. S.C. Cunnane, Childhood origins of lifestyle-related risk factors for coronary heart disease in adulthood, *Nutr Health* **9** (1993), pp. 107–115.

18. M.T. McGuire, P.J. Hannan, D. Neumark-Sztainer, N.H. Cossrow and M. Story, Parental correlates of physical activity in a racially/ethnically diverse adolescent sample, *J Adolesc Health* **30** (2002), pp. 253–261.

19. J.F. Sallis, J.J. Prochaska, W.C. Taylor, J.O. Hill and J.C. Geraci, Correlates of physical activity in a national sample of girls and boys in grades 4 through 12, *Health Psychol* **18** (1999), pp. 410–415.

20. R.J. Brustad, Attraction to physical activity in urban schoolchildren: parental socialization and gender influences, *Res Q Exerc Sport* **67** (1996), pp. 316–323.

21. L.B. Randsell, A. Taylor, D. Oakland, J. Schmidt, L. Moyer-Milleur and B. Schultz, Daughters and mothers exercising together: effects of home- and community-based programs, *Med Sci Sports Exerc* **35** (2003), pp. 286–296.

22. S.K. Kumanyika, E. Obarzanek, T.N. Robinson and B.M. Beech, Phase 1 of the Girls Health Enrichment Multi-site Studies (GEMS) conclusion, *Ethn Dis* **13** (2003) (suppl 1), pp. S88–91.

23. R. Baranowski, K.C. Anderson and C. Carmack, Mediating variable framework in physical activity interventions How are we doing? How might we do better? *Am J Prev Med* **15** (1998), pp. 266–297.

24. A. Jain, S.N. Sherman, D.L. Chamberlin, Y. Carter, S.W. Powers and R.C. Whitaker, Why don't low-income mothers worry about their preschoolers being overweight?, *Pediatrics* **107** (2001), pp. 1138–1146.

25. K.R. Ginsburg, P.M. Alexander, J. Hunt, M. Sullivan and A. Cnaan, Enhancing their likelihood for a positive future: focus groups reveal the voice of inner-city youth, *Pediatrics* **109** (2002), pp. 1136–1142.

26. M.E. Bentley, L. Gavin, M.M. Black and L. Teti, Infant feeding practices of low-income, African-American, adolescent mothers: an ecological, multigenerational perspective, *Soc Sci Med* **49** (1999), pp. 1085–1100.

27. M.E. Bentley, D. Dee and J.L. Jensen, Breastfeeding among low-income, African American women: power, beliefs, and decision making, *J Nutr* **133** (2003) 305S–9S.

28. L.E. Gavin, M.M. Black, S. Minor, Y. Abel, M.A. Papas and M.E. Bentley, Young, disadvantaged fathers' involvement with their infants: an ecological perspective, *J Adolesc Health* **31** (2002), pp. 266–276.

29. Ammerman A, Kelsey K. Girls Rule: church and home-based project for 6–9 year old African American girls. In: Kumanyika SK, Obarzanek E, eds. Proceedings from Investigators Workshop on Innovative Approaches to Prevention of Obesity, Pathways to Obesity Prevention. Arlington VA, August 12–13, 2002:42–54.

30. Katz ML, Gordon-Larsen P, Bentley ME, Kelsey K, Shields K, Ammerman A. "Does skinny mean healthy?" Perceived ideal, current, and healthy body sizes among African American girls and their female caregivers. Ethn Dis 2004. In press.

31. M.Q. Patton, Qualitative evaluation and research methods, Sage Publications, Newbury Park, CA (1990).

32. M.B. Miles and A.M. Huberman, Qualitative data analysis, Sage Publications, Thousand Oaks, CA (1994).

33. R.E. Andersen, C.J. Crespo, S.J. Bartlett, L.J. Cheskin and M. Pratt, Relationship of physical activity and television watching with body weight and level of fatness among children. Results from the Third National Health and Nutrition Examination Survey, *JAMA* **279** (1998), pp. 938–942.

34. Roberts DF, Foehr UG, Rideout VJ, Brodie M. Kids and media at the new millennium: a comprehensive national analysis of childrens' media use. Menlo Park, CA: Henry J. Kaiser Family Foundation, 1999.

35. C.J. Crespo, E. Smit, R.P. Troian, S.J. Bartlett, C.A. Macera and R.E. Andersen, Television watching, energy intake, and obesity in US children, *Arch Pediatr Adolesc Med* **155** (2001), pp. 360–365.

36. W.H. Dietz and S.L. Gortmaker, Do we fatten our children at the television set? Obesity and television viewing in children and adolescents, *Pediatrics* **75** (1985), pp. 807–812.

37. P. Gordon-Larsen, L.S. Adair and B.M. Popkin, US adolescent physical activity and inactivity patterns are associated with overweight: the National Longitudinal Study of Adolescent Health, *Obes Res* **10** (2002), pp. 141–149.

38. O.T. Raitakari, K.V. Porkka, S. Taimela, R. Telama, L. Rasanen and J.S. Viikari, Effects of persistent physical activity and inactivity on coronary risk factors in children and young adults The Cardiovascular Risk in Young Finns Study, *Am J Epidemiol* **140** (1994), pp. 195–205.

39. D.E. Bild, D.R. Jacobs Jr, S. Sydney, W.L. Haskell, N. Anderssen and A. Oberman, Physical activity in young black and white women. The CARDIA Study, *Ann Epidemiol* **3** (1993), pp. 636–644.

40. Kemper HC, Post GB, Twisk JW, van Mechelen W. Lifestyle and obesity in adolescence and young adulthood: results from the Amsterdam Growth and Health Longitudinal Study (AGAHLS). Int J Obes 1999; 23(suppl 3):S34–40.

41. B.G. Simons-Morton, R.J. McKenzie and E Stone *et al.*, Physical activity in a multiethnic population of third graders in four states, *Am J Public Health* **87** (1997), pp. 45–50.

42. S.G. Trost, R.R. Pate and J.F Sallis *et al.*, Age and gender differences in objectively measured physical activity in youth, *Med Sci Sports Exerc* **34** (2002), pp. 350–355.

43. J.F. Sallis, J.J. Prochaska and W.C. Taylor, A review of correlates of physical activity of children and adolescents, *Med Sci Sports Exerc* **32** (2000), pp. 963–975.

44. S.H. Kelder, C.L. Perry, K.I. Klepp and L.L. Lytle, Longitudinal tracking of adolescent smoking, physical activity, and food choice behaviors, *Am J Public Health* **84** (1994), pp. 1121–1126.

(continues)

RESEARCH EXAMPLE *(continued)*

45. N. Armstrong, J.R. Weisman and B.J. Kirby, Longitudinal changes in 11–13-year-olds' physical activity, *Acta Paediatr* **89** (2000), pp. 775–780.
46. Gordon-Larsen P, Nelson MC, Popkin BM. Longitudinal physical activity and sedentary behavior trends: Adolescents to adulthood. *Am J Prev Med* (in press).
47. H.W. Kohl, J.E. Fulton and C.J. Caspersen, Assessment of physical activity among children and adolescents: a review and synthesis, *Prev Med* **31** (2000), pp. S54–S76.
48. G. Egger and B. Swinburn, An "ecological" approach to the obesity pandemic, *BMJ* **315** (1997), pp. 477–480.
49. M. Nestle and M.F. Jacobson, Halting the obesity epidemic, *Public Health Rep* **115** (2000), pp. 12–24.
50. B. Swinburn, G. Egger and F. Raza, Dissecting obesogenic environments. The development and application of a framework for identifying and prioritizing environmental interventions for obesity, *Prev Med* **29** (1999), pp. 563–570.
51. J.F. Sallis, A. Bauman and M. Pratt, Environmental and policy interventions to promote physical activity, *Am J Prev Med* **15** (1998), pp. 379–397.
52. U.S. Department of Health and Human Services. The Surgeon General's call to action to prevent and decrease overweight and obesity. Rockville MD: U.S. Department of Health and Human Services, Public Health Service, Office of the Surgeon General, 2001.
53. P. Gordon-Larsen, R.G. McMurray and B.M. Popkin, Determinants of adolescent physical activity and inactivity patterns, *Pediatrics* **105** (2000), pp. 1–8.
54. R.C. Brownson, R.A. Houseman and D.R Brown *et al.*, Promoting physical activity in rural communities: walking trail access, use, and effects, *Am J Prev Med* **15** (2000), pp. 235–241.

SAMPLE CRITIQUE A Qualitative Study

STANDARD 1: DESCRIPTIVE VIVIDNESS

1. *Significance:* Both the "Introduction" and the literature review sections of the article demonstrate a paucity of research on African American girls who are at risk for being overweight (Gordon-Larsen et al., 2004).

No previous studies have included the perspectives of both girls and their female caregivers. This study focused on girls and their caregivers but did not present matched-pair results. In addition, responses for a given girl and her caregiver were not compared and contrasted. Responses of all of the girls and of all of the caregivers were reported, but a comparison of the responses of family members was not provided. It also would have been helpful to have the responses of the mothers compared and contrasted with those of the grandmothers. Likewise, it would have been interesting to hear whether the granddaughters' and daughters' responses were similar. Matched-pair comparisons would have added to the significance of the study.

The study does fill a significant gap in the literature and helps to identify interventions that could address the problem of barriers to physical activity in African American girls and their mothers/grandmothers. As the researchers point out, both health and psychosocial risks associated with being overweight as a young girl track into adolescence and adulthood, making this a significant area of study.

2. *Purpose:* The authors state that "the aim of this qualitative research is to explore perceptions of sedentary behaviors, barriers to, and facilitators of physical activity and directions for intervention factors in this high-risk population [African-American girls and their female caregivers]" (Gordon-Larsen et al., 2004, p. 481*).

*Page numbers in this critique refer to the version of the article reprinted in this book.

It was not clear whether another aim of the study was to explore eating patterns. The authors stated that the interviews focused on diet and its correlates, but they did not present results about diet. The researchers could have strengthened the article by including a clear statement about the study purpose and reiterating it consistently throughout the article.

3. *Interpretation and analysis:* Clearly, the girls preferred sedentary activities such as watching TV. The authors interpreted this preference as being influenced by caregiver's role modeling. Subtle aspects of how adult role modeling influences children's behavior could have been provided as the authors interpreted the significance of this finding. The authors also stated that TV was used as a "pick-me-up" or a sleep aid. However, were there other factors such as "being in the know" and being able to discuss a popular TV show with one's peers that made a difference in the girl's preferences? Why didn't caregivers and girls select to watch a Jazzercise or yoga exercise program on TV together? Additional interpretation and analysis would have helped to explain the quotes that were presented.

Two of the caregivers commented that they were not active because they (1) felt lazy from time to time and (2) enjoyed being alone and still. What meanings are associated with these comments? What did these comments have to say about the overall context of the caregivers' lives? Again, additional interpretation and analysis would have added depth to the research report (Huberman & Miles, 2002).

The quotes also indicated that not getting into a routine of walking kept caregivers and daughters from walking together on a regular basis. The authors did not explore what interfered with establishing such a routine other than traffic and lack of sidewalks. In general, more quotes than interpretations were provided in the article. Adding additional interpretation and analysis would have strengthened the article. The authors may have been limited in their interpretation and analysis by the number of pages allowed by the given journal. However, overall additional time spent on interpretation would have yielded richer understandings.

STANDARD 2: METHODOLOGICAL CONGRUENCE

Adequate Documentation of the Participants

1. *Description of study participants:* Twelve African American girls and their 11 female caregivers (8 mothers and 3 grandmothers) participated. Girls ranged in age from 6 to 9 years, with a median age of 7.8. The age ranges of the female caregivers were not provided, although this information would have been of interest. Female caregivers had a median age of 41.8 years. Everyone who met the inclusion criteria and volunteered to be interviewed was included. No mention was made of the caregivers' educational background or socioeconomic or employment status. It wasn't clear whether all the caregivers were single parents. It also wasn't clear whether the caregivers were responsible for any children other than the girls who were interviewed. Additional description of the participants would have strengthened the study.

2. *Selection of participants:* Obesity is a major health disparity affecting African American girls and female teens. A major strength of the study was the inclusion of African American girls. Studying matched-pair dyads of girls and female caregivers was another strength because it is likely that the female caregivers purchased the family food, gave their daughters or granddaughters permission to exercise or not, and served as role models for diet and exercise. A third strength of this study was the clear rationale for selecting African American girls and their female caregivers.

3. *Applicability to other settings:* Participants were recruited from North Carolina churches. The church members lived in suburban neighborhoods of median income. It would have been helpful to know whether the caregivers were single parents. The authors did not explicitly state whether the churches were primarily African American, although they were selected as sites for the Girls Rule! program for African American girls.

(continues)

SAMPLE CRITIQUE (*continued*)

It would have been helpful to have more of an objective description of the suburban neighborhood in terms of safety, availability of recreational facilities and parks, traffic patterns, sidewalks, lighting, and air quality. Problems in these areas can be assumed, because some of the participants described cancellation of parks and recreation classes because of lack of participation, bad traffic, no sidewalks, no street lights, and unrestrained dogs, as well as drinking and vagrancy issues. It isn't clear whether the entire neighborhood suffered these problems or only a few caregivers identified these concerns.

The authors did not specify whether the interviews took place at the church, in the homes of the participants, at the university, or at a location of the participant's choice. Generally, authors describe where interviews were conducted.

Careful Attention to Procedural Approach

1. *Articulation of assumptions:* The authors did not describe their assumptions; therefore, it cannot be determined whether the data collection procedures were congruent with the assumptions.

2. *Establishment of trust:* The authors did not mention whether any of the data collectors were African American or had an established relationship with this community. Because National Institutes of Health (NIH) funding for this study existed, it can be assumed that a strong letter of support was provided by the church, and indeed such a relationship did exist. Trust of researchers by the study community is extremely important in conducting qualitative studies. It would have been helpful in determining the level of trust to know how many potential subjects received the screening questionnaires from the pastor. How many total caregivers were contacted to yield the 11 who participated?

Because the interview guide and research questions used were not provided, it is not possible to assess whether an open dialogue and conversational approach were used during the interviews. Some of the published responses appeared to be succinct, possibly indicating that an easy conversational dialogue was not achieved. However, the interview guide, research questions, and detailed participants' responses were probably not included due to space limitations of the journal.

3. *Articulation of research questions:* Specific research questions were not listed. The authors state that the interviews focused overall on (1) diet and correlates, (2) activity, and (3) potential interventions. They also mention that the study focused on physical activity, neighborhood characteristics, and caregiver-daughter shared activities.

It may be that page limits prohibited the authors from including a list of the research questions. However, it would have significantly strengthened this study to provide a table of the actual research questions. It isn't possible to assess whether the questions were appropriate for the methodological approach used, age levels of participants, and study aims without such a list.

4. *Consistency of data collectors during the data collection process:* Were the same exact questions and follow-up inquiries used by the four different data collectors? Were there differences in depth of responses obtained among interviewers for certain questions?

Having a table of research questions would have been helpful because up to three interviews per dyad were scheduled. Some dyads completed only two interviews, with data missing for some questions. It is not clear how many dyads declined to answer certain questions and whether the depth of the responses was consistent among different interviewers.

The "Instruments" section of the study states that four interviewers worked in two pairs, but the acknowledgments section at the end of the article lists only the two authors as data collectors. Does this mean that two data collectors who were not authors were used? Clarity of who collected the data would have strengthen this article.

5. *Description of data collection process:* The authors clearly described some aspects of the data collection process but needed more detail in other areas. Interviews were conducted from April to October of 2000.

The researchers placed the girls and their caretakers in separate rooms and conducted 51 interviews with 23 participants. Respondents participated in a mean of 2.4 interviews, with interviews lasting approximately 1 hour each. The authors reported the interviews were recorded and transcribed, a strength of the study. It is not clear where the interviews were conducted, nor can the interviewers' levels of experience in qualitative research or familiarity with the population be determined.

The authors needed to indicate whether results differed for the first and subsequent interviews. How did different data collectors follow up to obtain missing data? Why does one section of the report state that four data collectors were used and another that only the two authors participated in data collection? Several questions about the data collection process remain unanswered.

6. *Time spent with participants:* The data collectors met with the participants on more than one occasion (a mean of 2.4 interviews each), which is a strength of this study. However, the authors mention that in spite of the use of multiple interviews, data were missing. The missing data were not identified.

The authors state that they based their interview schedule on pilot data that "indicated approximately 180 minutes of interview time, divided into three 60-minute parts, given caregiver schedules and the girls' attention spans" would be reasonable (Gordon-Larsen et al., 2004, p. 481). Because the authors had anticipated that three interviews might be needed for some dyads, and a mean of only 2.4 were conducted, it appears some participants ran out of things to say before others. The authors did not address whether the data were saturated (no new themes arising with additional interviews), with repeated themes showing up by the second interview. The discussion of whether saturation of data was reached is common in qualitative research and would have added to the clarity to the study findings.

7. *Similarity of approach:* Insufficient information is provided to know whether the approaches of multiple data collectors were similar. A list of interview questions and a description of how different interviewers approached follow-up questions should have been included. The authors did not compare the qualifications of the data collectors or discuss any previous experiences with this population. The authors state that some data were missing but not whether differences existed between data collectors in terms of the richness of data, length of interviews, or amount of missing data.

8. *Rationale for selection method:* The authors provide a good explanation of why African American girls and their female caretakers were selected as participants.

The researchers gained through "church pastors and liaisons that disseminated screening questionnaires in their churches" (Gordon-Larsen et al., 2004, p. 481). It is unclear how many questionnaires were distributed and how many were returned. It is also unclear if questionnaires were given out on more than one day. It is likely that the African American mothers and grandmothers trusted their pastor and were more willing to participate if he or she was supportive of the study. So contacting participants through churches is a strength of the study to gain an adequate sample for this study.

9. *Role of the researcher during the interview process:* The authors did not describe the role of the researchers in data collection and analysis. Did the researchers involve the participants in a conversational dialogue? Did they "bracket off" their own knowledge and beliefs (Husserlian phenomenology) or did they use those views to elicit a richer response from the participants (Heideggerian phenomenology)?

Adherence to Ethical Standards

Ethical standards—including acknowledgment of participant rights, informed consent, and protection of participant rights—must have been followed, because the data collection procedures adhered to those established by the University of North Carolina's School of Public Health Institutional Review Board. Because the study had NIH funding, all researchers were required to complete human subjects' protection training. It would have been helpful to know whether participants were compensated for participating in the study and, if so, in what manner. Additionally, the authors might have specified whether identifying information was eliminated from the transcribed interviews to protect the anonymity of the participants.

(continues)

SAMPLE CRITIQUE *(continued)*

Auditability

1. *Decision trail:* The authors describe using a matrix-based analysis but do not detail the specifics of this process. During data analysis, the researchers clearly indicated the categories developed to encompass their data.

"A total of six major categories related to physical activity were identified: (1) share activity (two subcategories); (2) barriers to activity (eight subcategories); (3) knowledge of health-promoting effects of activity (four subcategories); (4) need for change in activity (three subcategories); (5) facilitators to activity (six subcategories); and (6) control of behaviors related to activity by caregivers (three sub-categories). Three important themes (Table I, p. 482) identified through the six major thematic categories included: (1) sedentary behaviors, (2) barriers to physical activity, and (3) potential intervention strategies." (Gordon-Larsen et al., 2004, p. 482)

The researchers need to detail how the six thematic categories and three main themes are related. The subcategories within the thematic categories also need to be explained and more detail is needed to clarify how the six thematic categories were developed from the participants' original quotes.

2. *Sufficiency of quotations:* Participant quotations were included, but they were typically only one or two sentences long. It is hard to tell whether the quotations were shortened to adhere to the space limitations of the journal or whether the interviewers were not sufficiently experienced in eliciting detailed responses from participants.

When respondents gave quotations such as "my favorite thing to do is to lie down and watch TV," interviewers should have followed up with a question about what was enjoyable about lying down to watch TV. Why was this activity more fun than other activities? The girls' reports of using TV as a sleep aid or a "pick-me-up" called for a follow-up question about how TV worked to help them fall asleep or make them feel happier. Did the girls have other ways of relaxing or improving their mood? Most of the quotations leave the reader wanting to know more. Richer quotes would have been more informative but might have been limited by the space requirement of the journal.

3. *Sufficiency of data:* In the category of "sedentary behaviors," 15 of 17 quotations had to do with watching TV. Two quotations discussed the selection of computer activities if TV was denied. The entire category might be more accurately described as "TV viewing as a favorite sedentary behavior." The quotations the authors included did not all refer to possible sedentary behaviors; rather, they mentioned the primary sedentary behavior of TV viewing. In this case, the findings and supportive quotes were not perfectly aligned.

In the category of "barriers to physical activities," the authors provided sufficient quotations to support their conclusions regarding a lack of (1) affordable and available recreational activities, (2) safe places to walk and play, and (3) role modeling of an active lifestyle. This section used specific quotations and examples to document the conclusions.

In the category of "directions for intervention," the authors reported that girls identified liking hopscotch, jumping rope, dancing, swimming, bicycling, soccer, basketball, skating, and scooter riding. Because some of these activities, such as jumping rope and dancing, can be done inside the house and others, such as hopscotch and basketball, can be done in the safety of a suburban backyard, more quotations are needed to explain why the girls did not engage in these activities. The authors did not provide specific examples of when the girls last enjoyed these behaviors. The interventions suggested lacked the specific examples to support that the girls would try them rather than watching TV.

STANDARD 3: ANALYTICAL AND INTERPRETATIVE PRECISENESS

1. *Picture of phenomenon:* The "directions for intervention" results do not clearly link with the other findings. If the girls are able to identify liking hopscotch, jumping rope, dancing, swimming, bicycling,

soccer, basketball, skating, and scooter riding, why did they spend so much of their time watching TV? How could the girls pursue swimming, bicycling, soccer, skating, and scooter riding if the neighborhood did not have safe parks where such activities could be enjoyed? The interventions suggested require more supporting evidence that the girls would try them.

The themes of "barriers to physical activity," "sedentary behaviors," and "directions for intervention" did not yield a consistent, meaningful picture. Rather, results from one theme seem to undermine the results of another theme—probably because space limitations prohibited the inclusion of detailed quotations that would have addressed the inconsistencies. Alternatively, the authors could have included a detailed interpretation of why all of these results could simultaneously be true.

2. *Validation of findings:* No indication is provided that the authors validated their findings with the girls or their caretakers or with experts in the area of African American child obesity.

3. *Multiple researcher participation:* The acknowledgments section describes two authors as participating in the data analysis. In the "Data Analysis" section, the authors state that "individual researchers read all interviews and the team evaluated main codes and text samples" (Gordon-Larsen et al., 2004, p. 482). Half of the interviews were double-coded by two coders, as indicated by the statement "Cases of disagreement were discussed to generate consensus on coding" (p. 482). These descriptions of who participated in data analysis might have more detail.

STANDARD 4: PHILOSOPHICAL OR THEORETICAL CONNECTEDNESS

1. *Clear connection between data and nursing practice:* Although this was not a nursing study, the authors identified quality interventions that were derived from the research findings. They also emphasized the critical need for educational strategies targeting the disadvantages of watching TV. The need for educational sessions to sensitize caregivers to the amount of time their children spend watching TV also was detailed. In addition, the authors highlighted the need for affordable neighborhood recreational programs and facilities. Motivating caregivers to engage in physical activity was another intervention the researchers stressed, and they encouraged incorporating shared caregiver and daughter activities into the Girls Rule! intervention program. These are some excellent ideas to respond to the problems of TV watching and sedentary activities of the study participants.

2. *Identification of study basis:* It was not clear what philosophical or theoretical basis was used in the study because the authors did not cite their philosophical or theoretical sources. The researchers described their method as a qualitative approach but did not specify ethnography, grounded theory, Heideggerian phenomenology, Husserlian phenomenology, or some other qualitative approach. Sometimes these distinctions can be determined by looking at the reference section of the paper, but in this case the methodological approach is not clear.

3. *Consistency of study basis and analytical methods:* The authors did not clarify what philosophical or theoretical basis was used in the study. So it was difficult to determine if the assumptions, data collection, and methods of analysis were consistent. Nevertheless, these criteria are major factors to consider in evaluating qualitative research.

For example, in grounded theory, the purpose is to develop a theory based on participant perspectives. This would not be a reasonable goal in phenomenology. In Husserlian phenomenology, a typical assumption is that the researcher should distance himself or herself from any personal experience, knowledge, or understanding that could influence data analysis. An assumption of Heideggerian phenomenology is that it is not possible to block all of one's knowledge, beliefs, and values. A researcher who steps away from his or her background understandings will find it harder to conduct a sensitive interview and to produce a rich, nuanced interpretation of the phenomenon being studied (Benner, 1994). Being clear about the philosophical or theoretical approach used in a qualitative study is a critically important factor.

(continues)

SAMPLE CRITIQUE *(continued)*

STANDARD 5: HEURISTIC RELEVANCE

Intuitive Recognition

1. *Recognizability of phenomenon:* A strength of the study is that the findings match common understandings. It is reasonable that most children learn their activity preferences by role modeling the activity level of their caretakers. Any parent can relate to not allowing children to go outside to exercise unless the environment is safe and available parks and recreational facilities exist. Additionally, most parents have experienced not having sufficient time or the energy to be a perfect role model of an active lifestyle.

Relationship to Existing Body of Knowledge

1. *Examination of existing body of knowledge:* The researchers do an excellent job of linking their findings to those of other studies. In the "Discussion" section, the authors referenced their own research and the work of other investigators who have found that TV viewing is associated with being overweight (Andersen Crespo, Bartlett, Cheskin, & Pratt, 1998; Dietz, & Gortmaker, 1985; Gordon-Larsen, Adair, & Popkin, 2002). They discussed other studies that mentioned that inactive children are likely to remain inactive throughout life (Kemper, Post, Twisk, & van Mechelen, 1999; Kimm et al., 2002; Raitakari, Porkka, Taimela, Telama, Rasanen, & Viikari, 1994). The authors identified other researchers who have shown that African-American teens have low levels of physical exercise (Bandini, Must, Spadano, & Dietz, 2002; Gordon-Larsen, McMurray, & Popkin, 1999; Kimm et al., 2002). They listed other studies that have shown "parental enjoyment of physical activity is particularly important in encouraging girls to be active" (Brustad, 1996, p. 221). Finally, the authors identified other studies that point to environmental correlates between activity levels and safe recreational facilities (Brownson et al., 2000; Gordon-Larsen, McMurray, & Popkin, 2000).

2. *Comparison/contrast with other studies:* None of the study findings contradicted the results of other studies.

3. *Description of lacunae:* The unique aspect of this study is the focus on African American children and their care providers and their perception of sedentary behaviors, barriers to and facilitators of physical activity, and directions for interventions. This is significant because this population is at high risk for obesity. Previous research has focused on other populations, and the findings from this study support the findings from other studies (Davidson & Birch, 2002; McGuire, Hannan, Neumark-Sztainer, Cossrow & Story, 2002).

Applicability to Nursing Practice, Research, or Education

1. *Relevance to nursing practice, nursing research, or nursing education:* Although this is not a nursing study, the findings are relevant to the practice of school nurses, pediatric nurses, home health nurses, mental health nurses, public health nurses, pediatric nurse practitioners, and family nurse practitioners who make exercise and dietary recommendations to families and children. These study findings also are valuable as a basis for future research by nurses and other health professionals seeking to expand current understanding of and potential management for African American children experiencing obesity and sedentary lifestyle.

2. *Uniqueness of information:* The authors clearly identified the importance of lack of role modeling in terms of developing exercise patterns in African American girls. This addresses a very important gap in the literature and provides a basis for future research.

3. *Implications for related cases:* The findings have implications for any child who lives in an unsafe neighborhood or an area that lacks ample parks and affordable recreational activities. It is likely that most children are drawn to sedentary activities such as TV viewing in today's world. Children in all families learn to mimic the activity level of their caretakers. A strength of the study is that the implications are relevant for related cases.

4. *Suggestions for further study:* Most of the "Discussion" section focuses on intervention strategies, rather than on suggestions for future research. However, the authors do mention a need to examine individual barriers, such as lack of motivation to engage in exercise in subsequent studies.

In any critique, the summary of strengths will indicate the researcher's adherence to the standards; the summary of weaknesses will indicate the potential threats to the integrity of the study. If the overall study strengths outweigh the study weaknesses, a qualitative study can make a substantial contribution to the literature even if all of the evaluation criteria are not met. The study by Gordon-Larsen et al. demonstrates more strengths than weaknesses and does contribute to the understanding of African American girls and their care takers regarding their diet patterns and limited involvement in physical activities. The critique of a qualitative study increases understanding of the qualitative research process and provides direction for future research in the area of the study.

KEY CONCEPTS

- An intellectual critique of research requires careful examination of all aspects of a study to judge its strengths, weaknesses, meaning, and significance.
- Research is critiqued to broaden understanding, improve practice, and provide a background for conducting a study.
- All nurses, including students, practicing nurses, nurse administrators, nurse educators, and nurse researchers, need research critique expertise.
- The quantitative research critique process includes comprehension, comparison, analysis, and evaluation.
- The standards for critique of qualitative studies include descriptive vividness, methodological congruence, analytical and interpretative preciseness, philosophical or theoretical connectedness, and heuristic relevance.

TIPS FOR FURTHER STUDY

- To review the phases of the critique process, answer the questions in Chapter 13 of your Companion CD-ROM and in the Open-Book Quiz at http://evolve.elsevier.com/Burns/ understanding.
- Review the guidelines for conducting a critique in Table 13-1. This content will help you gain an overall understanding of the elements of the research critique process.
- Read the quantitative articles in the study guide that accompanies this text and conduct a critique of these studies using the quantitative research critique process that includes comprehension, comparison, analysis, and evaluation.
- Conduct a critique of the qualitative study in the study guide and use the standards for critique of qualitative studies, which include descriptive vividness, methodological congruence, analytical and interpretative preciseness, philosophical or theoretical connectedness, and heuristic relevance.

REFERENCES

Andersen, R. E., Crespo, C. J., Bartlett, S. J., Cheskin, L. J., & Pratt, M. (1998). Relationship of physical activity and television watching with body weight and level of fatness among children. Results from the Third National Health and Nutrition Examination Survey. *Journal of the American Medical Association, 279*(12), 938–942.

Bandini, L. G., Must, A., Spadano, J. L., & Dietz, W. H. (2002). Relation of body composition, parental overweight, pubertal stage, and race-ethnicity to energy expenditure among premenarcheal girls. *American Journal of Clinical Nutrition, 76*(5), 1040–1047.

Beck, C. T. (1993). Technical Notes: Qualitative research: The evaluation of its credibility, fittingness, and auditability. *Western Journal of Nursing Research, 15*(2), 263–266.

Benner, P. (1994). *Interpretive phenomenology: Embodiment, caring, and ethics in health and illness.* London: Sage Publications.

Benton, J. G., Brown, H., & Rusk, H. A. (1950). Energy expended by patients on the bedpan and bedside commode. *Journal of the American Medical Association, 144*(17), 1443–1447.

Brown, S. J. (1999). *Knowledge for health care practice: A guide to using research evidence.* Philadelphia: Saunders.

Brown, S. J. (2002). Focus on research methods. Nursing intervention studies: A descriptive analysis of issues important to clinicians. *Research in Nursing & Health, 25*(4), 317–327.

Brownson, R. C., Houseman, R. A., Brown, D. R., Jackson-Thompson, J., King, A. C., Malone, B. R., et al. (2000). Promoting physical activity in rural communities: Walking trail access, use, and effects. *American Journal of Preventive Medicine, 18*(3), 235–241.

Brustad, R. J. (1996). Attraction to physical activity in urban schoolchildren: Parental socialization and gender influences. *Research Quarterly for Exercise and Sport, 67*(3), 316–323.

Burns, N. (1989). Standards for qualitative research. *Nursing Science Quarterly, 2*(1), 44–52.

Burns, N., & Grove, S. K. (2005). *The practice of nursing research: Conduct, critique, and utilization* (5th ed.). Philadelphia: Saunders.

Cesario, S., Morin, K., & Santa-Donato, A. (2002). Evaluating the level of evidence of qualitative research. *Journal of Obstetric, Gynecologic, and Neonatal Nursing, 31*(6), 708–714.

Davidson, K. K., & Birch, L. L. (2002). Obesigenic families: Parents' physical activity and dietary intake patterns predict girls' risk of overweight. *International Journal of Obesity and Related Metabolic Disorders, 26*(9), 1186–1193.

DeKeyser, F. G., & Pugh, L. C. (1990). Assessment of reliability and validity of biochemical measures. *Nursing Research, 39*(5), 314–317.

Denzin, N. K., & Lincoln, Y. S. (Eds.) (2002). *The qualitative inquiry reader.* Thousand Oaks, CA: Sage Publications.

Dietz, W. H., & Gortmaker, S. L. (1985). Do we fatten our children at the television set? Obesity and television viewing in children and adolescents. *Pediatrics, 75*(5), 807–812.

Duffy, M. E. (1988). Statistics: Friend or foe? *Nursing & Health Care, 9*(2), 73–75.

Glaser, B., & Strauss, A. L. (1965). Discovery of substantive theory: A basic strategy underlying qualitative research. *American Behavioral Scientist, 8*(1), 5–12.

Gordon-Larsen, P., Adair, L. S., & Popkin, B. M. (2002). Ethnic differences in physical activity and inactivity patterns and overweight status. *Obesity Research, 10*(3), 141–149.

Gordon-Larsen, P., Griffiths, P., Bentley, M. E., Ward, D. S., Kelsey, K., Shields, K., et al. (2004). Barriers to physical activity: Qualitative data on caregiver–daughter perceptions and practices. *American Journal of Preventative Medicine, 27*(3), 218–223.

Gordon-Larsen, P., McMurray, R. G., & Popkin, B. M. (1999). Adolescent physical activity and inactivity vary by ethnicity: The National Longitudinal Study of Adolescent Health. *Journal of Pediatrics, 135*(3), 301–306.

Gordon-Larsen, P., McMurray, R. G., & Popkin, B. M. (2000). Determinants of adolescent physical activity and inactivity patterns. *Pediatrics, 105*(6), 1–8.

Guba, E. G., & Lincoln, Y. S. (1982). *Effective evaluation.* Washington, DC: Jossey-Bass.

Hamer, S., & Collinson, G. (1999). *Achieving evidence-based practice: A handbook for practitioners.* Edinburgh: Baillière Tindall.

Hawker, S. Payne, S., Kerr, C., Hardey, M., & Powell, J. (2002). Appraising the evidence: Reviewing disparate data systematically. *Qualitative Health Research, 12*(9), 1284–1299.

Huberman, A. M., & Miles, M. B. (2002). *The qualitative researcher's companion.* Thousand Oaks, CA: Sage Publications.

Kemper, H. C., Post, G. B., Twisk, J. W., & van Mechelen, W. (1999). Lifestyle and obesity in adolescence and young adulthood: Results from the Amsterdam Growth and Health Longitudinal Study (AGAHLS). *International Journal of Obesity and Related Metabolic Disorders, 23*(Suppl. 3), S34–S40.

Kimm, S. Y., Glynn, N. W., Kriska, A. M., et al., (2002). Decline in physical activity in black girls and white girls during adolescence. *The New England Journal of Medicine, 347*(10), 709–715.

Kirk, J., & Miller, M. L. (1986). *Reliability and validity in qualitative research.* Beverly Hills, CA: Sage.

Knafl, K. A., & Howard, M. J. (1984). Interpreting and reporting qualitative research. *Research in Nursing & Health, 7*(1), 17–24.

McGuire, M. T., Hannan, P. J., Neumark-Sztainer, D., Cossrow, N. H., & Story, M. (2002). Parental correlates of physical activity in a racially/ethically diverse adolescent sample. *Journal of Adolescent Health, 30*(4), 253-261.

Madison, G. B. (1988). *The hermeneutics of post modernity: Figures and Themes.* Bloomington, IN: Indiana University Press.

Mateo, M. A., & Kirchhoff, K. T. (1999). *Using and conducting nursing research in the clinical setting* (2nd ed.). Philadelphia: Saunders.

Melnyk, B. M., & Fineout-Overholt, E. (2005). *Evidence-based practice in nursing & healthcare: A guide to best practice*. Philadelphia: Lippincott Williams & Wilkins.

Miles, M. B., & Huberman, A. M. (1994). *An expanded sourcebook: Qualitative data analysis* (2nd ed.). Beverly Hills, CA: Sage.

Miller, M. A., & Babcock, D. E. (1996). *Critical thinking applied to nursing*. St. Louis: Mosby.

Munhall, P. L. (2001). *Nursing research: A qualitative perspective*. Sudbury, MA: Jones & Bartlett.

Munro, B. H. (2005). *Statistical methods for health care research* (5th ed.). Philadelphia: Lippincott/Williams & Wilkins.

Olsen, D. P. (2003). Methods: HIPAA privacy regulations and nursing research. *Nursing Research, 52*(5), 344–348.

Polit, D. F., & Beck, C. T. (2006). *Essentials of nursing research: Methods, appraisal, and utilization* (6th ed.). Philadelphia: Lippincott/Williams & Wilkins.

Raitakari, O. T., Porkka, K. V., Taimela, S., Telama, R., Rasanen, L., & Viikari, J. S. (1994). Effects of persistent physical activity and inactivity on coronary risk factors in children and young adults. The Cardiovascular Risk in Young Finns Study. *American Journal of Epidemiology, 140*(3), 195–205.

Roberts, W. D., & Stone, P. W. (2003). Ask an expert: How to choose and evaluate a research instrument. *Applied Nursing Research, 16*(1), 70–72.

Robinson, J. H. (2001). Mastering research critique and statistical interpretation: Guidelines and golden rules. *Nurse Educator, 26*(3), 136–141.

Sandelowski, M. (1986). The problem of rigor in qualitative research. *Advances in Nursing Science, 8*(3), 27–37.

Santacroce, S. J., Maccarelli, L. M., & Grey, M. (2004). Methods: Intervention fidelity. *Nursing Research, 53*(1), 63–66.

Schaefer, K. M., & Pond, J. B. (1991). *Levine's Conservation Model: A framework for nursing practice*. Philadelphia: F.A. Davis.

Singman, H., Kinsella, E., & Goldberg, E. (1975). Electrocardiographic changes in coronary care unit patients during defecation. *Vascular Surgery, 9*(1), 54–57.

Stevens, K. R. (2005). Critically appraising knowledge for clinical decision making. In B. M. Melnyk & E. Fineout-Overholt. (2005). *Evidence-based practice in nursing & healthcare: A guide to best practice* (pp. 73–78). Philadelphia: Lippincott Williams & Wilkins.

Stone, P. W. (2002). What is a systematic review? *Applied Nursing Research, 15*(1), 52–53.

van Manen, M. (1990). *Researching lived experience: Human science for an action sensitive pedagogy*. Albany, NY: State University of New York Press.

Winslow, E. H., Lane, L. D., & Gaffney, F. A. (1984). Oxygen uptake and cardiovascular response in patients and normal adults during in-bed and out-of-bed toileting. *Journal of Cardiac Rehabilitation, 4*(8), 348–354.

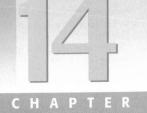

CHAPTER

Building an Evidence-Based Practice

Chapter Overview

Learning Outcomes

After completing this chapter, you should be able to:

1. Define research utilization and evidence-based practice in nursing.
2. Synthesize research findings for use in nursing practice.
3. Apply Rogers' Theory of Diffusion of Innovations to facilitate the use of research findings in your practice.
4. Describe the process for accessing and evaluating evidence-based guidelines for practice.
5. Implement research-based protocols and algorithms and national evidence-based guidelines to promote an evidence-based practice in nursing.

Key Terms

Algorithm, p. 523
Best research evidence, p. 500
Clinical expertise, p. 500
Cognitive clustering, p. 508
Evidence-based practice, p. 500
Innovations, p. 501
Innovators, p. 502
Integrative review of the literature, p. 508
Meta-analysis, p. 511
Metasummary, p. 511
Metasynthesis, p. 512
Research evidence, p. 508
Research utilization, p. 500

Rogers' Theory of Diffusion of Innovations, p. 501
Confirmation stage, p. 504
Continuance, p. 504
Discontinuance, p. 505
Disenchantment discontinuance, p. 506
Replacement discontinuance, p. 505
Decision stage, p. 503
Adoption, p. 503
Rejection, p. 503
Active rejection, p. 503
Passive rejection, p. 503
Implementation stage, p. 503

Direct application, p. 504
Indirect effect, p. 504
Reinvention, p. 504
Research-based protocol, p. 504
Knowledge stage, p. 501
Persuasion stage, p. 503
Compatibility, p. 503
Complexity, p. 503
Observability, p. 503
Relative advantage, p. 503
Trialability, p. 503
Systematic review of research, p. 510

STUDY TOOLS

Go to your Companion CD for interactive review questions related to this chapter. Also, be sure to visit http://evolve.elsevier.com/Burns/understanding for additional review questions, critiquing activities, and more. For additional content review and practice in critiquing, go to Chapter 14 of the *Study Guide for Understanding Nursing Research,* 4th edition.

Nursing research is conducted to generate knowledge for use in practice. The ultimate goal of this research is evidence-based nursing practice. The preceding chapters of this text describe the steps of the quantitative research process, discuss the different types of qualitative research, identify guidelines for critiquing studies, and present directions for summarizing research findings. Reading, critiquing, and synthesizing the research literature are essential for generating research evidence for use in practice. During the last 20 years, many high-quality clinical studies have been conducted and replicated, providing research knowledge that is useful for practice. Using evidence-based interventions enables nurses to provide high-quality care, improve patient outcomes, and decrease health care costs. Thus, patients, nurses, and health care agencies benefit when care is based on research.

The material presented in this chapter is intended to increase the use of research findings in practice and to facilitate the movement toward evidence-based care in nursing. The concepts of research utilization (RU) and evidence-based practice (EBP) are introduced. Rogers' Theory of Diffusion of Innovations, a guide for making changes in practice based on research, is explored. This theory provided direction for the early research utilization projects in nursing and is used today to facilitate implementation of research-based protocols in practice. Also addressed in this chapter is the importance of EBP in nursing, emphasizing the process for synthesizing research evidence for practical use. The Iowa Model for

Evidence-Based Practice provides direction for agencies to move toward evidence-based care. The chapter concludes with a discussion of the national EBP guidelines that have been developed by committees of experts to manage many acute and chronic illnesses. These guidelines are extremely important in the development of evidence-based health care.

What Are Research Utilization and Evidence-Based Practice?

Research utilization (RU) is the process of synthesizing, disseminating, and using research-generated knowledge to make an impact on or change in the existing practices in society. The time lag between generating and using knowledge by society has been a concern for many years. For example, the time lag between the discovery of citrus juice as a preventive measure for scurvy and its use on British ships was 264 years (Glaser, Abelson, & Garrison, 1983). Several studies over the last 20 years have documented the benefits of aspirin in protecting patients from myocardial infarction and stroke, but only recently has the U.S. Food and Drug Administration (FDA) approved the use of a baby aspirin (81 milligrams [mg]) as a preventive measure in persons at risk for cardiovascular disease (Marwick, 1997). Accordingly, the RU process was developed several years ago to address the problems of using research findings in practice. As a result of the emphasis on RU, the number of studies critiqued, synthesized, and used to change nursing practice has expanded.

During the past decade, however, the focus has expanded from RU to a goal of evidence-based practice for the profession of nursing and for health care. Evidence-based practice (EBP) is the conscientious integration of best research evidence with clinical expertise and patient values and needs in the delivery of quality, cost-effective health care (Sackett, Strauss, Richardson, Rosenberg, & Haynes, 2000). Best research evidence is produced by the conduct and synthesis of numerous, high-quality studies in a specific health area. In nursing, the best research evidence is focused on health promotion; illness prevention; and the assessment, diagnosis, and management of acute and chronic illnesses (American Nurses Association, 2004). Clinical expertise includes a practitioner's knowledge, skills, and past experience in accurately assessing, diagnosing, and managing an individual patient's health needs. Patient values and needs are the preferences, concerns, expectations, and health status that a person brings to a clinical encounter (Brown, 1999; Melnyk & Fineout-Overholt, 2005; Sackett et al., 2000). EBP has been emphasized in medicine for years and now is a major focus of nursing. The goal of EBP is the implementation of high-quality, cost-effective care to promote positive outcomes for patients, providers, and health care agencies. Thus, EBP has a broader focus than that of RU and is an essential requirement of high-quality health care delivery. For example, to be accredited, hospitals must provide evidence-based care. Funding for care is based on the implementation of EBP guidelines. The next section provides a historical overview of the RU process and the transition to EBP.

Historical Perspective on Research Utilization in Nursing

Most people believe that a good idea generated through research will sell itself—the word will spread rapidly and the idea will quickly be used. Unfortunately, this is seldom true. During most of the 20th century research findings were seldom used by nurses to improve practice. Thus, from the 1970s to 1990s, nursing focused on implementing the RU process to improve the use of research knowledge in practice. RU is a multiple-step process that involves (1) determining the research knowledge ready for use in practice, (2) persuading nurses to use this knowledge, (3) making a decision to use the knowledge in practice, (4) implementing the knowledge to change practice, and (5) determining the outcomes from making the research-based change in practice. Rogers (1995) developed the Theory of Diffusion of Innovations to promote the use of research findings in society. The steps to Rogers' theory are presented in this section to assist you in implementing RU projects in your agency.

Rogers' theory was used to guide the implementation of early RU projects implemented in nursing. Two major nursing projects that were undertaken to promote the use of research-based nursing interventions in practice were (1) the Western Interstate Commission for Higher Education (WICHE) Regional Nursing Research Development Project and (2) the Conduct and Utilization of Research in Nursing (CURN) Project. In these projects, nurse researchers, with the assistance of federal funding, designed and implemented strategies for using research in practice.

Strategy to Expand Research Use in Practice: Rogers' Theory of Diffusion of Innovations

RU was not a problem unique to nursing; many disciplines have experienced difficulties promoting change based on research. To address this problem, Rogers (1995) studied the processes for using research findings in society and developed a theory for communicating **innovations** or new ideas developed through research. **Rogers' Theory of Diffusion of Innovations** includes a five-stage process: (1) knowledge, (2) persuasion, (3) decision, (4) implementation, and (5) confirmation. The **knowledge stage** is the first awareness of the existence of an innovation or a new idea for use in practice. During the persuasion stage, nurses form an attitude toward the innovation. A decision is then made in the decision stage to adopt or reject the innovation. The implementation stage involves using the new idea to change practice. During the confirmation stage, nurses seek reinforcement of their decision and continue to adopt or reject the change in their practice. Figure 14-1 presents a model of Rogers' innovation-decision process to promote the use of research findings. Rogers' model guided the early RU projects in nursing and can provide direction in implementing research-based interventions in your practice.

Knowledge Stage

Knowledge of research findings can be obtained by formal communication through conference presentations, publications in clinical and research journals, Internet sites, and news releases on television and in newspapers. In addition, informal communication within an agency from one nurse to another or among different health professionals can be effective in increasing awareness of research knowledge. The strategies for communication of research findings to nurses and other health professionals have greatly expanded over the years. Research conferences have increased with more nurses attending these meetings. The studies published in professional journals have expanded, and now EBP journals exist for nursing and medicine. Many research studies are now available on the internet (Burns & Grove, 2005).

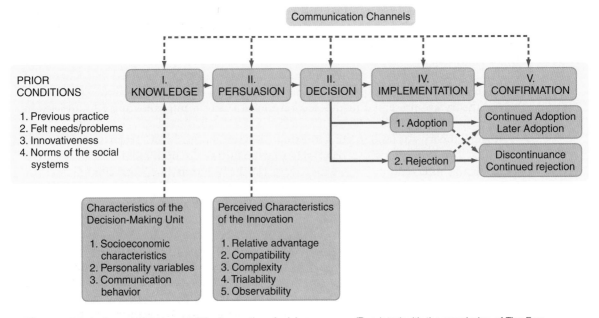

Figure 14-1. A model of stages of the innovation-decision process. (Reprinted with the permission of The Free Press, an imprint of Simon & Schuster. Rogers, E. M. (1995). *Diffusion of innovation* (4th ed.). New York: Simon & Schuster.

Certain conditions influence the knowledge stage, such as previous practice, acknowledged practices needs and problems, and innovativeness of the nurses and other health care providers, and the norms of the health care agency. Dissatisfaction with previous practice can lead to recognizing the needs or problems that require change. A need might create a search for an innovation to improve practice; knowledge of a new idea also might create a need for change. For example, knowledge of a new treatment for pressure ulcers might create the need to change the existing treatment protocol. Innovativeness is the degree to which a person or an agency is willing to adopt new ideas and make changes in practice (Rogers, 1995). People who read research and want to make changes in practice based on empirical evidence are **innovators**. They actively promote change and encourage others to change, but the degree and speed of change depend on the norms of the agency. Norms are the expected behavior patterns within an agency or social system. Norms can serve as barriers to change or can facilitate change. When the norms of the health care agency are oriented to change, the leaders in the agency tend to be innovative and facilitate change. When the norms are opposed to change, so are the agency leaders, thus creating barriers to change.

During the knowledge stage, it is necessary to examine the characteristics of the decision-making unit that is considering adoption of a research-based change. The decision-making unit might be an individual, a nursing unit, or the entire agency. The socioeconomic characteristics, personality variables, and communication behavior of the decision-making unit can support or interfere with the adoption of a new idea (see Figure 14-1). Can the agency afford the change? Will the change save money? Examination of personality variables often indicates an individual's innovativeness and whether he or she will facilitate or resist change.

Communication behavior, whether it is open and honest or closed and subversive, has a strong impact on the RU process. A health care agency that has innovative nurses, supports change, and promotes open, clear communication will facilitate RU.

Persuasion Stage

During the **persuasion stage**, an individual person or agency develops either a favorable or unfavorable attitude toward the change or innovation (Rogers, 1995). Characteristics of an innovation that determine the probability and speed of its adoption include relative advantage, compatibility, complexity, trialability, and observability (see Figure 14-1). **Relative advantage** is the extent to which the innovation is perceived to be better than current practice. **Compatibility** is the degree to which the innovation is perceived to be consistent with current values, past experience, and priority of needs. **Complexity** is the degree to which the innovation is perceived to be difficult to understand or use. If the innovation requires the development of new skills, complexity increases. **Trialability** is the extent to which an individual person or agency can try out the idea on a limited basis, with the option of returning to previous practices. **Observability** is the extent to which the results of an innovation are visible to others. An innovation with highly visible, beneficial results probably will be rapidly adopted. Innovations that have great relative advantage, are compatible within the agency, are not complex, have trialability, and are observable usually are adopted more quickly than those that do not meet these criteria.

In the persuasion stage, the proposed change is best communicated in small groups or one-to-one interactions. Innovative nurses will be attempting to convince others that they need to make changes in their practice based on research. They will be asked many questions about the change, such as: Have they used this intervention in their practice? How do they feel about it? What are the consequences of using it? What are the advantages and disadvantages of using it in my situation? Would they advise me to use it? Will I still be approved of and accepted if I use it? Extensive, honest communication usually increases the likelihood of adoption.

Decision Stage

At the **decision stage**, the innovation is either adopted or rejected (see Figure 14-1). **Adoption** involves full acceptance and the implementation of the innovation or intervention in practice. Adoption can be continued indefinitely or can be discontinued based on evaluation of the intervention's effectiveness for patients and the health care agency. **Rejection** of an intervention can be active or passive. **Active rejection** indicates that the intervention was examined and a decision was made not to adopt it. **Passive rejection** indicates that the intervention was never seriously considered. Over time, a health care agency might adhere to the decision to reject an intervention or might initiate adoption of the intervention when later research supports its value.

Implementation Stage

In the **implementation stage**, the intervention is put to use by an individual, a clinic, a hospital unit, many units in a hospital, or a group of hospitals. A detailed plan for implementation that addresses the risks and benefits of the intervention will facilitate change. The types of implementation include direct application, reinvention, and indirect effects.

Direct application occurs when an intervention is used exactly as it was developed. In fact, some researchers would not consider an intervention to have been adopted unless its original form was kept intact. For example, if a study demonstrated that a particular intervention, conducted in specifically defined steps, was effective in achieving an outcome, adoption requires that the nurse perform the steps of the intervention in exactly the same way in which they are described in the study. This expectation reflects the narrow, precise definition of an intervention that is necessary to the scientific endeavor. However, this preciseness is not compatible with typical practice behavior, and research indicates that maintenance of the original intervention does not always occur. A **research-based protocol** provides detailed guidelines that are documented with research sources for implementing an intervention in practice. These protocols promote direct application of an intervention in nursing practice (Haller, Reynolds, & Horsley, 1979). The Research-Based Protocol for Decreasing Discomfort with Intramuscular Injections is presented as an example in Figure 14-2. This protocol provides steps, which are documented with research, for positioning patients during intramuscular (IM) injections to reduce their discomfort. You can use this protocol when positioning your patients for IM injections.

Reinvention occurs when adopters modify the intervention to meet their own needs. Using this strategy, the steps of a procedure might be changed or deleted, or some of the steps might be combined with other care activities. Even with reinvention, nurses are using research findings to make changes in their practice. Nurses' use of research-based knowledge also can have indirect effects. For example, practicing nurses and researchers may discuss the findings, cite them in clinical papers and textbooks, and use them to strengthen arguments. Thus, the research knowledge has an **indirect effect** by being incorporated into people's thinking and combined with their experience, education, and current values. In such instances, determining if research knowledge is being used is more difficult; thus, the use of certain nursing research findings may be underestimated.

Confirmation Stage

During the **confirmation stage**, nurses evaluate the effectiveness of the change in practice and decide to either continue or discontinue it. Using the example of the intervention to decrease patient discomfort during an IM injection, the nurse might evaluate the effectiveness of the injection technique by asking patients how much discomfort they felt during the injection or by having patients complete a visual analogue scale. On a 100-mm line like the one shown below, patients are asked to mark the level of discomfort they felt during the injection.

No   Extreme
Discomfort _____ Discomfort

After one month of using the intervention, the data obtained from the pain scale can be analyzed and shared with other staff members. If the results indicate that the injection technique causes minimal discomfort, the intervention probably will be continued (**continuance**) and the protocol will be included in the procedure manual. If the IM injection protocol is

Research-Based Protocol for Decreasing Discomfort with IM Injections

1. Wash hands, gather necessary equipment for the injection, and put on gloves.

2. Explain to the patient that you will position him/her to decrease the discomfort of the IM injection based on research (Greenway, 2004; Keen, 1986; Kruszewski, Lang, & Johnson, 1979; Rettig & Southby, 1982).

3. Position the patient in the prone position or lying face down (Kruszewski et al., 1979; Rettig & Southby, 1982).

4. Identify the ventrogluteal (VG) site. A picture of the site would be provided in the protocol (Greenway, 2004; Rodger & King, 2000).

5. Have the patient turn his/her toes inward ("toe in"). This internal rotation of the femur causes relaxation of the gluteal muscle, which decreases the discomfort from the injection (Kruszewski et al., 1979; Rettig & Southby, 1982).

6. Give the injection, and reposition the patient for comfort after the injection (Beyea & Nicoll, 1995; Rodger & King, 2004).

7. Document how the injection was given and the patient's response or perceived level of comfort (Beyea & Nicoll, 1995; Rodger & King, 2004). (You might use the visual analogue scale presented in the selection titled "Confirmation Stage" to document the discomfort experienced with the injection.

References

Beyea, S. C., & Nicoll, L. H. (1995). Administration of medications via the intramuscular route: An integrative review of the literature and research-based protocol for the procedure. *Applied Nursing Research, 8*(1), 23–33.

Greenway, K. (2004). Using the ventrogluteal site for intramuscular injection. *Nursing Standard, 18*(25), 39–42.

Keen, M. F. (1986). Comparison of intramuscular injection techniques to reduce site discomfort and lesions. *Nursing Research, 35*(4), 207–210.

Kruszewski, A., Lang, S., & Johnson, J. (1979). Effect of positioning on discomfort from intramuscular injections in dorsogluteal site. *Nursing Research, 28*(2), 103–105.

Rettig, F. M., & Southby, J. R. (1982). Using different body positions to reduce discomfort from dorsogluteal injection. *Nursing Research, 31*(4), 219–221.

Rodger, M. A., & King, L. (2000). Drawing up and administering intramuscular injections: A review of the literature. *Journal of Advanced Nursing, 31*(3), 574–582.

Figure 14-2. Example of research-based protocol.

started on one hospital unit, it may then be used on all units in the hospital. If the data analysis indicates that most patients' levels of discomfort are still moderate to severe, the intervention probably will be discontinued.

Discontinuance can be of at least two types: replacement and disenchantment. With **replacement discontinuance**, the intervention is rejected to adopt a better idea. Thus innovations can occur in waves as new ideas replace outdated, impractical innovations. The computer is an excellent example; users can regularly upgrade their systems with new, more powerful interactive innovations in hardware and software. **Disenchantment discontinuance** occurs when an idea is rejected because the user is dissatisfied with its outcome. Rogers' theory provides guidance for implementing research-based changes in practice; and has served to organize the implementation of two important RU projects conducted in nursing.

Western Interstate Commission for Higher Education Regional Nursing Research Development Project

The Western Interstate Commission for Higher Education (WICHE) Project, initiated in the mid-1970s, was the first major nursing project to address RU. The 6-year project was directed by Krueger and colleagues (Krueger, 1978; Krueger, Nelson, & Wolanin, 1978) and was funded by the Division of Nursing. The initial goal of the project was to increase nursing research activities within the western region of the United States.

The WICHE Project, building on Rogers' Theory of Diffusion of Innovations, developed the Five-Phase Resources Linkage Model for using research findings in practice. Phase 1 of the model involved using resources to recruit members for the project and to prepare research-based materials. Phase 2 consisted of a workshop where participants were organized into dyads composed of a nurse educator and a clinician. The objective of the workshop was to help participants develop skills in critiquing research and applying utilization theory. Each dyad selected a research-based intervention that they were willing to implement within an institution. The dyad was to function as a change agent in phase 3, when the utilization projects were implemented in the participants' agencies for 5 months. Phase 4 was a second workshop for reports, analysis, and evaluation of the project; and phase 5 was the follow-up report on continuation of the utilization projects 3 and 6 months later.

The project staff and participants had difficulty identifying clinical studies with findings appropriate for implementation in practice. Findings that were identified tended to be merged with other activities by the dyad and then implemented as a package. Because the project staff expected the findings to be implemented in pure form, this strategy was viewed with disfavor. Three reports from this project were published: (1) Axford and Cutchen (1977) developed a preoperative teaching program, (2) Dracup and Breu (1978) devised a care plan for grieving spouses and tested its effectiveness, and (3) Wichita (1977) developed a program to treat and prevent constipation in nursing home residents by increasing the fiber in their diets.

Conduct and Utilization of Research in Nursing Project

The Conduct and Utilization of Research in Nursing (CURN) Project, directed by Horsley (Horsley, Crane, & Bingle, 1978; Horsley, Crane, Crabtree, & Wood, 1983), was awarded to the Michigan Nurses Association by the Division of Nursing. The 5-year (1975–1980) project was developed to increase the utilization of research findings by disseminating findings, facilitating organizational modifications necessary for implementation, and encouraging collaborative research that was directly transferable to clinical practice. RU was seen as an organizational process, rather than as a process to be implemented by an individual practitioner. Activities of the RU process included

Identification and synthesis of multiple research studies in a common conceptual area (research knowledge base),

Transformation of the knowledge derived from a research base into a solution or research-based clinical protocol,

Transformation of the clinical protocol into specific nursing actions (innovations) that are administered to patients (Rogers, 1995), and

Clinical evaluation of the new practice to ascertain whether it produced the predicted result (Horsley et al., 1983).

During this project, published clinical studies were critiqued for scientific merit, replication, and relevance to practice. The relevance of the research to practice involved examining (1) clinical merit or significance in addressing patient problems, (2) the extent to which clinical control belonged to nursing, (3) the feasibility of implementing a change in an agency, and (4) an analysis of the cost-benefit ratio. The following 10 areas were considered to have research of sufficient quality to warrant implementation: (1) structured preoperative teaching, (2) reducing diarrhea in tube-fed patients, (3) preoperative sensory preparation to promote recovery, (4) prevention of decubitus ulcers, (5) intravenous cannula change, (6) closed urinary drainage systems, (7) distress reduction through sensory preparation, (8) mutual goal setting in patient care, (9) clean intermittent catheterization, and (10) pain: deliberative nursing interventions (CURN Project, 1981, 1982).

Research-Based Protocol Development and Implementation

The CURN Project involved the development of protocols from research findings to implement and evaluate a change in practice (Horsley et al., 1983). Each protocol contained the following elements:

- Identification of the practice problem and the need for change
- Summary of the research base, including limitations of the research
- Design of the nursing practice innovation or intervention
- Description of the research-based principle to guide the innovation
- Description of the implementation of the innovation, or the clinical trial
- Evaluation of the effects of the innovation, including evaluation procedures and recording forms
- Summary and references

The protocols were implemented in clinical trials and evaluated for effectiveness. Based on the evaluations, a decision was made to reject, modify, or adopt the intervention (Rogers, 1995). Strategies could then be developed to extend the research-based intervention to other appropriate nursing practice settings.

The CURN Project was implemented on a test unit within a hospital, and baseline data and comparison groups were used to evaluate outcomes from the implementation. Follow-up questionnaires were sent to the 17 participating hospitals at intervals over a 4-year period to determine the long-term impact of the implementation on the organization. Pelz and Horsley (1981) reported that before the project, RU was low in both the comparison and experimental groups. One year after the intervention, significant differences were found, with experimental organizations having higher levels of utilization. The second year after the intervention, differences were still noted between the groups, but they were not significant for all 10 utilization activities. In the third year, experimental units continued to perform the protocols, but the rate of diffusion of the innovations to other units was not reported.

The clinical protocols developed during the CURN Project were published to encourage nurses in other health care agencies to use these research-based interventions in their practice (CURN Project, 1981, 1982). An important contribution of the CURN Project was the format for developing research-based protocols for nursing interventions. The WICHE and CURN projects were based on Rogers' Theory of Diffusion of Innovations (1995), which provided direction to nurses and health care agencies implementing RU projects in the 1980s and 1990s and today. The RU process provides a basis for developing an EBP for nursing.

Developing an Evidence-Based Practice for Nursing

EBP is a complex phenomenon that requires synthesizing study findings to determine the best research evidence. Findings from a study differ from **research evidence**, in that evidence is a synthesis of quality, relevant studies to form a body of empirical knowledge for a selected area of practice. The best research evidence is then integrated with clinical expertise and patient values and needs to deliver quality cost-effective care (Sackett et al., 2000). This section addresses the synthesis of research findings to determine the evidence or level of research knowledge that exists for use in practice. For some areas of practice, the research has been synthesized by experts and is ready to be implemented in practice. Models have been developed to promote the application of best evidence in practice and the Iowa Model of Evidence-Based Practice is presented as an example (Titler et al., 2001). This model is used to demonstrate how best research evidence can be used to manage patients' peripheral venous catheters.

Synthesis of Research Findings to Determine Evidence for Practice

Research or empirical knowledge is generated through the conduct of a variety of quality studies (quantitative, qualitative, and outcomes). Once extensive, quality studies have been conducted in a selected practice area, these studies' findings need to be synthesized for use in practice. The integration of findings from scientifically sound research to determine what is currently known or not known in a selected practice area is called **cognitive clustering**. Cognitive clustering is accomplished through integrative reviews of the literature, systematic reviews of research, meta-analyses, metasummaries, and metasyntheses of the research literature (Whittemore, 2005). The terms used to identify reviews in the published literature vary as does the quality and the rigor of the reviews conducted. In this text, the definitions provided by Whittemore (2005) are used to direct nurses in the conduct of reviews of the literature. Table 14-1 identifies the definition, purpose, scope, sampling frame, and analysis for the different research reviews commonly conducted and published in the nursing and health care literature.

Integrative Reviews of the Literature

Integrative reviews of the literature are rigorously conducted to identify, analyze, and synthesize results from independent quantitative and qualitative studies and theoretical and

| Table 14–1 | Methods of Nursing Research Reviews |

Type of Review (Exemplar)	Definition	Purpose	Scope	Sample Frame	Analysis
Integrative review (Redeker, 2000)	A summary of the literature on a specific concept or content area whereby the research is summarized, analyzed, and overall conclusions are drawn	To review methods, theories, and/or empirical studies around a particular topic	Narrow or broad	Quantitative or qualitative research; theoretical literature; methodological literature	Narrative
Meta-analysis (Clemmens, 2001)	A summary of past research using statistical techniques to transform findings of studies with related or identical hypotheses into a common metric and calculating the overall effect, the magnitude of effect, and subsample effects	To estimate the effect of interventions or relationships	Narrow	Quantitative research of similar methodology	Statistical
Systematic review (Forbes, 1998)	A summary of past research using an objective and rigorous approach of studies with related or identical hypotheses.	To summarize evidence regarding a specific clinical problem	Narrow	Quantitative research of similar methodology	Narrative or statistical
Metasummary Metasynthesis Formal grounded theory Metastudy (Beck, 2002)	A summary of past research combining the findings from multiple qualitative studies	To inform research or practice by summarizing processes or experiences	Narrow or broad	Qualitative research	Narrative

From Whittemore, R. (2005). Combining evidence in nursing research: Methods and implications. *Nursing Research, 54*(1), p. 57.

methodological literature to determine the current knowledge (what is known and not known) for a particular concept, measurement method, or practice topic (Conn & Rantz, 2003; Melnyk & Fineout-Overholt, 2005; Whittemore, 2005). The review includes multiple types of research designs, such as descriptive and correlational quantitative studies and qualitative studies, as well as theoretical and methodological literature. In the past, most integrative reviews have included quantitative studies but some major contributions can be made to the body of knowledge in selected areas by examining qualitative studies. Dixon-Woods, Fitzpatrick, and Roberts (2001) identified the following contributions to integrative reviews by qualitative studies:

> Identify and refine the question of the review
> Identify the relevant outcomes of interest
> Identify the relevant types of participants and interventions
> Augment the data to be included in a quantitative synthesis
> Provide data for a non-numerical synthesis of research
> Highlight inadequacies in the methods used in quantitative studies
> Explain the findings of a quantitative synthesis
> Assist in the interpretation of the significance and applicability of the review
> Assist in making recommendations to practitioners and planners about implementing the conclusions in the review (Dixon-Woods et al., 2001, p. 126).

An integrative review of the literature is best conducted by two or more health professionals to develop a quality synthesis of the research and theoretical literature in an area. Due to the breath of the literature reviewed, this is a complicated review to conduct but can result in an increase in the depth and breadth of the conclusions that can be drawn. It is also important that the integrative reviews be published. The *Annual Review of Nursing Research* books and research, clinical, and evidence-based journals provide excellent sources for publication of integrative reviews of the literature and systematic reviews of research.

Systematic Reviews of Research

A **systematic review of research** is a narrowly focused synthesis of the findings from quantitative studies focused on a particular practice intervention or problem. A systematic review focuses on studies of a similar methodology, such as a synthesis of quasi-experimental and experimental studies used to determine the best evidence for a particular intervention. The example presented later in this section includes both a systematic review of research and a meta-analysis to determine the best research evidence for selecting an irrigant (normal saline flush or heparin flush) to maintain the patency of peripheral venous catheters. Systematic reviews of research should be held to the same standards of clarity, rigor, and replication as primary research (Forrest & Miller, 2004; Whittemore, 2005). Frequently, systematic reviews are conducted to generate research evidence for use in practice and include the following steps:

1. Formulate the purpose of the review, which is usually a specific nursing intervention or clearly focused clinical problem.
2. Identify the scope of the review, which should be narrowly focused.
3. Develop specific questions to be answered by the review or hypotheses to be tested.

4. Establish criteria for inclusion and exclusion of studies in the review.
5. Conduct an extensive literature search including primarily research studies of similar methodology from a variety of authors.
6. Locate published and unpublished research sources.
7. Develop a questionnaire with which to gather data from the quantitative studies.
8. Contact authors for additional data and information.
9. Critique the scientific merit of the studies.
10. Identify rules of inference to be used in data analyses and interpretation.
11. Analyze data from the studies in a systematic fashion.
12. Interpret data with the assistance of others.
13. Report the review as clearly and completely as possible. (Melnyk & Fineout-Overholt, 2005; Whittemore, 2005)

Meta-analyses of the Research Literature

The next step beyond critique and integration of research findings is to conduct a meta-analysis on the outcomes of similar studies. **Meta-analysis** statistically pools the results from previous studies into a single quantitative analysis that provides the highest level of evidence for an intervention's efficacy (Conn & Rantz, 2003; Whittemore, 2005). This approach allows the application of scientific criteria to factors such as sample size, level of significance, and variables examined. Through the use of meta-analysis, the following can be generated:

- An extremely large, diverse sample that is more representative of the target population than the samples of the individual studies;
- The determination of the overall significance of pooled data from quality, confirmed studies;
- The average effect size determined from several quality studies that indicates the efficacy of a treatment or intervention; and
- The strength of relationship between variables (Conn & Rantz, 2003; Melnyk & Fineout-Overholt, 2005).

Meta-analyses make it possible to be objective rather than subjective in evaluating research findings for practice. The strongest evidence for using an intervention in practice is generated from a meta-analysis of multiple, controlled studies of the same methodology. However, the conduct of a meta-analysis is dependent on the quality, clarity, and completeness of information presented in studies. Stetler and colleagues (1998) provide a tool you can use to evaluate meta-analyses to determine the usefulness of the knowledge generated for practice. Conn and Rantz (2003) describe the steps for conducting a meta-analysis that could assist you, with the guidance of an expert researcher, in conducting your own meta-analysis in an area of interest.

Metasummaries and Metasynthesis of Qualitative Research

After 40 years of qualitative studies being conducted in nursing, metasummaries of these studies' findings are being developed for publication. **Metasummary** is a synthesis of multiple primary qualitative studies to produce a narrative about a selected phenomenon (Whittemore, 2005). These summaries are providing valuable knowledge for expanding our understanding of important aspects of practice. **Metasynthesis** is also conducted to synthesize qualitative research and involves the critical analysis of primary qualitative studies and synthesis of findings into a new theory or framework for the topic of interest. Beck (1999) and Dixon-Woods et al. (2001) provided detailed direction for the synthesis of qualitative research.

Best Evidence for Use in Practice

The empirical knowledge generated from integrative reviews of the literature, systematic reviews of research, meta-analyses, and metasummaries and metasyntheses of qualitative research provides the best evidence for making changes in practice. The strength of the research evidence is on a continuum, with the strongest evidence being generated from high quality meta-analyses. Figure 14-3 provides the continuum of evidence, with the strongest evidence on the left side of the continuum to the weakest evidence on the far right. A high-quality meta-analysis is conducted with well-designed, well-conducted, controlled clinical trials (random and nonrandom) with consistent, statistically significant results. Systematic reviews of research include a synthesis of high-quality studies (clinical trials and experimental and quasi-experimental studies) and provide the next strongest level of research evidence. One or two well-designed, well-conducted, controlled clinical trials and experimental studies provide the next strongest levels of research evidence (Craig & Smyth, 2002; Melnyk & Fineout-Overholt, 2005). Well-designed and well-conducted quasi-experimental studies provide the next level of strength in research evidence. Replication of these studies is needed to increase the strength of the research evidence. Integrative reviews of descriptive and correlational quantitative studies provide a basis for the development and implementation of quasi-experimental and experimental studies. More research is needed in these areas before evidence-based changes can be made in practice. Qualitative studies generate important evidence and theories for practice that can be tested through quantitative research. The qualitative research findings provide understanding of practice situations but are difficult to generalize from the sample to a larger population, which is important in developing guidelines for practice (Barbour, 2000). However, metasummaries and metasyntheses of qualitative research are being conducted to provide a stronger basis for the generalization of the findings to clinical situations. The strongest research evidence generated from meta-analyses and sometimes systematic reviews of research are used to develop evidence-based guidelines. Evidence-based guidelines are essential in developing EBP for nursing. As discussed next, the Iowa Model of Evidence-Based Practice was developed to facilitate the use of evidence-based guidelines in practice.

Strongest Evidence	Meta-analysis of Experimental Studies	Integrative Reviews of Experimental Studies	Experimental Studies	Quasi-experimental Studies	Correlational Studies	Qualitative Studies	Descriptive Surveys	Weakest Evidence

Figure 14-3. Strength of research evidence.

Iowa Model of Evidence-Based Practice

Nurses have been actively involved in implementing RU projects and have participated in the development of some of the evidence-based guidelines for practice. Thus, nurses have a strong commitment to EBP and can benefit by the direction provided by the Iowa model to expand their practice that is based on research. The Iowa Model of Evidence-Based Practice provides direction for the development of EBP in a clinical agency (Figure 14-4). This EBP model was initially developed by Titler and colleagues in 1994 and revised in 2001. In a health care agency, there are triggers that initiate the need for change, which is best made based on research evidence. These triggers can be problem focused and evolve from risk management data, process improvement data, benchmarking data, financial data, and clinical problems. The triggers can also be knowledge focused, such as new research findings, change in national agencies or organizational standards and guidelines, expanded philosophy of care, or questions from the institutional standards' committee. The triggers are evaluated and prioritized according to the needs of the clinical agency. If a trigger is considered an agency priority, then a group is formed to search for the best evidence to manage the clinical concern (Titler et al., 2001).

In some situations, the research evidence is inadequate to make changes in practice and additional studies are needed to strengthen the knowledge base. Sometimes the research evidence can be combined with other sources of knowledge (theories, scientific principles, expert opinion, and case reports) through an integrative review of the literature to provide fairly strong evidence for use in practice (see Figure 14-4). The strongest evidence is generated from meta-analyses of several controlled clinical trials. This is the type of evidence that is used to develop evidence-based guidelines. The research-based protocols or evidence-based guidelines would be pilot tested on a particular unit and then evaluated to determine the impact on patient care. If the outcomes are favorable from the pilot test, then the change would be made in practice and monitored over time to determine its impact on the agency environment, staff, costs, and the patient and family (Titler et al., 2001). If an agency strongly supports the use of the Iowa model, implements patient care based on the best research evidence, and monitors changes in practice to ensure quality care, then the agency is promoting EBP.

Application of the Iowa Model of Evidence-Based Practice

Preparing to use research evidence in practice raises some important questions. What are the most effective strategies for implementing research-based protocols, algorithm, or evidence-based guidelines in a clinical agency? What are the outcomes from using the research findings in practice? Do the risk management data, process improvement data, benchmarking data, and/or financial data support making the change in practice based on the research evidence? Is the proposed research-based change an agency priority? We suggest that effective strategies for using research findings in practice will require a multifaceted approach that takes into consideration the research findings, support of the nurses, the organization's philosophy, and national organizational standards and guidelines.

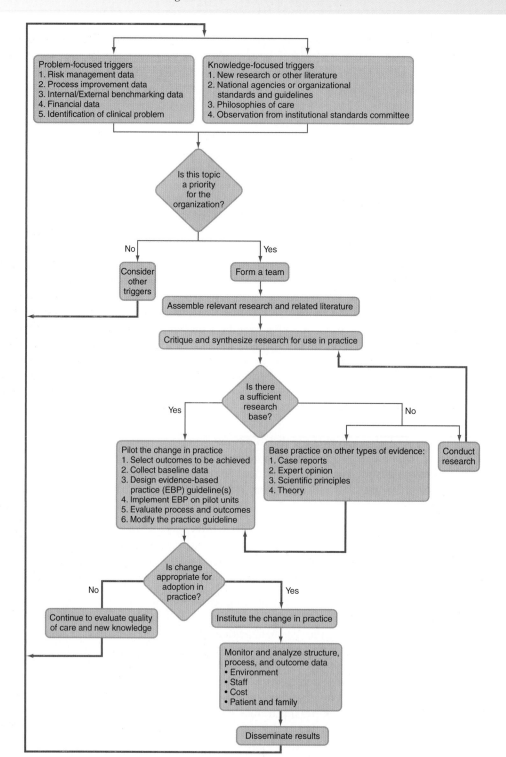

Figure 14-4. The Iowa Model of Evidence-Based Practice to Promote Quality Care. (From Titler, M. G., Kleiber, C., Steelman, V. J., Rakel, B. A., Budreau, G., Everett, L. Q., et al. [2001]. The Iowa Model of Evidence-Based Practice to promote quality care. *Critical Care Nursing Clinics of North America*, 13[4], 497–509.)

The steps of the Iowa model (see Figure 14-4) (Titler et al., 2001) were used as a guide for implementing a research-based protocol for saline flush irrigation of peripheral venous catheters. The research evidence focused on the effects of heparin flush versus saline flush for irrigating peripheral catheters. This section provides the details for making this evidence-based change in practice. Nurses who make the switch from heparin flush to saline flush using a research-based protocol are providing evidence-based care (Craig & Smyth, 2002; Sackett et al., 2000).

Synthesize Relevant Research

According to the Iowa Model of Evidence-Based Practice, the body of research and related literature needs to be assembled and critiqued for scientific merit (see Figure 14-4). All types of research, including clinical trials, quantitative studies, and qualitative studies need to be identified and critiqued when determining the research knowledge base for a selected intervention or practice problem (Melnyk & Fineout-Overholt, 2005). The scientific merit of nursing studies is determined by critiquing the following aspects of a study: (1) the conceptualization and internal consistency, or the logical links of a study; (2) methodological rigor, or the strength of the design, sample, measurement methods, data collection process, and analysis techniques; (3) generalizability of the findings, or the representativeness of the sample and setting and (4) the number of replications (Craig & Smyth, 2002). The critique processes for quantitative and qualitative research are presented in Chapter 13 to assist you in critiquing studies to determine the level of research knowledge in a practice area.

The next step in the Iowa Model of Evidence-Based Practice is to determine what synthesis of research has been conducted (see Figure 14-4).

RESEARCH EXAMPLE Synthesis of Research

Goode and colleagues (1991) conducted a meta-analysis "to estimate the effects of heparin flush and saline flush solutions on maintaining patency, preventing phlebitis, and increasing duration of peripheral heparin locks [peripheral venous catheters]" (p. 324). The meta-analysis was conducted on 17 high-quality studies, which the investigators summarized in a table (Table 14-A). The total sample size for the 17 studies was 4,153; the study settings included a variety of medical-surgical and critical care units. The small effect size values (most are less than 0.20) for clotting, phlebitis, and duration indicate that saline flush is as effective as heparin flush in maintaining peripheral venous catheters. Goode and colleagues summarized current knowledge on the use of saline versus heparin flushes:

> It can be concluded that saline is as effective as heparin in maintaining patency, preventing phlebitis, and increasing duration in peripheral heparin locks. Quality of care can be enhanced by using saline as the flush solution, thereby eliminating problems associated with anticoagulant effects and drug incompatibilities. In addition, an estimated yearly savings of $109,100,000 to $218,200,000 U.S. health-care dollars could be attained. (Goode et al., 1991, p. 324)

These investigators also provided a table (Table 14-B) to present evidence of cost savings from changing to saline.

(continues)

Table 14-A Studies Included in the Meta-analysis

Study	N	Subject	Assignment	Heparin Dose (U/cc)	Clotting Effect Size (d_c)	Phlebitis Effect Size (d_p)	Duration Effect Size (d_d)
Ashton et al., 1990	16 exp$_c$ 16 con$_c$ 13 exp$_p$ 14 con$_p$	Adult critical care	Random, double blind	10	0.3590	– 0.1230	
Barrett & Lester, 1990	59 experimental 50 control	Adult med-surg patients	Nonrandom double-blind	10	– 0.1068	– 0.4718	
Craig & Anderson, 1991	129 exp 145 con	Adult med-surg patients	Random double-blind crossover	10	0.0095	– 0.0586	
Cyganski et al., 1987	225 exp 196 con	Adult med-surg patients	Nonrandom	10	0.2510		
Donham & Denning, 1987	8 exp$_c$ 4 con$_c$ 7 exp$_p$ 5 con$_p$	Adult critical care	Random, double blind	10	0.0000	0.0548	
Dunn & Lenihan, 1987	61 experimental 51 control	Adult patients	Nonrandom	50	– 0.2057	– 0.2258	
Epperson, 1984	138 exp 120 con 138 exp 154 con	Adult med-surg patients	Random, double blind	10 100			– 0.1176 – 0.1232
Garrelts et al., 1989	131 exp 173 con	Adult med-surg patients	Random, double blind	10	– 0.1773	0.1057	0.2753
Hamilton et al., 1988	137 exp 170 con	Adult patients	Random, double blind	10	– 0.0850	– 0.1819	– 0.0604
Holford et al., 1977	39 experimental 140 control	Young adult volunteers	Nonrandom, double blind	3.3, 10, 16.5, 100, 132	0.6545		
Kasparek et al., 1988	49 exp 50 con	Adult med patients	Random, double blind	10	0.3670	– 0.5430	
Lombardi et al., 1988	34 experimental 40 control	Pediatric patients (4 wk to 18 yr)	Nonrandom, sequential double blind	10		– 0.2324	0.0000
Miracle et al., 1989	167 exp 441 con	Adult med-surg patients	Nonrandom	100	– 0.0042		
Shearer, 1987	87 exp 73 con	Med-surg patients	Nonrandom	10	– 0.1170	– 0.0977	

Table 14-A Studies Included in the Meta-analysis—cont'd

Study	N	Subject	Assignment	Heparin Dose (U/cc)	Clotting Effect Size (d_c)	Phlebitis Effect Size (d_p)	Duration Effect Size (d_d)
Spann, 1988	15 experimental 19 control	Adult telemetry step-down	Nonrandom, double blind	10	– 0.3163	– 0.3252	
Taylor et al., 1989	369 exp 356 con	Adult med-surg patients	Nonrandom, time series	10	0.0308	0.0288	– 0.1472
Tuten & Gueldner, 1991	43 exp 71 con	Adult med-surg patients	Nonrandom	100	0.0000	0.1662	

Modified from Goode, C. J., Titler, M., Rakel, B., Ones, D. S., Kleiber, C., Small, S., & Triolo, P. K. (1991). A meta-analysis of effects of heparin flush and saline flush: Quality and cost implications. *Nursing Research, 40*(6), 325. Copyright © 1991, The American Journal of Nursing Company. Used with permission.

TABLE 14-B Annual Cost Savings from Changing to Saline

Study	Cost Savings	Hospital
Craig & Anderson, 1991	$40,000/yr	525-bed tertiary care hospital
Dunn & Lenihan, 1987	$19,000/yr	530-bed private hospital
Goode et al., 1991 (this study)	$38,000/yr	879-bed tertiary care hospital
Kasparek et al., 1988	$19,000/yr	350-bed private hospital
Lombardi et al., 1988	$20,000–$25,000/yr	52-bed pediatric unit
Schustek, 1984	$20,000/yr	391-bed private hospital
Taylor et al., 1989	$30,000–$40,000/yr	216-bed private hospital

From Goode, C. J., Titler, M., Rakel, B., Ones, D. S., Kleiber, C., Small, S., & Triolo, P. K. (1991). A meta-analysis of effects of heparin flush and saline flush: Quality and cost implications. *Nursing Research, 40*(6), 325. Copyright © 1991, The American Journal of Nursing Company. Used with permission.

In 1994, the American Society of Hospital Pharmacists (ASHP) published a Therapeutic Position Statement on the institutional use of 0.9% sodium chloride (saline) flush to maintain patency of peripheral venous catheters versus heparin flush. Additional research continues to be conducted in this area, and in 1998, Randolph, Cook, Gonzales, and Andrew published a systematic review and meta-analysis of randomized controlled trials to determine the effectiveness of normal saline versus heparinized saline as a flush for peripheral venous and arterial catheters. These authors concluded: "Flushing peripheral venous catheters locked between use with heparinized saline at 10 U/ml [units/milliliter] is no more beneficial than flushing with normal saline" (Randolph et al., 1998, p. 969).

Determine Sufficiency of the Research Base for Use in Practice

The two meta-analyses and systematic review of controlled clinical trials provide sound scientific evidence for making a change in practice from heparin flush to saline flush for irrigating peripheral venous catheters or heparin locks in adults (Goode et al., 1991; Randolph et al., 1998). Clinical relevance is evident in that the use of saline to flush peripheral venous catheters promotes quality outcomes for the patient (patent heparin lock, fewer problems with anticoagulant effects, and fewer drug incompatibilities); the nurse (decreased time to flush the catheter and no drug incompatibilities with saline); and the agency (extensive cost savings and quality patient care).

The research evidence is extremely strong for making the EBP change from heparin to saline flush to maintain the patency of peripheral venous catheters in adults. However, additional research is needed to identify the best flush (saline or heparin) to use for maintaining the patency of peripheral venous catheters in neonates and children. In addition, initial clinical trials have demonstrated that heparin flush is better than saline flush in maintaining the patency of arterial pressure monitoring lines (American Association of Critical-Care Nurses, 1993) and peripheral artery catheters (Randolph et al., 1998). Thus, the evidence base for practice clearly indicates the population (adults) and type of catheter (venous) to irrigate with saline flush.

Pilot the Change in Practice

The relative advantages of using saline are the improved quality of care and cost savings, which are clearly documented in the research literature (Goode et al., 1991; Peterson & Kirchhoff, 1991; Randolph et al., 1998). (The cost savings for different sizes of hospitals are summarized in Table 14-B.) The compatibility of the change can be determined by identifying the changes that will need to occur in your agency. What changes will the nurses have to make in irrigating peripheral venous catheters with saline? What changes will have to occur in the pharmacy to provide the saline flush? Are the physicians aware of the research in this area? Are the physicians willing to order the use of saline to flush venous catheters?

The change in peripheral venous catheter flush from heparin to saline has minimal complexity. The only thing changed is the flush, so no additional skills, expertise, or time is required by the nurse to make the change. Because saline flush, unlike heparin flush, is compatible with any drug that might be administered through the peripheral venous catheter, the number of potential complications is decreased. As a practical consideration, the change can be started on one unit as a clinical trial and then evaluated. Once the quality of care and cost savings are documented for nurses, physicians, and hospital administrators, the change probably will spread rapidly throughout the institution. Changing from heparin flush to saline flush would be relatively simple on a trial basis, to demonstrate the positive outcomes for patients, nurses, and the health care agency.

The decision to use saline flush versus heparin flush as an irrigant requires institutional approval, physician approval, and approval of the nurses managing patients' peripheral venous catheters. When a change requires institutional approval, decision making may be distributed through several levels of the organization. Thus, a decision at one level may lead to contact with another official who must approve the action. In keeping with the guidelines of planned change, institutional changes are more likely to be effective if all those affected by the change have a voice in the decision. In your institution, who needs to approve the change? What steps do you need to take to get the change approved within your institution? Do the physicians support the change? Do the nurses on the units support the change? Who are the leaders in the institution, and can you get them to support the change? Try to get the nurses to make a commitment and take a public stand to make the change, because their commitment increases the probability that the change will be made. Contact the appropriate administrative people and physicians, and detail the pros and cons of making the change to saline flush for irrigating peripheral venous catheters. You need to clearly indicate to physicians and administrators that the change is based on extremely strong research evidence, provides extensive cost savings, and promotes high-quality patient care. Most physicians are positively influenced by research-based knowledge, and health care agencies will respond positively to cost savings and research-based changes.

Institute the Change in Practice

Implementing a research-based change can be simple or complex, depending on the change. The change may be implemented as indicated in the research literature or may be modified to meet the agency's needs. In some instances, implementation of the change after the decision is made may require a prolonged period of planning. In other instances, implementation can begin immediately. Usually, a great deal of support is needed during initial implementation of a change. As with any new activity, unexpected events often occur. Contact with a person experienced in the change can facilitate the change process.

The change from heparin flush to saline flush will involve the physicians' ordering saline for flushing peripheral venous catheters. You will need to speak with the physicians to gain their support for the change. You may be able to convince some key physicians to support the change, and they will convince others to make the change. The pharmacy will have to package saline for use as a flush. The nurses also will be provided information about the change and the rationale for the change. It may be best to implement the change on one nursing unit and give the nurses on this unit an opportunity to design the protocol and plan for implementing the change. The nurses may develop a protocol similar to the one in Figure 14-5. The protocol must include referencing from the research literature to document that the steps of the protocol are based on research. The evidence-based protocol directs you in preparing for irrigating a peripheral venous catheter, actually irrigating the catheter, and documenting your actions (see Figure 14-5).

Monitor Outcomes

After an evidence-based change has been implemented in practice, nurses and other health care professionals need to monitor appropriate outcomes to determine the effectiveness of the change. They need to document that the change improved quality of care, decreased the cost of care, saved nursing time, improved access to care, or any combination of these benefits. If the outcomes from the EBP change are positive, nurses, administrators, and physicians often will want to continue the change. Nurses usually seek feedback from those around them. Their peers' reactions to the change in nursing practice will influence continuation of the change.

You can confirm the effectiveness of the saline flush for peripheral venous catheter irrigation by examining patient care outcomes and cost-benefit ratios. Patient care outcomes can be examined by determining the number of clotting and phlebitis complications associated with peripheral venous catheters 1 month before the EBP change and 1 month after the change. If no significant difference is seen, the use of saline flush is supported. The cost

Evidence-Based Protocol for Irrigating Peripheral Venous Catheters in Adults*

1. Review the medical order for irrigation of the peripheral venous catheter. Order should indicate that the catheter be irrigated with normal saline (0.9% sodium chloride) (Goode et al., 1991; Randolph et al., 1998).

2. Obtain the saline flush for irrigation from the hospital pharmacy (ASHP, 1994).

3. Wash hands with chlorhexidine, collect equipment for irrigating the peripheral venous catheter, and put on gloves.

4. Evaluate the peripheral venous catheter site every 8 hours for complications of phlebitis. The symptoms of phlebitis include the presence of erythema, tenderness, warmth, and a tender or palpable cord (Goode et al., 1991; Randolph et al., 1998).

5. Cleanse the peripheral venous catheter prior to irrigation with alcohol.

6. Flush the peripheral venous catheter with 1cc of normal saline every 8 hours if no other medication is being given through the site (Goode et al., 1991; Randolph et al., 1998). Check the loss of catheter patency by noting any resistance in irrigating with 1cc of saline or by the inability to administer saline solution within 30 seconds (Geritz, 1992; Shoaf & Oliver, 1992).

7. If a patient is receiving IV medication, administer 1cc of saline, administer the medication, and follow with 1cc saline (Goode et al., 1991; Shoaf & Oliver, 1992).

8. Chart the date and time of the peripheral venous catheter irrigation and the appearance and patency of the catheter site.

*Note: All peripheral venous catheters for pediatric patients must be flushed with heparin flush unless otherwise ordered by physician (Randolph et al., 1998).

References

American Society of Hospital Pharmacists (ASHP) (1994). ASHP therapeutic position statement on the institutional use of 0.9% sodium chloride injection to maintain patency of peripheral indwelling intermittent infusion devices. *American Journal of Hospital Pharmacy, 51*(12), 1572–1574.

Geritz, M. A. (1992). Saline versus heparin in intermittent infuser patency maintenance. *Western Journal of Nursing Research, 14*(2), 131–141.

Goode, C. J., Titler, M., Rakel, B., Ones, D. S. Kleiber, C., Small, S., et al. (1991). A meta-analysis of effects of heparin flush and saline flush: Quality and cost implications. *Nursing Research, 40*(6), 324–330.

Randolph, A. G., Cook, D. J., Gonzales, C. A., & Andrew, M. (1998). Benefits of heparin in peripheral venous and arterial catheters: Systematic review and meta-analysis of randomized controlled trials. *British Medical Journal, 316*(7136), 969–975.

Shoaf, J., & Oliver, S. (1992). Efficacy of normal saline injection with and without heparin for maintaining intermittent intravenous site. *Applied Nursing Research, 5*(1), 9–12.

Figure 14-5. Example of evidence-based protocol.

savings can be calculated for 1 month by determining the cost difference between heparin flush and saline flush. This cost difference can be multiplied by the number of saline flushes conducted in 1 month. This cost savings can then be multiplied by 12 months and compared with the cost savings summarized in the table from Goode and colleagues' meta-analysis study (Table 14-B, p. 517). Nurses need to be given the opportunity to evaluate the change and indicate if it has saved nursing time and promoted high-quality care for management of peripheral venous catheters. If positive patient and nurse outcomes and cost savings are demonstrated, then the health care agency will probably support and extend the EBP of using saline flush for irrigating peripheral venous catheters.

Use of Evidence-Based Guidelines to Facilitate Evidence-Based Practice

EBP has been emphasized in medicine for years, and expert clinicians, professional organizations, and federal agencies have developed several evidence-based guidelines for the prevention of illness and the assessment, diagnosis, and management of acute and chronic diseases. This section describes the development of evidence-based guidelines, gives an example of an evidence-based guideline, and presents steps for implementing an evidence-based guideline in your practice.

Development of Evidence-Based Guidelines

Guideline development is initiated with a selection of a significant health topic. Since the 1980s, the AHRQ has had a major role in the identification of health topics and the development of evidence-based guidelines for these topics (http://www.ahrq.gov). Once the health topic is selected, a guideline development group or expert panel is formed. This group includes nationally recognized researchers in the subject area; expert clinicians, such as physicians, nurses, pharmacists, and social workers; health care administrators; policy developers; economists; government representatives; and consumers. The group designates the scope of the guidelines and conducts an extensive review of the literature including relevant meta-analyses, systematic reviews of research, and integrative reviews of the literature, individual studies, and theories. An excellent source of research publications is the Cochrane Library Collection, available online at http://www.cochrane.org.

The strongest research evidence is synthesized to develop recommendations for practice (see Figure 14-3). Most evidence-based guidelines include meta-analyses, systematic reviews of research, and individual clinical trials and quasi-experimental studies (Forrest & Miller, 2004; Whittemore, 2005). The guidelines are examined for their usefulness in clinical practice, impact on health policy, and cost-effectiveness (Stone, Curran, & Bakken, 2002). Often consultants, other researchers, and additional expert clinicians are asked to review the guidelines and provide input. On the basis of the experts' critique, the guidelines are revised and packaged for distribution to health care professionals. The guidelines are presented at a variety of professional meetings, published in health care journals, and distributed to individual physicians, nurses, and other health care providers. The health care professionals use the guidelines in their practice and examine the impact of the guidelines on their patients. Researchers and clinicians continue to conduct clinical trials and outcome studies to determine the impact of the guidelines on patient, provider, and agency outcomes (Craig & Smyth, 2002; Goode, 2000; Hamer & Collinson, 1999; Melnyk & Fineout-Overholt, 2005).

The AHRQ guidelines are extremely relevant to your own nursing practice. The practice areas with guidelines include (1) management of acute pain in infants, children, and adolescents; (2) prediction and prevention of pressure ulcers in adults; (3) identification and treatment of urinary incontinence in adults; (4) treatment of cataracts in adults; (5) management of functional impairment; (6) treatment of depression in primary care; (7) screening, diagnosis, and management of sickle cell disease in newborns and infants; (8) management of cancer-related pain; (9) treatment of low back problems; (10) treatment of pressure ulcers in adults; (11) quality determinants of mammography; (12) treatment of otitis media in children; (13) screening for Alzheimer's and related dementias; and (14) availability of cardiac rehabilitation services. The AHRQ provides access to numerous clinical practice guidelines on its website at http://www.ahrq.gov/. In addition to the evidence-based guidelines, the AHRQ has developed many tools to assess the quality of care that is provided by these guidelines. You can search a related website, http://www.qualitytools.ahrq.gov/, for an appropriate tool to measure a variable in a research project or to evaluate care in a clinical agency.

A resource that has provided the greatest access to evidence-based guidelines is the National Guideline Clearinghouse (NGC), sponsored by the AHRQ in partnership with the American Medical Association and the American Association of Health Plans in Care. The NGC was initiated in 1998 as an online database of 200 evidence-based guidelines for practice. Currently, the NGC has expanded to encompass more than a thousand clinical practice guidelines from greater than 165 health care organizations and other groups in the United States and other countries. The NGC website with guidelines can be viewed online at http://www.guideline.gov/. Many websites are available that include collections of research evidence and evidence-based guidelines. A partial listing of such websites follows:

- Academic Center for Evidence-Based Nursing: http://www.acestar.uthscsa.edu
- Agency for Healthcare Quality and Research (AHQR): http://www.ahrq.gov
- American College of Physicians: http://www.acponline.org/sci-policy/guidelines/index.html
- American College of Cardiology: http://aappolicy.aappublications.org/practice_guidelines/index.dtl
- American Association of Clinical Endocrinologists: http://www.aace.com/pub/guidelines/
- American Academy of Pediatrics: http://www.aap.org/policy/paramtoc.html
- American Psychiatric Association: http://www.psych.org/psych_pract/treatg/pg/prac_guide.cfm
- Centre for Health Evidence: http://www.cche.net/
- Health Web: Evidence-Based Health Care: http://www.healthweb.org
- HerbMed: Evidence-Based Herbal Database, Alternative Medicine Foundation: http://www.herbmed.org
- MD Consult: http://www.mdconsult.com/
- National Guideline Clearinghouse (NGC): http://www.guideline.gov/
- PIER: The Physicians' Information and Education Resource (authoritative, evidence-based guidance to improve clinical care; ACP-ASIM members only): http://pier.acponline.org/index.html

- U.S. Preventive Services Task Force: http://www.ahrq.gov/clinic/uspstfab.htm
- Primary Care Clinical Practice Guidelines: http://medicine.ucsf.edu/resources/guidelines
- University of Iowa Gerontological Nursing Interventions Research Center: http://www.nursing.uiowa.edu/centers/gnirc/protocols.htm

Example of an Evidence-Based Guideline

Use of evidence-based guidelines has become the standard for providing care to patients in the United States and other nations. A few nurses have participated on committees that developed these evidence-based guidelines and many nurses and advanced-practice nurses (nurse practitioners, clinical nurse specialists, nurse midwives, and nurse anesthetists) are using these guidelines in clinical practice.

An evidence-based guideline for the assessment, diagnosis, and management of high blood pressure is provided as an example. This guideline was developed from the seventh report of the Joint National Committee on Prevention, Detection, Evaluation, and Treatment of High Blood Pressure (JNC 7) and was published in *JAMA: The Journal of the American Medical Association* (Chobanian et al., 2003). The National Heart, Lung, and Blood Institute within the National Institutes of Health (NIH) of the U.S. Department of Health and Human Services (U.S. DHHS) developed educational materials to communicate the specifics of this guideline to promote its use by health care providers.

The guideline is presented in Figure 14-6 and provides clinicians with direction for (1) the classification of blood pressure as normal, prehypertension, hypertension Stage 1, and hypertension Stage 2; (2) the conduct of a diagnostic workup of hypertension; (3) the assessment of the major cardiovascular disease risk factors; (4) the assessment of the identification of causes of hypertension; and (5) the treatment of hypertension. An **algorithm**, or clinical decision tree, provides direction for the selection of the most appropriate treatment method(s) for each patient diagnosed with hypertension (U.S. Department of Health and Human Services [U.S. DHHS], 2003). This guideline will assist nurses in identifying patients with hypertension (HTN) for referral for treatment and also in identifying the common treatment plan for this illness.

Grove Model for Implementing an Evidence-Based Guideline in Practice

Health care providers need to assess the usefulness and quality of each evidence-based guideline before they implement it in their practice. Figure 14-7 provides a model for implementing an evidence-based guideline in practice. In the model, nurses identify a practice problem, search for the best research evidence to manage the problem in their practice, and note that an evidence-based guideline has been developed. The quality of the guideline is assessed by examining the following: (1) the authors of the guideline, (2) the significance of the health care problem, (3) the strength of the research evidence, (4) the link to national standards, and (5) the cost-effectiveness of using the guideline in practice.

The quality of the JNC 7 guideline is examined using the five criteria identified in the Grove Model for Implementing Evidence-Based Guidelines (see Figure 14-7). First, the authors were expert researchers, clinicians (medical doctors), policy developers, health care administrators, and the National High Blood Pressure Education Program Coordinating

EVALUATION

Classification of blood pressure (BP)*

Category	SBP mm Hg		DBP mm Hg
Normal	<120	and	<80
Prehypertension	120–139	or	80–89
Hypertension, Stage 1	140–159	or	90–99
Hypertension, Stage 2	≥160	or	≥100

**See Blood Pressure Measurement Techniques (reverse side)*

Key: SBP = systolic blood pressure
DBP = diastolic blood pressure

Diagnostic workup of hypertension

- Assess risk factors and comorbidities.
- Reveal identifiable causes of hypertension.
- Assess presence of target organ damage.
- Conduct history and physical examination.
- Obtain laboratory tests: urinalysis, blood glucose, hematocrit. and lipid panel, serum potassium, creatinine, and calcium. Optional: urinary albumin/creatinine ratio.
- Obtain electrocardiogram.

Assess for major cardiovascular disease (CVD) risk factors

- Hypertension
- Obesity (body mass index ≥30 kg/m^2)
- Dyslipidemia
- Diabetes mellitus
- Cigarette smoking
- Physical inactivity
- Microalbuminuria, estimated glomerular filtration rate <60 mL/min
- Age (>55 for men, >65 for women)
- Family history of premature CVD (men age <55, women age <65)

Assess for identifiable causes of hypertension

- Sleep apnea
- Drug induced/related
- Chronic kidney disease
- Primary aldosteronism
- Renovascular disease
- Cushing's syndrome or steroid therapy
- Pheochromocytoma
- Coarctation of aorta
- Thyroid/parathyroid disease

TREATMENT

Principles of hypertension treatment

- Treat to BP <140/90 mmHg or BP <130/80 mm Hg in patients with diabetes or chronic kidney disease.
- Majority of patients will require two medications to reach goal.

Algorithm for treatment of hypertension

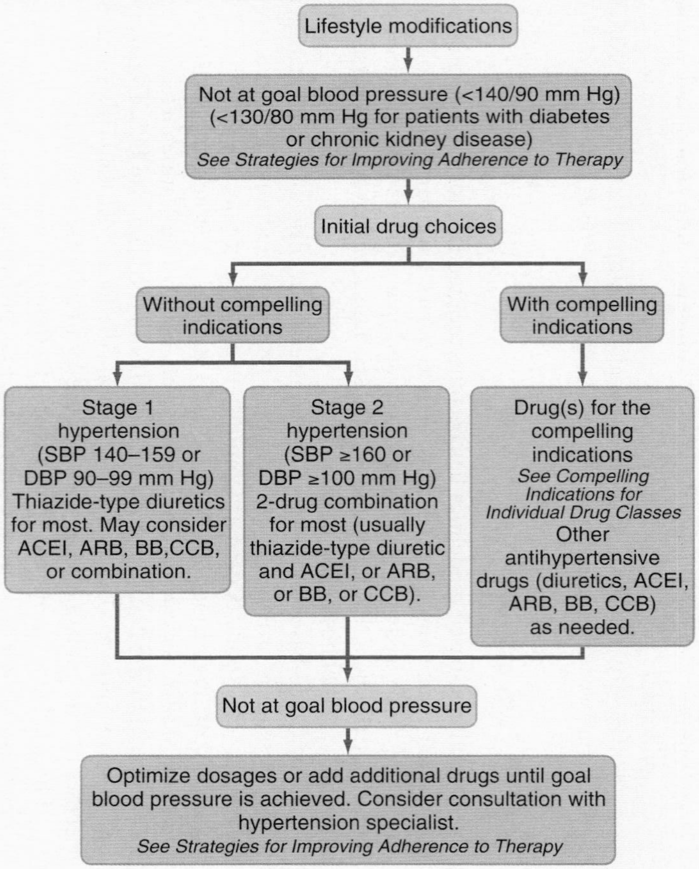

Figure 14-6. Reference card from the seventh report of the Joint National Committee on Prevention, Detection, Evaluation, and Treatment of High Blood Pressure [JNC 7]. (From U.S. Department of Health and Human Services. [2003]. Reference card from the Seventh Report of the Joint National Committee on Prevention, Detection, Evaluation, and Treatment of High Blood Pressure [JNC 7] [NIH Publication No. 03-5231]. Bethesda, MD: National Institutes of Health, National Heart, Lung, and Blood Institute. Retrieved January 25, 2004, from www.nhlbi.nih.gov/guidelines/hypertension/jnc7card.htm)

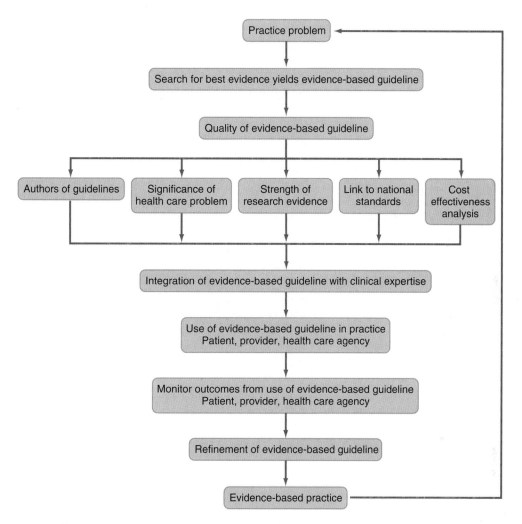

Figure 14-7. Grove Model for Implementing Evidence-Based Guidelines in Practice.

Committee. These professionals have the expertise to develop an evidence-based guideline for HTN.

Second, HTN is a significant health care problem because it affects

approximately 50 million individuals in the United States and approximately 1 billion individuals worldwide.... Hypertension is the most common primary diagnosis in the United States with 35 million office visits as the primary diagnosis.... Recent clinical trials have demonstrated that effective BP [blood pressure] control can be achieved in most patients with hypertension, but the majority will require 2 or more antihypertensive drugs. (Chobanian et al., 2003, p. 2562)

Third, the research evidence for the development of the JNC 7 guideline was extremely strong. The JNC 7 report included 81 references and 9 (11%) of the references were meta-analyses and 35 (43%) were randomized controlled trials, also known as experimental studies. Thus, 44 (54%) sources are considered extremely strong research evidence. The other references were strong and included retrospective analyses or case-control studies, prospective or cohort studies, cross-sectional surveys or prevalence studies, and nonrandom clinical intervention studies (quasi-experimental studies) (Chobanian et al., 2003).

Fourth, the JNC 7 provides the national standard for the assessment, diagnosis, and treatment of HTN. The recommendations from the JNC 7 are supported by the U.S. DHHS and disseminated through NIH Publication No. 03-5231. Finally, use of the JNC 7 guideline in practice is cost-effective because the clinical trials have shown that "antihypertensive therapy has been associated with 35% to 40% mean reductions in stroke incidence; 20% to 25% in myocardial infarction [MI]; and more than 50% in HF [heart failure]" (Chobanian et al., 2003, p. 2562).

The next step is for nurses and physicians to use the JNC 7 guideline in their practice (see Figure 14-7). Health care providers can assess the adequacy of the guideline for their practice and modify the hypertension treatments as indicated by the individual health needs and values of their patients. The outcomes for the patient, provider, and health care agency need to be examined. The outcomes are then recorded in the patients' charts and possibly in a database and will include blood pressure readings for patients; incidence of diagnosis of HTN based on the JNC 7 guidelines; appropriateness of the treatments implemented to manage HTN; and the incidence of stroke, MI, and HF over 5, 10, 15, and 20 years. The health care agency outcomes include the identification of patients with HTN, access to care by patients with HTN, patient satisfaction with care, and the cost related to diagnosis and treatment of HTN and the complications of stroke, MI, and HF. This EBP guideline is then refined according to clinical outcomes, outcome studies, and new controlled clinical trials. The use of this evidence-based guideline and additional guidelines promotes an EBP for nurses and physicians (see Figure 14-7).

We encourage you to visit the EBP websites provided in this textbook and note the guidelines that are available for use in your practice. You can use the algorithm in this chapter to determine the usefulness of the guideline for your practice. The frequent use of EBP guidelines moves nursing toward an evidence-practice profession.

KEY CONCEPTS

- RU is the process of communicating and using research-generated knowledge to make an impact on or a change in the existing practices in the health care system.
- Two major federally funded projects, the WICHE and CURN projects, were implemented to increase utilization of nursing research findings.
- The WICHE Project focused on critiquing research and using research findings to improve practice.
- The CURN Project was implemented to increase the utilization of research findings in the following ways: communicating findings, facilitating organizational modifications necessary for implementation, and encouraging collaborative research that is directly transferable to clinical practice.
- Rogers' Theory of Diffusion of Innovations is presented to direct your use of research findings in practice. Rogers proposes a five-stage process for RU: (1) knowledge, (2) persuasion, (3) decision, (4) implementation, and (5) confirmation.

- EBP is the careful and practical use of current best evidence to guide health care decisions. Current best evidence includes clinical practice guidelines, which usually are nationally developed by expert researchers, clinicians, and theorists in their areas of excellence.
- For selected practice interventions, evidence-based national guidelines have been developed to promote EBP in nursing and other areas of health care.
- EBP is a complex phenomenon, so an algorithm has been developed to help facilitate the movement of nurses toward EBP.

TIPS FOR FURTHER STUDY

- Use the Grove Model to assess the evidence-based guideline for prevention of pressure ulcers.
- Access the National Guideline Clearinghouse and identify a guideline for use in your practice.
- Clarify the difference between research utilization and evidence-based practice. If you are unclear on the difference, complete the Open-Book Quizzes at http://www.elsevier.com/Burns/understanding.
- Complete the *Study Guide* exercises to expand your understanding of evidence-based practice.

REFERENCES

American Association of Critical-Care Nurses [AACN]. (1993). Evaluation of the effects of heparinized and nonheparinized flush solutions on the patency of arterial pressure monitoring lines: The AACN Thunder Project. *American Journal of Critical Care, 2*(1), 3-15.

American Nurses Association. (2004). *Nursing: Scope and standards of practice.* Washington, DC: Author.

American Society of Hospital Pharmacists [ASHP]. (1994). ASHP Therapeutic Position Statement on the institutional use of 0.9% sodium chloride injection to maintain patency of peripheral indewelling intermittent infusion devices. *American Journal of Hospital Pharmacy, 51,* 1572-1574.

Ashton, J., Gibson, V., & Summers, S. (1990). Effects of heparin versus saline solution on intermittent infusion device irrigation. *Heart & Lung, 19*(6), 608–612.

Axford, R., & Cutchen, L. (1977). Using nursing research to improve preoperative care. *Journal of Nursing Administration, 7*(10), 16–20.

Barbour, R. S. (2000). The role of qualitative research in broadening the 'evidence base' for clinical practice. *Journal of Evaluation in Clinical Practice, 6*(2), 155-163.

Barrett, P. J., & Lester, R. L. (1990). Heparin versus saline flushing solutions in a small community hospital. *Hospital Pharmacy, 25*(2), 115–118.

Beck, C. T. (1999). Focus on research methods: Facilitating the work of a meta-analyst. *Research in Nursing & Health, 22*(6), 523-530.

Beck, C. T. (2002). Mothering multiples: A meta-synthesis of qualitative research. *American Journal of Maternal Child Nursing, 27*(4), 214–221.

Beyea, S. C., & Nicoll, L. H. (1995). Administration of medications via the intramuscular route: An integrative review of the literature and research-based protocol for the procedure. *Applied Nursing Research, 8*(1), 23–33.

Brown, S. J. (1999). *Knowledge for health care practice: A guide to using research evidence.* Philadelphia: Saunders.

Burns, N., & Grove, S. K. (2005). *The practice of nursing research: Conduct, critique, and utilization* (5th ed.). Philadelphia: Saunders.

Chobanian, A. V., Bakris, G. L., Black, H. R., Cushman, W. C., Green, L. A., Izzo, J. L., et al. (2003). The seventh report of the Joint National Committee on Prevention, Detection, Evaluation, and Treatment of High Blood Pressure: The JNC 7 report. *JAMA: The Journal of the American Medical Association, 289*(19), 2560-2572.

Clemmens, D. (2001). The relationship between social support and adolescent mothers' interactions with their infants: A meta-analysis. *Journal of Obstetric, Gynecologic, & Neonatal Nursing, 30*(5), 410–420.

Conn, V. S., & Rantz, M. J. (2003). Research methods: Managing primary study quality in meta-analyses. *Research in Nursing & Health, 26*(4), 322–333.

Craig, F. D., & Anderson, S. R. (1991). *A comparison of normal saline versus heparinized normal saline in the maintenance of intermittent infusion devices.* Unpublished manuscript.

Craig, J. V., & Smyth, R. L. (2002). *The evidence-based practice manual for nurses.* Edinburgh: Churchill Livingstone.

CURN Project. (1981, 1982). *Using research to improve nursing practice.* Series of Clinical Protocols: Clean intermittent catheterization (1982), Closed urinary drainage systems (1981), Distress reduction through sensory preparation (1981), Intravenous cannula change (1981), Mutual goal setting in patient care (1982), Pain: Deliberative nursing interventions (1982), Preventing decubitus ulcers (1981), Reducing diarrhea in tube-fed patients (1981), Structured preoperative teaching (1981). New York: Grune & Stratton.

Cyganski, J. M., Donahue, J. M., & Heaton, J. S. (1987). The case for the heparin flush. *American Journal of Nursing, 87*(6), 796–797.

Dixon-Woods, M., Fitzpatrick, R., & Roberts, K. (2001). Including qualitative research in systematic reviews: Opportunities and problems. *Journal of Evaluation in Clinical Practice, 7*(2), 125–133.

Donham, J., & Denning, V. (1987). Heparin vs. saline in maintaining patency, intermittent infusion devices: Pilot study. *The Kansas Nurse, 62*(11), 6–7.

Dracup, K. A., & Breu, C. S. (1978). Using nursing research findings to meet the needs of grieving spouses. *Nursing Research, 27*(4), 212–216.

Dunn, D. L., & Lenihan, S. F. (1987). The case for the saline flush. *American Journal of Nursing, 87*(6), 798–799.

Epperson, E. L. (1984). Efficacy of 0.9% sodium chloride injection with and without heparin for maintaining indwelling intermittent injection sites. *Clinical Pharmacy, 3*(6), 626–629.

Forbes, D. A. (2003). An example of the use of systematic reviews to answer an effective question. *Western Journal of Nursing Research, 25*(2), 179–192.

Forrest, J. L., & Miller, S. A. (2004). The anatomy of evidence-based publications: Article summaries and systematic reviews, Part I. *Journal of Dental Hygiene, 78*(2), 343–348.

Garrelts, J., LaRocca, J., Ast, D., Smith, D. F., & Sweet, D. E. (1989). Comparison of heparin and 0.9% sodium chloride injection in the maintenance of indwelling intermittent I.V. devices. *Clinical Pharmacy, 8*(1), 34–39.

Geritz, M. A. (1992). Saline versus heparin in intermittent infuser patency maintenance. *Western Journal of Nursing Research, 14*(2), 131–141.

Glaser, E. M., Abelson, H. H., & Garrison, K. N. (1983). *Putting knowledge to use.* San Francisco, CA: Jossey-Bass.

Goode, C. J. (2000). What constitutes the "evidence" in evidence-based practice? *Applied Nursing Research, 13*(4), 222–225.

Goode, C. J., Titler, M., Rakel, B., Ones, D. S., Kleiber, C., Small, S., & Triolo, P. K. (1991). A meta-analysis of effects of heparin flush and saline flush: Quality and cost implications. *Nursing Research, 40*(6), 324–330.

Greenway, K. (2004). Using the ventrogluteal site for intramuscular injection. *Nursing Standard, 18*(25), 39–42.

Haller, K. B., Reynolds, M. A., & Horsley, J. A. (1979). Developing research-based innovation protocols:

Process, criteria, and issues. *Research in Nursing & Health, 2*(2), 45–51.

Hamer, S., & Collinson, G. (1999). *Achieving evidence-based practice: A handbook for practitioners.* Edinburgh: Bailliére Tindall.

Hamilton, R. A., Plis, J. M., Clay, C., & Sylvan, L. (1988). Heparin sodium versus 0.9% sodium chloride injection for maintaining patency of indwelling intermittent infusion devices. *Clinical Pharmacy, 7*(6), 439–443.

Holford, N. H., Vozeh, S., Coates, P., Porvell, J. R., Thiercelin, J. F., & Upton, R. (1977). More on heparin lock. *The New England Journal of Medicine, 29*(22), 1300–1301.

Horsley, J. A., Crane, J., & Bingle, J. D. (1978). Research utilization as an organizational process. *Journal of Nursing Administration, 8*(7), 4–6.

Horsley, J. A., Crane, J., Crabtree, M. K., & Wood, D. J. (1983). *Using research to improve nursing practice: A guide.* New York: Grune & Stratton.

Kasparek, A., Wenger, J., & Feldt, R. (1988). *Comparison of normal versus heparinized saline for flushing of intermittent intravenous infusion devices.* Unpublished manuscript. Mercy Medical Center, Cedar Rapids, IA, pp. 1–18.

Keen, M. F. (1986). Comparison of intramuscular injection techniques to reduce site discomfort and lesions. *Nursing Research, 35*(4), 207–210.

Krueger, J. C. (1978). Utilization of nursing research: The planning process. *Journal of Nursing Administration, 8*(1), 6–9.

Krueger, J. C., Nelson, A. H., & Wolanin, M. O. (1978). *Nursing research: Development, collaboration, and utilization.* Germantown, MD: Aspen.

Kruszewski, A., Lang, S., & Johnson, J. (1979). Effect of positioning on discomfort from intramuscular injections in the dorsogluteal site. *Nursing Research, 28*(2), 103–105.

Lombardi, T. P., Gunderson, B., Zammett, L. O., Walters, J. K., & Morris, B. A. (1988). Efficacy of 0.9% sodium chloride injection with or without heparin sodium for maintaining patency of intravenous catheters in children. *Clinical Pharmacy, 7*(11), 832–836.

Marwick, C. (1997). Aspirin's role in prevention now official. *JAMA: The Journal of the American Medical Association, 277*(9), 701–702.

Melnyk, B. M., & Fineout-Overholt, E. (2005). *Evidence-based practice in nursing & healthcare: A guide to best practice.* Philadelphia: Lippincott Williams & Wilkins.

Miracle, V., Fangman, B., Kayrouz, P., Kederis, K., & Pursell, L. (1989). Normal saline vs. heparin lock flush solution: One institution's findings. *The Kentucky Nurse, 37*(3), 1, 6–7.

Pelz, D., & Horsley, J. (1981). Measuring utilization of nursing research. In J. Ciarlo (ed.), *Utilizing evaluation.* Beverly Hills, CA: Sage.

Peterson, F. Y., & Kirchhoff, K. T. (1991). Analysis of the research about heparinized versus nonheparinized intravascular lines. *Heart & Lung, 20*(6), 631–640.

Randolph, A. G., Cook, D. J., Gonzales, C. A., & Andrew, M. (1998). Benefit of heparin in peripheral venous and arterial catheters: Systematic review and meta-analysis of randomized controlled trials. *British Medical Journal, 316*(7136), 969–975.

Redeker, N. S. (2000). Sleep in acute care settings: An integrative review. *Journal of Nursing Scholarship, 32*(1), 31–38.

Rettig, F. M., & Southby, J. R. (1982). Using different body positions to reduce discomfort from dorsogluteal injection. *Nursing Research, 31*(4), 219–221.

Rodger, M. A., & King, L. (2000). Drawing up and administering intramuscular injections: A review of the literature. *Journal of Advanced Nursing, 31*(3), 574–582.

Rogers, E. M. (1995). *Diffusion of innovations* (4th ed.). New York: Free Press.

Sackett, D. L., Strauss, S. E., Richardson, W. S., Rosenberg, W., & Haynes, R. B. (2000). *Evidence-based medicine: How to practice and teach EBM* (2nd ed.). London: Churchill Livingstone.

Schustek, M. (1984). The cost effective approach to PRN device maintenance. *NITA, 7*(6), 527.

Shearer, J. (1987). Normal saline flush versus dilute heparin flush. A study of peripheral intermittent IV devices. *National Intravenous Therapy Association, 10*(6), 425–427.

Shoaf, J., & Oliver, S. (1992). Efficacy of normal saline injection with and without heparin for maintaining intermittent intravenous site. *Applied Nursing Research, 5*(1), 9–12.

Spann, J. M. (1988). Efficacy of two flush solutions to maintain catheter patency in heparin locks. *Dissertation Abstracts, 28*(1) 1337125, 1–58. *Dissertation Abstracts International, 42*(4), 1394B (University Microfilms No. 8120152).

Stetler, C. B., Brunell, M., Giuliano, K. K., Morsi, D., Prince, L., & Newell-Stokes, V. (1998). Evidence-based practice and the role of nursing leadership. *Journal of Nursing Administration, 28*(7/8), 45–53.

Stone, P. W., Curran, C. R., & Bakken, S. (2002). Economic evidence for evidence-based practice. *The Journal of Nursing Scholarship, 34*(3), 277–282.

Taylor, N., Hutchinson, E., Milliken, W., & Larson, E. (1989). Comparison of normal versus heparinized saline for flushing infusion devices. *Journal of Nursing Quality Assurance, 3*(4), 49–55.

Titler, M. G., Kleiber, C., Steelman, V. J., Goode, C., Rakel, B. A., Barry-Walker, J. et al. (1994). Infusing research into practice to promote the quality of care. *Nursing Research, 43*(5), 307–313.

Titler, M. G., Kleiber, C., Steelman, V. J., Rakel, B. A., Budreau, G., Everett, L. Q. et al. (2001). The Iowa Model of Evidence-Based Practice to promote quality care. *Critical Care Nursing Clinics of North America, 13*(4), 497–509.

Tuten, S. H., & Gueldner, S. H. (1991). Efficacy of sodium chloride versus dilute heparin for maintenance of peripheral intermittent intravenous devices. *Applied Nursing Research, 4*(2), 63–71.

U.S. Department of Health and Human Services. (2003). Reference card from the seventh report of the Joint National Committee on Prevention, Detection, Evaluation, and Treatment of High Blood Pressure (JNC 7) (NIH Publication No. 03-5231). Bethesda, MD: National Institutes of Health, National Heart, Lung, and Blood Institute. Retrieved December 14, 2005, from http://www.nhlbi.nih.gov/guidelines/hypertension/jnc7card.htm

Whittemore, R. (2005). Combining evidence in nursing research: Methods and implications. *Nursing Research, 54*(1), 56–62.

Wichita, C. (1977). Treating and preventing constipation in nursing home residents. *Journal of Gerontological Nursing, 3*(6), 35–39.

GLOSSARY

A

Abstract (adjective) Expressed without reference to any specific instance.

Abstract (noun) Clear, concise summary of a study, usually limited to 100 to 250 words.

Abstract thinking Thinking that is oriented toward the development of an idea, without application to or association with a particular instance; independent of time and space. Abstract thinkers tend to look for meaning, patterns, relationships, and philosophical implications. (*Compare* Concrete thinking.)

Academic library Library located within an institution of higher learning; contains numerous research reports in journals and books.

Acceptance rate The number or percentage of the subjects who agree to participate in a study. The percentage is calculated by dividing the number of subjects agreeing to participate by the number of subjects approached. For example, for a study in which 100 subjects are approached and 90 agree to participate, the acceptance rate is 90%: 90 ÷ 100 = 0.90 × 100% = 90%.

Accessible population Portion of the target population to which the researcher has reasonable access.

Accidental sampling *See* Convenience sampling.

Accuracy in physiological measures Addresses the extent to which a physiological instrument measures the concept defined in the study. Accuracy is comparable to validity.

Across-method triangulation Combining research methods or strategies from two or more research traditions in the same study.

Action application of research Use of research findings as a driving force for change, as an impetus for evaluation of services, and as a model for practice.

Active rejection Decision not to adopt an innovation that was examined.

Adoption Full acceptance and implementation of an innovation in practice.

Agency for Healthcare Research and Quality (AHRQ) Federal agency created in 1989 to carry out research, demonstration projects, evidence-based guideline development, training, and research dissemination activities with respect to health care services and systems. Focus of this agency is to promote evidence-based health care (website: www.ahrq.gov).

Algorithm Decision tree that provides a set of rules for solving a particular practice problem. Its development usually is based on research evidence and theoretical knowledge.

Alpha (α) Cutoff point used to determine whether the samples being tested are members of the same population or of different populations; alpha commonly is set at 0.05, 0.01, or 0.001.

Alternate forms reliability Degree of equivalence of two versions of the same paper-and-pencil instrument.

Analysis of covariance (ANCOVA) Statistical procedure in which a regression analysis is carried out before performing ANOVA; designed to reduce the variance within groups by partialing out the variance due to a confounding variable.

Analysis of variance (ANOVA) Statistical test used to examine differences among two or more groups by comparing the variability between groups with the variability within each group.

Analysis critique phase Phase of a critique in which the reader determines the strengths and limitations of the logical links between study elements.

Analytic induction Qualitative research technique that includes enumerative induction, in which a variety of instances are collected that verify the model, and eliminative induction, in which the hypothesis is tested against alternatives.

Analytical preciseness Precision obtained by transforming concrete data across several levels of abstraction to develop a theoretical schema that explains the phenomenon under study.

Analyzing research reports Critical thinking skill that involves determining the value of a study by breaking the contents of a study report into parts and examining the parts for accuracy, completeness, uniqueness of information, and organization.

Anonymity Conditions in which the subject's identity cannot be linked, even by the researcher, with his or her individual responses.

Applied (practical) research Scientific investigations conducted to generate knowledge that will directly influence clinical practice.

Approximate replication Operational replication that involves repeating the original study under similar conditions, following the original methods as closely as possible.

Ascendance to an open context Ability to see depth and complexity within the phenomenon examined; a greater capacity for insight than usually is found with the sedimented view. Requires deconstructing sedimented views and reconstructing another view.

Assent A child's affirmative agreement to participate in research.

Associative hypothesis Hypothesis that identifies variables that occur or exist together in the real world, such that when one variable changes, the other changes.

Associative relationship Relationship in which variables or concepts that occur or exist together in the real world are identified; thus when one variable changes, the other changes. Hypotheses can be developed to identify associative relationships.

Assumptions Statements taken for granted or considered true, even though they have not been scientifically tested.

Asymmetrical relationship Relationship in which the following are true: if A occurs or changes, then B will occur or change; but if B occurs or changes, A will not necessarily occur or change.

Auditability Rigorous development of a decision trail that can be applied by a second researcher to the original data. This process is done to determine if the second researcher's conclusions are similar to those of the original researcher.

Authority Person with expertise and power who is able to influence the opinions and behavior of others.

Autonomous agents Prospective subjects who are informed about a proposed study and who can voluntarily choose whether to participate.

B

Basic (pure) research Scientific investigations for the pursuit of "knowledge for knowledge's sake" or for the pleasure of learning and finding truth.

Benchmark Identified standard an agency wants to achieve in the provision of health care, such as having a 1% complication rate for intramuscular injections.

Benchmarking Process of measuring outcomes from a health care agency for comparison with identified national standards.

Beneficence, principle of Principle that encourages the researcher to do good and "above all, do no harm."

Benefit-risk ratio Ratio considered by researchers and reviewers of research as they weigh potential benefits (positive outcomes) and risks (negative outcomes) of a study; used to promote the conduct of ethical research.

Best research evidence Produced by the conduct and synthesis of numerous, high-quality studies in a health-related area. The best research evidence is generated in the areas of health promotion; illness prevention; and the assessment, diagnosis, and management of acute and chronic illnesses.

Between-group variance A source of variation of the group means around the grand mean.

Bias Influence or action in a study that distorts the findings or slants them away from the true or expected.

Bibliographical database Compilation of citations.

Bibliography List of publications for a specific topic or specialty area.

Bivariate analysis Statistical procedure in which the summary values from either two groups of the same variable or two variables within a group are compared.

Bivariate correlation Measure of the extent of the linear relationship between two variables.

Blocking System used in randomized block design in which subjects with various levels of an extraneous variable are included in the sample. The number of subjects are controlled at each level of the variable and are randomly assigned to groups within the study.

Body of knowledge Information, principles, and theories that are organized by the beliefs accepted in a discipline at a given time.

Bonferroni's procedure Parametric analysis technique that controls for escalation of significance and can be used if various *t*-tests must be performed on different aspects of the same data.

Borrowing Appropriation and use of knowledge from other disciplines to guide nursing practice.

Box-and-whisker plot Exploratory data analysis technique to provide fast visualization of some of the major characteristics of the data, such as the spread, symmetry, and identity of outliers.

Bracketing Qualitative research technique of suspending or setting aside what is known about an experience being studied.

Breach of confidentiality Accidental or direct action that allows an unauthorized person to have access to raw study data.

Byte Computer space for storing a single character, such as a number or a letter of the alphabet.

C

Canonical correlation Extension of multiple regression with more than one dependent variable.

Carryover effect Outcome observed when application of one treatment influences the response to subsequent treatments.

Case study In-depth analysis and systematic description of one patient or a group of similar patients to promote understanding of nursing interventions.

Case study design Intensive exploration of a single unit of study, such as a person, family, group, community, or institution.

Causal hypothesis Hypothesis that states the relationship between two variables, in which one variable (independent variable) is thought to cause or determine the presence of the other variable (dependent variable).

Causality Relationship that includes three conditions: (1) there must be a strong correlation between the proposed cause and effect, (2) the proposed cause must precede the effect in time, and (3) the cause must be present whenever the effect occurs.

Cell Intersection between the row and column in a table where a specific numerical value is inserted.

Central processing unit (CPU) Device that controls computer operations and includes the internal memory, control unit, and arithmetic and logic unit.

Centralized diffusion system System that involves group decision making within an organization; usually includes a change agent to promote utilization of research-based innovations.

Change agent A professional outside a social system who enters the system to promote adoption of a research-based innovation.

Chi-square test of independence Used to analyze nominal data to determine significant differences between observed frequencies within the data and frequencies that were expected.

Citation Information necessary to locate a reference. Citation for a journal article includes the author's name, year of publication, title, journal name, volume number, issue number, and page numbers.

Citation search indexes Link citations on the basis of the references at the end of articles.

Cleaning data Checking raw data to determine errors in data recording, coding, or entry.

Clinical decision analysis A systematic method of describing clinical problems, identifying possible diagnostic and management courses of action, assessing the probability and value of the various outcomes, and then calculating the optimal course of action.

Clinical expertise A practitioner's knowledge, skills, and past experience in accurately assessing, diagnosing, and managing an individual patient's health needs.

Clinical pathway Method used in health care that organizes, implements, and evaluates a comprehensive plan of care for a patient. Agencies develop clinical pathways to facilitate the implementation of quality cost-effective care.

Clinical significance Importance (significance) of research findings in answering a clinical question or solving a clinical problem.

Cluster sampling Sampling in which a frame is developed that includes a list of all the states, cities, institutions, or organizations (clusters) that could be used in a study; a randomized sample is drawn from this list.

Cochran Q test Nonparametric test that is an extension of the McNemar test for two related samples.

Code Symbol or abbreviation used to classify words or phrases in qualitative data.

Codebook Record that documents the location or the column(s) that represent each variable and other information entered in a computer file.

Coding Way of indexing or identifying categories in qualitative data.

Coefficient of determination (R^2) Computed from a matrix of correlation coefficients and provides important information on multicolinearity. This value indicates the degree of linear dependencies among the variables.

Coercion Overt threat of harm or excessive reward intentionally presented by one person to another in order to obtain compliance; an example is offering prospective subjects a large sum of money to participate in a dangerous research project.

Coefficient of multiple determination Statistical technique that involves the use of multiple independent variables to predict one dependent variable and is represented by R^2 statistic.

Cognitive application of research Process in which research-based knowledge is used to affect a person's way of thinking, approaching, or observing situations.

Cognitive clustering Comprehensive, scholarly synthesis of scientifically sound research that is evident in integrative reviews of research and meta-analyses.

Cohorts Samples in time-dimensional studies within the field of epidemiology.

Coinvestigators Two or more professionals conducting a study, whose salaries may be paid partially or in full by grant funding.

Communication of research findings Developing a research report and disseminating it to a variety of audiences with presentations and publications.

Comparative descriptive design Design used to describe differences in variables in two or more groups in a natural setting.

Comparison group The group of subjects in a study not receiving a treatment when nonrandom methods are used for sample selection. There are four types of comparison groups: (a) groups that receive no treatment, (b) groups that receive a placebo treatment, (c) groups that receive standard or usual health care, and (d) groups that receive a second experimental treatment or a different treatment dose for comparison with the first experimental treatment.

Comparison critique phase Phase or step of a critique in which the reader compares the ideal for each step of the research process with the real steps in a study.

Compatibility Degree to which an innovation is perceived to be consistent with current values, past experience, and priority of needs.

Complete observer Researcher who is passive and has no direct social interaction in the setting.

Complete participation Situation in which the researcher becomes a member of the group and conceals the researcher role.

Complete review Type of institutional review process for studies with risks that are greater than minimal. The review of a study is extensive or complete by an institutional review board.

Complex hypothesis Hypothesis that predicts the relationship (associative or causal) among three or more variables; thus, the hypothesis can include two (or more) independent and/or two (or more) dependent variables.

Complex search Search that combines two or more concepts or synonyms in one search. The concepts selected for search may be based on the results of previous searches.

Complexity Degree to which an innovation is perceived to be difficult to understand or use.

Comprehending research reports Critical thinking process used in reading a research report, in which the focus is on understanding the major concepts and the logical flow of ideas within a study.

Comprehension critique phase Step of a critique during which the reader gains understanding of the terms in a research report; identifies the study elements; and grasps the nature, significance, and meaning of these elements.

Computer search Process of using computer databases to scan literature citations and identify sources relevant to a selected topic.

Computerized database Structured compilation of information that can be scanned, retrieved, and analyzed by computer and can be used for decisions, reports, and research.

Concept Term that abstractly describes and names an object or phenomenon, thus providing it with a separate identity or meaning.

Concept analysis Strategy used to identify a set of attributes or characteristics that are essential to the connotative meaning or conceptual definition of a concept.

Concept derivation Process of extracting and defining concepts from theories in other disciplines.

Concept synthesis Process of describing and naming a previously unrecognized concept.

Conceptual clustering step of critique Step in which current knowledge in an area of study is carefully analyzed, summarized, and organized theoretically to maximize the meaning attached to research findings, highlight gaps in the knowledge base, generate research questions, and provide knowledge for use in practice.

Conceptual definition Definition that provides a variable or concept with connotative (abstract, comprehensive, theoretical) meaning; established through concept analysis, concept derivation, or concept synthesis.

Conceptual map Strategy for expressing a framework of a study that diagrammatically shows the interrelationships of concepts and statements.

Conceptual model Set of highly abstract, related constructs that broadly explains phenomena of interest, expresses assumptions, and reflects a philosophical stance.

Conclusions Syntheses and clarifications of the meanings of study findings.

Concrete thinking Thinking that is oriented to and limited by tangible things or events observed and experienced in reality. (*Compare* Abstract thinking.)

Concurrent relationship Relationship in which variables or concepts occur simultaneously.

Concurrent replication Simultaneous collection of data for both the original and replication study; the replication study provides a check of the reliability of the original study findings.

Confidence interval Range in which the value of the parameter is estimated to exist.

Confidentiality Management of private data in research in such a way that only the researcher knows the subjects' identities and can link them with their responses.

Confirmation stage Stage in Rogers' theory of research utilization in which nurses evaluate the effectiveness of the change in practice and decide whether to continue the change.

Confirmatory analysis Analysis performed to confirm expectations regarding data that are expressed as hypotheses, questions, or objectives.

Confounding variables Variables that cannot be controlled; they may be recognized before the study is initiated or may not be recognized until the study is in process.

Consent form Written form, tape recording, or videotape used to document a subject's agreement to participate in a study.

Consensus knowledge building Outcomes design that requires critique and synthesis of an extensive international search of the literature on the topic of concern, including unpublished studies, studies in progress, dissertations, and theses.

Constant comparison Methodological technique in grounded theory research in which every piece of data is compared with every other piece.

Construct validity Measure of how well the conceptual and operational definitions of variables match each other; determine whether the instrument measures the theoretical construct it purports to measure.

Constructs Concepts at very high levels of abstraction that have general meanings.

Consultants Persons hired for specific professional, specialized tasks during a study.

Content analysis Qualitative analysis technique used to classify words in a text into a few categories that were chosen for their theoretical importance.

Content-related validity Extent to which the method of measurement includes all the major elements relevant to the construct being measured.

Contingency table Cross-tabulation table that allows visual comparison of summary data output related to two variables within a sample.

Contingent relationship Relationship that occurs only when a third variable or concept is present.

Continuance Decision to continue using an innovation and include the protocol in the procedures manual.

Control Writing of a prescription to produce the desired outcomes in practice. In research, the imposing of rules by the researcher to decrease the possibility of error and increase the probability that the study's findings are an accurate reflection of reality.

Control group The group of elements or subjects not exposed to the experimental treatment in a study in which the sample is randomly selected.

Convenience sampling Including subjects in the study who happened to be in the right place at the right time, with addition of available subjects until the desired sample size is reached. Also referred to as "accidental sampling."

Correlation matrix Correlational results for a number of variables that are presented in table form.

Correlational analysis Statistical procedure conducted to determine the direction (positive or negative) and magnitude or strength (+1 to –1) of the relationship between two variables.

Correlational coefficient Statistical term used to indicate the degree of relationship between two variables; the coefficients range in value from +1.00 (perfect positive relationship) to 0.00 (no relationship) to –1.00 (perfect negative or inverse relationship).

Correlational design A study design for examining the relationships between or among two or more variables in a single group, which can occur at several levels.

Correlational research Systematic investigation of relationships between two or more variables to explain the nature of relationships in the world; does not examine cause and effect.

Cost-benefit analysis Analysis technique used in outcomes research that examines the costs and benefits of alternative ways of using resources as assessed in monetary terms and the use that produces the greatest net benefit.

Cost-effectiveness analysis Type of outcomes research in which costs and benefits are compared for different ways of accomplishing a clinical goal, such as diagnosing a condition, treating an illness, or providing a service. The goal of cost-effectiveness analyses is to identify the strategy that provides the most value for the money.

Costs, health-related Financial end points or outcomes of healthcare that are often examined to determine the most cost-effective way to deliver high-quality healthcare to patients and families.

Covered entity Public or private entity that processes or facilitates the processing of health information.

Covert data collection Data collection that occurs without subjects' knowledge or awareness.

Cramer's V Analysis technique for nominal data; a modification of phi for contingency tables.

Criterion-referenced testing Comparison of a subject's score with a criterion of achievement that includes the definitions of target behaviors. When the behaviors are mastered, the subject is considered proficient in these behaviors.

Critical analysis of studies Examination of the strengths, weaknesses, meaning, and significance of nursing studies using four steps: comprehension, comparison, analysis, and evaluation.

Critique Careful examination of all aspects of a study to judge its strengths, limitations, meaning, and significance.

Cross-sectional designs Designs used to examine groups of subjects in various stages of development simultaneously, with the intent of inferring trends over time.

Cultural immersion Strategy used in ethnographic research for gaining increased familiarity with aspects of a culture, such as language, sociocultural norms, and traditions.

Culture Way of life belonging to a designated group of people.

Current best evidence Includes clinical practice guidelines that usually are nationally developed by expert researchers, clinicians, and theorists in their areas of excellence.

Current sources Sources published within five years prior to acceptance of a respective manuscript for publication.

Curvilinear relationship Relationship between two variables that varies with the relative values of the variables.

D

Data Information that is collected during a study.

Data analysis Technique used to reduce, organize, and give meaning to data.

Data-based literature Consists of research reports, both published reports in journals and books and unpublished reports such as theses and dissertations.

Databased or empirical sources Relevant studies published in journals and books; also includes unpublished studies such as master's theses and doctoral dissertations.

Data coding sheet Sheet for organizing and recording data for rapid entry into a computer.

Data collection Identification of subjects and the precise, systematic gathering of information (data) relevant to the research purpose or the specific objectives, questions, or hypotheses of a study.

Data collection plan Plan specifying the details of how a study will be conducted.

Data storage and retrieval Process in which vast amounts of data collected for a study are stored, usually in a computer, and later retrieved for examination and analyses.

Data triangulation Collection of data from multiple sources in the same study.

Data use agreement Agreement that limits how the data set with health information may be used and how it will be protected in research.

Database *See* Computerized database.

Debriefing Complete disclosure of the study purpose and results at the end of a study.

Debugging Identifying and replacing errors in a computer program with accurate information.

Decentralized diffusion system System involving one-to-one communication and individual decisions regarding the use of research-based innovations.

Deception Misinforming subjects for research purposes. After a study is completed, subjects must be debriefed or informed of the true purpose and outcomes of a study so that areas of deception are clarified.

Decision stage Stage in Rogers' theory about research utilization in which nurses either adopt or reject an innovation or change in practice.

Decision theory Theory based on assumptions associated with the theoretical normal curve; used in testing for differences between groups, with the expectation that all of the groups are members of the same population. The expectation is expressed as a null hypothesis, and the level of significance (alpha) is often set at 0.05 before data collection.

Declaration of Helsinki Ethical code that distinguishes therapeutic from nontherapeutic research; based on the Nuremberg Code.

Deductive reasoning Reasoning from the general to the specific or from a general premise to a particular situation.

Degrees of freedom (df) The freedom of a score's value to vary, given the values of other existing scores and the established sum of these scores ($df = N - 1$).

Delphi technique Method of measuring the judgments of a group of experts for assessing priorities or making forecasts.

Demographic variables Characteristics or attributes of subjects that are collected to describe the sample.

Dependent groups Subjects or observations selected for data collection that are in some way related to the selection of other subjects or observations. For example, when subjects in the control group are matched for age or gender with the subjects in the experimental group, these groups are dependent groups.

Dependent (response or outcome) variable The response, behavior, or outcome that is predicted or explained in research; changes in the dependent variable are presumed to be caused by the independent variable.

Description Identification of the characteristics of nursing phenomena, or of the relationships among these phenomena.

Descriptive codes Terms used to organize and classify qualitative data.

Descriptive correlational design Design used to describe variables and examine relationships that exist in a situation.

Descriptive design Design used to identify a phenomenon of interest, identify variables within the phenomenon, develop conceptual and operational definitions of variables, and describe variables.

Descriptive research Research that provides an accurate portrayal or account of characteristics of a particular person, event, or group in real-life situations; research that is conducted to discover new meaning, describe what exists, determine the frequency with which something occurs, and categorize information.

Descriptive statistics Statistics that allow the researcher to organize the data in ways that give meaning and facilitate insight; examples are frequency distributions and measures of central tendency and dispersion.

Descriptive time dimensional designs Designs for examining sequences and patterns of change, growth, or trends over time.

Descriptive vividness Description of the site, subjects, experience of collecting data, and the researcher's thoughts during the qualitative research process. Information is presented clearly enough for the reader to have a sense of personally experiencing the event.

Design Blueprint for conducting a study; maximizes control over factors that could interfere with the validity of the findings.

Design validity Quality of the study design and the ability of the design to generate accurate findings. Types of design validity include statistical conclusion validity, internal validity, construct validity, and external validity.

Deterministic relationships Statements of what always occurs in a particular situation, such as a scientific law.

Developmental grant proposal Proposal written to obtain funding for the development of a new program in a discipline.

Dialectic reasoning Reasoning that involves a holistic perspective, in which the whole is greater than the sum of the parts; examining factors that are opposites and making sense of them by merging them into a single unit or idea greater than either alone.

Diary Type of measurement in research where a record of events is kept by a subject over time and is analyzed by a researcher.

Difference scores Deviation scores obtained by subtracting the mean from each raw score; measure of dispersion.

Diffusion Process of communicating research findings (innovations) through various channels over time to the members of a discipline.

Diminished autonomy Condition of subjects whose ability to give informed consent voluntarily is decreased because of legal or mental incompetence, terminal illness, or confinement to an institution.

Direct application Use of an innovation exactly as it was developed.

Direct measures Concrete variables that can be measured objectively with a specific measurement strategy, such as using a scale to measure weight.

Directional hypothesis Hypothesis stating the specific nature of the interaction or relationship between two or more variables.

Discomfort and harm Phrase used to describe the degree of risk for a subject participating in a study. These levels of risk include no anticipated effects, temporary discomfort, unusual levels of temporary discomfort, risk of permanent damage, or certainty of permanent damage.

Discontinuance Decision to stop or discontinue the use of an innovation. Two types of discontinuance are disenchantment and replacement discontinuance.

Discriminant analysis Analysis that allows the researcher to identify characteristics associated with group membership and to predict group membership.

Disenchantment discontinuance Decision to discontinue the use of an innovation because the user is dissatisfied with its outcome.

Dissemination of research findings The diffusion or communication of research findings.

Dissertation An extensive, usually original research project that is completed by a doctoral student as part of the requirements for a doctoral degree.

Distribution The spread of scores in a sample; includes the frequency and range of scores in the sample.

E

Early adopters of innovations Opinion leaders in a social system who learn about new ideas, rapidly utilize them, and serve as role models for their use in nursing practice.

Early majority in the use of innovations Individuals who are rarely leaders but are active followers and will readily follow in the use of a new idea in nursing practice.

Effect size The degree to which the phenomenon studied is present in the population or to which the null hypothesis is false.

Efficiency The least costly method of achieving a desired end or outcome with the maximum benefit to be obtained from available resources.

Electronic journals Journals that are published and available on the Internet.

Electronic mail (e-mail) Computer networking system that allows a user to rapidly exchange messages, files, data, and research reports using satellite networks.

Element of a study A person (subject), event, behavior, or any other single unit of a study.

Eligibility criteria *See* Sampling criteria.

Embodied The belief that the person is a self within a body.

Emic approach Anthropological research approach to studying behaviors from within a culture.

Empirical generalizations Statements that have been repeatedly tested through research and have not been disproved (scientific theories have empirical generalizations).

Empirical world The world that people experience through the senses; the concrete portion of human existence.

Environmental variables Types of extraneous variables composing the setting in which a study is conducted.

Error in physiological measures Error caused by environmental factors, variations in operation of equipment, machine instability and calibration, or misinterpreted electrical signals.

Error score Amount of random error in the measurement process.

Ethical inquiry Intellectual analysis of ethical problems related to obligation, rights, duty, right and wrong, conscience, choice, intention, and responsibility to obtain desirable, rational ends.

Ethical principles Principles of respect for persons, beneficence, and justice that are relevant to the conduct of research.

Ethnographic research Qualitative research methodology for investigating cultures. The research involves collection, description, and analysis of data to develop a theory of cultural behavior.

Ethnonursing research Type of research that emerged from Leininger's Theory of Transcultural Nursing; focuses mainly on observing and documenting interactions with people to determine how daily life conditions and patterns influence human care, health, and nursing care practices.

Etic approach Anthropological research approach to studying behavior from outside the culture and examining similarities and differences across cultures.

Evaluation critique phase Step of a critique in which the reader examines the meaning and significance of a study according to set criteria and compares it with previous studies conducted in the area.

Event partitioning designs Merger of the longitudinal and trend designs to increase sample size and avoid the effects of history on the validity of findings.

Event-time matrix Qualitative analysis technique for comparing events that occurred in different sites during particular time periods.

Evidence-based health care system Incorporates health care research evidence from a variety of disciplines, clinical expertise of the health care providers, views of the patients and families, and the resources available to deliver health care.

Evidence-based practice (EBP) The conscientious integration of best research evidence with clinical expertise and patients values and needs in the delivery of high-quality, cost-effective health care.

Evidence-based practice guidelines Patient care guidelines that are based on synthesized research findings from meta-analyses, integrative reviews of research, and extensive clinical trials; supported by consensus from recognized national experts; and affirmed by outcomes obtained by clinicians.

Evidence for best practices Synthesis of research findings to determine the best empirical knowledge to guide care delivery in a discipline.

Exact replication Precise or exact duplication of the initial researcher's study to confirm the original findings.

Exclusion sample criteria Sampling criteria or characteristics that can cause a person or element to be excluded from the target population.

Exempt from review Designation given to studies that have no apparent risks for the research subjects and thus are designated as exempt by an institutional review board.

Existence statement Declaration that a given concept or relationship exists.

Expedited review Institutional review process for studies that have some risks, but the risks are minimal or no greater than those ordinarily encountered in daily life or during the performance of routine physical or psychological examinations.

Experiment Procedure in which subjects are randomized into groups, data are collected, and statistical analyses are conducted to support a premise.

Experimental design Design that provides the greatest amount of control possible in order to examine causality more closely.

Experimental group Group of subjects receiving the experimental treatment.

Experimental research Objective, systematic, controlled investigation to examine probability and causality among selected variables for the purpose of predicting and controlling phenomena.

Explained variance Variation in values that is explained by the relationship between the two variables.

Explanation Clarification of relationships among variables and identification of reasons why certain events occur.

Explanatory codes Codes that are developed late in the data collection process after theoretical ideas from the qualitative study have begun to emerge.

Explanatory effects matrix Qualitative analysis technique that can assist in answering such questions as why an outcome was achieved or what caused the outcome.

Exploratory analysis Examining the data descriptively to become as familiar as possible with it.

External criticism Method for determining the validity of source materials in historical research; involves knowing where, when, why, and by whom a document was written.

External storage device Equipment for permanently storing data and programs outside a computer.

External validity Extent to which study findings can be generalized beyond the sample used in the study.

Extraneous variables Variables that exist in all studies and can affect the measurement of study variables and the relationships among these variables.

F

Fabrication in research A form of scientific misconduct in research that involves making up results and recording or reporting them.

Face validity Verification that the instrument measures the content desired.

Factor A category of several closely related variables that are considered together.

Factor analysis Analysis that examines interrelationships among large numbers of variables and disentangles those relationships to identify clusters of variables that are most closely linked. Two types of factor analysis are exploratory and confirmatory.

Factorial analysis of variance Analysis technique that is mathematically a specialized version of multiple regression; various types of factorial ANOVAs have been developed to analyze data from specific experimental designs.

Fair treatment Ethical principle that promotes fair selection and treatment of subjects during the course of a study.

Falsification of research A type of scientific misconduct that involves manipulating research materials, equipment, or processes, or changing or omitting data or results, such that the research is not accurately represented in the research record.

Fatigue effect Effect that occurs when a subject becomes tired or bored with a study.

Feasibility of a study Suitability of a study; determined by examining the time and money commitment; the researcher's expertise; availability of subjects, facility, and equipment; cooperation of others; and the study's ethical considerations.

Findings The translated and interpreted results from a study.

Focus groups Measurement strategy where groups are assembled to obtain the participants' perceptions in focused areas in settings that are permissive and nonthreatening in a qualitative study.

Foundational inquiry Research on the foundations for a science, such as studies that analyze the structure of a science and the process of thinking about and valuing certain phenomena held in common by the science. Debates related to quantitative and qualitative research methods emerged from foundational inquiries.

Framework Abstract, logical structure of meaning, such as a portion of a theory, that guides the development of the study, is tested in the study, and enables the researcher to link the findings to nursing's body of knowledge.

Fraudulent publication A type of scientific misconduct where published research reports do not reflect what was actually done in a study; indicated by documentation or testimony from coauthors.

Frequency distribution Statistical procedure that lists all possible measures of a variable and tallies each datum on the listing.

Friedman two-way analysis of variance by ranks Nonparametric test used with matched samples or in repeated measures.

Full-text databases Internet resource that provides full text and list of citations of journal articles for a specific topic.

G

Generalization Extension of the implications of the findings from the sample or situation that was studied to a larger population or situation.

General proposition A highly abstract statement of the relationship between two or more concepts that is found in a conceptual model.

Geographical analyses Used to examine variations in health status, health services, patterns of care, or patterns of use by geographical area.

Gestalt Organization of knowledge about a particular phenomenon into a cluster of linked ideas; the clustering and interrelatedness enhance the meaning of the ideas.

Grant Proposal developed to seek research funding from private or public institutions.

Grounded Theory that has its roots in the qualitative data from which it was derived.

Grounded theory research Inductive research technique based on symbolic interaction theory; conducted to discover the problems that exist in a social scene and the process that persons involved use to handle them; involves formulation, testing, and redevelopment of propositions until a theory is developed.

Grouped frequency distribution Means of grouping continuous measures of data into categories.

H

Hawthorne effect Psychological response in which subjects change their behavior simply because they are subjects in a study, not because of the research treatment.

Health Insurance Portability and Accountability Act (HIPAA) Federal regulations implemented in 2003 to protect an individual person's health information. The HIPAA Privacy Rule affects not only the health care environment but also the research conducted in this environment.

Heterogeneous sample A sample in which subjects have a broad range of values being studied, which increases the representativeness of the sample and the ability to generalize from the accessible population to the target population.

Heuristic relevance Standard for evaluating a qualitative study for criteria of intuitive recognition, relationship to the existing body of knowledge, and applicability.

Hierarchical statement set Specific proposition and a hypothesis or research question. If a conceptual model is included in the framework, the set also may include a general proposition.

Highly controlled setting Artificially constructed environment that is developed for the sole purpose of conducting research, such as a laboratory, research or experimental center, or test unit.

Historical research Narrative description or analysis of events that occurred in the remote or recent past.

History effect Event that is not related to the planned study but occurs during the time of the study and could influence the responses of subjects to the treatment.

Homogeneity in design Degree to which objects are elements in a study and affect the internal design validity are similar or share a form of equivalence, such as limiting subjects to only one level of an extraneous variable to reduce its impact on the study findings.

Homogeneity in instruments The correlation of various items within an instrument or multiple item scale that is calculated using the Cronbach alpha coefficient.

Homogeneous sample Sample in which subjects' scores on selected measurement methods in a study are similar, resulting in a limited or narrow distribution or spread of scores.

Homoscedastic Term describing data that are evenly dispersed above and below the regression line, indicating a linear relationship on a scatter diagram (plot).

Human rights Claims and demands that have been justified in the eyes of an individual person or by the consensus of a group of people and are protected in research.

Hypothesis Formal statement of the expected relationship between two or more variables in a specified population.

I

Implementation stage Stage in Rogers' theory of research utilization in which an individual practitioner or agency adopts a research-based change. The types of implementation include direct application, reinvention, and indirect effects.

Implications The meaning of research conclusions for the body of knowledge, theory, and practice.

Implicit framework Rudimentary ideas for the framework of a theory or portions of a theory expressed in an introduction or in a literature review in which linkages among variables found in previous studies are discussed.

Inclusion sample criteria Those sampling criteria or characteristics that the subject or element must possess to be considered part of the target population.

Incomplete disclosure Failure to fully inform subjects about the purpose of a study because of the possibility that knowledge might alter the subjects' actions; subjects need to be debriefed when the study is finished.

Independent groups Study groups chosen so that the selection of one subject is unrelated to the selection of other subjects. For example, if subjects are randomly assigned to a treatment group or a comparison group, the groups are independent.

Independent (treatment or experimental) variable Treatment or experimental activity that is manipulated or varied by the researcher to cause an effect on the dependent variable.

Index Library resource that can be used to identify journal articles and other publications relevant to a topic.

Indirect effects Use of research findings by citing them in clinical papers and textbooks and incorporating them to strengthen arguments.

Indirect measures Methods used with abstract concepts that are not measured directly; rather, indicators or attributes of the concepts are used to represent the abstraction and are measured in the study.

Individually identifiable health information (IIHI) "…any information, including demographic information collected from an individual that is created or received by healthcare provider, health plan, or healthcare clearinghouse; and related to past, present, or future physical or mental health or condition of an individual, the provision of healthcare to an individual, or the past, present, or future payment for the provision of healthcare to an individual, and identifies the individual; or with respect to which there is a reasonable basis to believe that the information can be used to identify the individual" (U.S. Department of Health and Human Services, 2003, *45 CFR*, Section 160.103).

Inductive reasoning Reasoning from the specific to the general, in which particular instances are observed and then combined into a larger whole or general statement.

Inference Generalization from a specific case to a general truth, from a part to the whole, from the concrete to the abstract, or from the known to the unknown.

Inferential statistics Statistics designed to allow inference from a sample statistic to a population parameter; commonly used to test hypotheses of similarities and differences in subsets of the sample under study.

Informed consent Agreement by a prospective subject to participate voluntarily in a study after he or she has assimilated essential information about the study.

Inherent variability Variability in which a few random observations can be naturally expected in the data in the extreme ends of the tail of the normal curve.

Interdisciplinary team A team comprising multiple health disciplines and involved in the care of the same patients. The team members share information and coordinate their services.

Innovation Idea, practice, or object that is perceived as new by an individual nurse, a nursing unit, an entire agency, or another decision-making unit.

Innovation-decision process Process that includes the steps of knowledge, persuasion, decision, implementation, and confirmation to promote diffusion or communication of research evidence to members of a discipline.

Innovators People who actively seek out new ideas.

Input device Device that enables the user to enter data and instructions into the computer system.

Institutional review Process of examining studies for ethical concerns by a committee of peers.

Institutional review board (IRB) A committee that reviews research to ensure that the investigator is conducting the research ethically.

Instrument validity Extent to which an instrument reflects the abstract construct being examined.

Instrumentation Component of measurement in which specific rules are applied to develop a measurement device or instrument.

Integrative review of the literature Rigorous analysis and synthesis of results from independent quantitative and qualitative studies and theoretical and methodological literature to determine the current knowledge (what is known and not known) for a particular concept, measurement methods, or practice topic.

Integrative review of research Review conducted to identify, analyze, and synthesize the results from independent studies to determine the current knowledge (what is known and not known) in a particular area.

Intellectual research critique Careful examination of all aspects of a study to judge the strengths, weaknesses, meaning, and significance of the study based on previous research experience and knowledge of the topic.

Interlibrary loan department Department that locates books and articles in other libraries and provides the sources within a designated time.

Intermediate end points Events or markers that act as precursors to the final outcome.

Internal criticism Criticism involving examination of the reliability of historical documents.

Internal validity Extent to which the effects detected in a study reflect reality rather than resulting from the effects of extraneous variables.

Internet Worldwide network that connects computers together.

Interpretation of research outcomes Process in which researchers examine the results from data analysis, form conclusions, consider the implications for nursing, explore the significance of the findings, generalize the findings, and suggest further studies.

Interpretative codes Organizational system developed late in the process of collecting and analyzing qualitative data, as the researcher gains insight into the existing processes.

Interpretative reliability Extent to which each judge assigns the same category to a given unit of data.

Interrater reliability Degree of consistency between two raters who are independently assigning ratings to a variable or attribute being investigated; also referred to as "equivalence."

Interrupted time series designs Designs similar to descriptive time dimensional designs, except that a treatment is applied at some point in the observations.

Interval estimate Range of values (identified by the researcher) on a number line where the population parameter is thought to be.

Interval-scale measurement Use of interval scales or methods of measurement with equal numerical distances between intervals of the scale; follows the rules of mutually exclusive categories, exhaustive categories, and rank ordering, such as temperature.

Intervention Treatment or independent variable that is manipulated during the conduct of a study to produce an effect on the dependent or outcome variables.

Interview Structured or unstructured oral communication between the researcher and the subject, during which information is obtained for a study.

Introspection Process of turning one's attention inward toward one's own thoughts, providing increased awareness and understanding of the flow and interplay of feelings and ideas.

Intuiting Process of looking at the phenomenon in qualitative research; all awareness and energy are focused on the subject of interest.

Intuition Insight or understanding of a situation or an event as a whole that usually cannot be logically explained.

Intuitive recognition Theoretical schema derived from the data of a qualitative study that has meaning within the reader's personal knowledge base.

Invasion of privacy Sharing private information with others without a person's knowledge or against his or her will.

Investigator triangulation Phenomenon that occurs when two or more research-trained investigators with divergent backgrounds explore the same phenomenon using different methods.

J

Justice, principle of Ethical principle stating that human subjects should be treated fairly.

K

Kendall's tau Nonparametric test used to determine correlations among variables that have been measured at the ordinal level.

Keywords Major concepts or variables of a research problem or topic that are used to begin a search of a database.

Knowledge Information that is acquired in a variety of ways, is expected to be an accurate reflection of reality, and is incorporated and used to direct a person's actions.

Knowledge stage Stage of Rogers' theory about research utilization in which nurses become aware of an innovation or new idea for use in practice.

Kolmogorov-Smirnov two-sample test Nonparametric test used to determine whether two independent samples have been drawn from the same population.

Kurtosis Degree of peakedness (platykurtic, mesokurtic, or leptokurtic) of the curve that is related to the spread or variance of scores.

L

Laggards People who are security oriented, tend to cling to the past, and often are isolated without a strong support system. Term used in the innovation-decision process to describe persons who are reluctant or refuse to adopt and use evidence-based interventions in practice.

Lambda Analysis technique that measures the degree of association (or relationship) between two nominal-level variables.

Landmark studies Major projects generating knowledge that influence a discipline and sometimes society in general.

Late majority People who are skeptical about new ideas and will adopt them only if group pressure is great. Term used in the innovation-decision process to describe persons who are reluctant to adopt and use research or evidence-based interventions in practice.

Leptokurtic Term used to describe an extremely peaked-shape distribution of a curve, which means that the scores in the distribution are similar and have limited variance.

Level of significance *See* Alpha (α).

Levels of measurement Organized set of rules for assigning numbers to objects so that a hierarchy in measurement from low to high is established. The levels of measurement are nominal, ordinal, interval, and ratio.

Library resources Library personnel, interlibrary loan department, circulation department, reference department, audiovisual department, computer search department, and photocopy services.

Library sources Sources for research, including journals, books, monographs, master's theses, doctoral dissertations, government documents, and other publications of research findings.

Likert scale Instrument designed to determine the opinion on or attitude toward a particular subject; contains a number of declarative statements with a scale after each statement.

Limitations Theoretical and methodological restrictions in a study that may decrease the generalizability of the findings.

Line of best fit Best reflection of the values on the scatterplot.

Linear relationship Relationship between two variables or concepts that remains consistent regardless of the values of each variable or concept.

Linking Activity that moves a computer user from one website to another.

Literature review Summary of theoretical and empirical sources to generate a picture of what is known and not known about a particular problem.

Logic A science in which valid ways of relating ideas are used to promote human understanding; includes abstract and concrete thinking and logistic, inductive, and deductive reasoning.

Logistic reasoning Reasoning used to break the whole into parts that can be carefully examined, as can the relationships among the parts.

Longitudinal designs Research designs used to examine changes in the same subjects over an extended time period.

M

Mainframe computer Computer with the largest memory and greatest speed; used in universities and large companies.

Manipulation Moving around or controlling a specific attribute (such as movement) of, as in the manipulation of a treatment.

Mann-Whitney U test Test used to analyze ordinal data (with 95% of the power of the *t*-test) to detect differences between groups of normally distributed populations.

Manual search Examination of catalogs, indexes, abstracts, and bibliographies for relevant sources.

Map *See* Conceptual map.

Matching Selecting subjects in the control group who are equivalent to subjects in the experimental group in important extraneous variables.

Maturation effect Unplanned and unrecognized changes subjects experience during a study, such as growing older, wiser, stronger, hungrier, or more tired, that can influence the findings of the study.

McNemar test Nonparametric test used to analyze the changes that occur in dichotomous variables.

Mean The value obtained by summing all the scores and dividing the total by the number of scores being summed.

Measurement Process of assigning numbers to objects, events, or situations in accordance with some rule.

Measurement error Difference between what exists in reality and what is measured by a research instrument.

Measures of central tendency Statistical procedures (mode, median, and mean) for determining the center of a distribution of scores.

Measures of dispersion Statistical procedures (range, difference scores, sum of squares, variance, and standard deviation) for examining how scores vary or are dispersed around the mean.

Median Score at the exact center of the ungrouped frequency distribution.

Memoing Method that is used by researchers to record insights or ideas related to notes, transcripts, or codes during qualitative data analysis.

Mentor Person who provides information, advice, and emotional support to a protégé.

Mentorship Intense form of role modeling in which an expert nurse serves as a teacher, sponsor, guide, exemplar, and counselor for a novice nurse.

Mesokurtic Term that describes a normal curve with an intermediate degree of kurtosis and intermediate variance of scores.

Meta-analysis Performing statistical analyses to integrate and synthesize findings from completed studies to determine what is known and not known about a particular research area.

Metasummary Synthesis of multiple primary qualitative studies to produce a narrative about a selected phenomenon (Whittemore, 2005).

Metasynthesis Synthesis of qualitative research involving the critical analysis of primary qualitative studies and synthesis of findings into a new theory or framework for the topic of interest.

Methodological congruence Standard for evaluating qualitative research, in which documentation rigor, procedural rigor, ethical rigor, and auditability of the study are examined.

Methodological designs Designs used to develop the validity and reliability of instruments to measure research concepts and variables.

Methodological limitations Restrictions in the study design that limit the credibility of the findings and the population to which the findings can be generalized.

Methodological triangulation The use of two or more research methods or procedures in a study (such as different designs, instruments, and data collection procedures).

Middle-range theories Theories that are relatively concrete and specific in focus and include a limited number of concepts and propositions. These theories are tested by empirical research.

Minimal risk Research subject's risk of harm anticipated in the proposed study that is not greater, considering probability and magnitude, than that ordinarily encountered in daily life or during the performance of routine physical or psychological examinations.

Mixed results Study results that include both significant and nonsignificant findings.

Modal percentage Percentage appropriate for nominal data; indicates the relationship of the number of data scores represented by the mode to the total number of data scores.

Modality Characteristic of distributions; symmetrical distributions usually are unimodal.

Mode Numerical value or score that occurs with the greatest frequency in a distribution but does not necessarily indicate the center of the data set.

Model testing designs Designs used to test the accuracy of a hypothesized causal model or map.

Monographs Sources that usually are written once, such as books, booklets of conference proceedings, or pamphlets, and may be updated with a new edition.

Mono-method bias Bias that occurs when more than one measure of a variable is used in a study, but all measures use the same method of recording.

Mono-operation bias Bias that occurs when only one method of measurement is used to measure a construct or concept.

Mortality rate, sample The percentage of subjects who drop out of a study before its completion, creating a threat to the internal validity of the study.

Multicausality Recognition that a number of interrelated variables can cause a particular effect.

Multicollinearity Phenomenon that occurs when the independent variables in a regression equation are strongly correlated.

Multilevel analysis Used in epidemiology to study how environmental factors and individual attributes and behavior interact to influence individual-level health behavior and disease risk.

Multimethod-multitrait technique Technique in which a variety of data collection methods are used, such as interview and observation; the same measurement methods are used for each concept.

Multiple regression Extension of simple linear regression; more than one independent variable is analyzed.

Multiple triangulation Use of two or more types of triangulation (theoretical, data, methodological, investigator, and analysis) in a study.

Multistage sampling Randomized selection that continues through several stages.

Multivariate analysis techniques Techniques used to analyze data from complex, multivariate research projects; they include multiple regression, factorial analysis of variance, analysis of covariance, factor analysis, discriminant analysis, canonical correlation, structural equation modeling, time series analysis, and survival analysis.

N

Natural (field) setting Uncontrolled, real-life setting where research is conducted, such as subjects' homes, work sites, and schools.

Necessary relationship Relationship in which one variable or concept must occur for the second variable or concept to occur.

Negative relationship Relationship in which one variable or concept changes (its value increases or decreases), and the other variable or concept changes in the opposite direction.

Network (or snowball) sampling Sampling technique that takes advantage of social networks and the fact that friends tend to have characteristics in common; subjects meeting the sample criteria are asked to assist in locating others with similar characteristics.

Networking Process of developing channels of communication among people with common interests.

Nominal-scale measurement Lowest level of measurement used when data can be organized into categories that are exclusive and exhaustive, but the categories cannot be compared, such as gender, race, marital status, and nursing diagnoses.

Nondirectional hypothesis Hypothesis that states that a relationship exists but does not predict the exact nature of the relationship.

Nonequivalent control group designs Designs in which the control group is not selected by random means, such as the one-group posttest-only design, the posttest-only design with nonequivalent groups, and the one-group pretest-posttest design.

Nonparametric statistics Statistical techniques used when the assumptions of parametric statistics are not met; most commonly used to analyze nominal and ordinal data.

Nonprobability sampling Sampling in which not every element of the population has an opportunity for selection, such as convenience sampling, quota sampling, purposive sampling, and network sampling.

Nonsignificant results Results that are negative or contrary to the researcher's hypotheses; the results may accurately reflect reality or may be caused by study weaknesses.

Nontherapeutic research Research conducted to generate knowledge for a discipline; the results might benefit future patients but will probably not benefit the research subjects.

Norm-referenced Term describing test performance standards that have been carefully developed over years with large, representative samples, using standardized tests with extensive reliability and validity.

Normal curve Symmetrical, unimodal, bell-shaped curve that is a theoretical distribution of all possible scores; no real distribution exactly fits the normal curve.

Null (statistical) hypothesis Hypothesis stating that no relationship exists between the variables being studied; a hypothesis used for statistical testing and for interpreting statistical outcomes.

Nuremberg code Ethical code of conduct to guide investigators in conducting research ethically.

Nursing process Subset of the problem-solving process. Steps include assessment, diagnosis, plan, implementation, evaluation, and modification.

Nursing research Scientific process that validates and refines existing knowledge and generates knowledge that directly and indirectly influences clinical nursing practice.

O

Observability Extent to which the results of an innovation are visible to others.

Observational measurement Use of structured and unstructured observation to measure study variables.

Observed score Score or value obtained for a subject on a measurement tool.

Observer-as-participant Researcher whose time is spent predominantly observing and interviewing subjects, with less time spent in the participant role.

One-tailed test of significance Analysis used with directional hypotheses, in which extreme statistical values of interest are thought to occur in a single tail of the normal curve.

Open context Condition that requires deconstructing a sedimented view, allowing the researcher to see the depth and complexity within the phenomenon being examined in qualitative research.

Operational definition Description of how variables or concepts will be measured or manipulated in a study.

Operational reasoning Identification and discrimination of many alternatives or viewpoints; focuses on the process of debating alternatives.

Opportunity costs Costs related to loss of opportunity for financial or other growth experiences by the patient, family member, or others.

Out-of-pocket costs Expenses incurred by the patient or family or both that are not reimbursable by the insurance company.

Ordinal-scale measurement Measurement yielding data that can be ranked, but the intervals between the ranked data are not necessarily equal, such as levels of coping.

Outcomes research Important scientific methodology that was developed to examine the end results of patient care. The strategies used in outcomes research are a departure from the traditional scientific endeavors and incorporate evaluation research, epidemiology, and economic theory perspectives.

Outliers Extreme scores or values due to inherent variability, errors of measurement or execution, or error in identifying the variables important in explaining the nature of the phenomenon under study.

P

Parallel forms reliability *See* Alternate forms reliability.

Parameter Measure or numerical value of a population.

Parametric statistical analyses Statistical techniques used when three assumptions are met: (1) the sample was drawn from a population for which the variance can be calculated, and the distribution is expected to be normal or approximately normal; (2) the level of measurement should be at least interval, with an approximately normal distribution; and (3) the data can be treated as random samples.

Paraphrasing Clearly and concisely restating the ideas of an author in the researcher's own words.

Partially controlled setting Environment that is manipulated or modified in some way by the researcher.

Participant observation Special form of observation in which researchers immerse themselves in the setting so that they can hear, see, and experience what the participants do; the participants are aware of the dual role of the researcher (participant and observer).

Passive rejection Decision not to adopt an innovation that was never seriously considered.

Pearson product-moment correlation Parametric test used to determine relationships among variables.

Percentage distributions Percentage of the sample whose scores fall into a specific group and the number of scores in that group.

Periodicals Literature sources such as journals that are published over time and are numbered sequentially for the years published.

Personal experience Knowledge gained through participation in rather than observation of an event, situation, or circumstance. Benner (1984) described five levels of experience in the development of clinical knowledge and expertise: (1) novice, (2) advanced beginner, (3) competent, (4) proficient, and (5) expert.

Persuasion stage Stage of Rogers' theory about research utilization in which an individual practitioner or agency develops a favorable or unfavorable attitude toward the change or innovation to be used in practice.

Phenomenological research Inductive, descriptive qualitative methodology developed from phenomenological philosophy for the purpose of describing experiences as they are lived by the study participants.

Phenomenon (*plural:* phenomena) An occurrence or a circumstance that is observed, something that impresses the observer as extraordinary, or a thing that appears to and is constructed by the mind.

Phi coefficient Analysis technique used to determine relationships in dichotomous, nominal data.

Philosophical analysis Use of concept or linguistic analyses to examine meaning and develop theories of meaning in philosophical inquiry.

Philosophical or theoretical connectedness Theoretical schema developed from a qualitative study; is clearly expressed, logically consistent, reflective of the data, and compatible with nursing's knowledge base.

Philosophical inquiry Research using intellectual analyses to clarify meanings, make values manifest, identify ethics, and study the nature of knowledge. Types of philosophical inquiry include foundational inquiry, philosophical analyses, and ethical analyses.

Philosophical stance Specific philosophical view held by an individual person or group of persons.

Philosophies Rational, intellectual explorations of truths; principles of being, knowledge, or conduct.

Physiological measurement Techniques used to measure physiological variables either directly or indirectly; examples are techniques to measure heart rate or mean arterial pressure.

Pilot study Smaller version of a proposed study conducted to develop and refine the methodology, such as the treatment, instruments, or data collection process to be used in the larger study.

Pink sheet Letter rejecting a research grant proposal, with a critique by the scientific committee that reviewed the proposal.

Plagiarism A type of scientific misconduct with appropriation of another person's ideas, processes, results or words without giving appropriate credit, including those obtained through confidential review of others' research proposals and manuscripts.

Platykurtic Term that indicates a relatively flat curve, with large variance among the scores.

Point estimate Single figure that estimates a related figure in the population of interest.

Population All elements (people, objects, events, or substances) that meet the sample criteria for inclusion in a study; sometimes referred to as a target population.

Population-based studies Important type of outcomes research that involves studying health conditions in the context of the community rather than the context of the medical system.

Positive relationship Relationship in which one variable changes (its value increases or decreases) and the second variable changes in the same direction.

Poster session Visual presentation of a study, with text, tables, and illustrations on a display board.

Posthoc analyses Statistical techniques performed in studies with more than two groups to determine which groups are significantly different. For example, ANOVA may indicate significant differences among three groups, but the posthoc analyses indicate specifically which groups are different.

Power Probability that a statistical test will detect a significant difference or relationship that exists; power analysis is used to determine the power of a study.

Power analysis Technique used to determine the risk of a Type II error so that the study can be modified to decrease the risk if necessary.

Practice effect Effect that occurs when subjects improve as they become more familiar with the experimental protocol.

Practice pattern profiling An epidemiological technique used in outcomes research that focuses on patterns of care rather than individual occurrences of care.

Practice theories Very specific theories that are developed to explain a particular element of practice. These theories can be generated through research and also tested by research.

Precision Accuracy with which the population parameters have been estimated within a study; also used to describe the degree of consistency or reproducibility of measurements with physiologic instruments.

Prediction Estimation of the probability of a specific outcome in a given situation that can be achieved through research.

Prediction equation Outcome of regression analysis.

Predictive correlational design Design developed to predict the value of one variable based on values obtained for other variables; an approach to examining causal relationships between variables.

Premise Proposition or statement of the proposed relationship between two or more concepts.

Preproposal Short document (generally four pages plus appendices) written to explore the funding possibilities for a research project.

Primary source Source whose author originated or is responsible for generating the ideas published.

Principal investigator Person who will have primary responsibility for administering a research grant and interacting with the funding agency.

Privacy Freedom to determine the time, extent, and general circumstances under which private information will be shared with or withheld from others.

Probability Chance that a given event will occur in a situation; addresses the relative rather than the absolute causality of events.

Probability sampling Random sampling technique in which every member (element) of the population has a probability higher than zero of being selected for the sample; examples include simple random sampling, stratified random sampling, cluster sampling, and systematic sampling.

Probability statement Statement expressing the likelihood that something will happen in a given situation; addresses relative rather than absolute causality.

Probability theory Theory addressing statistical analysis from the perspective of the extent of a relationship or the probability of accurately predicting an event.

Problematic reasoning Reasoning that involves identifying a problem, selecting solutions to the problem, and resolving the problem.

Problem-solving process Systematic identification of a problem, determination of goals related to the problem, identification of possible approaches to achieve those goals, implementation of selected approaches, and evaluation of goal achievement.

Problem statement Statement that concludes the discussion of a problem and indicates the gap in the knowledge needed for practice. The problem statement usually provides a basis for the study purpose.

Process Purpose, series of actions, and goal.

Process-outcome matrix Qualitative analysis technique that allows the researcher to trace the processes that led to differing outcomes.

Propositions (relational statements) When occurring within theories, statements expressed at various levels of abstraction.

Projective techniques Techniques for measuring persons' responses to unstructured or ambiguous situations as a means of describing attitudes, personality characteristics, and motives of the individuals (e.g., the Rorschach inkblot test).

Proposition Abstract statements that further clarify the relationship between two concepts in theories.

Prospective cohort study An epidemiological study in which a group of people are identified who are at risk for experiencing a particular event and are included as participants in a study.

Protection from discomfort and harm Ethical principle stating that

Public library Library that serves the needs of the community in which it is located; usually contains few research reports.

Purposive sampling Judgmental or selective sampling that involves the conscious selection by the researcher of certain subjects or elements to include in a study. This sampling strategy is used most frequently in qualitative research.

Q

Q-plots Displays of scores or data in a distribution by quartile for exploratory data analysis.

Q-sort Exploratory data analysis technique for comparative rating, in which a subject sorts cards with statements into designated piles (usually 7 to 10 piles in the distribution of a normal curve) that might range from best to worst.

Qualitative research Systematic, subjective methodological approach used to describe life experiences and give them meaning.

Quality of care Outcome examined in the conduct of outcomes research.

Quantitative research Formal, objective, systematic process used to describe variables, test relationships between them, and examine cause-and-effect interactions among variables.

Quantitative research process Conceptualizing, planning, implementing, and communicating the findings of a quantitative research project.

Quasi-experimental designs Types of designs developed to determine the effectiveness of interventions in quantitative quasi-experimental studies.

Quasi-experimental research Type of quantitative research conducted to explain relationships, clarify why certain events happen, and examine causality between selected independent and dependent variables.

Query letter Letter sent to a journal editor to determine interest in publishing an article or to a funding agency to determine interest in providing funds for a study.

Questionnaire Printed self-report form designed to elicit information that can be obtained through written or verbal responses of the subject.

Quota sampling Convenience sampling technique with an added strategy to ensure the inclusion of subjects who are likely to be underrepresented in the convenience sample, such as women, minority groups, and undereducated persons.

R

Random assignment Procedure used to assign subjects randomly to treatment or control groups; subjects have an equal probability of being assigned to either group.

Random error Error that causes individual subjects' observed scores to vary haphazardly around their true scores.

Random sampling Technique in which every member (element) of the population has a probability higher than zero for being selected for a sample, which increases the sample's representativeness of the target population.

Random variation The expected difference in values that occurs when the researcher examines different subjects from the same sample.

Randomized clinical trial Classic means of examining the effects of various treatments in which the effects of a treatment are examined by comparing the treatment group with the non-treatment group.

Range Simplest measure of dispersion; obtained by subtracting the lowest score from the highest score.

Rating scale Scale that lists an ordered series of categories of a variable and is assumed to be based on an underlying continuum.

Ratio-scale measurement Highest level of measurement form; meets all the rules of other forms of measure: mutually exclusive categories, exhaustive categories, rank ordering, equal spacing between intervals, a continuum of values, and an absolute zero. An example is measurement of weight.

Reading research reports Process used to learn about research studies; skills used include skimming, comprehending, and analyzing the content of the report.

Reasoning Processing and organizing ideas to reach conclusions; types of reasoning include problematic, operational, dialectic, and logistic.

Refereed journal Journal that uses referees or expert reviewers to determine whether a manuscript will be accepted for publication.

Referencing Comparing a subject's score against a standard; used in norm-referenced and criterion-referenced testing.

Reflexive thought Process in which a qualitative researcher explores personal feelings and experiences that may influence the study and integrates this understanding into the study.

Refusal rate The percentage of subjects who declined to participate in the study. The study should include their rationale for not participating. The refusal rate is calculated by dividing the number refusing to participate by the number of potential subjects approached. For example, if 100 subjects are approached and 15 refuse to participate, the refusal rate is $15 \div 100 = 0.15 \times 100\% = 15\%$.

Regression analysis Statistical procedure used to predict the value of one variable using known values of one or more other variables.

Regression line The line that best represents the values of the raw scores plotted on a scatter diagram; the procedure for developing the line of best fit is the method of least squares.

Reinvention Modification of an innovation by its adopters to meet their own needs.

Rejection Decision not to use an innovation; can be active or passive. *See* Active rejection; Passive rejection.

Relational statement Declaration that a relationship of some kind exists between two or more concepts.

Relative advantage Extent to which an innovation is perceived to be better than current practice.

Relevant sources Sources that are pertinent or highly important in providing the in-depth knowledge needed to make changes in practice or to study a selected problem.

Relevant studies Those investigations or studies that have a specific focus on in a researcher's area of interest.

Reliability Extent to which an instrument consistently measures a concept; three types of reliability are stability, equivalence, and homogeneity.

Reliability testing Measure of the amount of random error in the measurement technique.

Replacement discontinuance Decision to discontinue the use of an innovation in order to adopt a better idea.

Replication studies Studies that are reproduced or repeated to determine whether similar findings will be obtained.

Representative sample Sample that is like the population it is supposed to represent in as many ways as possible.

Representativeness Degree to which the sample, accessible population, and target population are alike.

Research Diligent, systematic inquiry or investigation to validate and refine existing knowledge and generate new knowledge.

Research-based protocol Document providing clearly developed steps for implementing a treatment or intervention in practice that is based on findings from studies.

Research design Blueprint for conducting a study; maximizes control over factors that could interfere with the validity of the findings; guides the planning and implementation of a study in a way that is most likely to achieve the intended goal.

Research evidence Knowledge generated from the synthesis of research findings from several quality studies.

Research hypothesis Alternative hypothesis to the null hypothesis; states that a relationship exists between two or more variables.

Research misconduct *See* Scientific misconduct.

Research objective Clear, concise, declarative statement expressed to direct a study; focuses on identifying and describing variables and relationships among variables.

Research outcomes Conclusions of findings, generalization of findings, implications of findings for nursing, and suggestions for further study presented in the discussion section of the research report.

Research problem An area of concern in which there is a gap in the knowledge base needed for nursing practice. Research is conducted to generate essential knowledge to address the practice concern, with the ultimate goal of providing evidence-based practice.

Research process Process that requires an understanding of a unique language and involves rigorous application of a variety of research methods.

Research proposal Written plan that identifies the major elements of a study, such as the problem, purpose, and framework, and outlines the methods that will be used to conduct the study.

Research purpose Concise, clear statement of the specific goal or aim of the study. The purpose is generated from the problem.

Research question Concise interrogative statement developed to direct a study; focuses on describing variables, examining relationships among variables, and determining the differences between two or more groups.

Research report Report summarizing the major elements of a study and identifying the contributions of that study to nursing knowledge.

Research topic Concept or broad problem area that provides the basis for generating numerous questions and research problems.

Research tradition A program of research that is important for building a body of knowledge related to the phenomena explained by a particular conceptual model.

Research utilization Process of communicating and using empirical or research-generated knowledge to affect or change the existing practices in the health care system.

Research variables or concepts The qualities, properties, or characteristics identified in the research purpose and objectives that are observed or measured in a study.

Researcher-participant relationships Relationships between the researcher and the individual subjects being studied in qualitative research.

Respect for persons, principle of Principle indicating that each person has the right to self-determination and the freedom to participate or not participate in research.

Results Outcomes from data analysis that are generated for each research objective, question, or hypothesis; results can be mixed, nonsignificant, significant and not predicted, significant and predicted, or unexpected.

Retrospective cohort study An epidemiological study in which a group of people are identified who have experienced a particular event; for example, studying occupational exposure to chemicals to determine cause-and-effect relationships.

Review of literature Summary of current theoretical and empirical sources to generate a picture of what is known and not known about a particular problem.

Review of relevant research literature Review of current studies conducted to generate what is known and not known about a problem and to determine whether the knowledge is ready for use in practice.

Rigor Excellence in research; attained through the use of discipline, scrupulous adherence to detail, and strict accuracy.

Robust Term describing an analysis procedure that will yield accurate results even if some of the assumptions are violated by the data being analyzed.

Rogers' Theory of Diffusion of Innovations Theory to direct research utilization or the use of research findings in practice; describes stages of knowledge, persuasion, decision, implementation, and confirmation.

Role modeling Process of teaching less experienced professionals by demonstrating model behavior.

S

Sample Subset of the population that is selected for a study.

Sample characteristics Demographic data analyzed to provide a picture of the sample.

Sample mortality rate Number of subjects who withdraw from or who are lost during a study. The mortality rate is calculated by dividing the number of subjects lost to the study by the sample size or 10 subjects lost ÷ by sample size = 0.10 × 100% sample mortality rate.

Sample size Number of subjects, events, behaviors, or situations that are examined in a study.

Sampling Process of selecting a group of people, events, behaviors, or other elements that are representative of the population being studied.

Sampling criteria List of the characteristics essential for inclusion or exclusion in the target population.

Sampling distribution Table of statistical values (such as the mean) of many samples obtained from the same population.

Sampling error Difference between a sample statistic used to estimate a parameter and the actual but unknown value of the parameter.

Sampling frame List of every member of the population; the sampling criteria are used to define membership in the population.

Sampling method Strategies used to obtain a sample, including probability and nonprobability sampling techniques; also called a sampling plan.

Saturation of data Phenomenon that occurs when additional sampling provides no new information, or there is redundancy of previously collected data. Sample size in a qualitative study is determined when saturation of data occurs.

Scale Self-report form of measurement composed of several items thought to measure the construct being studied; the subject responds to each item on the continuum or scale provided.

Scatterplot Diagram or figure showing the dispersion of scores on a variable from a study, or depicting the relationship of scores on one variable with scores on another variable. A scatterplot has two scales: horizontal (X-axis) and vertical (Y-axis).

Science Coherent body of knowledge composed of research findings, tested theories, scientific principles, and laws for a discipline.

Scientific community Cohesive group of scholars within a discipline who create new research ideas and develop innovative methodologies to conduct research.

Scientific method Approach to research comprising all procedures that scientists have used, currently use, or may use in the future to pursue knowledge; examples include quantitative research, qualitative research, outcomes research, and triangulation.

Scientific misconduct Intentional deviation from practices commonly accepted within the scientific community for proposing, conducting, or reporting research. May include fabrication, falsification, or plagiarism; does not include honest errors or honest differences in interpretation or judgment of data.

Scientific theory Theory that has been repeatedly tested through research with valid and reliable methods of measuring each concept and relational statement.

Search field Areas of research topics that are searched to identify relevant sources.

Secondary analysis design Design for studying data previously collected in another study; data are reexamined using different organizations of the data and different statistical analyses.

Secondary source Source whose author summarizes or quotes content from primary sources.

Sedimented view View from the perspective of a specific frame of reference, world view, or theory that gives a sense of certainty, security, and control.

Seeking approval to conduct a study Submitting a research proposal to a selected group for review and often verbally defending that proposal.

Selectivity of a physiological instrument Assessment of the accuracy of an instrument; the ability of the instrument to identify correctly the signal under study and to distinguish it from other signals.

Semantic differential scale Two opposite adjectives with a seven-point scale between them; the subject selects a point on the scale that best describes his or her view of the concept being examined.

Sensitivity of physiological measures Amount of change of a parameter that can be measured precisely.

Serendipity Accidental discovery of something valuable or useful during the conduct of a study.

Setting Location for conducting research; can be natural, partially controlled, or highly controlled.

Significant and unpredicted results Results that are opposite of those predicted by the researcher and indicate that flaws are present in the logic of both the researcher and the theory being tested.

Significant results Results that agree with those identified by the researcher.

Simple hypothesis Hypothesis stating the relationship (associative or causal) between two variables.

Simple linear regression Parametric analysis technique that estimates the value of a dependent variable based on the value of an independent variable.

Simple random sampling Random selection of elements from the sampling frame for inclusion in a study.

Situated Belief that the person is shaped by the language, culture, history, purposes, and values of his or her world and is constrained by that shaping in the ability to establish meanings.

Skewness Absence of symmetry in the curve formed by the distribution of scores; distribution can be positively or negatively skewed.

Skimming research reports Quickly reviewing a source to gain a broad overview of the content by reading the title, the author's name, the abstract or introduction, headings, one or two sentences under each heading, and the discussion section.

Small area analyses Geographical analyses used to examine variations in health status, health services, patterns of care, or patterns of use by geographical area.

Social system Set of interrelated persons (e.g., the nurses on a specific hospital unit, in one hospital, or in a corporation of hospitals) engaged in joint problem solving to accomplish a common goal or outcome.

Special library Library that contains a collection of material on a specific topic or specialty area.

Split-half reliability Technique used to determine the homogeneity of an instrument's items, in which the items are split in half and a correlational procedure is performed between the two halves.

Stability Type of measurement reliability that is concerned with the consistency of repeated measures; usually referred to as test-retest reliability.

Standard deviation Measure of dispersion that is calculated by taking the square root of the variance.

Standardized mortality ratio (SMR) The observed number of deaths divided by the expected number of deaths and multiplied by 100. SMR is regarded as a measure of the relative risk of the studied group to die of a particular condition.

Standardized scores Scores used to express deviations from the mean (difference scores) in terms of standard deviation units, such as Z-scores, in which the mean is 0 and the standard deviation is 1.

Standard of care A norm on which quality of care is judged.

Statements Express claims that compute to a theory; theories include existence and relational statements.

Statistic Numerical value obtained from a sample; it is used to estimate the parameters of a population.

Statistical conclusion validity Extent to which the conclusions about relationships and differences drawn from statistical analyses reflect reality.

Statistical regression Movement or regression of extreme scores toward the mean in studies using a pretest-posttest design.

Statistical significance Extent to which the results are probably not due to chance.

Stem-and-leaf display Type of exploratory data analysis in which scores are visually presented to obtain insights.

Story Time-bound event shared orally with others.

Storytakers People who listen to a story.

Storytellers People who share a story.

Storytelling Process used to share stories.

Stratification Design strategy used to distribute subjects evenly throughout the sample.

Stratified random sampling Technique used when the researcher knows some of the variables in the population that are critical to achieving representativeness; the sample is divided into strata or groups using these identified variables.

Structural equation modeling Analysis technique designed to test theories.

Structured interview Interview in which strategies are used that give the researcher increasing control over the content. An example is a questionnaire with structured responses.

Structured observation Clear identification of what is to be observed and precise definition of how the observations are to be made, recorded, and coded.

Structures of care The elements of organization and administration that guide the processes of care.

Subjects Individuals participating in a study (those being studied).

Substantive theory Theory recognized within a discipline as useful for explaining important phenomena.

Substitutable relationship Relationship in which a similar concept can be substituted for the first concept and the second concept will occur relatively unchanged.

Sufficient relationship Relationship in which, when the first variable or concept occurs, the second will occur, regardless of the presence or absence of other factors.

Summary statistics *See* Descriptive statistics.

Surfing the Web Following the links (underlined or highlighted names) on one website to reveal other websites.

Survey design Design used to describe a phenomenon by collecting data using questionnaires or personal interviews.

Survival analysis Set of techniques designed to analyze repeated measures from a given time (e.g., beginning of the study, onset of a disease, beginning of a treatment) until a certain attribute (e.g., death, treatment failure, recurrence of the phenomenon) occurs.

Symbolic interaction theory Explores how people define reality and how their beliefs are related to their actions.

Symmetrical This is a term used to describe the normal curve where both sides of the curve are mirror images of each other.

Symmetrical relationship Relationship in which, if A occurs or changes, B will occur or change, and if B occurs or changes, A will occur or change (A ↔ B).

Symmetry plot Exploratory data analysis technique designed to determine the presence of skewness in the data.

Synthesis of sources Clustering and interrelating ideas from several sources to form a gestalt or a new, complete picture of what is known and not known in an area.

Systematic bias *See* Systematic variation.

Systematic error Measurement error that is not random but occurs consistently in the same direction, such as a scale that inaccurately weighs subjects at 3 pounds heavier than their actual weight.

Systematic extension replication Constructive replication performed under distinctly new conditions, in which the researchers conducting the replication do not follow the design or methods of the original researchers; rather, the second investigative team begins with a similar problem statement but formulates new means to verify the first investigator's findings.

Systematic review of research Narrowly focused synthesis of the findings from quantitative studies focused on a particular practice intervention or problem.

Systematic sampling Selecting every *k*th individual from an ordered list of all members of a population, using a randomly selected starting point.

Systematic variation Phenomenon that occurs when the selected subjects' measurement values vary in some way from those of the population.

T

Tails Extremes of the normal curve where the significant statistical values fall.

Target population Population determined by the sampling criteria.

Tendency statement Deterministic relationship that describes what always happens if there are no interfering conditions.

Tentative theory Theory that is newly proposed, has had minimal exposure to critique by scholars in the discipline, and has undergone little testing.

Testable hypothesis Hypothesis containing variables that can be measured or manipulated in the real world.

Test-retest reliability Determination of the stability or consistency of a measurement technique by correlating the scores obtained from repeated measures.

Theoretical connectedness Theoretical schema developed from a qualitative study; is clearly expressed, logically consistent, reflective of the data, and compatible with nursing's knowledge base.

Theoretical limitations Weaknesses in the study framework and conceptual and operational definitions that restrict the abstract generalization of the findings.

Theoretical literature Concept analyses, maps, theories, and conceptual frameworks that support a selected research problem and purpose.

Theoretical sampling Sampling in which data are gathered from any individual subject or group that can provide relevant information for theory generation.

Theoretical triangulation Use of two or more frameworks or theoretical perspectives in the same study; the hypotheses are developed based on the different theoretical perspectives and are tested using the same data set.

Theory Integrated set of defined concepts, existence statements, and relational statements that present a view of a phenomenon and can be used to describe, explain, predict, and control that phenomenon.

Therapeutic research Research that provides a patient with an opportunity to receive an experimental treatment that might have beneficial results.

Thesis Research project completed by a graduate student as part of the requirements for a master's degree

Time-dimensional designs Designs used to examine the sequence and patterns of change, growth, or trends across time.

Time lag Time span between the generation of new knowledge through research and the use of this knowledge in practice.

Time-series analysis Technique designed to analyze changes in a variable across time and thus uncover patterns in the data.

Total variance The combination of the within-group variance and the between-group variance.

Traditions Truths or beliefs that are based on customs and past trends.

Trend designs Designs used to examine changes in the general population in relation to a particular phenomenon.

Trial and error Approach with unknown outcomes used in an uncertain situation when other sources of knowledge are unavailable.

Trialability Extent to which the results of an individual or agency allow an idea to be tried out on a limited basis, with the option of returning to previous practices.

Triangulation Use of two or more theories, methods, data sources, investigators, or analysis methods in a study.

True score Score that would be obtained if no measurement error occurred (but there is always some measurement error).

_t_-test Parametric analysis technique used to determine significant differences between measures of two samples.

Two-tailed test of significance Analysis technique used for a nondirectional hypothesis when the researcher assumes that an extreme score can occur in either tail of the normal curve.

Type I error Error that occurs when the researcher concludes that the samples tested are from different populations (a significant difference exists between groups) when, in fact, the samples are from the same population (no significant difference exists between groups); the null hypothesis is rejected when it is true.

Type II error Error that occurs when the researcher concludes that no significant difference exists between the samples examined when, in fact, a difference exists; the null hypothesis is regarded as true when it is false.

U

Unexpected results Study results that indicate relationships between variables or differences among groups that were not hypothesized and not predicted from the framework being used.

Unexplained variance Part of the variation between or among two or more variables that is the result of things other than the relationship.

Ungrouped frequency distribution Means of identifying and displaying all numerical values obtained for a particular variable from the subjects studied.

Unitizing reliability Extent to which each judge (data collector, coder, researcher) consistently identifies the same units within the data as appropriate for coding.

Ungrouped frequency distribution Categorical data in the form of a table that is developed to display all numerical values obtained for a particular variable.

Unpredicted significant results Results opposite those predicted, which indicate flaws in the logic of both the researcher and the theory being tested. However, if results are accurate, they constitute an important addition to the body of knowledge.

Unstructured interview Interview that is initiated with a broad question; subjects usually are encouraged to elaborate further on particular dimensions of a topic and often control the content of the interview.

Unstructured observation Spontaneous observation and recording of what is seen; planning is minimal.

Utilization of research findings Use of knowledge generated through research to guide nursing practice.

V

Validity Extent to which an instrument accurately reflects the abstract construct (or concept) being examined.

Variables Qualities, properties, or characteristics of persons, things, or situations that change or vary and are manipulated or measured in research.

Variance Measure of dispersion, where the larger the variance, the larger the dispersion of scores. Variance is calculated as one of the steps in determining standard deviation.

Variance analysis Outcomes research strategy to track individual and group variance from a specific critical pathway. The goal is to decrease preventable variance in process, thus helping patients and their families achieve optimal outcomes.

Virus, computer Program developed to alter and destroy information stored in a computer.

Visual analogue scale A 100-mm line, with right angle stops at either end, on which subjects are asked to record their response to a study variable.

Voluntary consent Decision made by a prospective subject, of his or her own volition, without coercion or any undue influence, to participate in a research study.

W

Wald-Wolfowitz runs test Nonparametric analysis technique used to determine differences between two populations.

Wilcoxon matched-pairs signed-ranks test Nonparametric analysis of changes that occur in pretest-posttest measures or matched-pairs measures.

Within-group variance Source of variation that reflects the individual scores in a group that vary from the group mean.

World Wide Web (www) An information service for access to Internet resources by content rather than file names.

X

X **axis** The horizontal scale of a scatterplot.

Y

Y **axis** The vertical scale of a scatterplot.

Z

Z-score Standardized score of the normal curve that is equivalent to the standard deviation of the normal curve.

INDEX

E